W9-ATW-062

Weight

Metric		Approximate apothecary equivalents		Metric		Approximate apothecary equivalents	
30	Gm.	1	ounce	30	mg.	½	grain
15	Gm.	4	drams	25	mg.	⅜	grain
10	Gm.	2½	drams	20	mg.	⅓	grain
7.5	Gm.	2	drams	15	mg.	¼	grain
6	Gm.	90	grains	12	mg.	⅕	grain
5	Gm.	75	grains	10	mg.	⅙	grain
4	Gm.	60	grains (1 dram)	8	mg.	⅛	grain
3	Gm.	45	grains	6	mg.	1/10	grain
2	Gm.	30	grains (½ dram)	5	mg.	1/12	grain
1.5	Gm.	22	grains	4	mg.	1/15	grain
1	Gm.	15	grains	3	mg.	1/20	grain
0.75	Gm.	12	grains	2	mg.	1/30	grain
0.6	Gm.	10	grains	1.5	mg.	1/40	grain
0.5	Gm.	7½	grains	1.2	mg.	1/50	grain
0.4	Gm.	6	grains	1	mg.	1/60	grain
0.3	Gm.	5	grains	0.8	mg.	1/80	grain
0.25	Gm.	4	grains	0.6	mg.	1/100	grain
0.2	Gm.	3	grains	0.5	mg.	1/120	grain
0.15	Gm.	2½	grains	0.4	mg.	1/150	grain
0.12	Gm.	2	grains	0.3	mg.	1/200	grain
0.1	Gm.	1½	grains	0.25	mg.	1/250	grain
75	mg.	1¼	grains	0.2	mg.	1/300	grain
60	mg.	1	grain	0.15	mg.	1/400	grain
50	mg.	¾	grain	0.12	mg.	1/500	grain
40	mg.	⅔	grain	0.1	mg.	1/600	grain

Pharmacology in nursing

Pharmacology in nursing

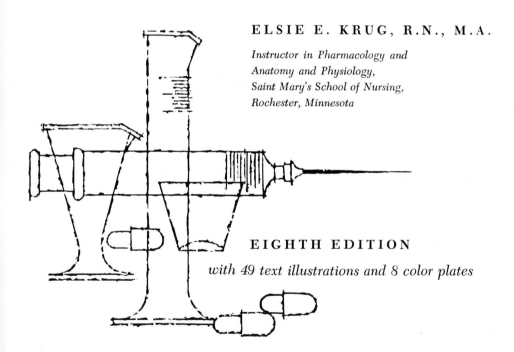

ELSIE E. KRUG, R.N., M.A.

*Instructor in Pharmacology and
Anatomy and Physiology,
Saint Mary's School of Nursing,
Rochester, Minnesota*

EIGHTH EDITION

with 49 text illustrations and 8 color plates

THE C. V. MOSBY COMPANY

St. Louis 1960

The use of portions of the text of *The United States Pharmacopeia*, Sixteenth Revision, official October 1, 1960, is by permission received from the Board of Trustees of the United States Pharmacopeial Convention. The said Board is not responsible for any inaccuracies of the text thus used.

Permission to use for comment parts of the text of *The National Formulary*, Eleventh Edition, in this volume has been granted by the Council of the American Pharmaceutical Association. The American Pharmaceutical Association is not responsible for any inaccuracy of quotation nor for any errors in the statement of quantities or percentage strengths.

Permission to use in this volume portions of the text of *New and Nonofficial Drugs 1960* has been authorized by the Secretary of the Council on Drugs of the American Medical Association, with the understanding that the Council is not responsible for any errors that may arise from such use.

Permission to include information relating to substances and preparations contained in the *British Pharmacopoeia* has been granted by the General Medical Council.

EIGHTH EDITION

Copyright © 1960 by The C. V. Mosby Company

All rights reserved

Second Printing

Previous editions copyrighted
1936, 1940, 1942, 1945, 1948, 1951, 1955

Printed in the United States of America
Library of Congress Catalog Card Number 60-12473
Distributed in Great Britain by Henry Kimpton, London

Preface

The eighth edition of this textbook represents considerable revision to bring it up to date and to include changes present in the sixteenth revision of *The Pharmacopeia of the United States* (1960), the *British Pharmacopoeia* (1958), and the list of admissions to the eleventh edition of *The National Formulary* (1960).

As was true of previous editions, this book is designed for the use of students at different levels of their nursing experience. No basic course in pharmacology is likely to include all the content of a student's textbook since the study of pharmacology is necessarily a continuous activity throughout the clinical experience of both students and graduates. In some instances the basic course in pharmacology includes only a selected number of drugs, each one representing a group of similar compounds. This arrangement provides for expedient use of time to develop concepts about a group of drugs through careful study of one or two of its members. Later study of other members of the group then may be made as the student encounters the need for broader and deeper understanding.

Older drugs that in medical practice have been replaced by better agents have, to a great extent, been deleted unless they have contributed to the advancement of pharmacology. Drugs that are well established and extensively used have received more attention than those undergoing investigation. Among the newer drugs that have been included in this edition are many that were included in the annual supplements to the seventh edition of *Pharmacology in Nursing*—for example, a number of nonbarbiturate sedatives and hypnotics, ataractics, analgesics, antibiotics, adrenocortical steroids, and many others. Some nonofficial drugs which are being used extensively have been included. The following drugs have been discussed in separate chapters: Histamine, Antihistamines, and Drugs Used for Motion Sickness; Antineoplastic Drugs; Enzymes.

An attempt has been made to place greater emphasis on drugs as chemical substances. Structural formulas have been included to a limited extent to help the student understand relationships among drugs and

5

also the relationship between the chemical structure of a drug and its action.

Certain additions have been made to make this edition useful to nursing students in Canada as well as in the United States—for example, some material on Canadian drug legislation and the inclusion of many preparations which are listed in the *British Pharmacopoeia*. However, if the preparation is listed in both *The United States Pharmacopeia* and the *British Pharmacopoeia* and the dosage or general description differs slightly in the two publications, the information provided in *The United States Pharmacopeia* is followed more closely.

The metric system of measurement has been indicated throughout in keeping with the general trend toward adoption of the metric system and exclusion of the apothecary system. The dosage of certain drugs that long have been ordered in apothecary units of measurement (for example, morphine, atropine, aspirin, etc.) is indicated in metric system and in the corresponding apothecary equivalent.

The chapters on Review of Arithmetic and Weights and Measures have been revised and again included in the book in response to wishes and opinions expressed by teachers of pharmacology.

The entire manuscript was submitted to Dr. Elijah Adams, Professor and Director, Department of Pharmacology, Saint Louis University School of Medicine, St. Louis, Mo. Grateful acknowledgment is made of his valuable suggestions, corrections, and additions.

The chapter on Anti-infectives—Antibiotics and the chapter on Serums and Vaccines were revised by Miss Jeanette Blake, R.N., member of the faculty of Saint Mary's School of Nursing, Rochester, Minn.

Grateful acknowledgment and warm appreciation is also hereby expressed to a number of others who read certain chapters of this revision and contributed valuable suggestions: John S. Lundy, M.D., formerly of the Section of Anesthesiology, Mayo Clinic, Rochester, Minn.; Gunnar B. Stickler, M.D., Consultant, Section of Pediatrics, Mayo Clinic, Rochester, Minn.; Sister M. Torello, Registered Pharmacist, Saint Mary's Hospital, Rochester, Minn.; Miss Jeanette Blake, R.N., Miss Mary Space, R.N., Sister Francis de Sales, R.N., and Sister M. Immaculata, R.N., members of the faculty of Saint Mary's School of Nursing, Rochester, Minn.; Sister M. Cecile, R.N., and Sister M. Declan, R.N., Department of Nursing, College of Saint Teresa, Winona, Minn.

I am also indebted to Sister Francis de Sales, R.N., and Sister M. Leota for several of the pen and ink drawings and to Miss Esther La Plant for her able typing assistance. Finally, I wish to recognize the contribution of Dr. Hugh A. McGuigan to the earlier editions that help to form the background of this edition.

Elsie E. Krug

Table of contents

1   Orientation and how to study pharmacology   13

2   Scope of pharmacology, definitions, drug standards, and drug legislation   18

3   Names, sources, active constituents, and pharmaceutic preparations of drugs   33

4   Review of arithmetic   47

5   Weights and measures   65

6   Administration of medicines   93

7   Action of drugs, sites of action, and factors that modify the action of drugs   126

8   Anti-infectives—antibiotics   137

9   Drugs that affect the central nervous system   171

10   Autonomic drugs   302

11   Skeletal muscle relaxants and their antagonists   348

12   Histamine, antihistamines, and drugs used for motion sickness   359

13   Drugs that affect the gastrointestinal organs   368

14 Drugs that affect the circulatory system   408

15 Drugs that affect the organs of the respiratory system   476

16 Drugs that affect the skin and mucous membranes
    (dermatologic agents)   492

17 Drugs that affect the kidney and organs
    of the urinary tract   510

18 Drugs that affect the eye   532

19 Drugs that act on the organs of the reproductive system   541

20 Anti-infectives other than antibiotics—sulfonamides   566

21 Systemic anti-infectives—drugs used in the treatment of
    tuberculosis, syphilis, leprosy, and certain protozoan diseases   577

22 Local anti-infectives—antiseptics and disinfectants   600

23 Anti-infectives—anthelmintics and amebicides   622

24 Minerals, vitamins, and hormones used as drugs   638

25 Antineoplastic drugs   704

26 Enzymes used as drugs   720

27 Serums and vaccines   726

28 Toxicology   736

29 History of materia medica   754

Glossary   768

Color plates

1   Areas stimulated and depressed by caffeine   174

2   *Papaver somniferum* (opium poppy)   188

3   Diagram of the autonomic nervous system   306

4   *Atropa belladonna* (deadly nightshade)   332

5   *Rhamnus purshiana*   398

6   *Digitalis purpurea* (foxglove)   416

7   Diagram representing the pathway of the portal-biliary circulation of bile salts   464

8   *Claviceps purpurea* (rye ergot)   542

Pharmacology in nursing

Chapter 1

Orientation
and how to study
pharmacology

Orientation to pharmacology

Among the many and interesting duties that arise in the preparation for and the practice of nursing, the administration of medicines holds a prominent position. From the first day on the hospital ward the young student is aware that medication is an essential part of patient care. She recognizes that safe administration of drugs is a real responsibility and may feel overwhelmed by what she does not know. The thoughtful and conscientious student welcomes the opportunity to build a sound foundation of knowledge and understanding of drugs, their administration, and their uses. This can be done in part in the classroom and can be richly supplemented by ward experiences.

The aura of importance that surrounds drug administration in the mind of the student has an important basis. Drugs have the power to help or to harm, and nurses entrusted with their administration carry a responsibility second only to that of the physician who prescribes them. The right medication in the right amount and at the right time is ensured only when the nurse is well prepared to assume her responsibility. This responsibility is, of course, shared by others on the ward, and this fact should be a source of support to the student, particularly when she is young and inexperienced.

Sufficient understanding of drugs for their safe administration involves more than mere memorizing of names. The nurse should know the action of the drug in the body, the correct dosage, the methods of administration, the symptoms of overdosage, and the abnormal reactions that may arise from individual differences in particular patients. To learn all this and more about each of the hundreds of drugs in common usage would be a tremendous undertaking were it not that drugs lend themselves to classification and that physiologic reactions tend to occur in related se-

Orientation and how to study pharmacology   13

quence. Hence, in the study of pharmacology, emphasis is placed on classes of drugs and their characteristic effects on various body systems both in health and in disease. Individual drugs can then be fitted into this general framework, and the special characteristics that differentiate them from others of their class can be more readily learned and remembered.

Even with this help, the study of pharmacology might still remain formidable if confined to a formal classroom with only exhibits of pills and powders, capsules and ampules, and charts and pictures to give it reality. Fortunately for the student nurse, pharmacology is not divorced from its practical application. The patient is never too far away, and the student may turn from the classroom to the ward to observe a nurse administer the very drug that is under consideration. With the nurse, the student can check the order for morphine sulfate, watch her write out the medication card, obtain the drug from the locked compartment, record the drug on the opiate record as required by federal law, prepare the hypodermic injection, and administer the drug. She has the opportunity to observe the symptoms which the patient may exhibit—restlessness, rapid pulse and respirations, severe pain, and possibly the look of approaching panic because of the pain. At intervals she can return and in this same patient note the relief of pain, the decreased emotional reaction, slowed respirations and pulse, and general relaxation. Now her knowledge of the drug's administration is not mere rote learning —it is the outgrowth of direct and directed observation.

As time goes on, the student continues to study and observe and finally is given the responsibility of administering medications to her own patients. This is now not like giving an aspirin tablet for a headache or giving her small brother a vitamin pill. Then she carried out mechanical instructions. Now she must select, interpret, organize, and observe, and on the strength of her carefully recorded observations the physician may base many of his conclusions regarding the patient's progress.

Again, a student may gain her first knowledge of a drug in a ward situation. She learns from the head nurse that a drug, still in the experimental stage, is being given to one of her patients. Perhaps it is identified only by a number, and the doctor himself administers it. He leaves, however, specific instructions about symptoms to be watched for in the patient, together with a blanket order to report any untoward reaction. This may go on for weeks, even years, until one day the headlines blazon a new success for medical science; a medicine has been found to combat another of the illnesses that disable man. What a thrill to the nurse who, even in her small way, has contributed to this discovery, to know that her work has helped make others healthier or more comfortable.

The constant advances in the field of drug therapy, the almost daily appearance of new drugs or new preparations of old drugs on the market and in the hospital, are a challenge to both the student and the graduate nurse to be always students. An examination passed and an R.N. acquired are no lasting guarantees of sufficient knowledge in the field of drugs to make a nurse helpful to the doctor or even safe for the patient. Drugs change and will continue to change. The nurse's pharmacology books become a permanent section of her library, and year by year as new editions or new books appear she must bring her library up to date. In addition, the official current literature on drugs must be followed carefully, as new drugs are slow in making their way into more permanent literature. For the nurse working in a hospital or health service, doctors, instructors, supervisors, and pharmacists will be on hand to help her. In more isolated practice, greater personal effort will be required to keep her abreast of current practices. In any case, a sustained interest in pharmacology will help to keep the nurse a well-informed and stimulating person as well as a valuable member of her profession.

The nurse's attitude toward drugs is an important factor in her use of them. Ideally, the body functions best when supported with adequate food, rest and recreation, and freedom from undue mental and emotional stress and strain. At times, because of physical and psychologic abnormalities, drugs must be resorted to to produce at least a semblance of normal body functions. As such, drugs deserve the respect of the nurse but that respect must be mingled with skepticism. Drugs, at best, are crutches, and undue dependence upon them can be dangerous. In giving drugs to patients, if the nurse has a friendly, matter-of-fact manner, assuming that under the circumstances drugs are necessary but that their use is temporary, a similar attitude is likely to develop in the patient. Only in rare instances, such as insulin for diabetes, should long-continued use of drugs be accepted as normal and reasonable.

In her personal life the nurse must be even more cautious and circumspect in taking drugs. Her invariable rule should be that she will take drugs only when necessary, on a doctor's prescription, and that she will never continue a drug a day beyond the period needed and prescribed. Since many nurses have almost constant access to potent, habit-forming drugs, this rule is an absolute necessity for safety.

Used respectfully and intelligently, drugs are a lifesaving boon. Used unwisely, they can produce irreparable tragedy. The nurse who combines diligent and intelligent observation with moral integrity and common sense in her use and administration of drugs will make many lasting contributions to her profession and to the patients for whom she cares.

How to study pharmacology

Many students are baffled by the study of a subject they find interesting but about which they frequently seem to learn relatively little. What can students themselves do to remedy this situation?

In pharmacology the student should think through what she hopes to achieve from the study of the subject. What does she need to know and what will she be expected to know about medicines when she is a graduate nurse? She will need the help of her instructor in formulating her objectives. A clear determination of what she wants to learn will help her decide how much effort will be necessary to achieve her goal.

Of primary importance is the understanding that learning is an active process and that learning does not take place without activity. Attending class and giving close attention constitutes a good beginning, and this alone may enable a few students to pass the examination over the formal part of the course, but unless there is more activity than this on the part of most students, little will be learned or retained. Furthermore, merely reading an assignment will not ensure learning. It is, rather, the amount and kind of cerebral activity that takes place when the student reads and after she has read, or when she discusses a problem associated with the subject matter of a lesson, that lays the basis for learning and remembering. Facts such as may be gleaned from a class discussion, at the bedside, from a doctor's comments, and from a textbook must be thought through and the parts mentally fitted together. The student must ask herself questions and then try to find the answers; e.g., "Why am I giving this medicine to Mrs. Smith? Is it helping her? How can I find out more about it? Why is the dosage larger for her than the dosage of this drug which we talked about in class yesterday?"

It is only in reasoning for herself how a drug affects the cells of human beings that the student develops understanding of its effect and uses. The student may, from her study of an assignment, learn that morphine depresses the central nervous system and that one of the parts of that system which is especially sensitive to morphine is the respiratory center. She may also have heard or read that individuals vary in the degree of response which they make to drugs such as morphine. Real understanding begins to dawn on her when she can relate this knowledge to an actual experience with a patient. Perhaps she can recall a specific instance; e.g., "Oh, that was why Mrs. Smith was breathing so slowly after her second hypodermic of morphine and I was asked to count her respirations so frequently. It also explains why everyone was so disturbed about her condition. She was really getting an unusual effect from that amount of the drug."

A number of facts about drugs and their administration must be memorized as the student progresses in her study of pharmacology, to make certain that she will be a safe person to care for patients. There is probably no way for the inexperienced student to "reason out" the usual dosage for drugs. She must memorize such things as dosage, abbreviations, and usual methods of administering certain preparations. This will provide her with a background of facts essential for thinking and reasoning. The student *must know* many facts about medicines and their administration even though she is expected to consult with her head nurse or supervisor when she is uncertain of what is correct procedure.

It is true, however, that certain facts, such as drug action, result of action in body tissues, uses of drugs, and symptoms of overdosage, can be recalled more readily if learned in an orderly manner. Drugs are frequently grouped according to their anatomic sites of action and according to the effects produced by them. Some drugs increase the activity of cells (stimulants) and some decrease cellular activities (depressants). If the student recalls the general functions of the sympathetic nervous system and is confronted with a list of drugs that behave in the body as stimulants of the sympathetic nervous system behave, she will know a good deal about this whole group of drugs and will be able to foretell many of their effects, even though many individual differences exist.

The whole field of pharmacology has undergone tremendous changes during the past few decades. Many new drugs are on the market and many are in the process of being evaluated. There is a fascination about the study of new drugs, even though they may soon be replaced by still newer ones. Although it is well for the student to learn all she can about new drugs, there is definite value in studying thoroughly those that have stood the test of time. A good understanding of the older drugs frequently constitutes a basis of understanding new synthetic compounds which are often chemically related to the older drugs. The repeated appearance of new medicines in the field of drug therapy means, however, that the student of nursing is confronted with the challenge of continuous study.

Chapter 2

Scope of pharmacology, definitions, drug standards, and drug legislation

Scope and definitions

Pharmacology is a broad science which includes all aspects of the subject of chemical substances that act upon cells. Practically speaking, it is a study of drugs and how they act. A *drug* is defined usually as a substance or mixture of substances used in the diagnosis, cure, treatment, or prevention of disease. The term comes from the Dutch, *droog*, meaning dry. This meaning probably originates from the early use of dried plants as a source of medicines. The terms drug and medicine are used interchangeably.

Present-day study of pharmacology can be subdivided into pharmacognosy, pharmacy, pharmacodynamics, pharmacotherapeutics, and toxicology.

Pharmacognosy is a subject concerned largely with the botanical sources of drugs. Many of the older drugs were obtained from plants and it was important to know something about the plants from which the drugs were extracted. Some of our present-day drugs are still obtained from plants. The term pharmacognosy has sometimes been used synonymously with materia medica.

Pharmacy is a body of technics involved in the preparation, compounding, and dispensing of drugs for medical use. It is also concerned with the preservation and storage of drugs. Most of the work formerly done by the individual pharmacist in the preparation of drugs has been taken on by the large drug companies, which send the preparations to local pharmacists in forms suitable for immediate use. This usually promotes economy as well as uniformity of dosage forms and ease of administration.

Pharmacodynamics is the study of the action of drugs in living tissues. It is concerned with the response of the tissues to the chemical agent being used and with the absorption, excretion, and fate of the chemical agent in the body. Pharmacodynamics is closely associated with other sciences, especially physiology, physiologic chemistry, microbiology, and pathology.

Pharmacotherapeutics is a study of the uses of drugs in the treatment of the sick.

Toxicology is the study of the poisonous effects that may be produced by drugs. It deals with the symptoms of poisoning, with treatment, and with the identification of poisons. Since the toxic effects of drugs are also part of their "pharmacodynamics," toxicology is really a special part of pharmacodynamics.

The need for drug standards

Drugs have been known to vary considerably in strength and activity. Drugs, such as opium and digitalis, obtained from plants have been known to vary in strength from plant to plant and from year to year, depending on where the plants are grown, their age conditions under which they are harvested, and how they are preserved. Occasionally one finds on the market drugs of low concentration or some that have been adulterated. Since accurate dosage and reliability of effect of a drug depend on uniformity of strength and purity, it has been necessary to find ways by which drugs can be standardized. *The technic by which the strength or potency of a drug is measured is known as assay.* The two general types of method used are chemical and biologic. Chemical assay really means chemical analysis to determine the ingredients present and their amount. A simple example would be the determination of the concentration of hydrochloric acid in a solution to be used medically. Thus the acid content of a solution might be measured by titration and then adjusted, for example, to a standardized tenth-normal solution.

Opium is known to contain certain alkaloids (active principles was the older term), and these may vary greatly in different preparations. Our official standard demands that opium must contain not less than 9.5 per cent and not more than 10.5 per cent of anhydrous morphine. Opium of a higher morphine content may be reduced to the official standard by admixture with opium of a lower percentage or with certain other pharmacologically inactive diluents such as sucrose, lactose, glycyrrhiza, or magnesium carbonate.

In the case of some drugs either the active ingredients are not known or there are no available methods of analyzing and standardizing them. These drugs may be standardized by biologic methods—"bioassay." Bioassay is performed by determining the amount of a preparation required to produce a definite effect on a suitable laboratory animal under certain standard conditions. For example, the potency of a certain sample of insulin is measured by its ability to lower the blood sugar of rabbits. The strength of a drug that is assayed biologically is usually expressed in units. For example, Insulin Injection, U.S.P., possesses a potency of not less than 95 per cent and not more than 105 per cent of the potency stated on the label, expressed in U.S.P. insulin units. Both the unit and the method of assay are defined, so that national and sometimes international standards exist.

Drug standards in the United States

In the United States an official drug is one which is included in *The Pharmacopeia of the United States of America, The National Formulary,* or the *Homeopathic Pharmacopoeia of the United States.* Drugs listed in these publications are official because they are so designated by the Federal Food, Drug, and Cosmetic Act.

The Pharmacopeia of the United States of America (usually referred to as the U.S.P.) is a book in which approved medicinal agents used in present-day medical practice are defined as to source, physical and chemical properties, tests for purity and identity, assay, method of storage, category (general type of drug), and dosage (range of dosage as well as the usual therapeutic dosage).

In most instances, preparations included in the U.S.P. are single drugs. They are listed under their official names. The purpose of the U.S.P. is to provide standards for the identification and purity of drugs and to ensure uniformity of strength. When a drug is prescribed by a physician anywhere in the United States, the pharmacist must fill the prescription with a preparation that meets pharmacopeial standards, if the drug is listed in the U.S.P. This assures the physician of uniform potency and purity of all official drugs which he prescribes for his patients.

The first pharmacopeia in the United States was published in 1820. The current edition, U.S.P. XVI, becomes official Oct. 1, 1960. At one time it was customary to revise the U.S.P. every ten years, but of late it has been revised every five years. Supplements to the U.S.P. are published between revisions to keep abreast of the rapid changes in this field.

The U.S.P. is revised by a special pharmacopeial committee headed by a full-time director. The committee is made up of outstanding pharmacologists, physicians, and pharmacists who donate their services to this important task. The main committee is assisted by many subcommittees and advisory boards. Drugs included in the U.S.P. are selected on the basis of their therapeutic usefulness and low toxicity. When drugs listed in the U.S.P. have been supplanted in practice by better drugs, the older ones are deleted and the newer or better drugs are added.

Sometimes a drug is deleted from the U.S.P. because after extensive use the incidence of toxic reactions is shown to be too high.

Drugs whose content or method of preparation is secret are not admitted to the U.S.P. Trade-marked or patented preparations of therapeutic merit may be included; when included they are listed under their official names, not the popular trade names by which they may be commonly known.

The National Formulary (N.F.) serves as a supplement to the U.S.P. It is sponsored by the American Pharmaceutical Association and is usually revised the same year as the U.S.P. The latest edition is the eleventh. Originally the National Formulary contained only formulas for drug mixtures. It now contains many single drugs as well as formulas for drug mixtures. Standards for those drugs listed in the Formulary but not included in the Pharmacopeia are indicated. The Pharmacopeia represents a more critical selection of drugs since they are more carefully screened as to their therapeutic value and toxic qualities. Drugs included in the National Formulary are selected not only on the basis of their therapeutic value but also on the basis of demand. Preparations deleted from the Pharmacopeia are often transferred to the National Formulary. It provides standards for many of the older remedies which the pharmacist continues to be called upon to dispense. As is true of the Pharmacopeia, drugs are listed in the Formulary under their official names only.

New and Nonofficial Drugs (N.N.D.), formerly known as New and Nonofficial Remedies (N.N.R.), is published annually under the direction and supervision of the Council on Drugs of the American Medical Association. The function of the Council on Drugs is to examine and evaluate evidence regarding the actions, uses, dosage, hazards, and other pertinent properties of drugs and to encourage rational therapy by timely informative reports to the medical profession. These reports of each evaluated drug are submitted in the form of monographs (written articles) to the editor of the American Medical Association for publication in *The Journal of the American Medical Association.* The monographs are subsequently included in the yearly publication of the N.N.D. The type of information supplied in the N.N.D. is not, for the most part, what is provided in the U.S.P. and N.F. Formerly drugs were *accepted* by the Council for inclusion in its annual publication provided certain rules of the Council were observed. Inclusion in the publication thus carried Council approval. Pharmaceutical companies could voluntarily submit their products for study by the Council or they could choose to ignore the Council.

Since 1955 the Council has changed its policy and studies all commercially available products about which it feels the medical profession should have as accurate information as it is possible to provide at the time of publication. Since neither approval nor official status is indicated when drugs appear in N.N.D., it is no longer appropriate to indicate the letters N.N.D. after the name of the drug.

The Council is particularly interested in protecting the public as well as the medical profession against fraud, undesirable secrecy, misleading advertising, and unjustifiable or premature conclusions appearing in medical literature.

The nurse should become acquainted with New and Nonofficial Drugs since it is a valuable source of authentic information. She is not likely to use the Pharmacopeia or the Formulary to any great extent, but she should be interested in knowing what these publications mean in terms of standards for drugs.

The Dispensatory of the United States of America is a large book which is encyclopedic in its scope. It contains comprehensive accounts of drugs old and new, official and nonofficial. It is sponsored by the American Pharmaceutical Association. It is a useful reference to consult in seeking a convenient digest of information about many drugs.

Hospital formularies are published by hospitals that handle and dispense large amounts of drugs from their pharmacies. They contain lists of drugs and dosage forms used in particular institutions. They may also contain statements of policy that relate to the dispensing of drugs, procedures for ordering drugs, etc.

Modern Drug Encyclopedia and *Physicians' Desk Reference to Pharmaceutical Specialties and Biologicals* contain short accounts of alphabetically listed drugs, which can be found under their trade names.

Drug standards in Great Britain and Canada

British Pharmacopoeia (B.P.) is similar to the U.S.P. in its scope and purpose. Drugs listed in it are considered official and subject to legal control in the United Kingdom and those parts of the British Commonwealth in which the British Pharmacopoeia has statutory force. The present revision became official September 1, 1958. It is published by the British Pharmacopoeia Commission under the direction of the General Medical Council. Dosage is expressed in metric system, although in some cases dosage is indicated in both metric and imperial systems.

The Pharmacopeia of the United States of America is used a great deal in Canada, and some preparations used in Canada conform to the U.S.P. instead of the B.P. because many of the drugs used in Canada are obtained from the United States.

British Pharmaceutical Codex (B.P.C.) is published by the Pharmaceutical Society of Great Britain. In general, it resembles the National Formulary.

Canadian Formulary (C.F.) is published by the Canadian Pharmaceutical Association. It contains formulas for preparations used extensively in Canada. It also contains standards for new drugs prescribed in Canada but not included in the British Pharmacopoeia. This publication has been given official status by the Canadian Food and Drug Act.

The *Physician's Formulary* contains formulas for preparations that are representative of the needs of medical practice in Canada. It is published by the Canadian Medical Association. New and Nonofficial Drugs is also used in Canada as a source of information about new drugs.

International standards

Various national pharmacopeias have been developed to meet the needs of medical practice in different countries. The Pharmacopeia of the United States has been translated into Spanish for the Spanish-speaking parts of the Americas. In addition, an international pharmacopeia has been published.

Pharmacopoeia Internationalis (Ph.I.) was first published in 1951. It was published by a committee of the World Health Organization and represents an important contribution to the development of international standards in drugs and unification of national pharmacopeias. The work done on this publication has resulted in better understanding of terms and in uniformity of strengths and composition of drugs throughout the world. It has also demonstrated that members of different nations can sit down together and come to agreement about matters that concern many people of the world.

The Pharmacopoeia Internationalis is published in English, Spanish, and French. The nomenclature is in Latin, and the system of measurement is metric. It is not intended to convey official status in any country, unless it is adopted by the appropriate authority of that country.

Drug legislation

Important though pharmacopeias, formularies and other publications are to the maintenance of standards for drugs, unless provision is made to enforce the standards the public can be defrauded, drugs adulterated, and the market flooded with unreliable and unsafe preparations. Enforcement of standards is partly a responsibility of individual states but federal legislation is needed to cover interstate commerce in drugs as well as other items.

United States drug legislation

Federal Food, Drug, and Cosmetic Act

The *Federal Food, Drug, and Cosmetic Act* was enacted by the Congress in 1906. This law designated the Pharmacopeia of the United States and the National Formulary as official standards and empowered the federal government to enforce these standards. It was "An act for preventing the manufacture of adulterated or misbranded or poisonous or deleterious foods, drugs, medicines, and liquors, and for regulating traffic therein, and for other purposes."

Before long it was evident that the law was inadequate to deal with the many problems arising from the rapid increase of preparations of drugs, foods, and cosmetics.

The *Federal Food, Drug, and Cosmetic Act (1938)* retained the worthy features of the 1906 law and added certain others. The enforcement of this law is the responsibility of the Food and Drug Administration of the Department of Health, Education, and Welfare. This Act conferred status on the drugs listed in the Homeopathic Pharmacopoeia of the United States as well as those in the Pharmacopeia of the United States and the National Formulary.

It was amended by the *Durham-Humphrey Law in 1952.* This provides a definition of certain types of drugs which may be sold by pharmacists only on the prescription of a practitioner licensed by law to administer such drugs, and it also clarifies the use of written and oral prescriptions. It was aimed at the tightening of control of the barbiturates by trying to restrict the refilling of prescriptions.

Provisions of the Federal Food, Drug, and Cosmetic Act. The provisions include many features which are designated to prevent misbranding and to ensure careful and accurate labeling. Labeling refers not only to the labels on the immediate container but also to circulars, pamphlets, and brochures that may accompany the preparations or in some manner reach the hands of the consumer. The Act prohibits certain statements from appearing on the label and insists upon certain others.

1. Statements on the label must not be false or misleading in any particular.
2. Drugs must not be dangerous to health when used in the dosage or with the frequency prescribed, recommended, or suggested on the label.
3. The label must indicate the name and the business address of the manufacturer, packer, or distributor, as well as an accurate statement of the contents.
4. The label must indicate quantitatively the presence of all habit-forming drugs, i.e., narcotics, hypnotics, or other habit-forming drugs or their derivatives. The label must also bear the statement "Warning—May Be Habit Forming."
5. Labels must designate the presence of official drugs by their official names, and if nonofficial they must bear the usual name of the drug or drugs, whether active or not.
6. The Act requires that official drugs be packaged and labeled as specified by the Pharmacopeia of the United States, National Formulary, or the Homeopathic Pharmacopoeia of the United States. Deviations in strength, quality, and purity are permitted, provided such deviations are clearly indicated on the label.
7. Labels must indicate the quantity, kind, and proportion of certain specified ingredients, including alcohol, bromides, atropine, hyoscine, digitalis, and a number of other drugs, the presence of which needs to be known for the safety of those for whom it is prescribed.

8. The label must bear adequate directions for use and adequate warnings against unsafe use (a) by children and (b) in pathologic conditions.
9. The label must bear adequate warning against unsafe dosage or methods or duration of administration or application in such manner and form as are necessary for the protection of the users.
10. The label must bear the following statement for all drugs considered unsafe for self-medication: "Caution—Federal Law Prohibits Dispensing Without Prescription." All drugs given by injection (with the exception of insulin) are considered prescription drugs, as well as the following groups of drugs:
    A. Hypnotic, narcotic, or habit-forming drugs or derivatives thereof as specified in the law.
    B. Drugs that because of their toxicity or because of the method of their use are not safe unless they are administered under the supervision of a licensed practitioner (physician or dentist).
    C. New drugs that are limited to investigational use or new drugs that are not considered safe for indiscriminate use by lay persons.
11. New drugs may not be introduced into interstate commerce unless an application has been filed with the Food and Drug Administration and the application has been permitted to become effective. Adequate scientific evidence must be presented to show that the drug is safe for use under the conditions proposed for its use. The applicant does not have to prove the efficacy of the drug in order to obtain an effective application. During the time that the drug is under investigation by experts, the label of the drug must bear the statement, "Caution: New Drug—Limited by Federal Law to Investigational Use."
    NOTE: When tests indicate that the requirements of the Food and Drug Administration have been met, the law permits a period of clinical testing by approved clinicians and clinical groups. Pertinent data are collected and submitted to the Food and Drug Administration for further evaluation. If the Administration is satisfied that the drug has therapeutic merit and is not unduly toxic, distribution and sale of the new drug is permitted.
12. Certain drugs must be obtained from a batch that has been certified by the Food and Drug Administration. This applies to insulin and the antibiotics. Samples of each batch of these drugs are examined, and if samples conform to standards set forth by the Food and Drug Administration, the batches are referred to as "Certified Drugs."
13. Provisions of the Act that refer to prescriptions include the following:
    A. The pharmacist cannot refill from the original prescription unless the physician has authorized him to do so either by designating the number of times or the intervals after which the prescription may be refilled.
    B. A physician may give a prescription for most drugs orally (over the telephone), but the pharmacist must convert the oral prescription to writing. This provision modifies a previous provision which recognized only written prescriptions. Authorization for refills may also be telephoned to the pharmacist.
    NOTE: Nothing in the Federal Food, Drug, and Cosmetic Act, including the Durham-Humphrey Amendment, modifies the law and regulations regarding prescriptions for narcotics.

The Act also contains provisions pertaining to foods and cosmetics as indicated in the name of the Act. The law is concerned with the prevention of misbranding, adulterating, and the incorporation of harmful substances into foods and cosmetics.

Food and Drug Administration. The Food and Drug Administration is charged with the enforcement of the Federal Food, Drug, and Cosmetic Act. Seizure of offending goods and criminal prosecution of responsible persons or firms in federal courts are among the methods used to enforce the Act.

Public Health Service. The Public Health Service is an agency which is also part of the United States Department of Health, Education, and Welfare. One of its many functions is the regulation of biologic products. This refers to "any virus, therapeutic serum, antitoxin, or analogous product applicable to the prevention, treatment or cure of diseases or injuries of man." The control exercised by the Public Health Service over these products is done by inspecting and licensing the establishments that manufacture the products and by examining and licensing the products as well.

Federal Trade Commission. The Federal Trade Commission is an agency of the federal government which is directly responsible to the President. Its principal control with respect to drugs lies in its power to suppress false or misleading advertising to the general public.

Harrison Narcotic Act

The Harrison Narcotic Act was originally passed in 1914. It has been amended several times. The Act regulates the importation, manufacture, sale, and use of opium and cocaine and all their compounds and derivatives. Marihuana and its derivatives are also subject to the Act, as are many synthetic analgesic drugs which have been shown to be addiction-forming or addiction-sustaining.

All persons who manufacture, sell, prescribe, or dispense these drugs must be licensed and registered with the Department of Internal Revenue and pay an annual registration fee. Those who are lawfully entitled to obtain and use narcotics for purposes of instruction, research, or analysis must also register and pay a yearly tax. All persons who handle these drugs must keep accurate records of the drugs that they handle or use and save the records for a period of at least two years, during which time they are subject to inspection at any time by a revenue official.

A prescription for preparations listed in the law must bear the physician's name, address, and registry number, as well as the name and address of the patient and the date on which the prescription was written. The pharmacist may not refill the prescription.

A prescription for an opiate may not be issued by a physician to satisfy the craving of an addict, unless it is done in the course of professional treatment of the addict.

Application of the Harrison Law in hospitals. Every hospital must register with the Department of Internal Revenue and conform to many of the same regulations as physicians. Hospital pharmacies order supplies of narcotics, as well as other drugs listed under the Harrison Narcotic Law, on special order blanks that bear the hospital registry number. A special record is kept on every hospital unit (ward) for every dose of the preparations mentioned. The nurse records the name of the patient receiving the drug, date of administration of the drug, the amount, the name of the physician who ordered the drug, and her own name. In this way nurses can account for the quantities of these drugs which have been dispensed from the pharmacy and help the pharmacists to account for the supplies which have been issued.

NOTE: Since the law designates that all derivatives of opium must be subject to the above-mentioned restrictions, it explains why a preparation like papaverine, which is essentially nonnarcotic but which is derived from opium, must be accounted for in the same manner as morphine.

Oral prescriptions for narcotics. A pharmacist may dispense certain narcotics on the verbal authority of a physician, e.g., via telephone. Narcotics that may be dispensed in this manner are those which are believed to have little or no addiction liability and include papaverine, apomorphine, nalorphine, codeine (in limited quantities and when combined with nonnarcotic ingredients or with one of the isoquinoline alkaloids of opium such as papaverine), limited amounts of dihydrocodeinone and ethylmorphine either alone or with other nonnarcotic ingredients, and certain others.

In case of emergency or in case of great necessity, telephone or verbal orders may be given by a physician to a nurse for a patient. The nurse must write the order on the doctor's order sheet, stating that it is a telephone order or an emergency order, give the doctor's name and sign her own name or initials. This written order must be signed by the doctor with his full name or initials within twenty-four hours.* The Bureau of Narcotics acceded to the latter with some reluctance but permits it because it recognizes that unusual situations arise in hospitals not common to other places. Individual hospitals may choose to adhere to more strict regulations regarding narcotic orders.

Preparations exempt from the Harrison Narcotic Law. Certain preparations (with or without a prescription) in small quantities are exempt from the Harrison Narcotic Law, provided the preparation does not contain more than any one of the following per ounce, fluid or solid: 2 grains of opium, ½ grain of morphine, 1 grain of codeine, or any salt or derivative of these drugs, and also contains certain active medicinal drugs (other than narcotics) that provide valuable medicinal qualities other than that possessed by the narcotics alone.

*Report of Committee on Narcotic Regulations, Ninth Annual Meeting of the ASHP, August, 1952; Interpretation of Regulations and Procedures, Revised and Coordinated with Comments by the Bureau of Narcotics.

Scope of pharmacology, definitions, standards, legislation

Some *state laws,* however, cause the sale of such preparations to be restricted just as for any narcotic. For example, camphorated opium tincture (paregoric) may be purchased in some states in small amounts without a prescription, whereas in others the laws are such that the same tight restrictions apply for small amounts as for larger amounts of any of the narcotics.

The Narcotic Control Act of 1956. This Act amended the Harrison Law by increasing the penalties for violation of the Harrison Law and by making it unlawful to have heroin in one's possession. No heroin can be lawfully used or distributed for purposes other than for scientific research. This amendment also makes the acquisition and the transportation of marihuana unlawful.

Possession of narcotics. It is important to know that federal and state laws make the possession of narcotics a crime, except in specifically exempted cases.[*] The laws make no distinction between professional and practical nurses in this respect. A nurse may give narcotics only under the direction of a physician or dentist who has been licensed to prescribe or dispense narcotics. She may not have narcotics in her possession unless she is giving them to a patient under a doctor's order, or she is a patient for whom the doctor has prescribed them, or she is the official custodian of a limited supply of narcotics on a ward or department of the hospital.

Narcotics ordered but not used for patients must be returned to the source from which they were obtained (the doctor or the hospital). Violation or failure to comply with the Harrison Narcotic Law is punishable by fine, imprisonment, or both.

Other problems in drug legislation

In addition to the federal laws discussed in the preceding pages it should be mentioned that many states have laws applicable to the sale and manufacture of drugs within the state. This refers to laws other than those applying to the sale of small amounts of narcotics. Outstanding among them are the regulations for the sale of barbiturates.

It is well to remember that the effectiveness of legislation will depend on the appropriation of adequate funds to enforce the laws, the vigor with which enforcement is pushed by proper authorities, and the interest and cooperation of professional and lay groups.

We continue to be plagued with many problems resulting from indiscriminate and unwise use of drugs, misunderstandings about vitamins, glandular preparations, drugs for obesity, and cancer "cures." Although the consumer is often led astray by attractive advertising, clever suggestion, and adroit mishandling of information, there are reliable

[*]Creighton, Helen: Law Every Nurse Should Know, Philadelphia, 1957, W. B. Saunders Co., p. 117.

sources of information concerning drugs, cosmetic preparations, depilatories (hair removers), obesity cures, laxatives, antiseptics, dentifrices, and numerous other things about which the public is often grossly misinformed. Organizations such as the American Medical Association, American Dental Association, American Society for the Control of Cancer, American Heart Association, and local, state, and county health departments will supply accurate information free of charge or for a very small fee, necessary to defray the expense of printing or mailing materials.

Canadian drug legislation

Canadian laws that pertain to drugs are administered by the Department of National Health and Welfare. In several instances they were enacted earlier than similar laws in the United States.

Canadian Food and Drug Act

"Part C of the regulations of this act deals with drugs and is concerned mainly in manufacturing and packaging. In a manner similar to a pharmacopeia it defines and gives the characters and the tests for identity and purity of a great number of drugs (notably biologicals and antibiotics) in use in Canada but not included in the British Pharmacopoeia. It also contains amendments affecting drugs in the B.P. and other recognized pharmacopeias which are necessary for their use in Canada. Section C. 01.021 contains a long list of drugs which no person shall sell to the general public unless the labels carry a statement of the recommended single and daily dose, and specifies that such doses shall not exceed the maximum stated in the appendix, or the drug must carry a warning on the labels and must not be advertised to the general public. Schedule F of the act contains lists of drugs which can be sold only on prescription. The regulations state that no person shall sell a drug or a preparation containing a drug named or included in Schedule F except on an oral or written prescription, nor shall any person refill such prescription unless the prescriber thereof has so directed."*

Canadian Opium and Narcotic Act

"The regulations of this act govern the importation, exportation, manufacture, and sale and use of opium, coca leaf and any other similar drugs included in the schedule of the act. Also included are preparations containing any of these drugs. From time to time any alkaloids, derivatives, or preparations of drugs or similar synthetic preparations are added to the act. The schedule includes opium and cocaine and their alkaloids and

*From Waud, Russell A.: Prescription Writing and Drug Preparations. In Drill, V. A. (editor): Pharmacology in Medicine, New York, 1958, Blakiston Division, McGraw-Hill Book Co., Inc., pp. 28-29.

derivatives, *Cannabis sativa,* and any other drugs having addicting properties similar to these, including all the new synthetic narcotics.

"By means of records which must be kept by the manufacturer and the retail druggist under the regulations, the Department of National Health and Welfare is able to follow these drugs from their importation or manufacture to the patient. Before a pharmacist legally may dispense a drug included in the schedule or medication containing such a drug, he must receive a prescription from a physician. A signed and dated prescription issued by a duly authorized physician is essential in the case of all narcotic medication prescribed as such or any preparation containing a narcotic which is in a form intended for parenteral administration. Oral medication containing a narcotic in combination with two nonnarcotics may be dispensed by a pharmacist on the strength of a verbal prescription received from a physician who is known to the pharmacist or whose identity is established. Prescriptions of any description calling for a narcotic may not be repeated.

"Proper records are required to be maintained by a pharmacist over all medication of this type which is dispensed. Moreover, a physician is required to furnish the Division of Narcotic Control of the Department with any information respecting the circumstances under which the material was purchased or distributed.

"There is only one exception to the prescription requirement. Certain codeine compounds with a small codeine content may be sold to the public by a pharmacist without a prescription. In such instances the narcotic content cannot exceed $\frac{1}{8}$ grain per unit in tablet, capsule or other solid form and $\frac{1}{3}$ grain per fl. oz. in liquid form. In products of this kind, codeine must be in combination with two or more nonnarcotic substances and in recognized therapeutic doses.

"Additionally, items of this nature are required to be labeled in such a fashion as to show the true formula of the medicinal ingredients, and the words 'It is unlawful to administer this preparation to a child under two years of age as it contains codeine and is dangerous to its life' must appear on the label.

"It should be pointed out that local, state or provincial laws modify to a certain extent regulations governing the sale and administration of narcotics."[*]

The Canadian nurse and the narcotic laws of Canada

Although the administration of the Canadian Opium and Narcotic Act is legally the responsibility of the Department of National Health and Welfare, the enforcement of the law has been made largely the respon-

[*]From Waud, Russell A.: Prescription Writing and Drug Preparations. In Drill, V. A. (editor): Pharmacology in Medicine, New York, 1958, Blakiston Division, McGraw-Hill Book Co., Inc., pp. 28-29.

sibility of the Royal Canadian Mounted Police. Prosecution of offenses under the Act is handled through the Department of National Health and Welfare by legal agents specially appointed by the Department of Justice.*

A nurse may be in violation of the Canadian Opium and Narcotic Act if she is guilty of illegal possession of narcotics. Ignorance of the content of a drug in her possession is not considered a justifiable excuse. Proof of possession is sufficient to constitute an offense. Legal possession of narcotics by a nurse is limited to times when she is administering a drug to a patient on the order of a physician, when she is acting as the official custodian of narcotics in a department of the hospital, or when she is a patient for whom a physician has prescribed narcotics. The nurse may be held liable if she engages in illegal distribution or transportation of narcotic drugs. Heavy penalties are imposed for violation of the Canadian Opium and Narcotic Act.

*Creighton, Helen: Law Every Nurse Should Know, Philadelphia, 1957, W. B. Saunders Co., p. 156.

Exercises and questions
for review and study

1 State the purpose of the Federal Food, Drug, and Cosmetic Act.
2 Name six specific features of the Federal Food, Drug, and Cosmetic Act which are of interest to medical groups.
3 To what extent do you think our present-day legislation ensures adequate control of commerce in drugs? Explain.
4 Preparations of what drugs are included in the federal narcotic laws?
5 How does a nurse account for narcotic drugs that she may have contaminated or lost?
6 How might a nurse be guilty of violating the narcotic laws of her country?
7 To which national organizations might you write to secure accurate information about cancer and heart disease?
8 Prepare a list of sources from which you would expect to secure accurate information about new drugs.
9 Bring to class several examples of drug, cosmetic, or dietary advertisements taken from current magazines. Be prepared to discuss what seems to you to be good or poor advertising from the standpoint of legitimacy of claims made.

10 May any physician who comes to your hospital write an order for a narcotic? Explain.

Single choice
Encircle the answer of your choice.

1 The study of the action of drugs in living tissues is called:
a. materia medica
b. posology
c. pharmacodynamics
d. pharmacognosy
2 The preparing and dispensing of drugs is known as:
a. therapeutics
b. pharmacotherapeutics
c. pharmacy
d. pharmacology
3 New and Nonofficial Drugs is issued under the direction and supervision of:
a. American Pharmaceutical Association
b. Council on Drugs of American Medical Association
c. American Association of Hospital Pharmacists
d. a pharmacopeial committee
4 The letters U.S.P. after the name of a drug provide what information about a drug?
a. source

b. therapeutic usefulness
c. legal status
d. classification

5 Drugs selected for inclusion in the N.F. are selected largely on the basis of their:
a. source
b. low toxicity
c. therapeutic merit
d. demand

6 The Pharmacopeia of the United States and the National Formulary are legal standards because they are made so by which of the following?
a. Council on Drugs
b. American Pharmaceutical Association
c. Federal Food, Drug, and Cosmetic Act
d. National Bureau of Standards

7 The publication in which reports of the Council on Drugs are made periodically is:
a. The American Journal of Nursing
b. The Journal of the American Medical Association
c. Supplements to the U.S.P.
d. American Journal of Medical Science

8 In the United States an official drug is one listed in the U.S.P., the N.F., or in:
a. The Dispensatory of the United States of America
b. New and Nonofficial Drugs
c. Homeopathic Pharmacopoeia of the United States
d. Physicians' Desk Reference

9 Which of the following best indicates what a drug really is?
a. an active substance extracted from a plant
b. a chemical substance
c. an organic compound
d. a therapeutic agent

10 Which of the following is the best source of authentic information about new drugs?

a. U.S.P.
b. N.F.
c. a hospital formulary
d. N.N.D.

References

Creighton, Helen: Law Every Nurse Should Know, Philadelphia, 1957, W. B. Saunders Co.

Drill, V. A. (editor): Pharmacology in Medicine, New York, 1958, Blakiston Division, McGraw-Hill Book Co., Inc.

Goodman, L., and Gilman, A.: The Pharmacological Basis of Therapeutics, New York, 1955, The Macmillan Co.

Official publications

Pharmacopoeia Internationalis, Geneva, Switzerland, vol. I—1952, Vol. II—1955, The World Health Organization.

British Pharmacopoeia, ed. 9, London, 1958, The Pharmaceutical Press.

The Canadian Formulary, ed. 7, Toronto, 1949, Canadian Pharmaceutical Association.

The National Formulary, ed. 11, Easton, Pa., 1960, The Mack Publishing Co.

The Pharmacopeia of the United States of America, rev. ed. 16, Easton, Pa., 1960, The Mack Publishing Co.

Nonofficial publications

Jordan, E. P. (editor): Modern Drug Encyclopedia and Therapeutic Index, ed. 7, New York, 1958, Drug Publications, Inc.

New and Nonofficial Drugs, Philadelphia, 1960, J. B. Lippincott Co.

Physicians' Desk Reference to Pharmaceutical Specialities and Biologicals, ed. 13, Oradell, N. J., 1959, Medical Economics, Inc.

Chapter 3

Names, sources, active constituents, and pharmaceutic preparations of drugs

Names of drugs

The present-day use of a variety of names for the same drug is cause for confusion not only for nurses but sometimes for physicians as well. One name under which a drug may appear is its official name, another is the generic name, another is its chemical name, and a fourth by which it may be known is its trade name.

The *official name* is the name under which it is listed in one of the official publications, e.g., the U.S.P. The official name may also have one or more synonyms by which it is known. Before a new drug becomes official it will have assigned to it a *generic name*. This name is more simple than the chemical name, although it may reflect the chemical family to which the drug belongs. The generic name is never changed and can be used in all countries. It is not protected by law. It is usually initiated or proposed by the company that develops the drug. When it is selected careful investigation is made to make certain that it does not conflict with already existing names. Then it is usually processed by way of the American Medical Association Council on Drugs and through the World Health Organization which has a committee on International Non-Proprietary Names. In that way the name may be adopted on a world-wide basis.

The *chemical name* is meaningful principally to the chemist, who sees in the name a very precise description of the chemical constitution of the drug and the exact placement of atoms or atomic groupings. For example, the chemical name of one of the antibiotics is 4-dimethyl-amino-1,4,4a,5,5a,6,11,12a-octahydro-3,6,10,12,12a-pentahydroxy-6-methyl-1,11-dioxo-2-naphthacenecarboxamide. Its generic name is tetracycline and it is known under a number of trade names—Achromycin, Panmycin, Polycycline, Tetracyn, and Tetracyn V.

Names, sources, active constituents, pharmaceutic preparations　33

A *trade-mark name* or a *brand name* frequently appears in the literature with the sign ® at the upper right of the name to indicate that the name is registered and its use is restricted to the manufacturer who is the legal owner of the name. The first letter of the trade name is capitalized but the generic name is not capitalized. Many times the generic name is stated and the trade name is given in parentheses.

The name of a drug is not patented but a patent may be issued by the United States Patent Office to cover the drug as a chemical entity, the method of manufacture, the method of use, or any combination of these. Patents expire after seventeen years; then other manufacturers may make the drug under its generic name but they must select a different trade name. Two or more drug companies may make the same drug under different trade or trade-mark names. Sometimes a single drug may be sold under ten or twenty different brand names, which results in a great deal of undesirable confusion.

In order to promote sales under the trade-mark name, extensive advertising is usually necessary. This involves considerable expense which is borne mainly by the consumer. On the other hand, much of the research in new drugs is done in laboratories of reputable drug firms, and in order that they realize a legitimate return for the cost of research, they need to patent their product and have exclusive rights of its manufacture and sale.

There is a real need to give more attention to generic and official names. Some hospital pharmacies in this country are labeling medications with their official or generic names and placing the trade name or trademark name at the bottom of the label. This would appear to place the emphasis properly.

Further confusion is fostered when mixtures or combinations of otherwise well-known drugs are sold under a name that does not reflect the content. For example, phenacetin, aspirin, and caffeine are sold under a variety of names such as Empirin compound, Anacin, APC, and PAC, as well as aspirin compound.

The word "proprietary" is also used in referring to drugs. This means that the drug is protected from competition in some manner. In other words, the drug or perhaps its name belongs to someone.

Sources of drugs

Drugs are derived from four main sources: (1) plants, examples of which are digitalis, opium, and belladonna; (2) animals, from which drugs such as epinephrine, insulin, and ACTH are obtained; (3) minerals or mineral products, such as iron, iodine, and Epsom salt; and (4) chemical substances made in the laboratory. These are pure drugs, and some of them are simple substances, such as sodium bicarbonate and magnesium hydroxide, whereas others are products of complex synthesis, e.g., the sulfonamides and the adrenocorticosteroids.

Active constituents of plant drugs

The leaves, roots, seeds, and other parts of plants may be dried or otherwise processed for use as medicine and, as such, are known as crude drugs. Their therapeutic effect is due to chemical substances contained in the crude preparation. When the pharmacologically active constituents are separated from the crude preparation, the resulting substances are more potent and usually produce effects more reliable than those of the crude drug. As might be expected, these "active principles" are also more poisonous, and the dosage must be smaller. Following are some of the types of pharmacologically active compounds found in plants, grouped according to their physical and chemical properties: alkaloids, glycosides, gums, resins and balsams, tannins, and oils.

Alkaloids. Alkaloids (alkali-like) are compounds composed of carbon, hydrogen, nitrogen, and oxygen. Alkaloids have a bitter taste; they are often poisonous and hence preparations of them are administered in small doses. They are, for the most part, white crystalline solids. The name of an alkaloid ends in "ine," for example, caffeine, atropine, and morphine. Alkaloids will combine with an acid to form a salt. The salts of alkaloids are used in medicine in preference to pure alkaloids because they are more soluble; for example, morphine sulfate is much preferred to morphine because the former compound is much more soluble in water. Increased solubility is important because it may make possible the administration of a particular preparation by injection. A number of alkaloids have been chemically synthesized in the laboratory.

Both alkaloids and their salts are precipitated by tannic acid and oxidized by potassium permanganate. Hence these substances can be used under certain circumstances as antidotes for poisoning from alkaloids.

Glycosides. Glycosides are active principles which upon hydrolysis yield a carbohydrate (a sugar) and some other chemical grouping such as an aldehyde, acid, or alcohol. The carbohydrate may be glucose, in which case the compound may be called a glucoside, but carbohydrates other than glucose may occur in the molecule; hence the use of the more general term glycoside. The carbohydrate molecule is usually not necessary for the action of the glycoside, and in the body it may be removed to liberate the active aglycone or genin. The presence of a sugar in the molecule of the glycoside is thought to modify activity by affecting solubility, absorption, permeability, and cellular distribution.* An important glycoside used in medicine is digitoxin.

Gums. Gums are exudates from plants. They are polysaccharides which vary in the degree of their solubility in water. Upon the addition of water some of them will swell and form gelatinous or mucilaginous masses. Some remain unchanged in the gastrointestinal tract, where they act as hydrophilic (water-loving) colloids; that is, they absorb water, form watery bulk, and exert a laxative effect. Agar and psyllium seeds are examples of natural laxative gums. Synthetic hydrophilic colloids such as methylcellulose and sodium carboxymethyl cellulose may eventually replace the natural gums as laxatives. Gums are also used to soothe irritated skin and mucous membranes. Tragacanth gum, upon the addition of water, forms an emulsion which is used as a basis for a greaseless catheter lubricant or for chapped skin. Acacia (Gum Arabic), U.S.P., B.P., and Acacia Mucilage, N.F., are used as suspending agents in making emulsions and mixtures.

Resins. Resins are sometimes crude drugs and sometimes they represent an extraction from a crude drug. The rosin used by violinists is an example of a solid resin. A few are devoid of color, and some give off an aromatic fragrance due to the admixture of a volatile oil. Resins form the sap of certain trees. They are insoluble in water but soluble in alcohol, ether, and various oils. Resins are local irritants and some have been used in medicine as cathartics. Podophyllum resin is a constituent of Aloin, Belladonna, Cascara, and Podophyllum Pills (Hinkle's Pills) and is a rather irritating cathartic.

Gum resins are mixtures of gums and resins of which myrrh and asafetida are examples. **Balsams** also contain resins in addition to benzoic or cinnamic acids. Benzoin, U.S.P., B.P., Peruvian Balsam, N.F., and Tolu Balsam U.S.P., B.P., are examples.

Tannins. Tannins are complex substances of widespread occurrence in plants. They are used largely for their astringent effect.

Oils. The term oil is applied to a large number of liquids characterized by being insoluble in water and highly viscous. Their greasy "feel" is due to these properties. Oils are of two kinds, volatile and fixed.

Volatile oils are liquids which impart an aroma to a plant. They evaporate easily and leave no greasy stain. Because of their pleasant odor and taste they are frequently used as flavoring agents. Because of their volatility and consequent power of penetration they may be irritating, mildly stimulating, and antiseptic in effect. Peppermint Oil, Wintergreen Oil, and Clove Oil are listed in the U.S.P. and are occasionally used in medicine. Peppermint Oil and Wintergreen Oil are in the B.P.

*Walton, R. P.: The Cardiac Glycosides. In Drill, V. A. (editor): Pharmacology in Medicine, Philadelphia, 1958, Blakiston Division, McGraw-Hill Book Co., Inc., chap. 31, p. 456.

Fixed oils are those which feel greasy and do not evaporate readily. They hydrolyze to form fatty acids and glycerin. Some fixed oils are used as food, for example, olive oil. Others are used in medicine, e.g., castor oil, and some as vehicles in which to dissolve other drugs, such as sesame oil.

Pharmaceutical preparations

Pharmaceutical preparations are the preparations that make a drug suited to various methods of administration to a patient. They may be made by the pharmacist or by the pharmaceutical company from which they are purchased. A nurse is likely to bring more understanding to the task of administering drugs if she has some knowledge of these preparations.

Solutions and suspensions

Aqueous solutions. Aqueous solutions have one or more substances dissolved in water. *Waters* are saturated (unless otherwise stated) solutions of volatile oils or other aromatic substances in distilled water. The volatile substance may be solid, liquid, or gaseous. Peppermint Water, U.S.P., and Concentrated Peppermint Water, B.P., are examples. Other aqueous solutions, sometimes referred to as *true solutions,* are made by dissolving a nonvolatile substance in water. Examples are Lugol's Solution, U.S.P., B.P., Epinephrine Solution, U.S.P., and Aluminum Subacetate Solution, U.S.P.

Syrups are sometimes used for their demulcent* effect on irritated membranes of the throat. A Simple Syrup U.S.P. is an aqueous solution of sucrose (85 per cent). Syrups may be flavored and used as a vehicle in which to disguise unpleasant-tasting medicines and also as a preservative. Examples of syrups listed in the U.S.P. and B.P. are Orange Syrup and Tolu Syrup. Cherry, Glycyrrhiza, and Raspberry Syrups are also listed in the U.S.P. Promethazine Hydrochloride Syrup, U.S.P., is an example of a syrup that reflects medicinal content, an iron compound.

Aqueous suspensions. Aqueous suspensions are defined in U.S.P. XVI as follows: "Preparations of finely divided drugs either intended for suspension in some suitable liquid vehicle prior to use or already in suspension in a liquid vehicle." Sterile suspensions are prepared by adding water for injection to the preparation, e.g., Sterile Chloramphenicol for Suspension, U.S.P. Others are sterile and already suspended in a suitable liquid vehicle and ready for use, e.g., Sterile Procaine Penicillin G Suspension, U.S.P. Sterile suspensions are intended for intramuscular or

*Demulcent is a substance that exerts a soothing effect.

subcutaneous injection, but they cannot be given intravenously or intrathecally. Oral suspensions may be prepared in much the same way, but they are not sterile and may not be injected. Suspensions for ophthalmic use are sterile suspensions in an aqueous medium which contains a suitable bacteriostatic agent. Hydrocortisone Acetate Ophthalmic Suspension, U.S.P.,* is a good example. Suspensions tend to settle slowly and should be shaken well before use to provide uniform distribution of the drug in the medium of the preparation.

Mixtures are aqueous preparations containing insoluble, nonfatty solid substances in suspension. No mixtures are listed in the U.S.P. The B.P. contains Mixture of Magnesium Hydroxide. There are several mixtures in the N.F., e.g., Chalk Mixture. The term mixture is also used to mean any preparation of several drugs, e.g., a cough mixture. However, the term is usually restricted to mean only preparations for internal use.

Emulsions are suspensions of fats or oils in water with the aid of an emulsifying agent (oil-in-water emulsion). This type of emulsion will mix with water. Emulsions are stabilized by agents such as acacia and gelatin which coat the tiny droplets of oil and prevent them from coming in direct contact with water. Thus the oily "feel" of oil-in-water emulsions is masked. Cod Liver Oil Emulsion is a well-known emulsion of this type.

Magmas are sometimes called milks because they are white and resemble milk. They are bulky suspensions of insoluble preparations in water. Magnesia Magma, U.S.P. (Milk of Magnesia), or Magnesium Hydroxide Mixture, B.P., is an example. Magmas tend to settle or separate upon standing and should be shaken well before they are poured.

Gels are aqueous suspensions of insoluble drugs in hydrated form. The particles suspended are approximately the size seen in colloidal dispersions. Magmas and gels are highly similar except that the particles suspended in a magma are larger; Aluminum Hydroxide Gel, U.S.P., is an example.

Spirits. Spirits are concentrated alcoholic solutions of volatile substances. They are also known as essences. The dissolved substance may be solid, liquid, or gaseous. Most spirits contain 5 to 10 or up to 20 per cent of the active drug. The alcohol serves as a preservative as well as a solvent. Peppermint Spirit, U.S.P., B.P., sometimes is used as a carminative or a flavoring agent.

Elixirs. Elixirs are aromatic, sweetened, alcoholic preparations, frequently used as flavored vehicles, such as Aromatic Elixir, U.S.P., or as active medicinal agents if they are medicated elixirs, such as Phenobarbital Elixir, U.S.P., or Cascara Elixir, B.P.

Tinctures. Tinctures are alcoholic or hydroalcoholic solutions prepared

*U.S.P., XVI Interim Admission.

38

usually from plant drugs or from chemical substances. Tinctures of potent drugs contain 10 Gm. of drug in 100 ml. of tincture. Most other tinctures contain 20 Gm. of drug in 100 ml. of tincture. Tinctures are prepared by extracting the drug from its crude source or by making an alcoholic solution of the drug. Iodine Tincture, U.S.P., is made by dissolving iodine in an alcoholic solution of sodium iodide. The alcoholic content of tinctures improves their keeping qualities and facilitates solution of drugs that are poorly soluble in water. Tinctures listed in the B.P. are preparations extracted from crude drugs, not simple solutions. The usual dose of a potent tincture is about 1 ml. (0.3 to 1 ml.) or 5 to 15 minims.

Fluidextracts. Fluidextracts are alcoholic liquid extracts of vegetable drugs made so that 1 ml. of the fluidextract contains 1 Gm. of the drug. They are the most concentrated of any of the fluid preparations, being of 100 per cent strength and ten times stronger than potent tinctures. Since many of them precipitate in light, they should be kept in dark bottles and not used if much precipitate has formed. Glycyrrhiza Fluidextract, U.S.P., is used as a flavoring agent, whereas Aromatic Cascara Sagrada Fluidextract, U.S.P., and Cascara Sagrada Liquid Extract, B.P., are used as cathartics.

Spirits, medicated elixirs, tinctures, and *fluidextracts* are preparations that tend to be potent and hence the dosage is likely to be small. A nurse would never expect to administer as much as 30 ml. (a fluid ounce) of any of them. A fraction of a milliliter (a few minims) up to as much as 2 to 4 ml. (1 to 2 fluidrams) is likely to be the range of dosage. Furthermore, these preparations are never injected, one reason being that they all contain alcohol. Most tinctures contain resins which make them incompatible with water.

Extracts. Extracts are concentrated preparations of vegetable or animal drugs obtained by removing the active ingredients of the drugs with suitable solvents and then evaporating all or part of the solvents. Extracts are made in three forms: semiliquids or liquids of syrupy consistency, plastic masses or pillular extracts, and dry powders known as powdered extracts. Extracts are intended to preserve the useful constituents of a drug in a form suitable for medication or for the making of other dosage forms such as tablets or pills. Liver Extract, N.F., is a dry extract. Cascara Dry Extract, B.P., is used to make Cascara Tablets, B.P.

Dosage forms

Capsules, Spansules, tablets, pills, troches, etc. are used to divide a drug or mixture of drugs into definite doses and avoid the inconvenience of preparing the dose from dry powders. They are therefore referred to as "dosage forms." Capsules and coated tablets are a convenient way of giving drugs that have an unpleasant taste. It has been true in the past and to some extent continues to be true that some patients are more impressed with a vile-tasting medicine than a pleasant-tasting or tasteless preparation. However, most patients appreciate preparations that are not unpleasant to take.

Capsules. Capsules are one of the most popular dosage forms for the oral administration of powders, oils, and liquids. Capsules are usually made of gelatin and may be hard or soft, depending on the amount of glycerin in the gelatin. Hard capsules are formed by two cylindrical halves, one of which fits into the other. They are used to dispense powdered drug. Soft capsules are sealed together. Ordinarily, gelatin capsules dissolve in the stomach to release the medication, although they may be coated with a substance which resists the action of the gastric juice and so will not disintegrate until they reach the alkaline secretions of the intestine. Such capsules are said to be *enteric coated.* Sizes of capsules range from 5 to 000 (see Fig. 1). Capsules filled in pharmaceutical houses are often of a distinctive color or shape to identify them with the manufacturer.

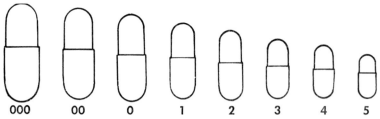

Fig. 1 Various sizes and numbers of gelatin capsules, *actual size.* (From Jackson, D. E.: Experimental Pharmacology and Materia Medica, St. Louis, The C. V. Mosby Co.)

Dosage forms which provide for gradual but continued release of drug are sold under a number of different names, e.g., Spansules, Gradumets, and Timespans.

Spansules are preparations usually contained in a capsule in which small particles of the drug are coated with materials that require a varying amount of time to dissolve. This provides for a long, continuous period of absorption and effect. Some particles dissolve and are absorbed almost immediately, others require a few hours, and some do not dissolve for six hours or more. An increasing number of drugs is available in one of these forms; e.g., Prochlorperazine, U.S.P. (Compazine), is available in Spansule form.

Tablets. Tablets are preparations of powdered drug which are compressed or molded into small disks. They may be made with or without a diluent (dextrose, lactose, starch, etc.), and they may differ greatly in size, weight, and shape. *Compressed tablets* are made with heavy machinery.

The granulated form of the preparation is formed, under great mechanical pressure, into tablets. Compressed tablets usually contain in addition to the drug a diluent, a binder, a disintegrator, and a lubricant. Binders are substances that give adhesiveness to the powdered drug. Diluents are used when the amount of active ingredient is small, and lubricants keep the tablet from sticking to the machines. A disintegrator, such as starch, helps the tablet to dissolve readily when it is placed in water, due to the fact that the starch expands when it gets wet. Tablets are sometimes scored (marked with an indented line across the surface) so that they can be broken easily if half a tablet is the dose required. Tablets may be coated with sugar or chocolate to enhance their palatability. They may be covered with a colored coating to make them more attractive to patients or for purposes of identification. Both tablets and capsules may be enteric coated either to protect the drug from the effect of the gastric secretions or to prevent irritation of the gastric mucosa by the drug. Compressed tablets are usually administered orally. *Molded tablets* or *tablet triturates* are made by mixing the moistened powdered drug with dextrose or lactose and powdered sucrose, so as to make a plastic mass suited for manual pressure into small molds. Later the tablets are ejected and dried. They disintegrate readily when placed in water. Molded tablets are administered orally, sublingually, or sometimes by inserting them in the buccal pouch (between the cheek and the teeth), depending on the type of medication which they contain and the purpose for which they are given. Hypodermic tablets are compressed or molded tablets that dissolve completely in water and are suitable for injection. They must be prepared under aseptic conditions and dissolved suitably before administration.

Troches. Troches or lozenges are flat, round, or rectangular preparations which are held in the mouth until they dissolve, liberating the drug or drugs involved. They usually contain water, sugar, and a mucilage in addition to the drug and are dried in hot air. They temporarily produce a high concentration of the drug in the oral cavity. They are held in the mouth until entirely dissolved. That which is swallowed may produce systemic effects.

Pills. Pills are mixtures of a drug or drugs with some cohesive material. The mass is molded into globular, oval, or flattened bodies which are convenient for swallowing. Pills are not suitable for injection. They have been replaced to a great extent by capsules and tablets. Although "pill" is a popular, general term for tablets or capsules, this is a misuse of the term. In fact, very few true pills are on the market today.

Powders. Powders are finely divided solid drugs or mixtures of drugs. Some are used externally and some are used internally. When prepared for internal use, the dose of the powder is dispensed in separate folded

How To Use
TUBEX®–Sterile Needle Units

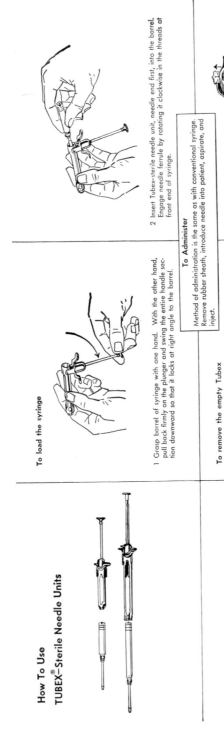

To load the syringe

1 Grasp barrel of syringe with one hand. With the other hand, pull back firmly on the plunger and swing the entire handle section downward so that it locks at right angle to the barrel.

2 Insert Tubex-sterile needle unit, needle end first, into the barrel. Engage needle ferrule by rotating it clockwise in the threads at front end of syringe.

To Administer

Method of administration is the same as with conventional syringe. Remove rubber sheath, introduce needle into patient, aspirate, and inject.

3 Swing plunger back into place and attach end to the threaded shaft of the piston. Hold the syringe barrel with one hand and rotate plunger until both ends of Tubex are fully, but lightly engaged. To maintain sterility, leave the rubber sheath in place until just before use. To aspirate before injecting, pull back slightly on the plunger.

To remove the empty Tubex

4 Disengage plunger from piston by rotating counterclockwise and open syringe as in step 1. Do not pull plunger back before disengaging or syringe will jam. Rotate Tubex-sterile needle unit counterclockwise to disengage at front end of syringe, remove from syringe, and discard.

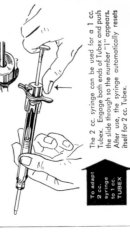

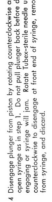

To adapt 2 cc. syringe to 1 cc. TUBEX

The 2 cc. syringe can be used for a 1 cc. Tubex. Engage both ends of Tubex and push the slide through so the number "1" appears. After use, the syringe automatically resets itself for 2 cc. Tubex.

Fig. 2 How to use Tubex-sterile needle units. (Courtesy Wyeth Laboratories, Philadelphia, Pa.)

papers or in gelatin capsules, or if the dose can be measured satisfactorily, it is sometimes given with a spoon.

Ampules and vials. Ampules and vials contain powdered or liquid drugs usually intended for injection. *Ampules* are sealed glass containers and usually contain one dose of the drug. *Vials* are glass containers with rubber stoppers and usually contain a number of doses of the drug. The powdered drug must be dissolved in sterile distilled water or in isotonic saline solution before administration.

Disposable syringes. Disposable syringes containing doses of drug preparations have become popular. Various antibiotic preparations are commonly given this way. Another dosage form which has been introduced is the "cartridge" type of container which is fitted into a metal framework and a needle attached, such as Tubex. The cartridge contains the drug which is given by injection. The whole resembles a hypodermic. (See Fig. 2.)

Additional preparations

Liniments. Liniments are liquid suspensions or dispersions intended for external application. They are applied to the skin by rubbing. In addition to one or more active ingredients they may contain oil, soap, water, or alcohol. The oil and the soap of liniments adhere to the skin and serve as lubricants while the preparation is being rubbed on. Liniments usually contain an anodyne (to relieve pain) or a rubefacient (to redden the skin). Liniments may temporarily relieve pain and swelling by counterirritation and by improving circulation of blood to the part.

Lotions. Lotions are liquid suspensions or dispersions intended for external application. Lotions usually should be patted on the skin and not applied by rubbing. This is particularly true if the skin is irritated or inflamed. Lotions can be protective, emollient, cooling, cleansing, astringent, or antipruritic, depending on their content and the purpose for which they are being used. Calamine Lotion, U.S.P., B.P., is an example of a lotion that has a soothing effect. Phenolated Calamine Lotion, U.S.P., is effective for the relief of itching.

Ointments are semisolid preparations of medicinal substances in some type of base and are intended for external application to the skin or mucous membranes. The usual bases used in ointments are petrolatum and lanolin. The base helps to keep the medicinal substance in prolonged contact with the skin. Ointments do not wash off readily unless surfactants have been added. A number of other bases can be used in ointments, some of which are miscible with water. Ointments are used for their soothing, astringent, or bacteriostatic effects, depending on the drug or drugs contained in the preparation. Sulfur Ointment, U.S.P., B.P., Rose Water Ointment, N.F., and Zinc

Oxide Ointment, U.S.P., or Zinc Ointment, B.P., are good examples.

Ophthalmic ointments are sterile, specially prepared ointments for use in the eye. The ointment base selected must be nonirritating to the eye, must permit free diffusion of the drug throughout the secretions of the eye, and must not alter or destroy the drug which it incorporates. Chloramphenicol Ophthalmic Ointment, U.S.P., is an example.

Pastes. Pastes are ointmentlike preparations suited only for external application. Many of them consist of thick stiff ointments which do not melt at body temperature. They tend to absorb secretions and they soften and penetrate the skin to a less extent than do ointments. Zinc Oxide Paste, U.S.P., and Compound Zinc Paste, B.P., are examples.

Plasters. Plasters are solid preparations which serve as either simple adhesives or counterirritants. When applied to the body the heat softens them and makes them adhere. The base is usually a rubber mixture called rubber plaster. Adhesive Plaster, U.S.P., and Salicylic Acid Plaster, U.S.P., are two examples.

Suppositories. Suppositories are mixtures of drugs with a firm base which can be molded into shapes suitable for insertion into a body cavity or orifice. The base may be glycerinated gelatin, a hard soap, cacao butter (cocoa butter), or carbowax (a polymer of ethylene glycol). These substances at body temperature dissolve in water or secretions of mucous membranes and allow the drug to come in contact with the mucous membrane to produce local or systemic effects. The shapes and sizes are suitable for insertion into the rectum, vagina, or urethra. Urethral suppositories are called *bougies.* Glycerin Suppositories, U.S.P., B.P., are official preparations. Aminophylline Suppositories and Carbarsone Suppositories are also listed in the U.S.P.

Fig. 3 Various forms of suppositories: rectal, vaginal, and urethral. (From Jackson, D. E.: Experimental Pharmacology and Materia Medica, St. Louis, The C. V. Mosby Co.)

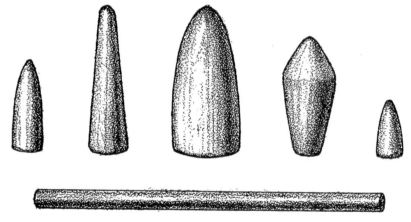

Poultices. Poultices are soft moist preparations, the purpose of which is to supply moist heat to a skin area. If applied too long they cause maceration of the skin. They tend to be regarded as home remedies. There are no poultices listed in the U.S.P., and the B.P. has only one, Kaolin Poultice.

Pharmaceutic accessories

Coloring substances. Coloring substances may be added to medicines to make them more acceptable to patients. Red and green colors seem to be favorites. The coloring agent must be either an official agent or one that has been certified under the Federal Food, Drug, and Cosmetic Act. Amaranth Solution, U.S.P., imparts a vivid red color to a preparation such as Phenobarbital Elixir, U.S.P. Compound Amaranth Solution is listed in the N.F.

Synthetic sweetening agents. Synthetic sweetening agents are useful to sweeten certain medicinal preparations, and they may be used advantageously for patients whose intake of carbohydrate is, for some reason, restricted.

Saccharin, U.S.P., B.P., when in dilute solution, is said to be 500 times sweeter than sugar (sucrose). Concentrated solutions of saccharin taste bitter and leave an aftertaste on the tongue. Saccharin has no food value.

Saccharin Sodium, U.S.P., B.P., has the advantage over plain saccharin of being much more soluble in water. It is available in 15, 30, and 60 mg. tablets.

Calcium Cyclamate, U.S.P. (Sucaryl Calcium), is a synthetic nonnutritive sweetening agent particularly useful to patients on a low-sodium diet. It is said to be essentially nontoxic, although excessive intake may cause diarrhea. Concentrated solutions tend to have a bitter taste. *Compound Calcium Cyclamate Solution,* U.S.P., and *Compound Calcium Cyclamate Tablets,* U.S.P., are preparations of calcium cyclamate and saccharin.

Cyclamate Sodium* (Sucaryl Sodium) is a stable synthetic nonnutritive sweetening agent. It is used for many of the same purposes as the preparations previously mentioned. It is stable in hot solutions, and no aftertaste is observed if dilute solutions are used. It is said to be about thirty times sweeter than sucrose. It is relatively nontoxic, although, like Cyclamate Calcium, it can produce a laxative effect if the intake is excessive. It is available in 50 mg. tablets and in a solution. Both the tablet and the solution are available which contain saccharin to overcome a bitter taste.

---

*Described in annual publication of A. M. A. Council on Drugs, N.N.D., 1960.

Questions
for study and review

1 What is meant by the generic name of a drug? How does it differ from a trade name?
2 What is the advantage of labeling drugs with both their generic and trade names?
3 How can you recognize a trade-mark name when it is used in medical literature?
4 From what source do most of our new drugs come? What advantages do they have from the standpoint of dosage and reliability of effect?
5 Define an active principle and name several.
6 What is meant by a crude drug? Why were so many of the early drugs used in this country as well as in other countries preparations of crude drugs?
7 What are the main differences between alkaloids and glycosides?
8 What seems to be the main role or function of a carbohydrate in the molecular make-up of a glycoside?
9 Name four medicinal preparations that contain alcohol. How would you expect to administer them to patients and why? What general statement could you make about their dosage?
10 What differences exist between compressed and molded tablets which are of significance to a nurse?
11 What is meant by an enteric-coated tablet? What is the purpose of the enteric coating? What colors have you observed in enteric coatings?
12 What preparation might be used to sweeten food for a diabetic patient who is on a diet which is restricted in both carbohydrate and sodium?

References

Council on Drugs of the American Medical Association: New and Nonofficial Drugs, Philadelphia, 1960, J. B. Lippincott Co.

Courchaine, A. J.: Chemistry Visualized and Applied, New York, 1950, G. P. Putnam's Sons.

Drill, V. A. (editor): Pharmacology in Medicine, New York, 1958, Blakiston Division, McGraw-Hill Book Co., Inc.

Reichert, P.: What's in a Name, Am. J. Nursing 59: 822, 1959.

Sollmann, T.: A Manual of Pharmacology, Philadelphia, 1957, W. B. Saunders Co.

Official drug compendia

British Pharmacopoeia, ed. 9, London, 1958, The Pharmaceutical Press.

The National Formulary, ed. 10, Philadelphia, 1955, J. B. Lippincott Co.

The National Formulary, ed. 11, Philadelphia, 1960, J. B. Lippincott Co. (List of Admissions).

United States Treasury Department, Bureau of Narcotics, Regulations No. 5, Washington, D. C., 1938, Government Printing Office.

The Pharmacopeia of the United States of America, rev. ed. 16, Easton, Pa., 1960, Mack Publishing Co.

Chapter 4

Review of arithmetic

Introduction

Students of nursing, like other persons, vary in their ability to comprehend mathematical principles. Some use arithmetical skills with ease and others have more or less difficulty. Some may never be entirely comfortable in dealing mentally with quantitative terms. This does not mean that such persons are lacking in intelligence or that they can never learn to work with numbers or quantitative ideas safely and satisfactorily. Fortunately, nurses do not have to deal in higher mathematics, only simple arithmetic which was studied in grade school. This includes addition, subtraction, multiplication, and division as these concepts are used in dealing with fractions, decimals, percentage, ratio, and proportion.

It is important that nurses know how to use simple mathematical skills quickly and accurately; therefore a certain amount of hard work and self-discipline may be called for if the students are to feel secure and safe in their roles as nurses. Each student needs to appraise her own ability or the lack of it and work accordingly.

Difficulty with arithmetic is due frequently to some form of carelessness, i.e., failure to read with comprehension, failure to add or subtract carefully, failure to work neatly so that what has been written can be read, etc. There are several things to which students should pay especial attention from the beginning of their review of arithmetic and study of metrology* in order to improve in accuracy.

1. When working a problem always treat the answer as if you suspected it to be wrong. Then check back over your work, preferably in a different way; e.g., if you have added a column of numbers from above downward, add the figures from below upward to see if you get the same answer.

2. Scrutinize your answer to see if it is plausible or if it "makes sense." For example, if

$$\frac{1}{2} X = 10$$
$$X = ?$$

*Metrology is the study of weights and measures.

If your answer is 20, you could say that is sensible because regardless of what X stands for, one half (½) of anything must be less than two halves (or a whole), and two halves must be twice one half.

3. Reread the statement of the problem (out loud if it helps you) and ask yourself if you have done what you were asked to do.

4. Draw pictures to clarify the problem to yourself or use examples that you can visualize. For example, if

$$4 X = 20$$
$$X = ?$$

X may mean very little to you and perhaps you cannot think whether you should divide 20 by 4 or 4 by 20. Say to yourself, "If four apples cost twenty cents, one apple would have to cost less than twenty cents (not more); therefore I would have to divide 20 by 4 which would make each apple cost 5 cents." Apples are things you have seen and felt and tasted and about which you know the cost. Then make certain that your answer is correct by checking in the following manner: If one apple cost 5 cents, 4 of them would cost 4 times 5 cents, or 20 cents. When dealing with a more difficult problem go back to a simple method like this, analyze how you arrived at your answer, and then apply the same method of procedure to the problem with which you are dealing. How would you solve the following?

$$\frac{2}{3} X = 0.5$$
$$X = ?$$

Your instructor will point out numerous other suggestions from time to time which will help you to help yourself.

Arabic and Roman numerals

There are two systems of expressing numbers in use in prescription writing, namely, the Arabic and the Roman. The Arabic system uses the figures 1, 2, 3, 4, 5, 6, 7, 8, 9, 10. The Roman system uses certain capital letters as follows:

I = 1	X = 10	C = 100	
V = 5	L = 50	D = 500	M = 1000

Roman numbers are expressed by combining the numerals in accordance with the following rules:

1. Repeating a numeral repeats its value: i.e., II = 2; XX = 20; CC = 200. But since doubling V, L, or D would give the equivalent of X, C, and M, respectively, these quantities are not doubled.

2. A numeral placed before a numeral of higher value is subtracted from the latter: i.e., IV = 5 – 1 or 4; IX = 10 – 1 or 9; XL = 40; XC = 90; CM = 900. Only one numeral can be so subtracted.

Table 1

Roman numerals and arabic equivalents

Roman	Arabic	Roman	Arabic
I	1	XIX	19
II	2	XX	20
III	3	XXX	30
IV	4	XL	40
V	5	L	50
VI	6	LX	60
VII	7	LXX	70
VIII	8	LXXX	80
IX	9	XC	90
X	10	C	100
XI	11	CC	200
XII	12	CD	400
XIII	13	D	500
XIV	14	DC	600
XV	15	CM	900
XVI	16	M	1000
XVII	17	MCMLX	1960
XVIII	18	MM	2000

3. Numerals placed after a numeral of higher value are added to the latter: i.e., VI = 5 + 1 or 6; XII = 10 + 2 or 12; LXV = 65; CXXIV = 124.

4. A numeral placed between two higher numerals is always read in connection with the one following: i.e., XIV = 14; XXIX = 29; LIX = 59.

See Table 1 for a list of Roman numerals and their Arabic equivalents.

Exercises Arabic and Roman numerals

1 Give the Arabic numbers for the following:

a. C   f. MCMXX
b. D   g. XXIX
c. M   h. XL
d. L   i. XC
e. LXI   j. XCIX

2 Give the Roman numerals for the following:

a. 76   f. 10
b. 54   g. 6
c. 20   h. 48
d. 85   i. 89
e. 19   j. 94

Common fractions, improper fractions, and mixed numbers

A common fraction is one or more of the equal parts of a unit. If a pie is cut into 6 equal parts, each part will be one sixth (⅙) of the pie. Two of the equal parts will be two sixths (²⁄₆); 3 of the equal parts will be three sixths (³⁄₆), and so on. A fraction is expressed by two numbers called the numerator and the denominator. The denominator of a fraction is the number of parts into which the unit is divided. In the fractions of the pie mentioned above the denominator is 6. The numerator of a fraction is the number of equal parts taken. In the fraction $\frac{1}{6}$, 1 is the numerator. The numerator and the denominator are called the terms of a fraction.

Proper fractions. A proper fraction is one in which the numerator is less than the denominator; e.g., $\frac{3}{4}$, $\frac{5}{8}$, $\frac{2}{3}$.

Different fractions of the same value. Suppose 3 pies are of equal size but one of them has been cut into 4 equal pieces, the second has been cut into 6 equal pieces, and the third has been cut into 8 equal pieces.

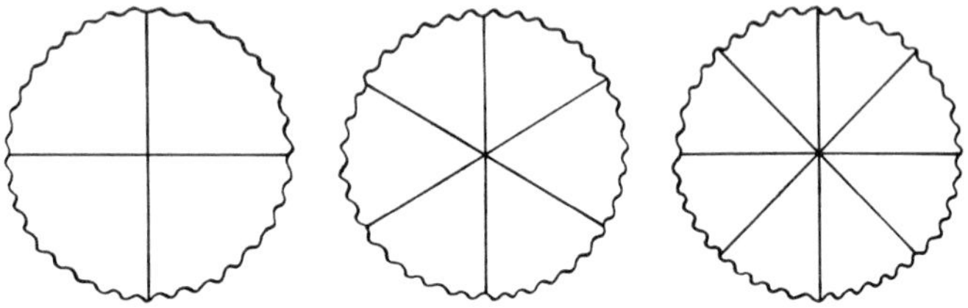

In each of these pies, which fraction equals $\frac{1}{2}$ of the pie? In other words, how many fourths equal one half? How many sixths equal one half and how many eighths equal one half? Likewise, how many eighths equal $\frac{3}{6}$? How many eighths equal $\frac{2}{4}$? How many eighths equal $\frac{4}{4}$? Thus it is apparent that a number of fractions can have the same value; e.g., $\frac{1}{2}$, $\frac{2}{4}$, $\frac{3}{6}$, and $\frac{4}{8}$ are *equivalent* fractions.

Changing a fraction to its simplest form is called reducing it to its lowest terms. The fraction $\frac{2}{4}$ can be changed to $\frac{1}{2}$ by dividing both the numerator and the denominator by 2. The proper fraction $\frac{3}{6}$ is reduced by dividing both terms by 3. The division of both terms of a fraction by the same number does not change its value.

Raising a common fraction to higher terms. To raise a common fraction to higher terms, multiply both terms of the fraction by the same number.

To change $\frac{5}{6}$ to twelfths, multiply both terms by 2. $\frac{5}{6} = \dfrac{5 \times 2}{6 \times 2} = \dfrac{10}{12}$; $\frac{3}{5}$ to tenths $\dfrac{3 \times 2}{5 \times 2} = \dfrac{6}{10}$; $\frac{3}{4}$ to sixteenths $\dfrac{3 \times 4}{4 \times 4} = \dfrac{12}{16}$; $\frac{2}{5}$ to tenths $= \dfrac{2 \times 2}{5 \times 2} = \dfrac{4}{10}$.

Improper fractions. Improper fraction is one in which the numerator is equal to, or greater than, the denominator; e.g., $\frac{5}{5}$, $\frac{6}{5}$, $\frac{9}{7}$, $\frac{250}{120}$.

Relationship between improper fractions and mixed numbers. A mixed number is an integer (or a whole number) and a fraction united; e.g., $4\frac{1}{4}$, $16\frac{2}{3}$, $9\frac{5}{6}$.

An *improper fraction* can be changed to a whole or mixed number by dividing the numerator by the denominator.

Examples:

$$\frac{16}{3} \; (16 \div 3) = 5\frac{1}{3} \qquad \frac{21}{8} \; (21 \div 8) = 2\frac{5}{8} \qquad \frac{20}{5} \; (20 \div 5) = 4$$

A *mixed number* can be changed to an improper fraction by multiplying the denominator of the fraction by the whole number, adding the numerator, and placing the sum over the denominator of the fraction.

Examples:

$$7\frac{1}{4} = \frac{4 \times 7 + 1}{4} = \frac{29}{4} \qquad\qquad 6\frac{2}{3} = \frac{6 \times 3 + 2}{3} = \frac{20}{3}$$

$$5\frac{1}{6} = \frac{5 \times 6 + 1}{6} = \frac{31}{6} \qquad\qquad 2\frac{2}{3} = \frac{2 \times 3 + 2}{3} = \frac{8}{3}$$

Multiplying a whole number by a fraction. To multiply a whole number by a fraction, proceed as follows.

Example: Multiply $4 \times \frac{2}{3}$

1. Multiply the whole number by the numerator of the fraction $2 \times 4 = 8$.

2. Place the product over the denominator thus $\frac{8}{3}$.

3. Change the improper fraction to a mixed number $\frac{8}{3} = 2\frac{2}{3}$.

Addition of common fractions. To add common fractions reduce fractions to equivalent fractions with a least common denominator, add the resulting numerators, and write the sum of them over the common denominator. Following are explanations:

1. To find the least common denominator it is necessary to find the smallest number that will contain all of the denominators concerned. For example, to find the least common denominator of $\frac{3}{4}$, $\frac{5}{6}$, and $\frac{7}{12}$ it is necessary to find the smallest number that will contain 4, 6, and 12. This obviously is 12.

2. To reduce fractions to equivalent fractions with a least common denominator, divide the least common denominator by the denominator of each fraction and multiply both terms of the fraction by the quotient. To reduce $\frac{3}{4}$, $\frac{5}{6}$, and $\frac{7}{12}$ to twelfths, divide 12 by the denominator of each fraction, and multiply both terms of the fractions by the quotients thus obtained:

$$12 \div 4 = 3; \; \frac{3 \times 3}{3 \times 4} = \frac{9}{12}$$

$$12 \div 6 = 2; \; \frac{2 \times 5}{2 \times 6} = \frac{10}{12}$$

$$12 \div 12 = 1; \; \frac{1 \times 7}{1 \times 12} = \frac{7}{12}$$

3. The addition of $\frac{9}{12}$, $\frac{10}{12}$, and $\frac{7}{12}$ equals $\frac{26}{12}$, or $1\frac{3}{6}$, or $2\frac{1}{6}$.

Subtraction of common fractions. To subtract common fractions it is again necessary to reduce the fractions concerned to equivalent fractions with a common denominator. Then subtract the smaller fraction from the larger.

Example: To subtract ¾ from ⅚—change both to twelfths.

$$\frac{5}{6} = \frac{10}{12}$$

$$\frac{3}{4} = \frac{9}{12}$$

$$\frac{10}{12} \text{ minus } \frac{9}{12} = \frac{1}{12}$$

When subtracting mixed numbers, the whole number which is to be subtracted always will be smaller than the whole number from which it is to be subtracted. If the same is true of the fractions, no difficulty arises. The least common denominator of the fractions is found and the lower fraction is raised as required. Then the whole number and the numerators are subtracted in separate operations.

Example: Subtract 6½ from 8¾

$$8\tfrac{3}{4} = 8\tfrac{3}{4}$$
$$6\tfrac{1}{2} = 6\tfrac{2}{4}$$
$$\overline{2\tfrac{1}{4}}$$

If the fraction to be subtracted is larger than the one from which it is to be subtracted, 1 must be borrowed from the whole number associated with the smaller fraction, and must be changed to a fraction having the same denominator as that fraction and added to it.

Example:

$$\begin{array}{ccc} 6\tfrac{1}{2} & 6\tfrac{2}{4} & 5\tfrac{6}{4} \\ -\tfrac{3}{4} & -\tfrac{3}{4} & -\tfrac{3}{4} \\ & & \overline{5\tfrac{3}{4}} \end{array}$$

Multiplication of fractions. To multiply a fraction by another fraction multiply the numerators together and the denominators together and reduce the resulting fraction to its lowest terms.

Examples:

$$\tfrac{2}{3} \times \tfrac{3}{4} = \frac{2 \times 3}{3 \times 4} = \frac{6}{12} \quad \frac{1}{2}$$

$$\tfrac{2}{3} \times \tfrac{7}{8} = \frac{2 \times 7}{3 \times 8} = \frac{14}{24} \quad \frac{7}{12}$$

The process may be shortened by cancelling common factors before multiplying, but care must be exercised that the numerator and denominator are divided by the same number.

Examples:

$$\frac{\cancel{3}^{1}}{5} \times \frac{2}{\cancel{3}_{1}} = \frac{2}{5}$$

$$\frac{\cancel{2}^{1}}{1} \times \frac{2}{\cancel{14}_{7}} = \frac{2}{7}$$

Multiplication of a whole number by a fraction or a fraction by a whole number. To multiply a whole number by a fraction or a fraction by a whole number it must be remembered that the unexpressed denominator of the fraction into which the whole number is mentally converted is 1.

Examples:

$$4 \times \tfrac{5}{6} = \frac{20}{6} \text{ or } 3\tfrac{1}{3} \qquad \tfrac{2}{3} \times 27 = \frac{54}{3} \text{ or } 18$$

$$8 \times \tfrac{3}{4} = \frac{24}{4} \text{ or } 6 \qquad \tfrac{1}{3} \times 20 = \frac{20}{3} \text{ or } 6\tfrac{2}{3}$$

Multiplication of mixed numbers. To multiply mixed numbers change the mixed numbers to improper fractions and multiply as for proper fractions. Do not forget what was said in the previous paragraph about the denominators of whole numbers (integers).

Examples:

$$3\tfrac{1}{5} \times 2\tfrac{1}{4} = \frac{16}{5} \times \frac{9}{4} = \frac{144}{20} \text{ or } 7\tfrac{1}{5}$$

$$12 \times 2\tfrac{2}{3} = 12 \times \frac{8}{3} = \frac{96}{3} \text{ or } 32$$

Divisions of whole numbers by fractions. To divide whole numbers by fractions or fractions by whole numbers invert (turn upside down) the divisor and multiply.

Examples:

$$6 \div \tfrac{1}{2} = 6 \times \frac{2}{1} = 12 \qquad \tfrac{1}{2} \div 6 = \frac{1}{2} \times \frac{1}{6} = \tfrac{1}{12}$$

$$10 \div \tfrac{1}{3} = 10 \times \frac{3}{1} = 30 \qquad \tfrac{1}{3} \div 10 = \frac{1}{3} \times \frac{1}{10} = \tfrac{1}{30}$$

Division of a fraction by a fraction. To divide a fraction by a fraction invert the terms of the divisor and proceed as in multiplication.

Examples:

$$\tfrac{1}{3} \div \tfrac{1}{2} = \frac{1}{3} \times \frac{2}{1} = \tfrac{2}{3}$$

$$\tfrac{4}{5} \div \tfrac{1}{10} = \frac{4}{5} \times \frac{10}{1} = 8$$

Comparison of sizes of fractions. It is sometimes very important for the nurse to recognize when one fraction is larger or smaller than another. For example, it is important to know and to recognize quickly that $\tfrac{1}{300}$ is a larger fraction than $\tfrac{1}{600}$ in spite of the fact that 600 is larger than 300. If the student will but recall some example from her own experience it becomes very simple. If a pie were cut into 300 pieces or into 600 pieces, of which pie would one piece be the larger? Both would be small, but the piece that comes from the pie cut into 600 pieces would be only one-half the size of the piece that represents $\frac{1}{300}$ of the pie. Likewise $\frac{1}{150}$ of a grain of a drug would be twice the dose of $\frac{1}{300}$ of a grain.

If the denominators of the fractions are the same, it is much easier to tell which fraction is the larger. For example, it is easy to tell which is the larger in the following: $\frac{9}{12}$ or $\frac{11}{12}$, $\frac{4}{6}$ or $\frac{5}{6}$, $\frac{3}{8}$ or $\frac{5}{8}$. Fractions with unlike denominators can be compared by changing them to the same denominator.

Examples:

$\frac{3}{4}$ or $\frac{2}{3}$? $\frac{3}{4} = \dfrac{9}{12}$; $\frac{2}{3} = \dfrac{8}{12}$ Therefore since $\dfrac{9}{12}$ is greater than $\dfrac{8}{12}$, $\dfrac{3}{4}$ is greater than $\dfrac{2}{3}$

$\frac{5}{6}$ or $\frac{7}{8}$? $\frac{5}{6} = \dfrac{20}{24}$; $\frac{7}{8} = \dfrac{21}{24}$ Therefore since $\dfrac{21}{24}$ is greater than $\dfrac{20}{24}$, $\frac{7}{8}$ is greater than $\frac{5}{6}$.

Division of a mixed number by a fraction. To divide a mixed number by a fraction change the mixed number to an improper fraction and proceed as with common fractions.

Examples:

(1) $3\frac{1}{4} \div \frac{1}{2}$ Change $3\frac{1}{4}$ to an improper fraction, which would be $\dfrac{13}{4}$

Divide $\dfrac{13}{4}$ by $\frac{1}{2}$, making certain to invert the divisor and multiply.

$$3\frac{1}{4} \div \frac{1}{2} = \frac{13}{4} \div \frac{1}{2} = \frac{13}{\underset{2}{\cancel{4}}} \times \frac{\overset{1}{\cancel{2}}}{1} = \frac{13}{2} \text{ or } 6\frac{1}{2}$$

(2) $2\frac{1}{8} \div \frac{1}{6}$ Change $2\frac{1}{8}$ to an improper fraction, which would be $\dfrac{17}{8}$

Divide $\dfrac{17}{8}$ by $\dfrac{1}{6}$ making certain to invert the divisor and multiply.

$$2\frac{1}{8} \div \frac{1}{6} = \frac{17}{8} \div \frac{1}{6} = \frac{17}{\underset{4}{\cancel{8}}} \times \frac{\overset{3}{\cancel{6}}}{1} = \frac{51}{4} \text{ or } 12\frac{3}{4}$$

Complex fractions

A complex fraction is one in which the numerator or the denominator, or both, are fractions; e.g., $\dfrac{\frac{2}{3}}{3}$, $\dfrac{5}{\frac{1}{2}}$, $\dfrac{\frac{1}{4}}{\frac{1}{8}}$, $\dfrac{\frac{1}{10}}{\frac{1}{100}}$

The expression $\dfrac{2}{3}$ means two divided by three; $\dfrac{1}{2}$ means one divided by two; $\dfrac{\frac{1}{4}}{\frac{1}{8}}$ means one-fourth divided by one-eighth.

To simplify complex fractions divide the number above the subordinate line by the number below the subordinate line.

Examples:

(1) $\dfrac{\frac{1}{10}/50}{100}$
First simplify 1/10/50

$$\frac{1}{10} \div 50 = \frac{1}{10} \times \frac{1}{50} = \frac{1}{500}$$

Then divide $\frac{1}{500}$ by 100

$$\frac{1}{500} \div 100 = \frac{1}{500} \times \frac{1}{100} = \frac{1}{50,000}$$

(2) $\dfrac{4\frac{1}{2}/100}{\frac{1}{50}}$
in like manner:

$$4\frac{1}{2} \text{ or } \frac{9}{2} \div 100 = \frac{9}{2} \times \frac{1}{100} = \frac{9}{200}$$

$$\frac{9}{200} \div \frac{1}{50} = \frac{9}{200} \times \frac{50}{1} = \frac{450}{200} \text{ or } 2\frac{1}{4}$$

Exercises Common fractions, improper fractions, complex fractions, and mixed numbers

1 Reduce the following fractions to their lowest terms:

a. $\dfrac{3}{6}$ b. $\dfrac{14}{16}$ c. $\dfrac{50}{100}$ d. $\dfrac{8}{24}$ e. $\dfrac{4}{12}$ f. $\dfrac{25}{50}$ g. $\dfrac{75}{125}$

h. $\dfrac{27}{72}$ i. $\dfrac{250}{1000}$ j. $\dfrac{500}{10,000}$ k. $\dfrac{60}{1500}$ l. $\dfrac{12}{16}$ m. $\dfrac{5}{15}$ n. $\dfrac{16}{18}$

2 Write the following improper fractions as mixed numbers:

a. $\dfrac{10}{3}$ b. $\dfrac{13}{5}$ c. $\dfrac{29}{12}$ d. $\dfrac{22}{3}$ e. $\dfrac{14}{5}$ f. $\dfrac{32}{6}$ g. $\dfrac{24}{5}$

h. $\dfrac{85}{12}$ i. $\dfrac{63}{8}$ j. $\dfrac{28}{3}$ k. $\dfrac{35}{4}$ l. $\dfrac{31}{6}$ m. $\dfrac{50}{7}$ n. $\dfrac{49}{4}$

3 Change the following mixed numbers to improper fractions:

a. $2\frac{7}{8}$ b. $3\frac{2}{5}$ c. $4\frac{3}{7}$ d. $5\frac{1}{3}$ e. $6\frac{3}{4}$ f. $8\frac{1}{6}$ g. $14\frac{2}{7}$

4 Add the following and reduce to lowest terms:

a. $\frac{1}{2} + \frac{2}{3}$	d. $\frac{2}{3} + \frac{3}{5}$	g. $6\frac{1}{4} + 4\frac{1}{8}$	j. $1\frac{1}{2} + \frac{3}{4}$
b. $\frac{1}{3} + \frac{3}{4}$	e. $16\frac{2}{3} + 12\frac{1}{2}$	h. $3\frac{1}{5} + \frac{1}{2}$	k. $1\frac{1}{3} + 3$
c. $\frac{1}{4} + \frac{1}{3}$	f. $2\frac{1}{2} + 3\frac{1}{2}$	i. $\frac{2}{4} + \frac{2}{4}$	l. $\frac{1}{2} + \frac{1}{6} + 2\frac{1}{3}$

5 Subtract the following fractions and reduce to lowest terms:

a. $\frac{5}{8} - \frac{1}{4}$	d. $\frac{3}{4} - \frac{1}{2}$	g. $2\frac{1}{8} - \frac{1}{12}$	j. $12\frac{5}{8} - 11\frac{7}{8}$
b. $\frac{5}{9} - \frac{1}{3}$	e. $4\frac{1}{3} - 1\frac{1}{3}$	h. $20\frac{1}{2} - 2\frac{3}{4}$	k. $\frac{1}{8} - \frac{1}{16}$
c. $\frac{1}{6} - \frac{1}{9}$	f. $6\frac{3}{4} - 2\frac{1}{2}$	i. $16\frac{2}{3} - 12\frac{1}{6}$	l. $\frac{1}{3} - \frac{1}{4}$

6 Multiply the following and reduce answers to lowest terms:

a. $4 \times \frac{3}{4}$	e. $\frac{1}{5} \times 25$	i. $\frac{1}{5} \times \frac{2}{3}$	m. $1\frac{7}{8} \times 1\frac{1}{3}$
b. $3 \times \frac{2}{3}$	f. $\frac{2}{3} \times 10$	j. $\frac{2}{3} \times \frac{9}{10}$	n. $2\frac{5}{6} \times 1\frac{3}{5}$
c. $8 \times \frac{4}{9}$	g. $\frac{7}{8} \times 60$	k. $\frac{1}{4} \times \frac{3}{5}$	o. $6 \times 2\frac{1}{4}$
d. $120 \times \frac{3}{10}$	h. $\frac{3}{4} \times 20$	l. $\frac{2}{3} \times \frac{5}{6}$	p. $7\frac{1}{4} \times 2$

7 Divide and reduce answers to lowest terms:

a. $12 \div \frac{1}{4}$	e. $5 \div \frac{1}{5}$	i. $6\frac{2}{3} \div 10$	m. $\frac{1}{200} \div \frac{1}{2}$
b. $1 \div \frac{1}{3}$	f. $4 \div \frac{2}{3}$	j. $4\frac{1}{2} \div \frac{3}{4}$	n. $10\frac{1}{2} \div \frac{1}{3}$
c. $\frac{1}{2} \div \frac{1}{4}$	g. $\frac{1}{4} \div \frac{1}{2}$	k. $8\frac{1}{3} \div 1\frac{3}{5}$	o. $\frac{1}{75} \div \frac{3}{4}$
d. $\frac{4}{5} \div \frac{3}{4}$	h. $\frac{3}{5} \div 9$	l. $\frac{2}{5} \div 2\frac{1}{4}$	p. $\frac{1}{100} \div \frac{1}{2}$

8 Solve the following problems containing complex fractions:

a. $\dfrac{1/2}{50}$	b. $\dfrac{\frac{2/3}{100}}{1/50}$	c. $\dfrac{1/2}{1/50}$	d. $\dfrac{\frac{1/100}{50}}{1/50}$
e. $\dfrac{1/10}{100} \times 5000$	f. $\dfrac{2\frac{1}{2}}{100} \times 200$	g. $\dfrac{1/5}{1/10} \times 100$	h. $\dfrac{\frac{1/2}{1/4}}{100} \times 100$

9 Indicate which of the following are the larger fractions; encircle your answer:

a. $\frac{5}{8}$ or $\frac{3}{4}$	e. $\frac{1}{75}$ or $\frac{1}{150}$	i. $\frac{1}{4}$ or $\frac{1}{8}$
b. $\frac{5}{6}$ or $\frac{7}{8}$	f. $\frac{1}{10}$ or $\frac{1}{5}$	j. $\frac{1}{300}$ or $\frac{1}{600}$
c. $\frac{3}{5}$ or $\frac{7}{10}$	g. $\frac{1}{150}$ or $\frac{1}{300}$	k. $\frac{1}{120}$ or $\frac{1}{150}$
d. $\frac{2}{3}$ or $\frac{5}{6}$	h. $\frac{1}{6}$ or $\frac{1}{8}$	l. $\frac{1}{10}$ or $\frac{15}{100}$

Decimal fractions

Definitions and explanations. A decimal fraction is one or more of the tenth parts of a unit. It results from the division of a unit into tenths, tenths into hundredths, hundredths into thousandths, etc., called the *decimal division.* The denominator of a decimal fraction is 10, 100, 1000, etc. Decimal fractions may be expressed in three ways:

1. By words: e.g., three tenths, fifteen hundredths, one hundred twenty-five thousandths.

2. By writing the denominator under the numerator: e.g., $\frac{3}{10}$, $\frac{15}{100}$, $\frac{125}{1000}$.

3. By omitting the denominator and writing the numerator in decimal form: e.g., .3, .15, .125.

The *decimal form* is so called because only decimal fractions can be thus expressed. When a decimal fraction is written in the decimal form, it is called a *decimal*.

The *decimal point* is a period placed at the left of the order of tenths, to designate the decimal orders. The orders on the left of the decimal point are integral and those on the right are decimal. The decimal orders are called *decimal places*.

Following are the names of six integral and six decimal orders:

Hundred-thousands	Ten-thousands	Thousands	Hundreds	Tens	Units	Decimal Point	Tenths	Hundredths	Thousandths	Ten-thousandths	Hundred-thousandths	Millionths
6	5	4	3	2	1	.	1	2	3	4	5	6

The successive decimal orders decrease in value from left to right, and increase from right to left in the same manner as integral orders. Hence, the removal of a decimal figure one order to the left multiplies its value by 10, and its removal one order to the right divides its value by 10. Annexing ciphers to a decimal, or decimal ciphers to an integer, does not change its value. Removing ciphers from the right of a decimal, or decimal ciphers from the right of an integer, does not change its value.

Examples:

.1	one-tenth
.25	twenty-five hundredths
.255	two hundred and fifty-five thousandths
.0165	one hundred and sixty-five ten-thousandths
.0025	twenty-five ten-thousandths
8.26	eight and twenty-six hundredths

Annexing zeros to the decimal does not change its value, e.g.,

.25	.25000

But moving the decimal point does change the value, e.g.,

.25	2.5 (increases the value ten times)

In the number 8.26, moving the decimal point to the left one place, .826, decreases its value ten times.

Addition and subtraction of decimals. In the addition and subtraction of decimals place the decimal fractions in such a manner that the decimal points are in a vertical column and the numerical values are in proper order; that is, tenths to the right of the decimal point, hundredths next, etc. (See examples.) Then add or subtract as in the case of integers and place the decimal point at the left of the tenths order in the answer.

Examples:

(1) Add .25, 3.75, .0045, .01, and .001

   .25
3.75
  .0045
  .01
  .001

4.0155 sum

(2) Subtract 1.65 from 4.85

4.85
1.65

3.20   result

(3) Subtract .25 from .5

.5   = .50
.25   .25

       .25 result

Multiplication of decimals. To multiply one decimal by another, multiply as in the multiplication of whole numbers and point off from the right as many places in the product as there are in both the multiplicand and the multiplier.

Examples:

.425 × 2.6

  .425 multiplicand
2.6   multiplier

2550
850

1.1050 product

3.82 × 50

3.82
 50

191.00

It is of utmost importance that the nurse verify and verify again all arithmetic to avoid error. It is advisable when doing problems such as these to reverse the multiplicand and the multiplier and multiply again. Thereby an error may be detected. The answer should be viewed skeptically and examined with an eye to its reasonableness.

It is possible to be so concerned with the details of solving the problem that an answer is accepted although it does not make sense.

For example, in multiplying 4.25 × 2.06 the following answers were obtained from three different persons: 87.550, 8.7550, and 875.50. Considering the fact that the multiplication of the whole numbers 2 and 4 yields 8, which answer appears reasonable?

Division of decimals. In division of decimals, move the decimal point in the divisor enough places to the right to convert the divisor into a whole number. Next move the decimal point in the dividend the same number of places to the right, adding zeros if necessary to supply the required decimal places. Then proceed as in the division of whole numbers and point off as many decimal places in the quotient as the number of decimal places in the dividend exceeds the number in the divisor.

Moving the decimal point one place to the right is the same as multiplying by ten; moving it another place to the right multiplies by 10 a second time. This moving of the decimal points the same number of places in dividend and divisor is similar to multiplying both terms of a fraction by the same number; that is, the relative values are unchanged.

Example:

$$\text{Divide } 205.65 \text{ by } 4.5 \quad 4.5 \ \overline{\smash{)}205.65} \text{ adjusted } 45. \ \overline{\smash{)}\begin{array}{r} 45.7 \\ 2056.5 \\ 180 \\ \hline 256 \\ 225 \\ \hline 315 \\ 315 \\ \hline \end{array}}$$

In the above problem

4.5 is the divisor
205.65 is the dividend
45.7 is the quotient

It was not necessary, in this problem, to add zeros to supply the required number of decimal places.

To verify the accuracy of the calculation, multiply the quotient by the divisor; the result should equal the dividend.

Changing fractions to decimals. Fractions may be changed to the decimal form by dividing the numerator by the denominator.

Example:

$$\frac{1}{2} \text{ means } 1 \div 2 \qquad 2 \ \overline{\smash{)}\begin{array}{r} .5 \\ 1.0 \end{array}}$$

Likewise decimals may be expressed as fractions.

Examples:

.3 may be expressed as $\frac{3}{10}$
.03 may be expressed as $\frac{3}{100}$

Exercises Decimals

1 Express as decimals:

a. $\frac{9}{10}$	e. $\frac{425}{1000}$	i. $8\frac{3}{100}$
b. $\frac{25}{100}$	f. $\frac{5}{10.000}$	j. $10\frac{7}{10}$
c. $\frac{6}{100}$	g. $3\frac{3}{4}$	k. $\frac{65}{1000}$
d. $\frac{25}{1000}$	h. $2\frac{5}{10}$	l. $15\frac{5}{100}$

2 Express in words:

a. .4	e. 1.25	i. 400.004
b. .06	f. .0025	j. 0.00125
c. .025	g. .020	k. 7.5
d. .4215	h. .2456	l. 1.75

3 Add the following sets of decimals:

    a. .5, .05, 1.65, .005
    b. 65.54, .96, .006, 8.02, 2.265
    c. .25, 1.75, .0065, 10.0

4 Subtract the following sets of decimals:

    a. 1.335 minus .08
    b. 70.2 minus 18.025
    c. 25 minus .25

5 Multiply the following decimals and whole numbers:

a. 5.65 × 4	**e.** .25 × 4	**i.** .145 × 2
b. .05 × 2	**f.** 500 × .005	**j.** .25 × 15
c. 1645 × .02	**g.** 12 × .06	**k.** 2.45 × 45
d. 75 × .05	**h.** 9 × .08	**l.** 250 × .035

6 Multiply the following sets of decimals:

a. .55 × .4	**e.** 1.78 × 5.1	**i.** 19.3 × 5.75
b. .05 × .05	**f.** .08 × .04	**j.** 10.5 × 2.25
c. .065 × 1.5	**g.** 21.1 × .1	**k.** 1.85 × 20.9
d. .875 × .25	**h.** 1.25 × .4	**l.** .15 × .5

7 Make the following indicated divisions:

a. 12 by .625	**e.** .9975 by 2.5	**i.** 25 by 3.25
b. 25 by 3.25	**f.** 1.025 by .012	**j.** 39.6 by 2.75
c. .84 by 6	**g.** 4.50 by 55	**k.** 3.25 by .6
d. 20 by .8	**h.** .496 by .09	**l.** .49 by .7

8 Comparison of decimals: Indicate in each of the following sets which is the larger decimal:

a. .5 or .15	**e.** .25 or .125	**i.** .42 or .428
b. .1 or .2	**f.** .05 or .15	**j.** 1.7 or 1.75
c. .025 or .25	**g.** .325 or .035	**k.** .064 or .8
d. .8 or .64	**h.** .08 or .16	**l.** .1 or .15

9 Convert into decimals the following fractions:

a. $\frac{1}{2}$	**e.** $\frac{1}{6}$	**i.** $\frac{3}{4}$
b. $\frac{1}{4}$	**f.** $\frac{1}{50}$	**j.** $\frac{3}{8}$
c. $\frac{1}{20}$	**g.** $\frac{1}{15}$	**k.** $\frac{2}{3}$
d. $\frac{1}{100}$	**h.** $\frac{1}{5}$	**l.** $\frac{2}{5}$

10 Express as common fractions in their lowest terms:

a. .02	**e.** .125	**i.** .0025
b. .065	**f.** .075	**j.** .00025
c. .4	**g.** .175	**k.** .24
d. .05	**h.** .005	**l.** .65

Percentage

Per cent is an *abbreviation of per centum* which means *by the hundred*. When we write "5 per cent" we may use the symbol "%"; we mean 5 parts of every 100 parts, or $\frac{5}{100}$, or $\frac{1}{20}$. Five hundredths may also be written (.05).

With reference to solutions, per cent means the number of parts of solute (the substance dissolved) in 100 parts of solution. Thus a 5% solution of sugar means $5/100$, or $1/20$, of the total solution is sugar.

Changing per cent to decimal fractions. To change per cent to a decimal fraction, omit the per cent sign and express as hundredths decimally (or divide by 100).

Examples:

$$5\% = .05 \qquad\qquad 12\tfrac{1}{2}\% = .125$$
$$2\% = .02 \qquad\qquad 150\% = 1.50$$
$$15\% = .15 \qquad\qquad \tfrac{1}{4}\% = .00\tfrac{1}{4} \text{ or } .0025$$

In other words a per cent can be changed to a decimal by moving the decimal point two places to the left and dropping the per cent sign. If the per cent is a mixed number it is well first to express the fraction as a decimal and then change the per cent to a decimal by moving the decimal point two places to the left.

Examples:

$$12\tfrac{1}{2}\% = 12.5\% \text{ or } .125 \qquad \tfrac{1}{4}\% = .25\% \text{ or } .0025$$

Changing per cent to a common fraction. To change per cent to a common fraction, omit the symbol and write the per cent as the numerator and 100 as the denominator of the fraction.

Examples:

$$5\% = \tfrac{5}{100} = \tfrac{1}{20} \qquad 12\tfrac{1}{2}\% = \tfrac{12.5}{100} = \tfrac{1}{8}$$
$$2\% = \tfrac{2}{100} = \tfrac{1}{50} \qquad 150\% = \tfrac{150}{100} = \tfrac{3}{2} = 1\tfrac{1}{2}$$
$$15\% = \tfrac{15}{100} = \tfrac{3}{20} \qquad \tfrac{1}{4}\% = \tfrac{1}{4}/100 = \tfrac{1}{400}$$

Changing common fractions to per cent. To change a common fraction to a per cent, divide the numerator by the denominator and multiply the resulting decimal by 100.

Examples:

$$\tfrac{1}{4} = 4\,\overline{\big)\,1.00}^{\;.25} = .25 \times 100 = 25\%$$

$$\tfrac{1}{50} = 50\,\overline{\big)\,1.00}^{\;.02} = .02 \times 100 = 2\%$$

$$\tfrac{1}{8} = 8\,\overline{\big)\,1.00}^{\;.125} = .125 \times 100 = 12\tfrac{1}{2}\%$$

$$\tfrac{1}{400} = 400\,\overline{\big)\,1.0000}^{\;.0025} = .0025 \times 100 = .25\% \text{ or } \tfrac{1}{4}\%$$

To change a decimal fraction to per cent multiply by 100 and write as a whole number with the per cent sign. Thus $.2 \times 100 = 20\%$; $.02 \times 100 = 2\%$. Or a simple way to change a decimal fraction to per cent is to move the decimal point two places to the right and add the per cent sign.

Examples:

$$.25 = 25\% \qquad\qquad .125 = 12.5\% \text{ or } 12\tfrac{1}{2}\%$$
$$.02 = 2\% \qquad\qquad 1.50 = 150\%$$
$$.15 = 15\% \qquad\qquad .0025 = .25\% \text{ or } \tfrac{1}{4}\%$$

To find a certain per cent of any number, multiply the number by the per cent expressed as a decimal fraction.

Examples:

5% of 200 =	200 .05 10.00	$\frac{1}{4}$% of 75 =	75 .0025 375 150 .1875
25% of 2.00 =	2.00 .25 1000 400 .5000	$\frac{1}{2}$% of 200 =	200 .005 1.000

Exercises Percentage

1 Change the following per cents to decimal fractions:

a. 10%	**e.** 18%	**i.** $\frac{1}{50}$%
b. 50%	**f.** 200%	**j.** $2\frac{1}{2}$%
c. 1.5%	**g.** $\frac{1}{5}$%	**k.** 150%
d. 20%	**h.** $\frac{4}{5}$%	**l.** $2\frac{3}{4}$%

2 Change to a common fraction and reduce to lowest terms:

a. 1%	**e.** 60%	**i.** 90%
b. 6%	**f.** 75%	**j.** $\frac{1}{5}$%
c. 10%	**g.** $33\frac{1}{3}$%	**k.** $\frac{2}{3}$%
d. 25%	**h.** $\frac{1}{3}$%	**l.** $\frac{1}{25}$%

3 Change the following fractions to percentages:

a. $\frac{1}{2}$	**e.** $\frac{1}{5}$	**i.** .2
b. $\frac{2}{3}$	**f.** $\frac{1}{6}$	**j.** .5
c. $\frac{7}{8}$	**g.** $\frac{3}{4}$	**k.** .25
d. $\frac{4}{5}$	**h.** $\frac{1}{7}$	**l.** .125

4 Give the following per cents of the corresponding whole numbers:

a. 2% of 100	**e.** $\frac{1}{4}$% of 400	**i.** $\frac{3}{4}$% of 150
b. 5% of 1000	**f.** 2.5% of 500	**j.** 30% ot 30
c. .5% of 2000	**g.** 10% of 1000	**k.** $12\frac{1}{2}$% of 320
d. 20% of 2	**h.** 4% of 500	**l.** $\frac{1}{10}$% of 100

Ratio and proportion

Ratio means the relation which one quantity bears to another. The ratio 1:20 means that for every twenty parts of one substance there is one part of another substance; e.g., in a 1:20 solution of physiologic saline there is one part of salt in every twenty parts of solution. In any quantity of the solution, the amount of solute would be in the same relation to the whole as 1 bears to 20, or, in other words, the ratio shows the relation between the solute and the whole solution.

The ratio of one amount to an amount expressed in terms of the same unit is the number of units in the first divided by the number of units in the second. The ratio of 2 ounces of Lysol to 10 ounces of water is 2 to 10 or 1 to 5 or $\frac{1}{5}$. The ratio may be written $\frac{1}{5}$ or 1:5. The two numbers compared are called the terms of the ratio. The first term of a true ratio is always one (1); this is the simplest form of a ratio.

To change ratio to per cent, make the first term of the ratio the numerator of a fraction whose denominator is the second term of the ratio. Divide the numerator by the denominator and multiply by 100.

$$1:5 = \frac{1}{5} \times 100\% = 20\%$$
$$5:1 = \frac{5}{1} \times 100\% = 500\%$$

To change per cent to ratio, change the per cent to a fraction, which is reduced to its lowest terms. The numerator of the fraction is the first term of the ratio, and the denominator is the second term of the ratio.

$$50\% = \frac{50}{100} = \frac{1}{2} = 1:2$$
$$2\% = \frac{2}{100} = \frac{1}{50} = 1:50$$
$$\frac{1}{2}\% = \frac{1}{2}/100 = \frac{1}{200} = 1:200$$

A proportion is an expression of the equality between two ratios. For example, 1:2 as 5:10 or $\frac{1}{2} = \frac{5}{10}$. The first and last terms are called the extremes; the second and third terms are called the means. In any proportion the *product of the means equals the product of the extremes.* In the above proportion $1 \times 10 = 10$ and $2 \times 5 = 10$.

When one of the extremes in a proportion is not known, it can be found by dividing the product of the means by the extreme that is known. If one of the means is not known, it can be found by dividing the product of the extremes by the mean that is known.

Exercises Ratio and proportion

1 Express each of the following ratios in its simplest form:

a. 5:10	e. 75:100	i. $\frac{1}{3}$:30
b. 4:12	f. $\frac{15}{20}$	j. 10:5
c. 3:9	g. $\frac{1}{2}$:50	k. 12:15
d. 25:100	h. $\frac{1}{4}$:100	l. 5:15

2 When two quantities are to be compared they must be expressed in the same units of measure. For example, if the ratio of six inches and six feet is to be determined, both units must be in inches or both must be in feet, i.e., 6 inches:72 inches or $\frac{1}{2}$ foot:6 feet. What would be the true ratio for the following?

a. 2 pints to 2 quarts	d. 8 ounces to 4 pounds
b. 1 dime to 1 dollar	e. 1 dollar to 25 cents
c. 1 quarter to 2 dollars	f. 1 cent to 1 dollar

3 Express the following percentages as common fractions, as decimals, and as ratios:

Per cent	Common fraction	Decimal	Ratio
5%			
50%			
2%			
20%			
1%			
30%			
16%			

Per cent	Common fraction	Decimal	Ratio
10%	———————————	———————	———————
300%	———————————	———————	———————
⅕%	———————————	———————	———————
¼%	———————————	———————	———————
⅛%	———————————	———————	———————
1/100%	———————————	———————	———————
2½%	———————————	———————	———————
66⅔%	———————————	———————	———————
12½%	———————————	———————	———————

4 If a person can walk 9 miles in 3 hours, how far can he walk in 4 hours if he continues to walk at the same rate?

5 Property valued at $10,000 is taxed $450. What would be the tax on a piece of property assessed at $75,000 at this rate?

6 X : 50 :: 3 : 5   What is the value of X?

7 X : 8 :: 7½ : 15   What is the value of X?

Chapter 5

Weights and measures

Brief history of weights and measures

The science of weights and measures is known as metrology. Many measures used by English-speaking nations grew out of Egyptian, Roman, and Greek measures which were based on the human hand, finger, or foot. The Egyptian cubit was the distance from the elbow to the tip of the middle finger. The Roman mile was 1000 paces, a pace being 5 Roman feet. King Henry I of England is said to have made the yard (cloth yard) the distance from his nose to his outstretched thumb. The drachma (dram) is from the Greek and meant a handful.* The hand meant the breadth of the palm.

Measures based on everyday objects or parts of the body were highly variable although useful to meet the simple everyday needs of people at one time. The ruling monarch of a country frequently decided on the amount of a measure in order that some conformity could prevail in his country. The King of England adopted the avoirdupois pound as an outgrowth of trade relations with France where the pound was 16 ounces. This resulted in two weights for pounds in England and later in the United States, the apothecary pound (12 ounces) and the avoirdupois pound (16 ounces). The apothecary pound is the one used for weighing drugs, precious metals, and jewels.

Englishmen and Americans are not referring to the same measurement when they speak of gallons. The United States quart is really a quarter-gallon and contains 32 ounces. The British quart contains 40 ounces. Both the English gallon and the American gallon contain 4 quarts, however.

Slight variation in measurement makes little difference until scientists begin to reach out into the universe or probe the nucleus of the atom, in which case there is need for almost infinitesimal measures of length and weight.

There are two systems of weighing and measuring drugs in the United States. These are the apothecaries' system and the metric system. There is a growing tendency to use the metric system entirely, but until such

*This Ancient Greek unit of measurement had several values.

time when the change to metric system is complete, nurses will need to know something about both. Moreover, since these systems are often used interchangeably, the nurse needs to be able to change from one system to the other.

The apothecaries' system

The apothecaries' system of weights and measures was a part of the system used in England at the time of colonization in the United States. It has been superseded in England by the imperial system, which is official in Great Britain.

The unit of weight is the grain, which originally meant a grain of wheat. The other units are the scruple, the dram, the ounce, and the pound. The scruple is seldom used and therefore is not included in Table 2. Quantities less than 1 dram are usually expressed in grains. The abbreviation lb. is for libra, the Latin word meaning pound.*

The unit of fluid measure is a minim (Table 3), approximately the quantity of water that would weigh a grain. The symbol O is the abbreviation of the Latin word *octarius*, meaning an eighth (eighth of a gallon), and C, for the Latin word *congius*, meaning a vessel holding a gallon.

*The imperial system of weights and measures as well as the metric system is used in the *British Pharmacopoeia* and the *Canadian Formulary*. The imperial system is being replaced gradually by the metric system.

1 pound (lb.)	= 16 ounces = 7000 grains
1 ounce (℥)	= 437½ grains
1 dram (ℨ)	= 60 grains (unofficial)—officially 1 grain is 1/7000 part of a pound
1 pint (O)	= 20 fluidounces (f℥)
1 fluidounce (f℥)	= 8 fluidrams (fℨ)
1 fluidram (fℨ)	= 60 minims (min.)

Table 2
Weight

60 grains	= 1 dram (ℨ)
480 grains or 8 drams	= 1 ounce (℥)
12 ounces	= 1 pound (lb.)

Table 3
Fluid measure

60 minims (♏)	= 1 fluidram (fℨ)
8 fluidrams or 480 minims	= 1 fluidounce (f℥)
16 fluidounces	= 1 pint (pt. or O)
2 pints	= 1 quart (qt.)
4 quarts	= 1 gallon (C)

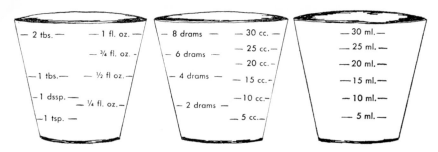

Fig. 4 Disposable medicine glasses made of plastic material. Metric, apothecary, and household measures are indicated.

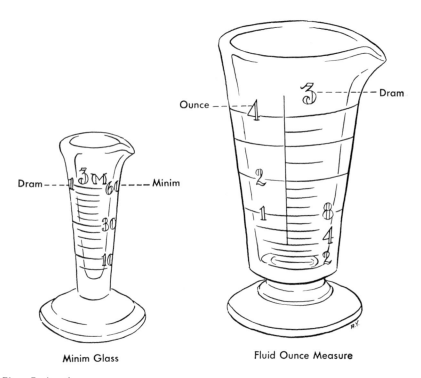

Minim Glass   Fluid Ounce Measure

Fig. 5 Apothecary measures.

When the symbols are used, the quantity is expressed in Roman numerals which are placed after the symbols: e.g., three grains are written, gr. iii; five drams, ℨ v; ten ounces, ℥ x. Fractions are expressed in Arabic numerals; gr. ¼, gr. ⅛, gr. ½; the symbol "ss" may be used for ½; thus, two and one-half grains, gr. iiss.

The *minim* (♏) is often assumed to be identical with the drop (gtt. from L. *gutta*), but such measurement is inaccurate. A minim of water or of an aqueous solution is approximately equal to a drop; a minim of an alcoholic solution such as digitalis tincture equals approximately two drops; a minim of ether contains three drops and a minim of chloroform equals approximately four drops. A minim of a gummy substance is less than a drop. Minims should always be measured when minims are ordered and a minim glass or minim pipette used to measure accurately. When drops are ordered, they may be measured by means of a medicine dropper.

Exercises Apothecaries' system

1 Read the following:

    a. ℥ iiss   **c.** ℈ ss   **e.** ♏ viii   **g.** ℥ iv   **i.** ♏ xxiv

    b. gr. xiii   **d.** ℥ xviii   **f.** gr. xxx   **h.** ℨ vi   **j.** O v

2 Write the following expressions as they should be written in a prescription: 15 minims, 3 fluidrams, 7 fluidounces, 1 pint, 2½ drams, 20 grains, 12 minims, 5 ounces, ½ ounce.

3 How many grains are there in:

    a. ℥ iii   **c.** ℈ i   **e.** lb. i   **g.** ℨ ss   **i.** ℈ iv

    b. ℨ viii   **d.** ℨ viss   **f.** ℥ v   **h.** ℥ iss   **j.** ℨ ix

4 How many minims are there in:

    a. fℨ i   **c.** fℨ ss   **e.** 1 qt.   **g.** O iii   **i.** f℥ iiss

    b. f℥ iv   **d.** f℥ 1½   **f.** f℥ iii   **h.** f℥ iv   **j.** O ss

5 What part of a dram is gr. xv, gr. xx, gr. xxx, gr. xiv, gr. i?

  What part of an ounce is ℨ iv, ℨ ii, ℈ iii, ℨ ss, ℨ vii?

  What part of a fluidram is ♏ xv, ♏ xx, ♏ xxx, ♏ xiv, ♏ i?

  What part of a fluidounce is f℥ ii, f℥ ss, f℥ iv, f℥ vi, f℥ v?

6 Add the following and express in fluidrams: O ss, ♏ xx, f℥ vi, ♏ 480.

7 A physician's prescription calls for gr. xxiv of a drug. This would be what part of an ounce?

8 One headache powder contains gr. v of the drug; how many drams of this drug would be required to make up 60 powders?

9 How much morphine sulfate would be required to make up two fluidounces of solution if every 20 minims of the solution is to contain gr. ¼?

10 If a pint of solution contains ℨ ii of drug, how many grains in each fluidounce of solution?

Laboratory suggestions

Materials for use. Apothecaries' scales and measures; colored solution and salt.

1 With a minim measure determine the number of minims in:

    a. 1 fluidram _ _ _ _ _ _

    b. 2 fluidounces _ _ _ _ _ _

    c. 1 fluidounce _ _ _ _ _ _

Why would a minim glass be unsuitable to measure out several fluidounces of a solution? **d.** Observe the various apothecaries' measures set out for your use. Note the amount of their content. Measure out 1 fluidram, 1 fluidounce, 60 minims, 1 pint, and so on. Try to form a mental picture of various quantities and how they compare with each other; e.g., compare the amount of water in 15 minims with the amount in 1 fluidram or 1 fluidounce. Compare the weight of 1 grain with 15 grains, with 1 ounce, and with 1 pound.

2 With a fluidram measure determine how many fluidrams there are in 1 fluid-ounce _____; in 1 pint _____. What kind of an apothecary measure would you select to measure out ½ pint of a solution if you had the following to choose from: minim glass; fluidram measure; fluidounce measure? Why?

3 Weigh out 60 grains of salt on an apothecary scale. This corresponds with how many drams?

4 Dissolve ℥ i of salt in f℥ iv of water. How many grains of salt are there in each fluidounce of solution? In each fluidram?

5 Dissolve gr. xxx of salt in f℥ iiss of water. How many grains of salt would there be in 40 ℳ of the solution?

6 Using the colored solution to represent alcohol, add 1 fluidram of alcohol to 4 fluidrams of water. What part of the solution will be alcohol? How many minims of alcohol would there be in 60 ℳ of the solution?

7 Add f℥ ii of alcohol to f℥ iv of water. What part of the solution is alcohol? How many minims of alcohol in each fluidram of solution?

Metric system

The metric system is the system prescribed by law in most European countries, and several legislative attempts have been made to render its use obligatory in the United States. It is now used in the sciences and pharmacy, in weighing foreign mail, in weighing at the mints and in certain other governmental departments, particularly the medical department of the Army and Navy.

History of metric system

The metric system of weights and measures was invented by the French in the latter part of the eighteenth century. For this purpose a committee of the Academy of Sciences, consisting of five men, was appointed under authority of the government. They had two preconceived ideas regarding the proposed system: (1) that the standards should be based upon some unalterable object in nature, so that the correctness of the measures accepted as models might be redetermined, if necessary; (2) that the system should employ the decimal scale. Of the three natural linear bases proposed, namely, the length of a second's pendulum, a fourth of the earth's circumference measured along the equator, and a fourth of the earth's circumference measured across the poles, the committee recommended the last, one ten-millionth of which should be the standard unit of linear measure. They calculated the distance from the equator to the North Pole from surveys made along the meridian which passes through Paris, and this distance, divided by 10,000,000, was chosen as the unit of length, the meter. The meter is the fundamental unit of the metric system. A bar of platinum of this length was constructed and deposited in the French Archives to serve as a model for the meter measures intended for actual use. There was also constructed and deposited in the Archives a weight of platinum of such size as to counterpoise in vacuo one cubic decimeter of water at its greatest density. This weight constituted the fundamental standard of mass and was to serve as the model for the kilogram weights (and indirectly for the other weights) intended for actual use.

The metric standards were adopted in France in 1799. In 1875 the International Metric Convention met in Paris. Seventeen countries including the United States participated. This convention resulted in the foundation of the International Bureau of Weights and Measures, whose first work was the preparation of an international standard meter bar and an international standard kilogram weight and duplicates for each of the countries that had contributed to the support of the bureau. For the international standard meter, a bar of platinum iridium was selected and two lines drawn on its surface at a distance from each other equal to one meter measured when the bar was at the temperature of melting ice (0° C.). The distance between these lines is the official unit of the metric system. The international standards were placed in the custody of the International Bureau of Weights and Measures near Paris. The duplicates were distributed by lot, the United States drawing meters No. 21 and No. 27 and kilograms No. 4 and No. 20. Meter No. 27 and kilogram No. 20 were selected as our national standard and are carefully preserved in the United States Bureau of Standards at Washington, D.C. Meter No. 21 and kilogram No. 4 are used as working standards.

Metric units of measurement

Metric units of measurement are the meter, the liter, and the gram. The *meter* is the unit for linear measurement, the *liter* for capacity or volume, and the *gram* for weight.

The metric system is a decimal system, i.e., the basic unit can be divided into 10, 100, or 1000 parts, or the basic unit may be multiplied by 10, 100, or 1000 and thus form secondary units which differ from each other by 10 or some multiple of 10. The names of the secondary units are formed by joining Greek and Latin prefixes to the names of the primary unit. Subdivisions of the basic unit can be made by moving

Table 4

Metric linear measurement

1 meter	=	10 decimeters (dm.)
	=	100 centimeters (cm.)
	=	1000 millimeters (mm.)
10 meters	=	1 dekameter (Dm.)
100 meters	=	1 hectometer (Hm.)
1000 meters	=	1 kilometer (Km.) (approx. ⅝ mile)

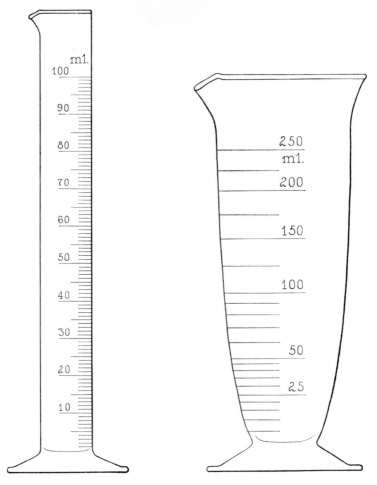

Fig. 6 Metric measures suited to the measurement of volume. The cylindrical graduate on the left is marked so that small amounts can be measured more accurately than with the graduate on the right.

the decimal point to the left, and multiples of the basic unit are indicated by moving the decimal point to the right.

The prefixes used to designate subdivisions of the unit, deci (0.1), centi (0.01), and milli (0.001), are from the Latin; those used to designate multiples, deka (10), hecto (100), and kilo (1000), are from the Greek. Thus the subdivisions of a meter are known as decimeters, centimeters, and millimeters; and the multiples of the meter are known as dekameters, hectometers, and kilometers.

The meter. The meter is the unit from which the other metric units were derived (Table 4). The meter is comparable to the yard although it is several inches longer (39.37 inches).

The first part of Table 4 is most frequently used and is similar to the system of money used in the United States: one dollar = 10 dimes, or 100 cents, or 1000 mills.

Centimeters and millimeters are the chief linear measures used in hospital work. Measurement of the size of body organs is made in centimeters and millimeters, and students will recall that the sphygmomanometer used in measuring of blood pressure is calibrated in millimeters. Microns, which are one millionth of a meter, are used in measuring minute distances, e.g., the length or size of bacteria. There are 2.5 centimeters (25 millimeters) in 1 inch (approximately).

The liter. The liter is the unit of capacity (Table 5). The contents of a cube whose sides measure a decimeter or 10 centimeters constitute the unit of capacity. It was originally intended that the liter and a cubic decimeter should be exactly the same. Because of the difficulty of measurement, however, it is found to be 1.000028 cubic decimeter. This is from a recent recomputation of the Bureau of Weights and Measures. For a long time 1.000027 was the accepted figure.

The liter, therefore, is 28 parts per 1,000,000 larger than intended. The difference is so small that it is of no importance except in determinations of great precision. The weight of a liter of water at 4° C. is 1 kilogram.

If the liter contained exactly 1000 cc., the cubic centimeter and the milliliter would be exactly the same volume and each the one thousandth part of the liter. However, since the liter in common use is 1000.028 cc., the cubic centimeter is less than the milliliter by 0.000028 cc. *In practice the cubic centimeter and the milliliter are considered equal.* The change in the U.S.P. from cubic centimeter to milliliter (ml.) is not because of inaccuracy but merely to conform with the general practice. The Pharmacopeias of all other countries use milliliter.

Fractional parts of a liter are usually expressed in milliliters or cubic centimeters. For example, 0.6 L. would be expressed as 600 ml. or 600 cc. Multiples of a liter are similarly expressed: 2.4 L. would be 2400 ml. or cc.

Table 5

Capacity

1 liter (L.)	=	10 deciliters	(dl.)
	=	100 centiliters	(cl.)
	=	1000 milliliters	(ml.)
10 liters	=	1 dekaliter	(Dl.)
100 liters	=	1 hectoliter	(Hl.)
1000 liters	=	1 kiloliter	(Kl.)

Table 6

Weight

1 gram (Gm.)	=	10 decigrams (dg.)
	=	100 centigrams (cg.)
	=	1000 milligrams (mg.)
	=	1,000,000 micrograms (μg.)
10 grams	=	1 dekagram (Dg.)
100 grams	=	1 hectogram (Hg.)
1000 grams	=	1 kilogram (Kg.)

A gram. A gram is the metric unit of weight which is used in weighing drugs and various pharmaceutical preparations. Originally the unit of measurement of weight was the kilogram but this proved too large to meet the practical needs of the pharmacist. The gram is the weight of 1 milliliter of distilled water at 4° Centigrade. The official abbreviation of gram is Gm.*

In studying Table 6 it becomes apparent that 1 decigram is 10 times greater than a centigram and 100 times greater than a milligram. To change decigrams to centigrams one would therefore multiply by 10; to change decigrams to milligrams one would multiply by 100. To change milligrams to centigrams one would divide by 10; to change milligrams to decigrams one would divide by 100; and to change milligrams to grams one would divide by 1000.

In reading a whole number expressing a metric quantity only one unit is used, however large the number, i.e., 2750 Gm. is read twenty-seven hundred and fifty grams, not two kilograms, seven hectograms, five dekagrams; 7500 ml. is read seven thousand five hundred or seventy-five hundred milliliters.

In expressing a fraction of a gram, the terms decigram and centigram are seldom used. The quantity is expressed in its equivalent grams or milligrams; e.g., 6 decigrams, written 0.6 Gm., is called six-tenths gram; 5 centigrams, written 0.05 Gm., is called preferably fifty milligrams. The thousandth part of a gram and multiples or fractions of it are commonly expressed as milligrams; i.e., 0.001 Gm. may be expressed as 1 mg.; 0.003 Gm. as 3 mg., etc., and 0.0005 Gm. as 0.5 mg., etc. 0.001 mg. is a microgram.

Multiples of the gram are not used in medical work except the kilogram. Nurses will observe that this measure is used in weighing patients and in calculation of dosage in terms of kilograms of body weight (1 kilogram = 2.2 lbs. avoirdupois weight).

*The abbreviation for gram has a capital G (Gm.) to avoid confusion with gr. for grain.

To ensure accuracy in reading, a zero always should be used before the decimal point in writing a fractional part of a metric unit; i.e., 0.5 Gm., 0.6 ml., or 0.001 L. The misplacement of the period or point is the most usual cause of danger and poisoning. When the abbreviations for gram, milliliter, and cubic centimeter are omitted, it is taken for granted that 1.0 means 1 gram when expressing weight or 1 ml. when expressing liquid quantity. When metric abbreviations are used, the numerals are always expressed in Arabic and precede the abbreviation; e.g., 20 Gm., 50 ml., 250 mg.

The metric system has many advantages over the apothecaries' system, chief of which are as follows: all the standard units of weight and measure bear a simple relation to the fundamental unit, the meter; the prefixes deci, centi, milli, deka, hecto, and kilo have a numerical significance and have other applications in our language, which makes them readily understood; the uniform decimal scale of relation between the successive units makes the use of the decimal notation possible; the system is a universal one.

Exercises Metric system

1 **a.** What part of a gram is a decigram?
  b. What part of a gram is a milligram?
  c. What part of a gram is a centigram?
2 **a.** How many dekagrams in a kilogram?
  b. How many centigrams in a kilogram?
  c. How many dekagrams in a hectogram?
3 In the statement of calculation of the following problems, state the process of reasoning
  Example: Change 5000 milligrams to grams.
      From Table 6: 1000 mg. = 1 Gm.
               5000 mg. ÷ 1000 = 5 ∴* 5 Gm.
  *The three dots = "therefore."
  a. Convert the following to milligrams: 5 Gm., 3 dg., 50 cg., 100 mg.
  b. Add and express the sum in grams: 500 mg., 300 cg., 20 dg., 10 Gm.
  c. Add and express the sum in centigrams: 250 mg., 2.5 Gm., 20 dg., 0.5 cg.
  d. Add and express in milligrams: 0.6 Gm., 0.25 cg., 0.125 Gm., 0.5 dg.
4 A preparation of medicine is made by dissolving 15 mg. of drug in 240 ml. of water. If 3 mg. is the dose, how many milliliters must be given for each dose?
5 If the dose of cascara sagrada is 4 ml., how many doses will there be in ½ liter?
6 If 4 Gm. of drug are added to 400 ml. of water, how many milligrams of drug are there in each milliliter of solution?
7 If 20 ml. of alcohol are added to 80 ml. of water to make a certain desired strength of solution, how much alcohol would be required to make a liter of solution?

Laboratory suggestions

Materials for use. Glass measures marked in milliliters, gram scales, salt, water, and colored solution for alcohol.

1 Study the gram scale. Balance it and note how the scale is marked to indicate the subdivisions of the gram.

2 Study the various metric measures which can be used to measure liquids. Note the amount of water contained in 4 ml., 30 ml., and 500 ml. Try to build a mental concept of these quantities. Many of the graduates are also marked in the apothecaries' system. Compare the above quantities with the corresponding amounts in the apothecaries' system. How many minims in a milliliter? in 4 ml.?

3 Weigh out 2 Gm. of salt and add it to 20 ml. of water; notice how much constitutes each of these amounts. Is the volume of the liquid noticeably changed? Why? How much salt is there in each milliliter of solution?

4 Normal salt solution is made by adding 9 Gm. of salt to 1000 ml. of water; weigh out the amount of salt needed for ½ liter of normal salt solution.

5 Add 5 ml. of alcohol to 25 ml. of water. Is the volume of the liquid increased? Why? What part of the finished solution is alcohol? How much alcohol would be needed to make 1½ liters of solution of the same strength?

6 Add 20 ml. of alcohol to 60 ml. of water. How much alcohol is there in each milliliter of solution?

Conversion from one denomination to the other within same system

In the apothecaries' system it is often expedient to convert the units on hand to units that are more usable or more easily measured. The change may need to be made to a higher or lower denomination, e.g., 15 minims is more easily measured than ¼ fluidram. The measurement of 2500 minims with a minim glass is almost like trying to empty a lake with a teaspoon. The large number of minims would be more easily measured if converted to fluidounces.

In the metric system the weight of a substance is usually expressed in terms of grams, decimal fractions of a gram, milligrams, or decimal fractions of a milligram. A large number of milligrams might better be expressed in grams, in which case the decimal point would be moved three places to the left, e.g., 5000 mg. = 5 Gm.; 200 mg. = 0.2 Gm. In converting grams to milligrams move the decimal point three places to the right, e.g., 0.004 Gm. = 4 mg.; 0.0001 Gm. = 0.1 mg. The same procedure applies to measures of volume, the liter and milliliter.

Conversion from one system to another

Since nurses have occasion to use both the apothecaries' and the metric systems in computing dosage of drugs to be given orally or hypodermically as well as in preparing solutions for external use, it is essential that they know how to use these systems interchangeably.

A fraction is expressed as a common fraction in the apothecaries' system and as a decimal fraction in the metric system; morphine sulfate gr. ¼ (apothecaries') when changed to metric would be stated morphine sulfate 0.015 Gm. or 15 mg.

Although these systems are used interchangeably, greater emphasis is being placed on the metric system, as its convenience is increasingly appreciated. *Nevertheless it is advisable for nurses to learn the tables of weights and measurements and at least some of the approximate equivalents as thoroughly as they learned the multiplication tables.*

Although it is well to know how to calculate the change from one system to the other, often the accepted equivalent is not the same as the exact amount in the other system, and confusion results. For the most part, exact equivalents are used only by the pharmacist in compounding prescriptions or in converting a pharmaceutical formula from one system to the other (Table 7). When dosage forms such as tablets and capsules of a drug are prescribed in the metric system the nurse may administer the apothecary approximate equivalent and vice versa.

It is therefore worth while to memorize certain approximate equivalents that are commonly used (Table 8), to be assured of a quick recall when there is need for it. The approximate equivalents are also a convenience to the physician when prescribing. They are used in the *Pharmacopeia of the United States of America*, the *National Formulary*, and *New and Nonofficial Drugs*, and they have the approval of the Federal Food and Drug Administration.

Table 7
Examples of exact equivalents*

1 fluidounce	= 29.5729 ml.	1 liter	= 33.815 fluidounces
1 ounce†	= 29.5729 Gm.	1 ml.	= 16.23 minims
1 grain	= 0.0648 Gm.	1 Gm.	= 15.4324 grains

°U.S.P. XVI, p. 1106.

†The imperial ounce is 28.350 grams (exact equivalent), and 30 grams is the approximate equivalent. B.P. official spelling is "grammes."

Table 8
Commonly used approximate equivalents

Weight		Volume	
1 Gm. = 15 grains		1 ml. = 15 minims	
0.06 Gm. = 1 grain		1 cc. = 15 minims	
4 Gm. = 1 dram		0.06 ml. = 1 minim	
30 Gm. = 1 ounce		4 ml. = 1 fluidram	
1 Kg.* = 2.2 pounds (imperial or avoirdupois)		30 ml. = 1 fluidounce	
		500 ml. = 1 pint	
		1000 ml. (1 L.) = 1 quart	

°1 Kg. is equivalent to 2.6 apothecary pounds; however, the nurse has little or no occasion to use the apothecary pound.

Table 9
Additional approximate equivalents (weight)

gr. xv	= 1.0	Gm. =	1000 mg.	gr. $\frac{1}{20}$	= 0.0032	Gm. =	3 mg.
gr. x	= 0.6	Gm. =	600 mg.	gr. $\frac{1}{30}$	= 0.0022	Gm. =	2 mg.
gr. viiss*	= 0.5	Gm. =	500 mg.	gr. $\frac{1}{40}$	= 0.0016	Gm. =	1.6 mg.
gr. v	= 0.3	Gm. =	300 mg.	gr. $\frac{1}{50}$	= 0.0013	Gm. =	1.3 mg.
gr. iii	= 0.2	Gm. =	200 mg.	gr. $\frac{1}{60}$	= 0.001	Gm. =	1 mg.
gr. 1½	= 0.1	Gm. =	100 mg.	gr. $\frac{1}{100}$	= 0.0006	Gm. =	0.6 mg.
gr. 1	= 0.06	Gm. =	60 mg.	gr. $\frac{1}{120}$	= 0.0005	Gm. =	0.5 mg.
gr. ¾	= 0.05	Gm. =	50 mg.	gr. $\frac{1}{150}$	= 0.0004	Gm. =	0.4 mg.
gr. ½	= 0.03	Gm. =	30 mg.	gr. $\frac{1}{200}$	= 0.0003	Gm. =	0.3 mg.
gr. ¼	= 0.015	Gm. =	15 mg.	gr. $\frac{1}{300}$	= 0.0002	Gm. =	0.2 mg.
gr. ⅙	= 0.010	Gm. =	10 mg.	gr. $\frac{1}{600}$	= 0.0001	Gm. =	0.1 mg.
gr. ⅛	= 0.008	Gm. =	8 mg.				
gr. $\frac{1}{12}$	= 0.005	Gm. =	5 mg.				
gr. $\frac{1}{15}$	= 0.004	Gm. =	4 mg.				

*ss = semis (Latin) = one-half.

It is important to know how to change from one system to the other in the event that one forgets the corresponding equivalent or no table is available that includes the desired equivalent. It must be remembered, of course, that 1 gram is the equivalent of 15 grains and that 1 ml. is the equivalent of 15 minims. One gram (1 Gm.) divided by 15 is 0.06 Gm., the equivalent of 1 grain, and 0.06 ml. is the equivalent of 1 minim.

Method of converting metric to apothecaries' system

1. To convert grams to grains, multiply by 15, since there are approximately 15 grains in 1 gram.

Example: Convert 15.0 Gm. to grains.

$$1.0 \text{ Gm.} = 15 \text{ gr.}$$
$$15.0 \text{ Gm.} = 15 \times 15 = 225 \text{ gr.}$$

2. To convert milliliters into minims, multiply by 15 since there are 15 minims in 1 ml.

3. To convert grams or milliliters into drams, divide by 4, since there are 4 grams or milliliters in 1 dram.

4. To convert grams or milliliters into ounces, divide by 30, since there are approximately 30 grams or milliliters in 1 ounce.

Method of converting apothecaries' to metric system

1. To convert grains or minims into grams or milliliters, divide by 15.

2. To convert drams into grams or milliliters, multiply by 4.

3. To convert ounces into grams or milliliters, multiply by 30.

Exercises *Converting from one system to another*

Indicate the process whereby you arrive at an answer.

1 Convert the following to their apothecary equivalents:

a.	30 Gm.	f.	0.6 ml.	k.	500 ml.	p.	15 mg.
b.	4 Gm.	g.	0.6 Gm.	l.	1000 ml.	q.	10 mg.
c.	4 ml.	h.	0.1 Gm.	m.	250 ml.	r.	100 mg.
d.	1 ml.	i.	0.03 Gm.	n.	120 ml.	s.	0.1 mg.
e.	45 Gm.	j.	0.010 Gm.	o.	15 ml.	t.	30 mg.

2 Change to metric:

a.	℥ i	f.	♏ xv	k.	gr. ⅙	p.	gr. v
b.	℥ iv	g.	gr. viiss	l.	gr. ½	q.	f℥ i
c.	℥ ii	h.	gr. 1½	m.	gr. 1	r.	♏ lx
d.	O ss	i.	gr. ⅙	n.	gr. ⅟₆₀₀	s.	f℥ iv
e.	C i	j.	gr. ¼	o.	gr. ¾	t.	qt. 1

3 Without consulting the text, practice giving metric equivalents for:

a.	gr. xv	f.	♏ viiss	k.	gr. ⅟₆₀	p.	gr. viiss
b.	gr. x	g.	♏ x	l.	℥ 1	q.	gr. ⅛
c.	♏ v	h.	gr. ⅙	m.	gr. ½	r.	gr. ⅟₁₅₀
d.	gr. v	i.	1 qt.	n.	gr. ¼		
e.	gr. 1½	j.	♏ xv	o.	1 qt.		

4 In the same way, give apothecaries' equivalents for:

a.	1.0 Gm.	f.	0.03 Gm.	k.	500.0 ml.	p.	0.065 Gm.
b.	0.3 Gm.	g.	4.0 ml.	l.	0.0006 Gm.	q.	0.008 Gm.
c.	0.004 Gm.	h.	1000 ml.	m.	30.0 ml.	r.	250.0 Gm.
d.	1.0 ml.	i.	0.5 Gm.	n.	0.015 Gm.		
e.	1½ ml.	j.	0.1 Gm.	o.	2.0 Gm.		

5 Change:

a.	3 ounces to minims	g.	1 liter to ounces (fluidounces)
b.	1 liter to pints	h.	36 drams to grams
c.	6.0 ml. to fluidrams	i.	5.0 ml. to minims
d.	75 grains to grams	j.	3 pints to milliliters
e.	7.0 Gm. to grains	k.	75.0 ml. to ounces (fluidounces)
f.	2 gallons to milliliters		

6 If the dose of milk of magnesia is 15 ml., how many fluidounces would be necessary to give 10 doses?

7 If there are 7½ grains of drug in each 5 ml. ampule of the preparation, how many grams of the drug in 4 ampules?

8 If the dose of a certain medication is 0.5 Gm. and the tablets are marked 7½ grains, how many tablets will be given for each dose? How many tablets will be required for 10 doses?

9 If the dose of a medication is 4 ml., how many fluidounces would you order from the pharmacy in order to have 60 doses?

10 If a physician orders 15 mg. of a drug and the preparation comes marked "Tab. gr. ⅛," how many tablets or what part of a tablet will you give?

Household measures

When nursing is done in a home, a graduate for accurate measurement may not be available and some household article may be used to measure, approximately, the amount required. Household measures include glasses, cups, tablespoons, teaspoons, and drops. Pints and quarts seem to belong to a "household," but they are apothecary measures. Household measures are not accurate and their use should be avoided in the administration of medicines. A teaspoon is said to hold a dram, but the average present-day teaspoon often holds 5 ml. or more.* Drops and minims are also said to be equivalent, but when the physician orders a certain number of minims of a drug, the dose should be measured in minims. If he orders drops, the dose should be measured with a medicine dropper. The volume of a drop varies with the viscosity of the liquid to be dropped, the diameter of the dropper used, the angle at which the dropper is held, and sometimes the temperature of the solution. Approximate equivalents (Table 10) are not absolutely accurate, but they are sufficiently accurate for practical purposes.

The following statement of equivalents is sometimes easier to remember than Table 10.

Household	Apothecaries'	Metric
1 t. = ¼ T. = 60 gtt.	= M 60 = gr. 60 = ℥ i = ℥⅛	= 4 ml. = 4 Gm.

Exception: In calculating the equivalent of a fluidounce in milliliters the above statement will give 32 instead of 30. The latter, however, is the accepted equivalent of a fluidounce.

*An American standard teaspoon has been established by the American Standards Association as containing approximately 5 ml. and is accepted as such in U.S.P. XVI.

Table 10
Approximate equivalents

60 drops (gtt.)	=	1 teaspoonful (t.)
4 teaspoonfuls	=	1 tablespoonful (T.)
2 tablespoonfuls	=	1 fluidounce
6 fluidounces	=	1 teacupful
8 fluidounces	=	1 glassful

Household	Apothecaries'	Metric
1 drop	1 minim	0.06 ml.
1 teaspoonful	1 fluidram	5 (4) ml.*
1 tablespoonful	4 fluidrams	15 ml.
2 tablespoonfuls	1 fluidounce	30 ml.
1 teacup	6 fluidounces	180 ml.
1 glassful	8 fluidounces	240 ml.

*A scant teaspoon is generally accepted as an equivalent of 4 ml. (cc.) or f℥ i.

Exercises Approximate equivalents

1 Using household measures, how would you measure:

a. gr. xxx	e. f℥ iii	i. qt. ss	m. 120 ml.
b. ℨ i	f. 30 ml.	j. 0.3 ml.	n. C ss
c. f℥ i	g. 1000 ml.	k. 4 ml.	o. gr. xv
d. 2 Gm.	h. ℳ xxx	l. ℥ ss	p. f℥ iv

2 Change to the approximate apothecary equivalents:

a. 1 T.	d. 2 T.	g. 60 drops	j. ½ teacupful
b. 2 t.	e. 1 teacupful	h. 4 glassfuls	k. ½ T.
c. ½ t.	f. 1 glassful	i. ½ glassful	l. 15 drops

3 Give the approximate metric equivalents:

a. 1 teacupful	d. 1 t.	g. 2 T.	j. ½ T.
b. 1 glassful	e. 60 gtt.	h. ¼ t.	k. 2 teacupfuls
c. 1 T.	f. ½ t.	i. 20 gtt.	l. 2 glassfuls

Laboratory suggestions

Materials for use. Apothecaries' measures, metric measures, household measures of various sizes and shapes, medicine droppers, water, and oil.

1 Determine the capacity of the household measures provided for you, using apothecaries' and metric measures. Compare the sizes of three or four cups, glasses, teaspoons, and tablespoons. Do you find any discrepancy? What can you say about the reliability of household measures?

2 With a medicine dropper, drop 20 drops of water into a minim glass. How many minims are there? Do the same with a water faucet instead of a medicine dropper. How many minims? Under what circumstances would a medicine dropper measure minims accurately?

3 Drop 20 drops of oil into a minim glass. How many minims? What factors determine the size of a drop?

The preparation of solutions and doses

Methods of making solutions

There are three methods of making solutions. One is on the weight-to-weight basis, commonly designated as W/W. This means that a given part by weight of solute is dissolved in a given number of parts by weight of solvent. This method is used chiefly where a high degree of accuracy is essential, such as in highly technical work.

A second method is the weight-to-volume method, designated W/V, in which a given part by weight of drug (solute) is placed in a graduate and a sufficient amount of solvent added to make the required amount of solution. This method is commonly used in medicine and pharmacy. Many of the intravenous fluids given to patients, e.g., the glucose and saline solutions, are prepared on a weight-to-volume basis and are so indicated on the label.

The third method is the volume-to-volume method in which a liquid solute is added to the liquid solvent and is designated V/V.

The difference in expressing the strength of a solution on a weight-to-volume (W/V) basis or on a volume-to-volume (V/V) basis is very apparent when one considers the difference in weight of two liquids such as alcohol and water. Alcohol weighs considerably less than water so the amount of alcohol in a 50 per cent solution prepared on a weight-to-volume basis would be quite different than if it were prepared on a volume-to-volume basis.

The strength of solutions is frequently spoken of in terms of molarity or normality. A *normal solution* is one that contains 1 gram equivalent weight of solute in each 1000 ml. of solution. An equivalent combining weight is the weight of an element in grams which will combine with 1.008 grams of hydrogen or 8 grams of oxygen. It is obtained by dividing the atomic weight by the valence. Normal solution of sodium chloride contains 58.454 grams of sodium chloride per liter of solution. The atomic weight of sodium is 22.997 and the atomic weight of chlorine is 35.457, making a total of 58.454. Since the valence of both sodium and chlorine is 1, the atomic weight and the equivalent weight of each is the same.

Normal solution of sodium chloride should not be confused with physiologic saline solution, particularly since the physiologic saline solution is sometimes referred to as normal saline. The former is 5.8 per cent solution of sodium chloride, whereas the latter is approximately 0.9 per cent strength.

Solutions may be designated as normal (1 N), half normal (0.5 N), tenth normal (0.1 N) etc.

A *molar solution* is one that contains a mole (gram molecular weight) of the solute in 1000 ml. of solution. Thus each liter of molar solution of sulfuric acid contains 98.08 grams of hydrogen sulfate (H_2SO_4). Since the equivalent weight would be half this amount, a normal solution of sulfuric acid would contain 49.04 grams of solute. Solutions containing one tenth of a gram molecular weight of solute in 1 liter of solution are designated as (0.1 M) or M/10.

Solutions are made from pure drugs, tablets, or stock solutions. *Pure drugs* are unadulterated substances in solid or liquid form. They are 100 per cent pure unless otherwise stated. Powders and crystalline substances, such as boric acid, magnesium sulfate, sodium chloride, sodium bicarbonate, etc., and a few liquids, such as cresol, alcohol and glycerin, are pure drugs.

Tablets containing a definite known quantity of drug may be used in making solutions. They also save the inconvenience of weighing the pure drug. The tablet is essentially a preparation of pure drug.

Stock solutions are relatively strong solutions from which weaker solutions may be made. It is customary to have stock solutions on hand so that dilutions of various strengths may be made without the inconvenience and delay of weighing the pure drug. Examples of stock solutions commonly used are bichloride of mercury, phenol, potassium permanganate and magnesium sulfate.

Solutions from pure drugs

To prepare a solution of a given strength of a pure drug, it is necessary to determine the amount of drug to use to make a given quantity of solution. If ratio and proportion is the method of calculation, the proportion may be expressed as follows: The amount of drug is to the finished solution as the strength in per cent is to 100 (or equivalent ratio expression):

Amount of drug : finished solution :: % : 100

The first ratio expresses the relationship between the drug or solute and the solvent containing the solute (finished solution). Both must be expressed in the same denomination or the equivalent:

Right way	*Wrong way*
(X) Gm. of drug are to ml. of solution	(X) gr. of drug are to ml. of solution
(X) ml. of drug are to ml. of solution	(X) ℔ of drug are to ml. of solution
(X) gr. of drug are to ℔ of solution	(X) ml. of drug are to ℔ of solution
(X) f℥ of drug are to f℥ of solution	(X) f℥ of drug are to f℥ of solution

Examples (using the above rule):

(1) Prepare 500 ml. of a 5 per cent solution of boric acid. Since no strength of solute is indicated, boric acid crystals or powder are considered 100 per cent pure drug.

$$X \text{ (Gm. of drug) : 500 ml. (finished solution) :: 5 (\%) : 100 (\%)}$$
$$100 \ X = 2500$$
$$X = 25 \text{ Gm. of drug}$$

In any proportion the product of the means equals the product of the extremes.

Proof: $25 \times 100 = 2500$
$5 \times 500 = 2500$

Another method which can be used to solve this problem or to prove the answer is as follows:

Five per cent means that $\frac{5}{100}$ of the solution is boric acid. 500 ml. weigh 500 Gm. Hence $\frac{5}{100} \times 500$ (Gm.) $= 25$ Gm. It is necessary to use 25 Gm. of pure drug. To prepare the solution, place 25 Gm. of boric acid in a graduate, add enough water to dissolve it and then add water up to 500 ml.

(2) How much drug is needed to make 1 fluidounce of a 1:25 sodium chloride solution?

Amount of drug : finished solution :: % : 100
The ratio 1:25 = 4%

Since so small an amount is to be made it is well to change the fluid-ounce to minims.

$$X \text{ (gr.)} : 480 \text{ (M)} :: 4 \text{ (\%)} : 100 \text{ (\%)}$$
$$100 \text{ X} = 1920$$
$$X = 19.2 \text{ gr. of the drug}$$

Note that since the finished solution is in minims the amount of drug represented by X in the proportion must be in an equivalent denomination. Hence the answer is in grains.

Another method of solving the problem is similar to that mentioned under (1); i.e., the ratio 1:25 means that $\frac{1}{25}$ of the solution is sodium chloride. One fluidounce weighs 480 gr.

$$\frac{1}{25} \times 480 = 19.2 \text{ gr.}$$

Dissolve 19.2 gr. of sodium chloride in a quantity of water so that the total amount of solution measures 1 fluidounce.

(3) Prepare a gallon of 1:1000 bichloride of mercury from tablets of 7½ gr.

$$X \text{ (Gm.)} : 4000 \text{ (ml.)} :: 1 : 1000$$
$$1000 \text{ X} = 4000$$
$$X = 4 \text{ Gm. of the drug}$$

Each tablet contains 7½ gr. or ½ Gm. Since 4 Gm. of the drug are needed, $4 \div \frac{1}{2} = 8$, or 8 tablets.

(4) If 2 f℥ of alcohol are added to 4 f℥ of water, what is the percentage strength of the resulting solution? State the strength also as a ratio.

Amount of drug : finished solution :: % : 100
$$2 \text{ (f℥)} : 6 \text{ (f℥)} :: X : 100$$
$$6 \text{ X} = 200$$
$$X = 33\frac{1}{3}\%$$

When a liquid drug is added to a given amount of water, the finished solution is the sum of the two. Addition of a dry drug to the water of a solution will not increase the volume appreciably since it will be soluble.

$33\frac{1}{3}\%$ means $33\frac{1}{3}$ parts in 100 parts or 1:3 ratio

(5) How much water would you add to a pint of pure alcohol to make it an 80 per cent solution?

Amount of drug : finished solution :: % : 100
$$500 : X :: 80 : 100$$
$$80 \text{ X} = 50,000$$
$$X = 625 \text{ ml. finished solution}$$
$$625 \text{ ml. minus } 500 \text{ ml.} = 125 \text{ ml. water}$$

Since the alcohol is a liquid, to determine the amount of water needed, the liquid drug must be subtracted from the finished solution.

(6) How much potassium permanganate solution 1:100 could you make from fifteen 5 gr. tablets?

Since it is convenient and customary to measure solutions of this type in milliliters, it will be necessary to convert the known available drug to grams. One 5 gr. tablet is $\frac{5}{15}$ or $\frac{1}{3}$ of a gram. Fifteen tablets would therefore be 15 times $\frac{1}{3}$ Gm., or 5 Gm. Since you now know the amount of drug with which you have to work, you can ascertain the amount of solution this quantity of drug will make by following the same rule.

Amount of drug : finished solution :: % : 100 or (ratio of strength)

5 (Gm.) :   X (ml.)   ::   1:100

X = 500; therefore 500 ml. of finished solution

Exercises *Solutions from pure drugs*

1 How much salt would be required to make the following:
  a. 1 gallon of a 0.9% solution?
  b. 250 ml. of a 1% solution?
  c. O ss of a ½% solution?
  d. 1 liter of 1:20 solution?
2 How much drug would be required to make up the following:
  a. 4 fluidounces of a 2% Lysol solution?
  b. 1000 ml. of a 4% vinegar solution?
  c. 2 liters of ⅕% soda bicarbonate solution?
  d. 1 liter of 5% glucose solution?
3 Express the strength of the following in per cent:
  a. 200 ml. of solution containing gr. xv of mercuric cyanide.
  b. 1 pint of solution containing 50 ml. of glycerin.
  c. 1000 ml. of solution containing 4 fluidounces of alcohol.
  d. If you add 500 ml. of alcohol to a liter of water what will the percentage strength be?
4 Express the strength of the following in ratio:
  a. 500 ml. of solution containing 20 Gm. of boric acid.
  b. 4 fluidounces of solution containing 60 gr. of a drug.
  c. 120 ml. of solution containing 1½ fluidrams of a drug.
  d. O ss containing 1 ounce of a drug.
5 How many tablets would you need for each of the following:
  a. 1 liter of 1:1000 mercuric cyanide, using 7½ gr. tablets?
  b. 2 quarts of 1:100 potassium permanganate solution, using 5 gr. tablets?
  c. 1 fluidounce of 2% ammonium chloride solution, using 3 gr. tablets?
  d. 1 gallon of bichloride of mercury 1:5000, using 0.5 Gm. tablets?
6 How much water would be required:
  a. to prepare a ½% solution from gr. x of soda bicarbonate?
  b. to prepare a 40% solution from 200 ml. of pure alcohol?
  c. to prepare a 1:10 solution from f℥ iii of glycerin?
  d. to prepare a 2% solution from 1 level teaspoon of soda bicarbonate?

Solutions from stock solutions

Stock solutions are relatively concentrated solutions which are kept on hand and from which weaker solutions can be made. The problem is always how much stock solution of a given strength is needed to make a certain amount of solution of a lesser strength. The rule is much the same as the one used in the previous lesson.

> *The amount of drug (stock solution) : the finished solution :: the ratio of strength of the two solutions (lesser to the greater)*

Examples:

(1) How would you prepare a quart of a 2 per cent solution of formaldehyde from a stock solution labeled 40 per cent?

$$X \text{ (ml. of stock sol.)} : 1000 \text{ (ml.)} :: 2 \text{ (\%)} : 40 \text{ (\%)}$$
$$40 \text{ X} = 2000$$
$$X = 50 \text{ ml. stock solution}$$

Fifty milliliters of stock solution would be measured in a graduated container and to this amount would be added 950 ml. of water.

(2) How would you prepare two liters of a 1:2000 potassium permanganate solution from a 1 per cent stock solution?

In this case, the strength of the stock solution is expressed in per cent and the strength of the solution to be made is in terms of a ratio. In order to be able to compare the strengths, both must be ratios or both must be in percentage.

$$X \text{ (ml. of stock sol.)} : 2000 \text{ (ml.)} :: \tfrac{1}{20}\% : 1\%$$
$$X = 100 \text{ ml. of stock solution}$$
or
$$X \text{ (ml. of stock sol.)} : 2000 \text{ (ml.)} :: 100 : 2000$$
$$2000 \text{ X} = 200{,}000$$
$$X = 100 \text{ ml. stock solution}$$

In each case the balance of the 2 liters would be water (1900 ml. water). The smaller percentage is to the larger percentage and the smaller ratio is to the larger ratio.

Exercises *Solutions from stock solutions*

1 How much of a 5 per cent solution would be needed to prepare 1 L. of a 2 per cent solution?

2 How much of a 1:5 solution would be needed to prepare 1 pint of a 10 per cent solution?

3 How much water would be needed to prepare 1 gallon of a 3 per cent solution from a 10 per cent solution?

4 How many milliliters of a 20 per cent stock solution would be needed to prepare f℥ ii of a 4 per cent solution?

5 How much water should be added to 50 ml. of a 15 per cent solution to make it a 1:24 solution?

6 How much of a 1:5 stock solution would be needed to prepare 1 gallon of a 1:20 solution?

7 How much of a 25 per cent stock solution would be needed to prepare 10 fluid-ounces of a 1:25 solution?

8 How much of a ½ per cent solution would be needed to make 20 minims of a ⅕ per cent solution?

9 How much stock solution 1:10 would be needed to prepare f℥ ivss of a 1:80 solution?

10 How many milliliters would be needed to prepare 5 fluidrams of a 15 per cent solution from a 1:4 solution?

11 How many fluidounces of a 5 per cent glucose solution could be prepared from 2 fluidrams of a 1:4 solution?

12 How many minims of a 1 per cent solution would be needed to prepare f℥ ss of a ⅒ per cent solution?

13 How much of a 1:2000 solution would be needed to prepare 1 gallon of a 1:10,000 solution?

14 How much of a 12 per cent solution could be made from a fluidounce of a 20 per cent solution?

15 How much stock solution 1:3 would be needed to prepare f℥ v of a 1:5 solution?

Doses from stock solutions

In some hospitals, drugs for hypodermic use are kept in solutions of various strengths. The strength is expressed either by percentage or as the number of minims that contain a certain dose, as ℳ x = gr. ⅛. The problem for the nurse is to determine how many minims of the stock solution contain the dose she is required to give.

Examples:

(1) How would you give morphine sulfate gr. ¼ from a stock solution labeled "ℳ 15 contains gr. ⅙"?

(a) *Amount of drug : finished solution as the ratio of strength or as the strength is to 100.*

¼ gr. : X (unknown number of minims) :: ⅙ gr. : 15 ℳ
⅙ X = 3¾
X = 22½ ℳ

(b) *Another way of reasoning the problem is:*

If ⅙ gr. is contained in 15 ℳ
1 gr. will be contained in 6 × 15 or 90 ℳ
¼ gr. will be contained in ¼ of 90 or 22½ ℳ

(2) How would you give atropine sulfate gr. ¹⁄₁₅₀ from a 1 per cent solution?

¹⁄₁₅₀ gr. : X (unknown number of minims) :: 1:100
X = ⅔ ℳ

To obtain a fraction of a minim, dissolve 1 minim of the stock solution in a number of minims of water so that the total number of minims of the new solution can be divided evenly by the denominator, and take the amount indicated by the fraction. To prepare the above dose, dissolve 1 minim of stock solution in 14 minims of water. This gives a total of 15 minims of which two thirds, or 10 minims, contain atropine sulfate gr. ¹⁄₁₅₀.

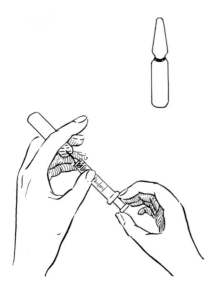

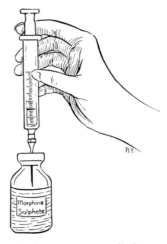

Fig. 8 Inserting hypodermic needle into a stoppered vial. When a hypodermic needle is inserted into a vial of this type, it is important that air be injected first to facilitate withdrawal of the liquid medication. Note that the plunger has been withdrawn and is supported by the index finger. After the plunger has been pushed down to the end of the barrel, the vial can be turned and held much like the ampule in Fig. 7. The desired amount is then drawn into the syringe.

Fig. 7 Withdrawing medication from an ampule. An ampule may be made like the one in the upper right part of this illustration, i.e., it will break easily when pressure is exerted at the constricted portion; or the ampule may be made so that a metal file must be used at the neck to secure a clean break.

Exercises *Doses from stock solutions*

1 If the bottle of morphine sulfate is labeled mg. 15 = 1 ml., how would you give the following, i.e., how many minims would you need in order to give:
   a. gr. $\frac{1}{6}$?
   b. gr. $\frac{1}{8}$?
   c. gr. $\frac{1}{12}$?
   d. gr. $\frac{1}{4}$?

2. If the solution of Demerol Hydrochloride is labeled mg. 50 = 1 ml., how many minims would be required to give:
   a. 100 mg?
   b. gr. i?
   c. gr. ss?
   d. gr. ii?

3 If the solution of codeine phosphate is labeled gr. i = 1 ml., how many minims would be required to give:
   a. 0.03 Gm.?
   b. 0.015 Gm.?
   c. 60 mg.?
   d. 8 mg.?

4 If a solution of atropine sulfate is labeled gr. $\frac{1}{150}$ = 1 ml., how many minims would be needed to give:
   a. gr. $\frac{1}{200}$?
   b. gr. $\frac{1}{300}$?
   c. gr. $\frac{1}{20}$?
   d. gr. $\frac{1}{75}$?

5 How would you give gr. $\frac{1}{200}$ of atropine sulfate from a $\frac{1}{20}$% solution?
6 How would you give gr. $\frac{1}{4}$ of morphine sulfate from a solution labeled 1:50?
7 How would you give eserine sulfate gr. $\frac{1}{60}$ from a $\frac{1}{2}$% solution?
8 How much of a 25% solution would you measure in order to give gr. viii of sodium bromide?

Doses from tablets

Potent drugs such as alkaloids and glycosides usually come in tablets of definite doses designed for hypodermic use. If the dose which the nurse is called upon to give is not the same as that of the tablet, it is necessary for her to calculate how many tablets, or what part of a tablet, will contain the required dose.

The rule is: *Divide the desired dose by the dose on hand to determine the part of a tablet or the number of tablets required.*

Example: The physician orders atropine sulfate gr. $\frac{1}{300}$ (H), and the tablets in the medicine cupboard are labeled gr. $\frac{1}{150}$. The letter (H) means that the medication is to be administered hypodermically. It is obvious that gr. $\frac{1}{300}$ is half as much as gr. $\frac{1}{150}$ and that $\frac{1}{2}$ tablet will be required; the arithmetic involved would be:

$$\tfrac{1}{300} \div \tfrac{1}{150} = \frac{1}{300} \times \frac{150}{1} = \frac{150}{300} \text{ or } \tfrac{1}{2} \text{ (tablet)}$$

It is important to label the answer of this part of the calculation in terms of a tablet or tablets. But in this instance and in most others in which drugs are given hypodermically, the nurse does not cut the tablet. Since the drug is to be given hypodermically, the tablet gr. $\frac{1}{150}$ will be dissolved in a suitable number of minims of water and $\frac{1}{2}$ of the solution will be administered to the patient. The volume of solution given hypodermically is usually between 10 and 20 minims. More than this can make the patient uncomfortable and less than this increases the margin of error should some of the solution be lost. In this example, 30 would be a good choice of minims in which to dissolve the stock tablet, gr. $\frac{1}{150}$, because $\frac{1}{2}$ of 30 minims is 15 minims and the patient will get $\frac{1}{2}$ of gr. $\frac{1}{150}$ or gr. $\frac{1}{300}$. The remaining 15 minims would be discarded.

Examples:

(1) The physician orders morphine sulfate gr. $\frac{1}{6}$ (H) and the tablets in the stock supply are labeled gr. $\frac{1}{8}$.

$$\tfrac{1}{6} \div \tfrac{1}{8} = \frac{1}{6} \times \frac{8}{1} = \frac{8}{6} \text{ or } 1\tfrac{1}{3} \text{ (tablets)}$$

Dissolve one tablet gr. $\frac{1}{8}$ in 30 minims of water and take $\frac{1}{3}$ of it or 10 minims. This will now contain $\frac{1}{3}$ of a tablet. To this 10 minims add the other tablet.

The above manner of preparation is practical only if one has a container other than a hypodermic in which to prepare the solution.

Another way of dealing with the problem of dosage in which more than one tablet will be needed is to determine what part of the total number of tablets (in this case, two) will be required to give the dose ordered. Since the previous calculation of the problem shows that two tablets or gr. ⅓ (⅙ + ⅙ = 2/6 or ⅓) is what one must have on hand, revert to the rule previously stated: Divide the desired dose by the dose on hand to determine the part of a tablet or the number of tablets required. Therefore, ⅛ divided by ⅓ = ⅛ × 3/1 = 3/8 of two tablets. Dissolve two tablets (gr. ⅙) in a number of minims of water so that 3/8 of the total number of minims will be a suitable amount to administer hypodermically; e.g., dissolve the two tablets in 32 minims of water and discard all except 12 minims, which will contain the dose gr. ⅛.

(2) The physician orders codeine phosphate 15. mg. (H), and the stock tablets are labeled 60 mg.

$$15 \div 60 = \frac{15}{60} \text{ or } \frac{1}{4} \text{ (tablet)}$$

Dissolve 1 tablet (60 mg.) in 40 minims of water and give 10 minims.

Exercises Dosage from tablets

1 How would you calculate and prepare the following doses:
   a. Atropine sulfate gr. 1/200 from tablets gr. 1/100?
   b. Atropine sulfate gr. 1/600 from tablets gr. 1/150?
   c. Atropine sulfate gr. 1/350 from tablets gr. 1/150?
   d. Morphine sulfate gr. 1/16 from tablets gr. ⅙?
   e. Morphine sulfate gr. 1/64 from tablets gr. ⅙?
   f. Codeine sulfate gr. ¼ from tablets gr. ½?
2 How would you calculate and prepare the following:
   a. Dilaudid Hydrochloride gr. 1/60 from tablets gr. 1/30?
   b. Pantopon gr. 1/12 from tablets gr. ⅓?
   c. Morphine sulfate 15 mg. from tablets gr. ⅙?
   d. Codeine sulfate mg. 60 from tablets gr. ¼?
   e. Morphine sulfate 0.01 Gm. from tablets gr. ⅛?
   f. Hyoscine Hydrobromide gr. 1/150 from tablets gr. 1/200?
3 How would you prepare 3 gr. of a drug from a 5 gr. tablet? How would you expect to administer it?

Dosage for children

Dosage for children as well as dosage for adults is determined by the physician. Certain time-honored rules have been used in calculating the dosage for infants and children although some pediatricians give little heed to rules per se but calculate dosage on the basis of weight and the amount of skin surface of the child.

The following rules are sometimes followed, however.

Clark's rule

Clark's rule is based on the weight of the child as compared to the weight of the average adult.

$$\frac{\text{Weight of child in pounds}}{150 \text{ lb. (average adult weight)}} \times \text{Adult dose}$$

Example: If a child weighs 50 pounds and the usual adult dose of the drug to be administered is 600 mg., the dose of the child would be:

$$\frac{50}{150} \times 600 \text{ mg.} = 200 \text{ mg.}$$

Fried's rule for infants

Fried's rule presupposes a relationship between age of an infant and the dose.

$$\frac{\text{Age in months}}{150} \times \text{Adult dose}$$

Example: If the adult dose of a drug is 60 mg., the dose for an infant of 10 months would be:

$$\frac{10}{150} \times 60 \text{ mg.} = 4 \text{ mg.}$$

Young's rule

Young's rule is based on the assumption that there is a relationship between the dose and the age of the child and this rule is used especially for children between the ages of 3 and 12 years.

$$\frac{\text{Age of child}}{\text{Age plus 12}} \times \text{Adult dose}$$

Example: If the adult dose is 100 mg., the dose for an 8-year-old child is:

$$\frac{8}{8 \text{ plus } 12} \times 100 \text{ mg.} = 40 \text{ mg.}$$

Exercises Dosage for children

The nurse is often called upon to calculate children's doses from standard dosage forms.

1 How would you prepare 250,000 units of crystalline penicillin from a vial that contains 300,000 units per milliliter?

2 The label on a bottle of digoxin reads 0.05 mg. per milliliter. How many milliliters would be needed to give 0.15 mg.?

3 How many minims of Demerol would you expect to withdraw from a vial labeled 50 mg. per milliliter if you wish to give 5 mg.?

4 An oral preparation of an antibiotic drug is labeled 1 Gm. per 5 ml. (cc.). The child is to have 500 mg. How many teaspoons or what part of a teaspoon would you give?

5 If an oral antibiotic preparation is labeled 125 mg. per fluidram, how many milliliters are needed to give 100 mg.?

6 How many minims of liquid preparation of morphine would you need to give 4 mg. if the label indicates there is gr. ¼ in each milliliter?

7 How would you prepare 4 mg. of morphine from tablets gr. ⅙?

8 How would you give 50 mg. of a drug from a vial in which there is 0.4 Gm. per milliliter (cubic centimeter)?

9 How would you prepare gr. ⅟₃₀₀ of atropine from tablets gr. ⅟₂₀₀?

10 If a bottle of antibiotic suspension is labeled 5 mg. per drop, how many drops should be administered to give 50 mg.?

Exercises Weights and measures

Change to appropriate metric equivalents	Change to appropriate apothecary equivalents	Change to appropriate household equivalents
a. f℥ iv _____	**a.** 30 Gm. _____	**a.** 4 Gm. _____
b. ℥ ii _____	**b.** 0.5 Gm. _____	**b.** 30 ml. _____
c. ℳ xv _____	**c.** 1 L. _____	**c.** quart 1 _____
d. ½ cup _____	**d.** 30 mg. _____	**d.** f℥ i _____
e. C ii _____	**e.** 0.2 mg. _____	**e.** f℥ i _____
f. lb. 2.2 _____	**f.** 1 cup _____	**f.** ℳ xxx _____
g. gr. ⅛ _____	**g.** 1 T. _____	**g.** ℥ iv _____
h. gr. ¹⁄₁₂₀ _____	**h.** 1 t. _____	**h.** gr. lx _____
i. gr. 7½ _____	**i.** 15 gtt. _____	**i.** O ii _____
j. f℥ ii _____	**j.** 500 ml. _____	**j.** 1 L. _____

For the following problems, state the rule by which you solve the problem, indicate the equation you use, and label all answers. Additional information may be indicated in some instances.

1 How many 5 gr. tablets would you need to make a gallon of 1:100 potassium permanganate solution?

2 How many 7½ gr. tablets of mercuric cyanide would you need to make 2 L. of 1:1000 solution?

3 How would you prepare 1 L. of potassium permanganate solution from a stock solution labeled 1:100?

4 How would you prepare a gallon of 1:2000 solution from a stock solution labeled 1/10 per cent?

5 If Sodium Pentothal solution is made by adding 400 ml. of distilled water to 10 Gm. of drug, what is the percentage strength of the solution? The ratio of strength?

6 If 4 fluidrams of drug are added to 4 fluidounces of water, what is the strength of the resulting solution? Express strength also as a ratio.

7 How much water would you add to a pint of 95 per cent alcohol to make a 70 per cent solution?

8 How much salt (sodium chloride) would be required to make a quart of physiologic saline solution (0.9 per cent)?

9 If you have on hand tablets of morphine gr. ⅙ and the doctor orders gr. ⅛ how would you prepare the dose?

10 If you have on hand tablets of morphine gr. ¼ and wish to give gr. ⅙, how would you prepare the dose?

Change to appropriate metric equivalents	Change to appropriate apothecary equivalents	Change to appropriate household equivalents
1 f℥ i _____	**1** 250 ml. _____	**1** 1 L. _____
2 f℥ ii _____	**2** 1 mg. _____	**2** 45 ml. _____
3 C ss _____	**3** 10 mg. _____	**3** f℥ iv _____
4 O ii _____	**4** 30 ml. _____	**4** f℥ vi _____
5 2 T. _____	**5** 500 mg. _____	**5** ℳ xv _____
6 gr. ¹⁄₆₀₀ _____	**6** 300 mg. _____	**6** 120 ml. _____
7 gr. x. _____	**7** 10 gtt. _____	**7** 4 Gm. _____
8 gr. ¹⁄₁₅₀ _____	**8** 8 mg. _____	**8** 45 Gm. _____
9 ½ cup _____	**9** 0.6 Gm. _____	**9** ℳ lx _____
10 1 t. _____	**10** 0.3 Gm. _____	**10** O i _____

For the following problems, state the rule by which you plan to solve the problem, state the equation, and label all answers.

1 How would you prepare a gallon of 1:2000 solution from a stock solution labeled ⅕ per cent?
2 How would you make 2 L. of 1:2000 solution from tablets containing 7½ gr. of drug in each tablet?
3 How much water is needed to make a 70 per cent solution from a pint of pure alcohol?
4 How much soda bicarbonate is needed to make 1½ L. of 2 per cent solution?
5 If a physician ordered 2 Gm. of drug to be given in four equally divided doses and the drug is available in 250 mg. capsules, how many capsules would you give per dose?
6 How much water would you add to a pint of 95 per cent alcohol to make a 50 per cent solution?
7 If the container of Demerol Hydrochloride solution reads 50 mg. per milliliter (cubic centimeter), how many minims would be required to give 1½ gr.?
8 If a bottle of codeine sulfate solution is labeled 60 mg. per milliliter (cubic centimeter), how many minims would you need to give gr. ¼?
9 How would you prepare 2 quarts of a 2 per cent vinegar douche for a patient?
10 If a fluidounce of glycerin is added to 120 ml. of water, what is the strength of the solution?
11 How would you prepare 1½ quarts of a physiologic saline solution to be used for a throat irrigation?
12 How much water is needed to make a ⅒ per cent solution from 2 gr. of a drug?

Questions
for review and study

1 Explain how you would prepare 1 L. of a 5 per cent solution from a stock solution labeled 12 per cent.
2 How would you prepare 2 L. of 1:10,000 solution of potassium permanganate from a stock solution labeled 1:100?
3 How would you prepare 2 gallons of a 1:1000 mercuric cyanide solution from 7½ gr. tablets? How many tablets would you use?
4 How would you give gr. i of sodium phenobarbital from a tablet containing 0.12 Gm.?
5 A 2 ml. ampule of caffeine with sodium benzoate contains 7½ gr. of drug; how much would be necessary to give 5 gr.?
6 Explain how you would give morphine sulfate gr. 1/64 from tablet gr. ¼.
7 What is the ratio of strength of a solution in which 10 fluidounces contain 2 drams of drug? What is the percentage strength?
8 How much salt is needed to make 2 quarts of normal saline solution?

9 If ♏ xx of solution contain gr. ¼ of a drug, how much of the solution would you use to give gr. ⅙?
10 How would you prepare 1500 ml. of a 7 per cent solution, using 5 gr. tablets?
11 How would you give atropine gr. 1/150 from tablets marked gr. 1/200?
12 If 2 fluidounces of alcohol are added to a liter of water, what is the percentage strength of solution? What part of the total solution is alcohol?
13 If a physician orders 100 mg. of Demerol Hydrochloride and your stock bottle is marked in grains, how much would you give?
14 If a physician orders 10 mg. of morphine sulfate and the liquid narcotic bottle is labeled 1 ml. and contains ¼ gr., how many minims will you give?
15 How many minims of a 1/10% solution would you use to give gr. 1/100 of atropine sulfate?
16 How much 1:1000 solution could be made from ten 7½ gr. tablets of a drug?

Chapter 6

Administration of medicines

The role of the nurse

The administration of medicines is a unique responsibility of the nurse. To be sure, some medicines are administered by physicians, but the greater number, by far, are given by nurses. The nurse carries out the orders given by the physician, but many times she has responsibilities which extend beyond the following of orders. She would not be considered a good nurse if this were not the case. Often she must help the patient to accept the medicine; sometimes she must re-enforce his confidence in the physician who prescribed it, as well as try to meet his various needs at the time of administration. Medicine tends to be very meaningful to the patient. If it is administered later than usual, if it is diluted more or less than the previous dose, if a different nurse brings it, or if it is not producing the effects as rapidly as he thinks it should, the patient may be disturbed about it. If the drug is given by means of a needle the injection may be a terrifying experience regardless of the age of the patient. The memory of a previous unpleasant experience or comments made by other persons about injections may cause him to dread the administration of anything with a needle. Understanding and accepting the feelings of the patient is essential to the establishment of rapport with the patient. Time spent explaining, simply, what must be done is usually time well spent.

If the nurse is to help the patient and also cooperate effectively with the physician, she needs to know why a patient is receiving a certain medicine, what effects to expect, what unusual effects may develop or what symptoms of overdosage may occur, the amount of the drug usually given, and the usual channel of administration. New drugs appear on the market so rapidly today it is sometimes difficult to secure authentic information about them. Occasionally only the physicians who order the drugs know much about them because the preparations may be so new they are known only by a number and little or no printed information is available. This is particularly true in hospitals connected with research institutions.

Major channels of administration

Certain drugs are suited only to one method of administration, whereas others can be given in a number of ways, depending on the preparation used and the purpose for which it is given. It is important to know the channel of administration that will afford optimum effects of the drug. As a rule, we are concerned with two main types of administration: *local*, in which the effects are confined to the site of application, and *systemic*, in which the results are realized after the drug is absorbed into the blood and diffuses into one or more tissues of the body. Some drugs are given locally but they may produce both local and systemic effects if they are partly or entirely absorbed. Other drugs may be swallowed or given by needle, but their effects are confined to the tissues with which they have immediate contact, so that their action is essentially local. Certain antibiotics are given orally, but because they are poorly absorbed they exert their major effects in the intestine. A drug may be injected into a joint cavity and have little or no effect beyond the tissues of that structure. Few drugs are absorbed from the skin; absorption is much more likely to occur from a mucous membrane.

Administration for local effect

Application to the skin. Medications are applied to the skin chiefly as antiseptics, astringents, and emollients (soothing agents). The skin may be painted with a drug such as iodine tincture or some other antiseptic. Lotions may be applied to the skin to relieve itching and irritation. Ointments are sometimes applied for prolonged effect on lesions of various kinds. Wet dressings, local baths or soaks, and plasters and poultices are usually used for their effect at the site of application.

Application to mucous membranes. Preparations of drugs are applied to mucous membranes of the nose, throat, mouth, respiratory tract, eye, and genitourinary tract. They may be painted or swabbed on the surface, instilled, sprayed, or administered by way of a douche or irrigation.

Sprays or nebulae are fine particles of drug suspended or dissolved in oil or water and administered with a nebulizer. Oily preparations should be applied only to the upper part of the respiratory tract because fine droplets are carried easily to the deeper respiratory passages where untoward effects from the oil can result. (Some physicians do not like to use any kind of an oily preparation in the nose or respiratory passages.) Aerosols are dry, powdery drugs which may be drawn into the respiratory passages by means of a flow of air or oxygen under pressure. Intermittent positive pressure combined with nebulization is being used in the treatment of certain respiratory disorders.

Drugs in suppository form can be used for their local effects on the mucous membrane of the vagina, urethra, or rectum. Packs and tampons may be impregnated with a drug and placed in a body cavity. They are used particularly in the nose, ears, and vagina. Powders are sometimes blown on a mucous membrane. This method of local application is called insufflation and the applicator used, an insufflator.

Administration for systemic effects

Drugs that produce a systemic effect must be absorbed and carried to the cells or tissues capable of responding to them. The channel of administration used depends upon the nature and amount of the drug to be given, the desired rapidity of effect, and the general condition of the patient. The usual channels selected for systemic effect include the following: oral, sublingual, rectal, inhalation, and parenteral (injection)— intradermal, subcutaneous, intramuscular, intravenous, intraspinal, and sometimes intracardiac, intrapericardial, and intraosseous.

Oral. The oral channel of administration is the safest, most economic, and most convenient way of giving medicines. Hence they should be given orally unless some distinct advantage is to be gained by giving them another way.

Certain disadvantages, however, may be encountered with some drugs when given orally. Certain drugs have an objectionable odor or taste. A few drugs are known to be harmful to the teeth and must be administered with a glass tube or straw. Drugs irritating to the gastric mucosa may produce nausea and emesis. Oral administration may not be satisfactory if a patient is excessively nauseated, vomiting, uncooperative, or so sick that aspiration is a hazard. Some drugs cannot be given orally because they are subject to change by digestive enzymes. Absorption from the alimentary tract is always subject to a number of irregularities and therefore the effects may be less predictable than when drugs are given by injection.

Sublingual. Drugs given sublingually are placed under the patient's tongue where they must be retained until they are dissolved and absorbed. The epithelium on the underside of the tongue is relatively thin, and the drug soon finds its way into the rich network of blood capillaries. Rapid action can thus be secured and the effects of gastric and intestinal enzymes avoided. Furthermore, the patient can be spared the services of a person to administer the drug by injection. The number of drugs that can be given sublingually is limited. The drug must dissolve readily, and the patient must be able to cooperate, i.e., the patient must understand that the drug is not to be swallowed and he must not take a drink until the drug has been absorbed. Tablets of nitroglycerine are usually administered sublingually.

Rectal. Rectal administration can be used advantageously when the stomach is nonretentive, when the medicine has an objectionable taste or odor, and when it can be changed by digestive enzymes. It is a reasonably convenient and safe method of giving drugs when the oral method is unsuitable, e.g., when the patient is unconscious.

The rate of absorption is likely to be uncertain. In the event that some of the drug is expelled, it is difficult to determine how much has been retained. Absorption from the rectum may be satisfactory, provided the organ is empty and is not excessively irritable. An evacuant enema prior to the administration of the medication is usually advisable. The amount of solution that can be given rectally is usually small. The dosage form used for rectal administration is usually a suppository.

Inhalation. The respiratory tract offers an enormous surface of absorbing epithelium. If the drug is volatile and capable of being absorbed and if there is more in the inspired air than in the blood, a large amount of drug may be rapidly absorbed to produce an almost immediate effect. This fact is of significance in situations of emergency. Amyl nitrite, ether, oxygen, and carbon dioxide are examples of volatile and gaseous agents that are given by inhalation.

Parenteral. The term parenteral literally means "beside the intestine." It refers to all the ways by which drugs are administered with a needle. The drug may be injected into the tissues or fluids of the body. Drugs given parenterally must be readily soluble, sterile, and rapidly absorbed and should not cause pain or irritation at the site of injection. There are certain dangers associated with all forms of parenterally administered medications. Whenever the skin is broken, it is possible for an infection to develop. Drugs given by injection often act rapidly, and rapid action can save a life but it can also result in the loss of one, since an error in dosage or too rapid injection cannot easily be corrected. Injections may cause trauma and soreness in the tissues, and if a spinal nerve is injured paralysis can be one of the results. Parenteral administration calls for special equipment, skill, and a suitably prepared form of medication which is often more expensive than the oral form. Some types of parenteral administration are done only by the physician and others by the nurse.

Intradermal. Intradermal or intracutaneous injection means that the injection is made into the upper layers of the skin. The amount of drug given is small and absorption is slow. This method is used to advantage when testing for allergic reactions of the patient. Minute amounts of the solution to be tested are injected just under the outer layers of the skin. The medial surface of the forearm and the skin of the back are the sites frequently used. A physician is usually responsible for this procedure.

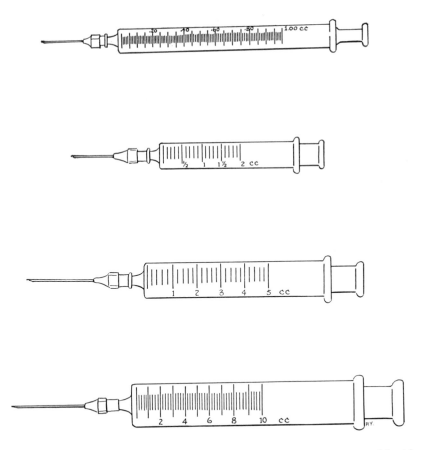

Fig. 9 These syringes are used to measure accurately varying amounts of liquids and liquid medications. The uppermost syringe is known as a tuberculin syringe and is graduated in 0.01 cc. (ml.). It is a syringe of choice for administration of very small amounts. The 2 cc. syringe is the one commonly used to give a drug subcutaneously (hypodermically). It is graduated in 0.1 cc. The larger syringes are used when a larger volume of drug is to be administered.

Subcutaneous. Small amounts of drug in solution are given subcutaneously (synonym: hypodermically) by means of a hypodermic syringe and needle. The needle is inserted through the skin with a quick movement, but the injection is made slowly and steadily. The angle of insertion should be 45 to 60 degrees and should be made preferably on the outer surface of the upper arm or on the anterior surface of the thigh. In these locations there are fewer large blood vessels, and sensation is less keen than on the medial surfaces of the extremities. After the injection of the drug and the withdrawal of the needle, the site of injection should be massaged gently. Disposable syringes and needles so popular

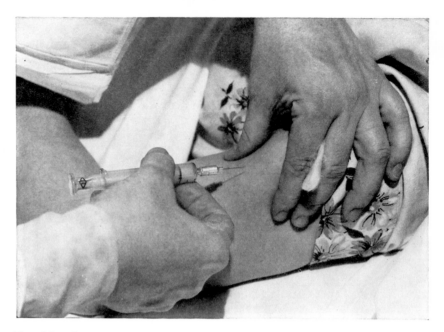

Fig. 10 Subcutaneous injection. **A,** The skin surface has been cleansed and the hypodermic is held at the angle at which it will penetrate the tissue. The left hand is used to pinch the arm gently but firmly.

today contribute to accuracy and safety of the procedure. Hypodermically injected medicines are limited to the administration of drugs that are highly soluble and nonirritating and to solutions of limited volume (0.5 to 2 ml.).

Irritating drugs given subcutaneously can result in the formation of sterile abscesses and necrotic tissue. Infection can also occur more easily following subcutaneous administration than when drugs are given intravenously. Care should be exercised to avoid contamination.

Large amounts of solution given into subcutaneous tissue is known as *hypodermoclysis*. Isotonic solutions of sodium chloride or glucose are administered this way. The needle is longer than that used for a hypodermic injection and it is inserted into areas of loose connective tissue such as that under the breasts, in the groin, and into the subscapular region of the back. Fluids must be given slowly to avoid overdistention of the tissues. Hyaluronidase is sometimes added to the solution to facilitate the spread and absorption of the fluid by decreasing the viscosity of the ground substance in connective tissues. Some physicians prefer intravenous infusion of fluids to hypodermoclysis because the amount of absorption is more readily determined.

Intramuscular. Injections are made through the skin and subcutaneous

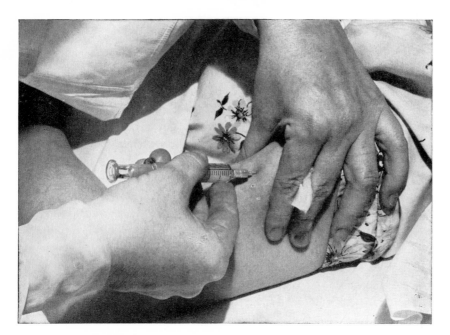

Fig. 10 (cont'd) B, The needle has been inserted.

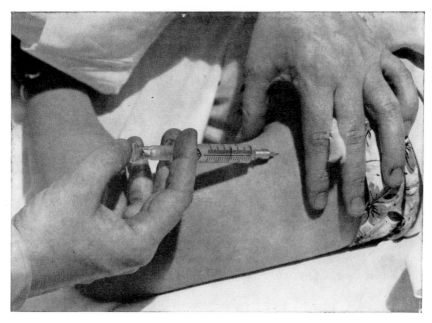

Fig. 10 (cont'd) C, The tissue of the arm is released (left hand) and the solution is steadily injected.

Administration of medicines 99

tissue into the muscular tissue of the body when prompt absorption is desirable and the drug is too irritating to be given subcutaneously. Larger doses can be given intramuscularly than subcutaneously (1 to 10 ml.). Muscles into which injection can usually be made conveniently are those of the buttock, the lateral side of the thigh, and the deltoid region of the arm. The gluteal muscles are usually thick and well suited to the injection of the larger intramuscular doses. The drug spreads along the muscle fibers and along the fasciae. This affords a large absorbing surface and relatively few sensory nerves.

A drug may be given intramuscularly in an aqueous solution, an aqueous suspension, or in a solution or suspension of oil. Suspensions form a depot of drug in the tissue, and slow gradual absorption usually results. Two disadvantages are sometimes encountered when preparations in oil are used: the patient may be sensitive to the oil or the oil may not be absorbed. In the latter case, incision and drainage of the oil may be necessary.

The type of needle used for intramuscular injection depends upon the site of the injection, the condition of the tissues, and the nature of the drug to be injected. Needles from 1 to 3 inches in length may be used. The usual gauge is 19 to 22 (the larger the number, the finer is the needle). Fine needles can be used for thin solutions and heavier needles for suspensions and oils. Needles for injection into the deltoid area should be 1 to 1½ inches in length, the gauge again depending on the material to be injected. For many intramuscular injections the preferable site of injection is the buttock. The needle must be long enough to avoid depositing the solution of drug into the subcutaneous or fatty tissue. The buttock should be divided into four parts and the injection made into the upper outer quadrant. The crest of the ilium serves as a good landmark and should be palpated to confirm the location of the upper outer quadrant, and then the needle should be inserted straight in, with a firm bold pressure, about 2 to 3 inches below the iliac crest. In this region the muscle is thick and the nerve supply is less profuse than in an area near the middle of the buttock or in the region closer to the rectum. Nurses sometimes make the mistake of giving intramuscular injections too near the rectum or too near the middle of the buttock, where it is possible to cause the patient unnecessary discomfort or actually to injure the sciatic nerve and cause a paralysis of the lower extremity.

After the needle is inserted the plunger should be pulled up to aspirate for a few seconds to make certain that the needle is not in a blood vessel. Although this probably seldom occurs when the injection is made in the sites mentioned, it is not justifiable to take a chance of injecting a drug into a blood vessel when this is not the route of administration selected for the drug. In certain instances, injection of oily or particulate

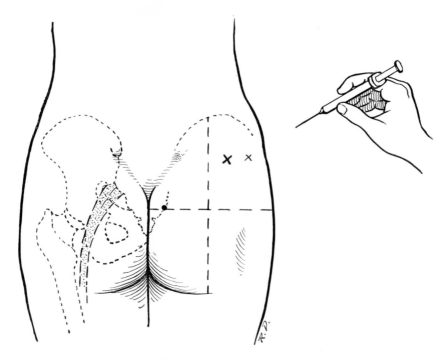

Fig. 11 In determining the location of the upper outer quadrant, it is important to locate the crest of the ilium above and the inferior gluteal fold below before marking the buttock into fourths. The checks indicate two of a number of sites which may be used in the upper outer quadrant, although it is well to keep in the general area of about 2 inches below the iliac crest. An injection near the middle of the buttock may result in an injury to the sciatic nerve. It is, of course, important to vary the sites of injection, preferably using alternate buttocks.

medicines, killed bacteria, etc. by inadvertent intravenous administration could result in a serious emergency.

When giving an intramuscular injection, it is usually preferable to have the patient in a prone position, with his head turned to one side and with a pillow under the legs just below the knees. He should be instructed to "toe inward"; this will help to promote relaxation of the gluteal muscles. If this is not a convenient position for the patient to take, he may be placed on his side with the leg flexed at the knee.

When injection is made in the upper extremities, the deltoid is the muscle of choice. Injections of small bulk are given here. To prevent excessive scar formation or tissue irritation, no two injections should be made in the same spot during a course of treatments. When injection is made into the buttocks, it should be given first on one side and then on the other.

Administration of medicines 101

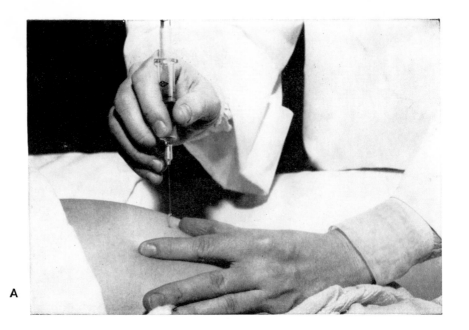

A

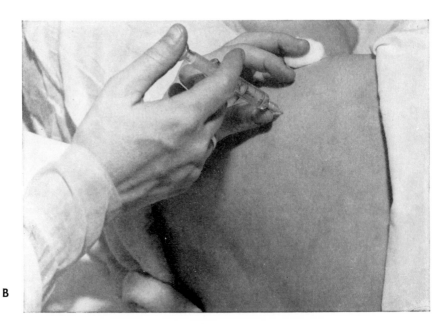

B

Fig. 12 Intramuscular injection. **A,** If a patient is unable to lie face downward, the intramuscular injection must be given when the patient is lying on the side. The needle is inserted "straight in" with a quick, firm movement. **B,** After aspirating to make certain that the needle is not in a blood vessel, the solution is injected slowly and steadily.

Penicillin, streptomycin, Demerol, and whole blood are examples of preparations that may be given by intramuscular injection.

Intravenous. When an immediate effect is desired or when for any reason the drug cannot be injected into the other tissues, it may be given directly into a vein as an *injection* or *infusion.* The technic of this method requires skill and perfect asepsis, and the drug must be highly soluble and capable of withstanding sterilization. It should therefore be used carefully and not too frequently. The method is of great value in emergencies. The dose and amount of absorption can be determined with accuracy, although the rapidity of absorption and the fact that there is no recall once the drug has been given constitute dangers worthy of consideration. From this standpoint it is one of the least safe methods of administration. However, irritating drugs may sometimes be given this way when they cannot be tolerated by any other method. This is possible because the drug is rapidly diluted with the blood and the vessel wall is relatively insensitive.

There continues to be considerable controversy as to whether nurses should or should not administer medications intravenously. Laws defining certain procedures as medical practice are not specific. In some hospitals, licensed professional nurses are expected to give intravenous medications and fluids under the direction of a physician, and in other hospitals the nurse is limited to adding prescribed doses of vitamins to the intravenous fluids of the patient.

INTRAVENOUS INJECTION. In intravenous injection a comparatively small amount of solution is given by means of a syringe. The drug is dissolved in a suitable amount of normal saline or other isotonic solution. The injection is made usually into the median basilic or the median cephalic vein at the bend of the elbow. However, any vein that is accessible may be used. Factors that determine the choice of a vein are related to the thickness of the skin over the vein, the closeness of the vein to the surface, and the presence of a firm support under the vein (bone). A vein that is normally distended with blood is much easier to enter than a partially collapsed vein. If a vein of the arm has been chosen, a tourniquet is drawn tightly around the middle of the arm to distend the vein, the air is expelled from the syringe, and the needle is introduced, pointing upward toward the heart. A few drops of blood are aspirated into the syringe to make sure the needle is in the vein; the tourniquet is then removed and the solution is injected very slowly. The needle, syringe, and solution must be sterile, and the hands of the doctor and nurse and the skin of the patient at the point of insertion of the needle must be clean. Intravenous injection is employed when immediate action is necessary, when the drug is too irritating to be injected into the other tissues, or when the circulation is so poor that absorption is much retarded.

INTRAVENOUS INFUSION. In intravenous infusion a larger amount of fluid is usually given, varying from 1 to 5 pints, and the method differs somewhat. The solution is made to flow by gravity or siphonage from a graduated glass flask through tubing, connecting tip, and needle into the vein.

Infusions are most commonly given to relieve tissue dehydration, to restore depleted blood volume, to dilute toxic substances in the blood

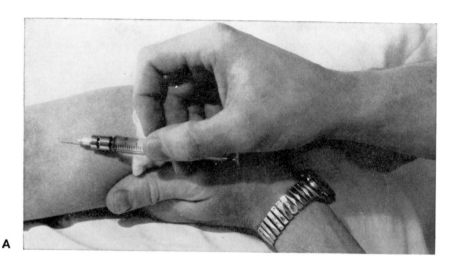

A

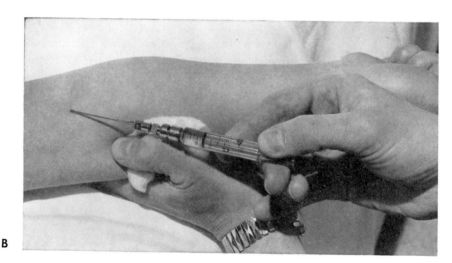

B

Fig. 13 Insertion of a plastic needle for intravenous infusion. Although here a vein of the arm had been used, other veins are also used such as veins of the hand or foot. **A,** The skin area of the arm has been cleansed with a solution of alcohol, and a small amount of local anesthetic is administered prior to the insertion of the plastic needle. **B,** Insertion of a combination of steel and plastic needles (a steel

and tissue fluids, and to supply electrolytes, drugs, and foods.

During the administration of the intravenous infusion, the patient must remain very quiet to prevent the displacement of the needle. The fluid must be given very slowly, however, to prevent reaction or loss of important constituents by way of the kidney. Ordinarily 3 to 4 hours are required for every 1000 ml. of fluid, depending on the condition of the patient, the nature of the solution, and the reasons for giving it.

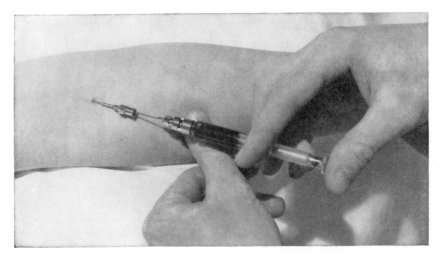

C

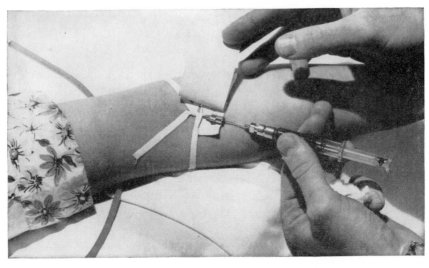

D

needle is inside the plastic needle). **C,** Withdrawal of blood indicates that the needles are in the vein, after which the steel needle is withdrawn, leaving the plastic needle in the vein. **D,** The plastic needle is fastened securely with adhesive tape, after which the tubing connected to the intravenous solution is attached to the needle and the flow of the solution is regulated.

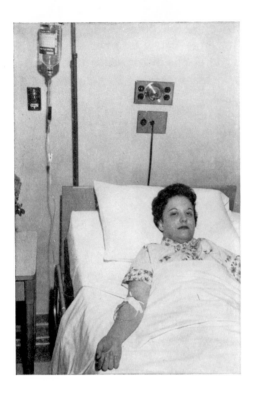

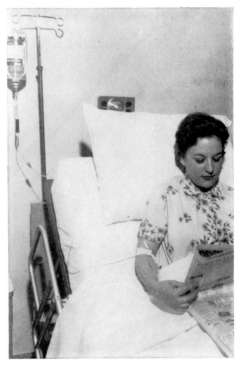

Fig. 14 Intravenous infusion. Drugs such as vitamins, minerals, and hormones are sometimes added to the intravenous infusion.

Fig. 15 Intravenous infusion. The use of a plastic needle instead of a steel needle permits the patient to move around with greater ease.

INTRAVENOUS INFUSION: SOLUTIONS USED. Sodium chloride (0.9 per cent) solution, commonly known as physiologic salt solution, is the fluid of choice for intravenous infusion to relieve any case of dehydration that is not complicated by acidosis. Physiologic salt solution may be sterilized by boiling, and it is isotonic with normal body fluids.

Five per cent dextrose solution is frequently administered and is of value because it provides a means of administering water and a sugar which is a food. A concentration of 5.5 per cent is approximately isotonic with normal body fluids. Dextrose in physiologic saline solution is sometimes given.

A special gelatin solution may be given intravenously as an infusion colloid to support blood volume in the management of various types of shock.

A number of commercial solutions are on the market at present which are used in intravenous replacement therapy. Some contain not only salts of sodium and potassium but also salts of calcium and magnesium. Vitamins are also added to intravenous fluids when their need is indicated.

Whole blood and blood plasma are likewise given intravenously and are ideal to restore depleted blood volume, as well as constituents of the blood.

Intraspinal. Intraspinal injection is also known as intrathecal (into a sheath), subdural, subarachnoid, or lumbar injection. The technic is the same as that required for a lumbar puncture. A needle is inserted into the subarachnoid space, some cerebrospinal fluid is withdrawn, and the drug is injected. The drug exerts more of a local effect than a systemic one because the effect of the drug is on the spinal cord, the meninges, or the nerve roots and is used only when for some reason drugs fail to reach the nerve tissue by diffusion from the blood. Antibiotics, antisera, and local anesthetics are sometimes administered this way. Serious neurologic complications have been known to occur following intra-spinal injection; hence more than the usual amount of danger is associated with this type of injection. Nurses do not administer drugs intraspinally.

Intracardiac, intrapericardial, and intraosseous. There are a number of other ways by which drugs may be introduced into specific tissues. *Intracardiac* injection is occasionally made directly into the myocardium to resuscitate the heart when, for some reason, it has stopped beating. *Intrapericardial* injection makes possible the introduction of medication into the pericardial sac from which absorption into the heart muscle is said to be rapid. *Intraosseous* injection is made directly into bone marrow. The effect is rapid since the marrow is highly vascular. The danger and consequences of infection are possible disadvantages which must be considered when this method of administration is used.

Orders for medications

The procedure used for ordering medicines for a patient depends on whether the patient is in the hospital, in his home, in the doctor's office, or in some institution other than a hospital. On the ward of the hospital there is usually a book or file in which the physician writes his orders. Sometimes orders are written on the patient's chart. In an emergency there may be no time to write an order and it is given verbally. Sometimes the physician gives an order over the telephone. It is customary for the nurse to write the order which she has been given verbally. She indicates the name of the physician who gave the order and how it was given (verbally or by telephone), and the physician later confirms the order by signing his name or initials.

Written orders are a form of protection to every one concerned with medicines—the patient, the physician, and the nurse. They constitute permanent records which can be referred to as often as necessary. No nurse may modify or in any way alter a physician's order. If she has reason to think that an error has been made she should ask the physician about it. If inquiry is made courteously, the physician is usually pleased that the nurse is alert and conscientious. If the head nurse is available she will appreciate being asked regarding an order about which there is question. She may be able to explain something about the order which will clarify matters and save the student the embarrassment that may result from questioning an order that is not wrong. *However, the nurse should not go ahead and give a medicine if she believes there is an error involved.* On the other hand, she may not disregard the order.

Prescriptions

Outside the hospital the physician will write a prescription when he wishes to order a drug. Nurses do not write prescriptions, but they need to understand what is involved and who may write them. Pharmaceutical supply houses have succeeded in preparing drugs in a form both attractive and practical so that much less is required of the pharmacist in the way of preparing and compounding medicines. The present-day pharmacist often has merely to dispense the medicine with due attention to proper measurements, labeling, etc. Only persons legally licensed—physicians, dentists, and veterinarians—may write prescriptions.

A number of medicinal agents may be purchased over the counter without a prescription, but an amendment to the Federal Food, Drug, and Cosmetic Act (as mentioned in Chapter 2) requires that all drugs which can be used safely and effectively only under the supervision of a physician must have a prescription. Such prescriptions can be refilled only if authorization is granted by the prescriber. Authorization may be made in writing by indicating on the written prescription the number of times or the frequency with which the prescription may be refilled, or the physician may authorize the pharmacist by telephone. Sometimes the pharmacist telephones the physician if a patient requests that a prescription be refilled and no previous authorization has been given. Prescriptions for narcotics cannot be refilled; they must be rewritten.

A typical prescription is a written formula given by a physician to a pharmacist for the preparation of a medicine for a patient. It consists of four parts:

1. The superscription, which includes the patient's name, address, the date and the symbol ℞, an abbreviation for "Recipe" meaning "Take Thou."

2. The inscription, which states the names and amounts of the ingredients to be used.

3. The subscription, which contains the directions to the pharmacist. Sometimes this is confined to the word or symbol meaning "Mix."

4. The signature, which is abbreviated "S" or "Sig." and means "Write on the label." This indicates the directions for the patient who is to take the medicine.

The physician's name is also indicated. His name, address, and registry and telephone numbers are frequently printed on his prescription blanks. The prescription is usually written in English, although Latin and English may still be used by some physicians. Quantities are expressed in either the apothecaries' or metric system. The following is an example of a prescription.

Superscription	Mr. James Wiley	Age:	Date 7/1/60
	210 Elmwood Pl., Minneapolis, Minn.		
Inscription	℞	Gm. or ml.	
	Ammonium Chloride	15.	
	Syrup Citric Acid	48.	
	Syrup Glycyrrhiza to make	120.	
Subscription	Mix		
Signature	Sig: one teaspoonful every 3-4 hours		
		J. B. Tanner, M.D.	
		(address)	

If the prescription is for a narcotic or any other drug listed in the Harrison Narcotic Law, the physician's registry number as well as his address must appear on the prescription form. If the patient is a child, the age is sometimes included.

If the patient is in the hospital and a medicine is ordered for him, prescription blanks are sometimes used to copy the order for the preparation. The nurse copies the order and sends it to the pharmacist. The form is similar to the prescription, although it is usually for some drug that is ready for use and requires no special preparation.

The abbreviations in Table 11 are used in written orders, prescriptions, and labels on medicines, and it is necessary for the nurse to know what they mean. A difference exists between the abbreviation s.o.s. and p.r.n. The former, when used in connection with medicines, means "if necessary" and refers to one dose only. The latter, p.r.n., means when required, as often as necessary, or according to circumstances. The nurse is expected to use her judgment about repeating the dose. For example, a physician may leave an order for a patient which reads:

For Mrs. Smith, Room 210, Elixir Terpin Hydrate drams i q. 3 h. p.r.n. for cough.
John Doe, M.D.

Table 11

Abbreviations for orders, prescriptions, and labels

Abbreviation	Derivation	Meaning
a͞a	ana	of each
a.c.	ante cibum	before meals
ad	ad	to, up to
ad lib.	ad libitum	freely as desired
aq.	aqua	water
aq. dest.	aqua destillata	distilled water
b.i.d.	bis in die	two times a day
b.i.n.	bis in noctis	two times a night
c.	cum	with
caps.	capsula	capsule
comp.	compositus	compound
dil.	dilutus	dilute
elix.	elixir	elixir
ext.	extractum	extract
fld.	fluidus	fluid
Ft.	fiat	make
Gm.	gramme	gram
gr.	granum	grain
gtt.	gutta	a drop
h.	hora	hour
h.s.	hora somni	hour of sleep (bedtime)
M.	misce	mix
m.	minimum	a minim
mist.	mistura	mixture
non rep.	non repetatur	not to be repeated
noct.	nocte	in the night
O	octarius	pint
ol.	oleum	oil
o.d.	omni die	every day

The order means that the patient may have a dose of cough medicine every three hours. However, if the patient is not coughing and has no need for the medicine, the nurse may allow longer intervals to elapse between doses.

"Morphine sulfate 10 mg. q. 4 h. p.r.n." means that the dose of morphine sulfate may be given every four hours if the patient has need of it. If the nurse thinks that the patient has no need for it, i.e., the patient seems to have no pain, is resting comfortably, is asleep most of the time, etc., she will allow a longer interval than four hours to elapse before repeating the dose. If, however, the order read "Morphine sulfate 10 mg. s.o.s.," the nurse would give one dose of the drug if the patient seemed to need it and then would give no more. If a dose of the drug is to be given immediately, it would read "Morphine sulfate 10 mg. stat."

Table 11—cont'd
Abbreviations for orders, prescriptions, and labels

Abbreviation	Derivation	Meaning
o.h.	omni hora	every hour
o.m.	omni mane	every morning
o.n.	omni nocte	every night
os	os	mouth
oz.	uncia	ounce
p.c.	post cibum	after meals
per	per	through or by
pil.	pilula	pill
p.r.n.	pro re nata	when required
q.h.	quaque hora	every hour
q. 2 h.		every two hours
q. 3 h.		every three hours
q. 4 h.		every four hours
q.i.d.	quatour in die	four times a day
q.s.	quantum sufficit	as much as is required
℞	recipe	take
s	sine	without
Sig. or S.	signa	write on label
Sol.		solution
s.o.s.	si opus sit	if necessary
sp.	spiritus	spirits
ss	semis	a half
stat.	statim	immediately
syr.	syrupus	syrup
t.i.d.	ter in die	three times a day
t.i.n.	ter in nocte	three times a night
tr. or tinct.	tinctura	tincture
ung.	unguentum	ointment
vin.	vini	wine

Nursing responsibilities relative to medicines and their administration

The care of medicines

Regulations vary in different hospitals, but, regardless of the place, certain principles of organization should be observed in the care of drugs and associated equipment.

1. All medicines should be kept in a special place, which may be a cupboard, closet, or room. It should not be freely accessible to the public.

2. Narcotic drugs and those dispensed under special legal regulations must be kept in a locked box or compartment.

3. In some hospitals each patient's medicines are kept in a designated place on a shelf or compartment of the medicine cupboard or room.

Such an arrangement means that the nurse must be careful to keep the patient's medicines in the right area and to make certain that when the patient leaves the hospital his medicines are returned to the pharmacy, unless the patient is taking his medicines with him. It is imperative that the medicines have the patient's full name on the label of the container. In some hospitals the medicines are dispensed wholly or in part from a stock supply kept on the ward.

4. If stock supplies are maintained they should be arranged in an orderly manner. Preparations for internal use should be kept separate from those used externally.

5. Some preparations, e.g., sera, vaccines, certain suppositories, certain antibiotics, as well as insulin, need to be kept in the refrigerator.

6. Labels of all medicines should be clean and legible. If they are not, they should be sent to the pharmacist for relabeling. *Nurses should not label or relabel medicines.*

7. Bottles of medicines should always be stoppered.

8. The medicine closet or room should be kept clean and orderly. Misplaced medicines and equipment can contribute to errors in handling and administration.

Policies and regulations regarding the administration of medicines

Experience has demonstrated that it is wise to abide by established policies and regulations pertaining to the administration of medicines. Such regulations vary from hospital to hospital, but over-all policies are probably more alike than unalike. They have been established usually to protect patients and also to save nurses from the traumatizing effects of errors that other nurses have had the misfortune to experience. This does not mean that deviation from the rule or regulation under special circumstances is always bad judgment. The nurse must consider the situation carefully before departing from established policy. If possible she should consult with a more experienced person such as her head nurse or supervisor. Policies and regulations are protective guides to live by, not to be followed so blindly that thinking and good sense do not enter into the making of decisions. The following are policies or regulations which have been found to be sound relative to the administration of medicines.

1. When preparing or giving medicines concentrate your whole attention on what you are doing. Do not permit yourself to be distracted while working with medicines.

2. Make certain that you have a written order for every medication for which you assume the responsibility of administration. (Verbal orders should become written orders as soon as possible.)

3. Develop the habit of reading the label of the medicine three times:

Fig. 16

Read the label three times

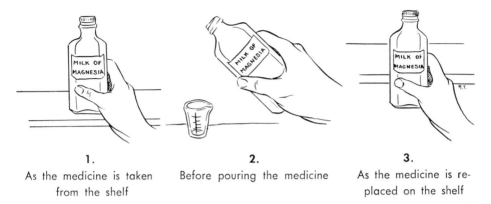

1.	2.	3.
As the medicine is taken from the shelf	Before pouring the medicine	As the medicine is re-placed on the shelf

(a) before taking the medicine from the shelf, (b) before removing the dose from the container, and (c) before returning the container to its proper place.

4. Make certain that the data on your medicine card corresponds exactly with the doctor's written order and with the label on the patient's medicine. A medicine card should accompany each medicine.

5. Never give a medicine from an unlabeled container.

6. Do not administer medicines that have been prepared by some other person.

7. If you must in some way calculate the dosage for a patient from the preparation on hand and you are uncertain of your calculation, verify your work by checking with some responsible person, e.g., the head nurse, the pharmacist, or an instructor.

8. Measure quantities as ordered, using the proper apparatus, graduated containers for milliliters, fluidounces, or fluidrams, minim glasses, or calibrated pipettes for minims and droppers for drops. When measuring liquids, hold the container so that the line indicating the desired quantity is on a level with the eye. The quantity is read when the lowest part of the concave surface of the fluid is on this line.

9. Take pains to identify your patient. Call each patient by name. If there is the least doubt of his identity, ask him to state his name. If you say to a patient, "Will you tell me your name, please?" he will more than likely respect your concern for accuracy and safety. Patients have been known to answer to names other than their own, but they are not likely to give the wrong name when asked to state their name. If the patient wears an identification band, check with the band.

10. Remain with the patient until the medicine has been taken. Most patients are very cooperative about taking medicines at the time that the

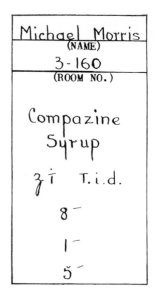

Fig. 17 Samples of medicine cards used to accompany medications. Cards should bear the following information: name and room of patient; name of medicine; dosage; time of administration; route of administration if there is any question about how it might be given; and special precautions.

nurse brings them. However, sometimes patients are more ill than they appear and have been known to hoard medicines until they had accumulated a lethal amount and then have taken the entire amount, with fatal results.

11. Never return an unused dose of medicine to a stock bottle.

12. Never chart a medicine as having been given until it has been administered.

Additional suggestions relative to the giving of medicines. The following suggestions constitute habits of thought and behavior developed by experienced professional nurses which the nursing student will also be expected to develop.

1. Dosage forms such as tablets, capsules, pills, etc. should be handled in such a way that the fingers will not come in contact with the medicine. Use the cap of the container or a clean medicine card to guide or lift the medicine into the medicine glass or container you will be taking to the bedside of the patient.

2. When pouring liquid medicines, hold the bottle so that the liquid does not run over the side and obscure the label. Wipe the rim of the bottle with a clean piece of paper tissue before replacing the stopper or cover.

3. Assist weak or helpless patients to take their medications.

4. Most liquid medicines should be diluted with water. This is espe-

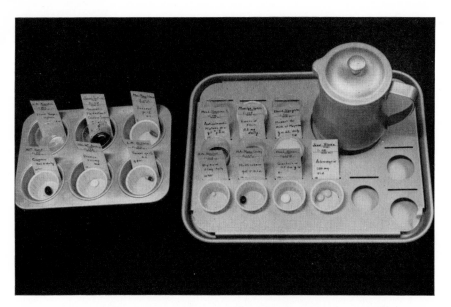

Fig. 18 Two medicine trays with cards. The small tray at the left may be used for a number of patients, as in a double room or a small ward. Soufflé cups instead of medicine glasses may be used for capsules or tablets. The large tray is arranged for the administration of medications to a group of patients.

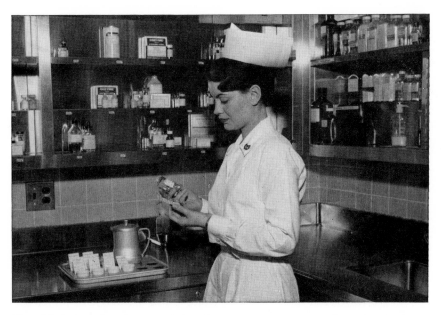

Fig. 19 It is well to have medicines kept in a separate unit where the nurse may work with a minimum of disturbance. Careful checking of labels and medicine cards helps to prevent errors.

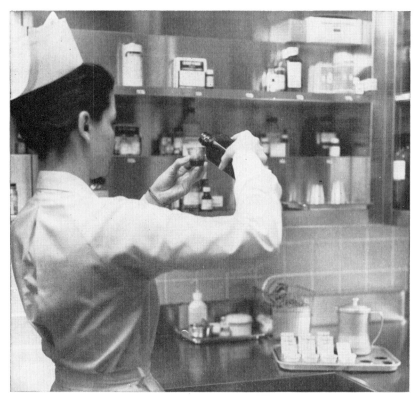

Fig. 20 When pouring liquid medicine, the thumbnail is placed at the mark on the medicine glass and the medicine is poured on a level with the eye. The bottle should be held so that the medication is not poured over the label.

cially desirable when medicines have a bad taste. Exceptions to this rule would include oils and cough medicines which are given for a local effect in the throat. The patient should be supplied with an ample amount of fresh water after swallowing solid dosage forms such as tablets or capsules, unless for some reason the patient is allowed limited fluids.

5. Medicine glasses should be thoroughly washed with hot soapy water and scalded with hot water. Glasses used for oils should be washed separately. Disposable medicine containers provide a more sanitary means of dispensing medicines than glasses and are used in many hospitals.

6. The nurse should avoid waste of medicines. Medicines tend to be expensive; in some instances a single capsule may cost the patient several dollars. Dropping a medicine on the floor is one way of wasting it.

7. If a patient expresses doubt or concern about a medication or the dosage of the medication, the nurse should do everything possible to

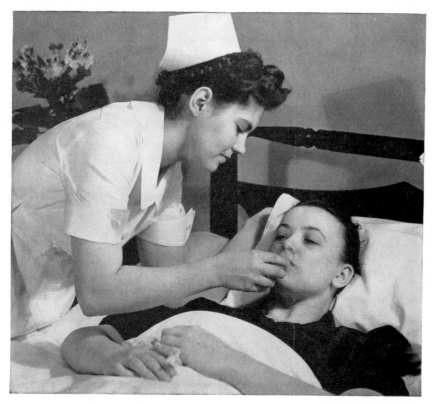

Fig. 21 Weak patients or those who are very ill should be given special assistance in taking their medications.

make certain that no mistake has occurred. Occasionally the patient may be right. The nurse should reassure the patient as well as herself by rechecking to make certain that there is no error. She may need to recheck the order, the label on the medicine container, the patient's chart, etc.

8. Do not leave a tray of medicines unattended. If you are in a patient's room and must leave, take the tray of medicines with you.

9. As a rule nurses should not prepare mixtures of drugs. They should be prepared by the pharmacy.

10. Record all medicines. The manner of recording, too, varies from hospital to hospital. Sometimes all medications are charted in one place on the patient's chart and sometimes they are charted in more than one place. The name of the drug, the dosage, the time of administration, and the channel of administration, as well as the patient's reaction to the medication (if any), should be indicated.

The nurse's approach. The reaction of a patient to the nurse who brings a medicine or to the medicine itself is sometimes an expression of the patient's feelings of fear, frustration, or hostility. The brief interval during which the nurse may be at the bedside of the patient to give him his medicine may have been preceded by many incidents that disturbed him or in some way affected him. The nurse may have no knowledge of this. After she leaves the patient there may continue to be major or minor crises with which the patient must come to grips. For example, a physician calls upon a patient to discuss the possibility of doing a serious type of surgery which he thinks will benefit the patient. The proposition leaves the patient rather shaken. He also knows that sometime during the day he must make some kind of financial arrangement for continued hospitalization. The latter has been worrying him for some time. In the midst of this morning of problems and worries the nurse walks in with a medicine he does not like anyhow and "bang," seemingly for no reason at all he flatly refuses to take it.

The understanding nurse is not content to simply chart on the nurse's notes that the patient refused his 10 o'clock medication. She will probably try to draw him out to discover what happened to make him feel like reacting this way. She may encourage him to talk about the things that are concerning him so deeply and thus make him feel that she is able to accept his reaction whatever it may be. Recognition of the patient's right to have feelings can lead to greater security for the patient and deeper insight for the nurse.

Most patients are assured by the nurse who goes about the task of giving medicines in a pleasant but businesslike manner. The patient likes to feel that here is someone who knows what she is doing and why she is doing it. To see her carefully check a medicine with the medicine card and hear her say, "This is your medicine, Mr. Smith," helps to assure Mr. Smith that there is no doubt in the nurse's mind as to whom this medicine should be given.

The medicine containers from which the patient is served his medicine should be scrupulously clean, and the water supplied immediately after the medicine should be fresh and cold. Orange slices which may accompany a medicine tray on which there are glasses of mineral oil can, by the neat way they are arranged and the deft way they are handled, help to make the whole matter of taking the oil as pleasant as possible. Carelessly prepared medicines and the lack of consideration in the way a medicine is handed to a patient can disgust him in the same way that poor food, cracked dishes, and inefficient service affect him in a restaurant.

The nurse who refers to intramuscular injections as "shots" may, in the thinking of the patient, make the whole procedure seem crude and gruesome.

When giving a medicine with an unpleasant taste it is better to admit that it is unpleasant and thereby agree with the patient than to make him feel that his perfectly normal reaction is grossly exaggerated or silly.

Administration of medicines on the psychiatric ward

The giving of medicines on a psychiatric unit automatically assumes symbolic meanings present in lesser degree on any hospital ward. All individuals need and seek meaningful interpersonal relationships; most individuals find such relationships outside medical situations. Psychiatric patients, however, are universally starved for affection and yearn for some person to whom they may look for security and interest. Frequently this emotional deprivation is concealed by an appearance of hostility or disdain.

In addition, the immediate personal needs of the patient, the current symptoms against which the patient is fighting, must be considered. Overwhelming anxiety, depression to the point of suicide, pain of an uncanny nature, or distortions of thought which constantly separate the patient from his fellows demand of the nurse much care in the handling of any contact, particularly that of the medication. To the patient in a state of psychologic disequilibrium, that which is taken by mouth or given by injection may hold threats and symbolic meanings rarely felt by the medical or surgical patient. The fear of poisons or supernatural effects of capsules or the suggestion of witchcraft inherent in a needle often reaches the degree of catastrophe unless the nurse is able to inter-relate her action and the thought processes of the patient. The psychiatric patient's tendency toward impulsiveness and his high titer of emotional sensitivity must constantly be kept in mind.

No practical suggestions can ever take the place of the technics practiced by the psychiatrically oriented nurse, but the following factors should be considered in the general handling of medications for the psychiatric patient:

1. The actual contents of the medicine cupboard in a psychiatric station should be kept at a minimum. Nurse stations and cupboards are routinely kept locked, but unforeseen difficulties may be avoided by stocking only a bare minimum of the necessary medications. On the other hand, the need of various drugs used in an emergency must be anticipated and such drugs must be made available.

2. Medicines should be given in metal or paper, not glass, containers. The psychiatric patient is often so impulsive that all possible precautions must be taken to avoid accidents, and glass is always a potential suicide weapon.

3. The giving of medications, especially on a disturbed ward, is best done on an individual basis. Walking down the corridor with a trayful of medications invites the uninhibited individual to an impulsive over-

throw of the tray and the suicidal patient to a quick ingestion of the medications.

4. *The nurse must remain with the patient until the oral medications have been swallowed.* This principle is basic in the giving of all medications but one of particular importance to the depressed and suicidal patient; such patients may secrete capsules in the mouth for long periods, only to hoard them until a lethal supply has been accumulated. Frequently measures such as the piercing of the capsule case and staying with the patient until the drug is dissolved or the practice of using liquid preparations will enforce the actual ingestion of the drug.

5. It is often necessary not only to urge the psychiatric patient to take medication but also to insist upon its acceptance. The psychiatric patient is frequently an indecisive, emotionally confused individual who tends to doubt everything. He often presses the nurse for detailed information about the drug prescribed and frequently rebels because of minor discrepancies in information. Paradoxically, however, he complies quickly if a positive yet interested attitude is presented without undue explanation.

6. It is of utmost importance to report all drug refusals to the physician in charge. But in the meantime it is frequently also of importance to persuade the patient to take the medicine. Omission of doses may cause the blood level of sedatives to be lowered so that larger doses than usual may eventually be needed.

A word should be said about placebos because of their unique psychologic implications. Occasionally on nonpsychiatric services, for purposes of temporary control or diagnosis, it may be necessary to give such medications. From a psychiatric point of view it is imperative to look behind the medication to the basic needs which are being satisfied. In all psychiatric treatment, and particularly in the handling of drugs, honesty always pays. If placebos are ordered, the nurse has no choice but to carry out the order, but she should constantly be searching in her own mind for the meaning of this medication to the patient. If placebo medication is symptomatically successful, it is by virtue of the psychologic implications inherent in the interpersonal relationships involved.

Administration of medicines to children

By the time the nursing student is given the responsibility of drug administration to her patients on the pediatric ward, she will already have had some experience in giving medications to adult patients. Many of the principles of this aspect of good nursing apply to all age groups, but to children the nurse has certain added responsibilities.

Development of cooperation on the part of the child. It is important to secure the cooperation of the child, and to do this it is highly desirable that the nurse's initial contact with the child be a favorable one, since future cooperation during his stay in the hospital is often dependent on this first experience.

Cooperation on the part of the child should at first, at least, be taken for granted. "Good morning, Johnny; I've brought your medicine for you," or "Elizabeth, here is what Dr. Smith wants you to have to make you feel better," are statements which may bring forth the desired response. Hesitancy or indication of dislike of a medicine on the part of the nurse or some older child will often provoke a similar attitude in the patient. Walter was a child who apparently enjoyed his daily dose of cod-liver oil until one day his older brother made a wry face at seeing Walter swallow the oil; ever after Walter insisted that he detested it.

Most children are courageous or like to be considered so, and appealing to their courage is sometimes effective. It often pleases a child to hold his own medicine glass, to drink unassisted, and to take his pills from the container without help from the nurse. Because of the sense of achievement which follows, he may like to save the pill cups to show his mother. Children are also intrigued by the novelty of taking liquids through a straw.

It is important to be honest with children. Each child has a right to some explanation for each procedure that concerns him. The explanation should of course be within his range of understanding. The nurse should by all means know what a medicine tastes like in order to answer such questions as, "Is it bad tasting?" A suggested reply might be: "It tastes like black cherry to me; tell me if you think it tastes like that to you." The suggestion to taste it and find out is often accepted. However, if the medicine is "bad" tasting, there is no point in denying the fact. Children never like to be deceived. If a vehicle is used to disguise the taste of a medicine, the child should, nonetheless, realize that he is receiving a medicine.

Physical force is seldom necessary, but if and when it is, it should be used with dispatch and firmness. It is important not to combine force with anger, however. Nor should force be resorted to because of one nurse's failure to administer the medicine. Careful consideration should be given to such factors as: Why does the child resist? Does he disapprove only of this one nurse? Has he been frightened by other hospital experiences which were traumatizing to him and thus he fears all approaches to him? Will forcing a medication and the accompanying struggle counteract desirable effects of the drug if the drug is some type of sedative?

The use of force, when necessary, should be explained to the child in such a way that he gets the idea that this form of treatment is necessary for his well-being. An attempt should be made to help him understand that the nurses realize that his fears may be ungrounded but that he will gradually get over them and will then be able to cooperate in this matter of taking his medicine. Cooperation of the child cannot be gained, and often his confidence in all personnel will be lost forever, if he feels that force was used as a punishment for his inability to cooperate. A child may be helped if he is permitted the security of having someone's hand to hold during the prick of a needle. And it is well to spend a few minutes with the child after an unpleasant episode, to give him support in regaining control of his feelings.

Selection of a suitable vehicle. Disagreeable-tasting medicine should be disguised if at all possible. The following are suggestions which may prove helpful:

1. Avoid the use of essential foods such as milk, cereal, orange juice, etc., as the child may be conditioned against the future acceptance of the food in his diet.

2. Never underestimate the reaction of a child; he may require no addition to his medicine other than water.

3. A sip of fruit juice or a peppermint before and after administration may dull the unpleasant taste of a medicine.

4. Avoid using syrups with unpalatable fluids because sweet syrups tend to prolong the taste of the medicine.

5. Sticky vehicles such as honey and syrup are ideal for suspending drugs that do not dissolve in water.

6. Sugarless vehicles should be used as disguises for medications given to diabetic children or those on a ketogenic diet. They may have aromatic waters (peppermint, wintergreen, spearmint, etc.).

7. Children tend to take syrup flavoring agents well and to show preference for certain ones, such as syrup of lime, syrup of peppermint, syrup of anise, or mint cooler syrup. Chocolate syrup is also a favorite.

8. Fruit syrups are usually acid in reaction and should not be used for medicines that react in an acid medium (soda bicarbonate, soluble barbiturates, and salicylates).

Channels of administration. Medication may be administered orally, rectally, intravenously, subcutaneously, and intramuscularly.

Oral. The foregoing discussion relates principally to precautions and technics important in the oral administration of drugs. In addition it must be remembered that the oral method is probably the easiest way to give a medication to a child because it is the easiest understood and accepted by the child and results in the least amount of unpleasant recollection. When medicines are given to infants they should be given from a spoon or with a plastic medicine dropper rather than in milk or water from their bottle. It is important to give the medicine slowly to avoid choking.

Pills and tablets should be crushed and powders suspended in a heavy syrup, in applesauce, or fruit purée when given to infants, young children, or children whose condition does not favor their swallowing the medicine in its original form. Many drugs are now available in the form of syrups or elixirs which are palatable and well suited for administration to children.

Rectal. When oral administration is difficult or contraindicated, the rectal route is often advised. The rectum of the child, as well as the adult, will absorb the drug best when it is empty. The medication may be dissolved or suspended in approximately 8 ml. of tap water (100° F. but not over) and followed by about half this amount of clear tap water of the same temperature. Following the procedure the buttocks should be taped together to relieve pressure on the rectal sphincter and thereby help to ensure retention and absorption of the medicine. The procedure should be performed with the smallest catheter possible, depending on the size of the child, but at no time should an enema tip be used. The fluid should be introduced slowly, preferably by gravity. A number of drugs are available for rectal administration in suppository form.

Intravenous. Older children may be given fluids or drugs intravenously in the same way as that used for adults. The younger and smaller the child, the greater the difficulty of administration and the greater the danger associated with it. Injection into a scalp vein may be quite satisfactory, or surgical dissection of a vein may be done to make the vein accessible.

Subcutaneous. Hypodermic injections are preferably made into the buttock of a small child rather than into an extremity. Restraint is likely to be necessary, and help should be secured when the drug is given this way. Never fill the syringe or prepare it in front of the child.

Intramuscular. Intramuscular injections are best given into the buttock. Swift skillful insertion of the needle helps to lessen the anxiety felt about subsequent injections. If the thigh must be used, injections should be made into the lateral side.

Children must be observed carefully for reactions to drugs; they do not understand that changes in their feelings are associated with the action of the medication and therefore do not comprehend the need to report these changes.

Children often react more rapidly and more violently to drugs than do adults. Toxic symptoms or symptoms of idiosyncrasy may appear suddenly. Drugs which children are frequently able to tolerate in disproportionately large amounts include cathartics, atropine, arsenic, vaccines, sera (even when given in almost adult dosage), and bromides. Drugs to which children are sensitive include the opiates, especially morphine, and the hypnotics.

Questions

for study and review

1 How would you attempt to secure the co-operation of a patient who tells you to leave his medication on the bedside table and he will take it later in the day?

2 What are some of the habits that you think would help you to develop safety and accuracy in the administration of drugs?

3 Make a list of precautions which should be observed in a home to prevent accidents in the care and handling of medicines.

4 Write out a plan of instruction for one of your patients who expects to go home and will continue to take several of the medicines which he has been taking while in the hospital. What explanation does the patient need, to help him understand what to do, how to do it, and when to do it?

5 How would you interpret the following orders?

Sherry Wine ℥ ii t.i.d. a.c.
Nitroglycerin gr. 1/100 stat. and p.r.n.
Mineral Oil and Milk of Magnesia ℥ ss āā b.i.d. and p.r.n.
Phenobarbital gr. ss q.i.d.

6 Mrs. Jones received a prescription from her physician for some "sleeping pills." When she attempted to have the prescription refilled at the end of a month the pharmacist told her that he was unable to refill it. Mrs. Jones was disturbed and angry with the pharmacist. What explanation and suggestion could you make which would probably be helpful?

7 Select the answer which in your opinion is the one best answer.

A. If a drug is injected into the cavity of a joint where its effect is limited to the tissue of the joint, its action is said to be:
   a. general   c. systemic
   b. local   d. selective

B. Drugs administered by which of the following channels are likely to be the least costly?
   a. orally   c. subcutaneously
   b. intravenously d. intraspinally

C. Which of the following channels of administration is likely to afford least dependable absorption?
   a. oral   c. intravenous
   b. intraspinal   d. rectal

D. Which of the following must be characteristic of a drug if it is to be administered by inhalation?
   a. volatile   c. nontoxic
   b. sterile   d. water soluble

E. Irritating drugs given for rapid effect are usually given:
   a. orally   c. intravenously
   b. subcutaneously d. by inhalation

F. Which of the following channels of administration is the nurse likely to use most often?
   a. intravenous   c. subcutaneous
   b. intramuscular   d. intradermal

G. If when you bring a patient her medicine she says to you, "Oh, I have already had one of those red tablets this morning," which of the following statements is likely to be most reassuring to the patient?
   a. "Well, maybe you are right. I will have to check with the other nurses."
   b. "Oh no, you must be mistaken. I have checked and double-checked these medicines this morning."
   c. "I believe that this is a different medicine than what you received earlier but I will recheck so that we will both feel certain."
   d. "Lots of medicines are red, Mrs. Smith. I am sure that this is right for you."

H. A 3-year-old child is to receive 5 ml. of an antibiotic syrup. In which of the following measures would you choose to give it?
   a. a calibrated   c. a medicine glass
      medicine drop-   d. a minim glass
      per
   b. a teaspoon

I. If a patient tells you that he can swallow liquids but insists that he cannot swallow tablets and capsules and the physician has ordered a dose of sedative that comes in capsule form, which of the following is probably the simplest way of solving the difficulty?
   a. Explain to the patient that he can swallow the capsules if he will drink adequate fluid at the same time.
   b. Ask the doctor for an order to give the drug parenterally.
   c. Dissolve the drug and give it rectally.
   d. Ask the pharmacy to send the drug in a liquid flavored form.

124

J. If one of your patients is a 3-year-old child for whom 3 gr. of aspirin has been ordered and the stock supply of aspirin is in 5 gr. tablets, which of the following would you consider the best solution?

   a. Cut the 5 gr. tablet in two and give the child one half tablet.

   b. Dissolve a 5 gr. tablet in 50 ml. of water and give 30 ml.

   c. Try to get 1 gr. tablets from the pharmacy and give three tablets.

References

Beckman, H.: Drugs, Their Nature, Action and Use, Philadelphia, 1958, W. B. Saunders Co.

Byrne, A. K.: Errors in Making Medications, Am. J. Nursing 53: 829, 1953.

Cadmus, R. R.: Medication Cost Study, Mod. Hosp. 75: 68, Sept., 1950.

Capps, R. B.: A Syringe-Transmitted Epidemic of Infectious Hepatitis, J. A. M. A. 136: 819, 1948.

Clatsworthy, H. W., and Stewart, M.: Intravenous Therapy for Infants and Children, Am. J. Nursing 57: 630, 1957.

Jeans, P. C., Wright, F. H., and Blake, F. G.: Essentials of Pediatrics, Philadelphia, 1958, J. B. Lippincott Co.

Lowe, C. A.: Principles of Parenteral Fluid Therapy, Am. J. Nursing 53: 963, 1953.

Shallowhorn, G.: Intramuscular Injections, Am. J. Nursing 54: 438, 1954.

Sollmann, T.: A Manual of Pharmacology and Its Application to Therapeutics and Toxicology, Philadelphia, 1957, W. B. Saunders Co.

Stephan, P. J.: Nebulization Under Intermittent Positive Pressure, Am. J. Nursing 57: 1159, 1957.

Thompson, N.: Nurses and Venipuncture, Nursing Outlook 3: 392, 1955.

Wessler, S., and Rogers, W. R.: Intermittent Intravenous Therapy, New England J. Med. 255: 22, 1956.

Whiting, J. F.: Patient's Needs, Nurses Needs, and the Healing Process, Am. J. Nursing 59: 661, 1959.

Chapter 7

Action of drugs,
sites of action, and factors
that modify the action of drugs

Empiric versus rational medicine

Early medicines could be described frequently as empiric remedies; that is, experience with them revealed that they were sometimes useful but that very little was actually known about the basis of their helpful effects. Lack of knowledge and understanding sometimes resulted in the use of weird combinations and mixtures of drugs in the hope that an effective one would somehow be included in the mixture. This type of remedy has been replaced by drugs whose effects are often highly predictable and whose action in the body has to a great extent been substantiated by scientific research.

Quinine was at one time used empirically in the form of infusion of Peruvian bark. Natives knew that this preparation would relieve some cases of chills and fever, but knowing nothing of chemistry they had no understanding of the therapeutically active ingredient in the infusion, and knowing little of the etiologic classification of fevers, they could not know why some persons were benefited and others were not. Since that time, quinine has been isolated from Peruvian bark, or the bark of the Cinchona tree, and its effectiveness against the asexual forms of the malarial parasite has been demonstrated. When a physician prescribes for a malarial patient today, he is able to predict with reasonable accuracy just what the drug will do for his patient. Treatment of patients ill with malaria has progressed from the era of empiricism to that of rational medicine. This implies that much has been learned about the disease as well as about drugs used in treatments, since rational therapy depends on both.

On the other hand, while much has been learned about drugs and how they behave in the body, there is still much that is unknown. Not enough is known either about cells or about drugs to know whether drugs introduce new functions in cells or alter old ones.

Present-day knowledge about the chemical structure of drugs enables the scientist to predict to some extent what a drug will do and in certain instances what the results will be. It has been found, for example, that drugs containing a certain molecular structure are prone to produce allergic reactions in patients; hence any new drug having this general type of molecular structure may have a tendency to produce hypersensitivity in some patients. It must be admitted, however, that scientists still do not have any general theoretic picture which allows them to predict what chemical groupings will have specific desired physiologic effects.

Chemists, pharmacologists, and other scientific workers are attempting to discover the biochemical and physical changes that drugs exert upon the molecular structures of cells. The advances made in knowledge regarding the chemistry of proteins, the nature and behavior of enzymes, and the metabolism of microbes have contributed greatly to our understanding of the responses that living systems make to drugs. The electron microscope has also contributed immeasurably to scientific advancement.

Sites of drug action

There is reason to believe that the effect of a drug may be induced on the surface of cells, within the structure of the cell, or in the extracellular fluid of the body. In most cases the *exact* site of action in the cell is unknown. Under some conditions the organ in which a drug acts may be distant from the tissue that ultimately responds; e.g., nikethamide stimulates the respiratory center of the brain, but it is the muscles of respiration that bring about increased respiratory movements.

Local action. Drugs may act at the site of application on the skin or mucous membrane, e.g., the effect produced by the application of an antiseptic to a small abrasion or the application of cold cream to the skin of the face. Drugs act locally to produce antiseptic, astringent, soothing, counterirritant, irritant, or neutralizing effects, depending upon the preparation and the purpose for which it is used. Drugs that act within the gastrointestinal tract but are not absorbed are considered to have a local action; e.g., neomycin sulfate is used to suppress the bacteria in the colon prior to surgery on that organ because the drug is poorly absorbed after oral administration and exerts mainly a local action in the bowel.

Systemic action. Systemic action is the action of a drug after it is absorbed. Absorption usually means absorption into the blood stream and distribution to all parts of the body by means of the blood stream. A hypodermic dose of morphine may be injected into the tissues of the arm, but the systemic effect of the drug is obtained only after it is absorbed and carried to those tissues capable of responding to the drug —in this instance, chiefly the cells of the brain.

The following terms are used to describe systemic action or effects of drugs.

stimulation the action whereby the activity of cells is increased. For example, caffeine increases the activity of cells in the central nervous system. Caffeine is therefore called a stimulant. It is of significance that prolonged overstimulation of cells can result in depression.

depression the action of a drug that results in decreased power of the cells to function. A drug that decreases the ability of the respiratory center to send out nerve impulses to the muscles of respiration would be called a respiratory depressant.

irritation the action that produces slight temporary damage to tissues. Castor oil irritates the mucosa of the intestine and therefore is said to act as a chemical irritant. Mild irritation usually results in increased activity of cells, whereas prolonged irritation produces depression of cellular activity. Marked irritation can produce inflammation and death of tissue.

selective action the action of a drug that is usually greater on some tissues than on others. Morphine acts on the respiratory center of the brain, even if given in very small doses. Posterior pituitary hormone has a highly selective action on the function of tubular cells of the kidney. Selective action is probably explained on the basis that certain cells contain some chemical substance or molecular structure for which the drug has a marked affinity.

physiologic action the action of a drug on normal healthy tissues.

therapeutic action the action of a drug in diseased tissues or in the sick individual. The effect of a drug in a well person and in the sick individual may be very different. Thyroid extract may relieve distressing symptoms of hypothyroidism in the patient with myxedema, but the same drug in a normal person may precipitate a severe toxic reaction.

side effect (side action) any effect of a drug other than the one for which it is administered. The therapeutic effect of a drug given for one condition may become a side effect when given for a different purpose. Morphine sulfate is often given to relieve pain, not for its ability to constrict the pupil of the eye. The latter would be called a side effect.

untoward effect (untoward action) a side effect regarded as harmful to the patient. The effect of morphine which results in nausea and vomiting, constipation, and habit formation is usually undesirable and harmful. They are then untoward effects. Side effects are frequently spoken of in such a manner as to include untoward effects.

cumulation the action or effect which may be produced when drugs are excreted or destroyed more slowly than they are absorbed and thereby accumulate in the body. Unless dosage is adjusted, a sufficiently high concentration can be reached to produce toxic effects. Inconsistant absorption and irregularity of excretion may at times be responsible for the "stock-piling" effect.

synergism, potentiation, and additive effects imply that drugs may work together but in different ways. The exact words are not as important as the concepts. Certain drugs which produce the same general kind of effect when given together may produce an exaggerated effect out of proportion to the amount of each drug given. Such drugs are said to be synergistic.

128

When two drugs are given together and one intensifies the action of the other by the same mechanism of action or a different one, the one drug is said to potentiate the other. For example, when epinephrine is given with the local anesthetic procaine, it intensifies the effect of the procaine not because of its anesthetizing action but because it produces vasoconstriction and holds the procaine in the area where its action is desired.

When two or more drugs are given together and their effects represent the action of one plus the action of the other (others), their effects are said to be additive. An additive effect is the effect obtained when, for example, one-half a dose of one drug plus one-half a dose of a similarly acting drug will produce the effect of a full dose of either drug alone. The term *potentiation* has come to be used more or less synonymously with synergism, although some authorities reserve it for the situation in which one drug exerts no appreciable effect on cells but exaggerates the response made by these cells to some other drug. Promethazine (Phenergan) potentiates the depressant effects of narcotics, i.e., it intensifies their effects so that the dose of morphine and related depressants can be reduced by one fourth to one half when given with promethazine.

antagonism drugs that have an opposite effect in the body are said to be pharmacologically antagonistic. They may be valuable in counteracting one another in the case of poisoning; e.g., a central nervous system stimulant, such as picrotoxin, can be used to counteract the effects of a central nervous system depressant, such as one of the barbiturates. There are various ways by which antagonistic reactions take place in the body, some of which are complicated and not well understood.

idiosyncrasy any abnormal or peculiar response to a drug. It may manifest itself by (1) overresponse or abnormal susceptibility, (2) underresponse, showing abnormal tolerance, (3) a qualitatively different effect than the usual one, such as excitement or delirium instead of relaxation and sleep after a dose of morphine, and (4) unexpected symptoms which are unexplainable. This bears out the idea that patients can be expected to react to drugs differently even though they may be treated for the same disorder.

hypersensitivity an allergic response to a drug (sometimes confused with idiosyncrasy but not the same). This means that at some time the patient has become sensitized, and thereafter a minute dose of the drug can produce an allergic reaction which may vary from a slight reaction to a very severe one. This is one of the real problems encountered in drug therapy. Many times the patient is merely uncomfortable with hives, itching, and a skin rash; at other times acute anaphylaxis and death result.

tolerance an acquired reaction to a drug that necessitates an excessive increase of dosage to maintain a given therapeutic effect. Drugs to which tolerance is readily developed are nitrites, opiates, and alcohol. Exposure to certain drugs is likely to result in tolerance to chemically related drugs having a similar action. This is known as *cross tolerance*. Patients who are chronic heavy users of ethyl alcohol have a tolerance to certain anesthetics such as ether, requiring more ether for anesthesia than the usual nonalcoholic patient.

habituation a psychic craving for a drug when it is withheld. If the psychic influence is strong, individuals may become habituated to almost anything; e.g., if a patient believes that a little white tablet makes it possible for him to sleep at night he probably will not sleep until he has swallowed it. It makes no difference that the tablet is made of sugar if the patient is habituated to white tablets.

addiction a condition that develops after continued administration of certain drugs. It is characterized by altered physiologic processes and psychic craving when the drug is withheld. Tolerance is also manifest in true addiction. Somehow the drug has become essential to the maintenance of ordinary cellular activities. Morphine is a well-known example of a drug to which persons may become addicted and may then suffer a variety of withdrawal symptoms when the drug is denied them.

How drugs act

The above terms are commonly used to describe the action of drugs or the effects produced by their action. It is another matter to think about the mechanism of action in terms of molecular biology. If one were to use an example of a well-known drug such as aspirin, one would probably find that many persons have some idea of how this remedy acts. It is well known that it relieves pain and lowers the temperature in case of fever. When asked how does aspirin do this, some persons could probably explain its action in terms of depression of the brain and the heat-regulating center. But this still would not describe how this drug accomplishes this effect. A neurophysiologist might throw further light on the subject by saying that aspirin raises the threshold of excitability of certain nerve tracts or nuclei in the hypothalamus. This would add to our information about the drug and the site of its action but would not tell us what the drug does to bring about the characteristic response. These explanations are something like peeling an onion, since there is no core but always a deeper layer. The most complete answer now visualized would probably reveal a series of chemical reactions between aspirin and some particular chemical part or parts of specific nerve cells, reactions of which govern the physiologic activity of heat regulation by the brain.

There are a number of ways by which drugs are known to act or bring about cellular responses. Some types of action seem relatively simple and easy to understand and some are exceedingly complex. Many are unknown. Fundamentally the reaction of all drugs is chemical, but the nature of the chemical action is extremely variable. The chemical action may be relatively simple, e.g., the neutralization of gastric acid with sodium bicarbonate. Other chemical reactions are much less easily understood. There is a growing belief that drugs induce effects in cells because of particular features of their molecular structure which have an attraction for particular "receptor" groups in or on the surface of cells. What these receptor groups are or how they regulate the activity of the cell is not known; they are believed to exist in order to explain the marked molecular specificity of most drugs. One of the basic areas of pharmacology in which great progress can be anticipated is this area, in which answers are sought to questions about the chemical nature and the functions of these mysterious drug receptors. A generation ago it was believed that all drug receptors were enzymes, i.e., that specific enzymes were the "targets" of specific drugs. Today many pharmacologists believe that some more subtle and less well-understood class of cell substances than the enzymes are involved, perhaps the specific substance or substances that regulate the permeability of the cell membrane, about which very little is yet known in detail.[*]

*Adams, Elijah: Personal communication.

It is recognized that characteristic actions of drugs are related to their chemical structure. This understanding has resulted in the synthesis of many valuable compounds. However, it is also true that slight variations in structure may alter greatly the effects of two otherwise similar compounds, and sometimes drugs which differ greatly in chemical structure may produce highly similar effects. It is clear that full understanding regarding these features about structural specificity of drugs will not be known until more is known about the receptors on which they act.

Other drugs may act by interfering chemically with the way in which the cell utilizes some essential substance. This is referred to as competitive inhibition. The sulfonamides as a group of drugs are thought to exert an antibacterial action by competing with para-aminobenzoic acid, a substance which they structurally resemble, for the essential enzyme systems of the bacterial cell. Since para-aminobenzoic acid is essential to the metabolism of many bacteria and since the sulfonamides deprive the bacterial cells of this substance which they need, their growth is inhibited. The following formulas show the similarity of structure mentioned.

$$COOH \qquad\qquad SO_2 - NH_2$$

$$NH_2 \qquad\qquad\qquad NH_2$$

Para-aminobenzoic acid   Sulfanilamide

The studies of Woods further revealed that the action of the sulfonamides can be slowed by making available to the bacteria additional amounts of para-aminobenzoic acid.

In noncompetitive inhibition the drug is believed to inhibit an enzyme directly rather than by competing with something essential to the cell. For example, disulfiram (Antabuse) is a drug that increases the toxicity of ethyl alcohol by inhibiting the enzyme which helps promote the oxidation of acetaldehyde, an intermediate product in the metabolism of alcohol. Failure to oxidize acetaldehyde permits this toxic substance to accumulate and thereby causes the individual to become ill.

Other types of chemically explainable action may be through osmotic effects, e.g., the action of a nonabsorbable saline cathartic in the intestinal tract. Water then remains within the intestinal tract to increase the volume of the bowel contents even though there may be no direct effect on the intestinal cells.

The restoration of normal physiologic function by the replacement of essential biologic substances is another way by which drugs act, e.g., the use of adrenocortical hormone in the treatment of patients with Addison's disease or the effect of thyroid extract in patients with hypothyroidism. It must be pointed out in this case, however, that no explanation of the action of the drug is being given. Recognition is simply made that the drug replaces a natural constituent of the body which is lacking.

Factors that influence or modify the actions of drugs

The dose of the drug. Posology is the study of dosage, and a dose is defined as that amount of drug which is given for a therapeutic effect. Under some conditions and within limits, the larger the dose the greater the response. Since it is conceived that drugs probably combine with receptor groups in or on the surface of cells, the degree of response depends in part on the extent as well as on the effectiveness of the combinations. A number of terms are applied to the amount of drug in a dose:

minimal dose the smallest amount of drug that will produce a therapeutic effect.
maximal dose the largest amount of drug that will produce a desired effect without accompanying symptoms of toxicity.
toxic dose the amount of drug that will produce untoward effects or symptoms of poisoning.
lethal dose the amount of drug that will cause death.

The responsibility of prescribing the dosage of drugs rests with the physician, but the nurse shares a responsibility in relation to dosage. She may not alter a prescribed dose, but if an error seems to have been made, she is responsible for seeing that the order is verified or corrected. If she has had the opportunity to become informed about dosage she shares a responsibility to see that error is avoided. This is a way in which she can cooperate intelligently with the physician.

A number of factors may be taken under consideration when dosage is prescribed. It helps the nurse to understand deviations from the usual or average when she knows some of the factors that the physician has in mind when he orders a certain dose for a certain patient.

Age. It is generally recognized that for certain drugs there is a relationship between the effect produced and the age of the individual. Children, as a rule, are more sensitive to some drugs than are adults. Young children are particularly susceptible to central nervous system depressants. Aged individuals may respond to drugs differently than younger adults. This may be due in part to changes in their blood vessels, which cause functional deterioration of their organs. Altered response to the usual dosage of drugs may also be due to change in weight. Modification of dosage must be made on an individual basis.

Weight. The nurse will observe that dosage is frequently determined on the basis of a certain amount of drug per kilogram of body weight.

This is particularly desirable when a definite concentration of drug in the blood is desired. In general, small individuals require lesser amounts of drug than large individuals. However, large numbers of drugs are administered to adults, with little or no consideration of the weight of the individual. Both age and weight probably affect the response made to drugs, but usually no general rule is followed to modify dosage for adults.

Sex. For the female, consideration is given to dosage of drugs that may be harmful to the fetus in utero or to the infant of a nursing mother. Some authorities are of the opinion that women respond sufficiently differently than men to some drugs that dosage should be modified; others believe that such differences are negligible and unimportant.

The condition of the patient. The presence of pathology (disease) and the severity of symptoms may call for an adjustment of dosage. Larger doses than usual of morphine may be required to control severe pain. Larger doses than usual of insulin may be required by the diabetic patient whose condition is complicated by fever or infection. Psychiatric patients who are disturbed and hyperactive may need large amounts of sedatives. Patients with hyperthyroidism may not tolerate well even small doses of epinephrine or central nervous system stimulants.

Temperament. Nervous, unstable, and easily excited individuals seem to require smaller amounts of stimulants and larger amounts of depressants than so-called average individuals. Phlegmatic persons may require larger amounts of stimulants and smaller doses of depressants.

Route of administration. The dose of a drug depends in part on the channel of administration. This is due to the rate at which it enters the circulation, and dosage must sometimes be adjusted to take this factor into account. The intravenous dose is often smaller than the subcutaneous dose, and the subcutaneous dose in turn may be smaller than the oral dose. No hard and fast rule is followed. Dosage for rectal administration may not be larger necessarily than the oral dose of the same drug, provided the rectum is empty and the circulation is normal. Appreciably more penicillin G must be given by mouth than is given by intramuscular injection because the drug is subject to a certain amount of destruction in the digestive tube. Digitoxin, on the other hand, is given in the same quantity whether orally or intravenously because it is quickly and almost (if not entirely) absorbed from the intestine. In this instance a given dose produces the same effect regardless of whether it is given by mouth or by injection.

Time of administration. The time of administration refers particularly to oral administration of drugs in relation to meals. Absorption is delayed by the presence of food in the stomach and intestine and proceeds more rapidly when these organs are comparatively empty, thus modifying the dose necessary to produce a given therapeutic effect. It can be readily noted that the amount of drug needed to relieve the discomfort of a headache needs to be greater if the medication is taken after a full meal than before the meal, when the stomach is empty. Large doses of irritating drugs, however, are more easily tolerated if there is food in the stomach.

Absorption and excretion. Drugs are often administered every three or four hours during the day. By the end of that time most drugs have begun to be excreted and the blood level begins to fall. If the drug is excreted slowly, the dosage may need to be decreased or administered less frequently or both.

Relative safety of the drug. Individual drugs show great variability in their safety; e.g., true toxic reactions to penicillin (not allergic reactions) are rare and millions of units have been given in treatment of severe infections without untoward effects. As a result the dosage of penicillin tends to be generous when the infection seems to warrant large dosage. When streptomycin (another antibiotic) is given, however, the dosage tends to be conservative because of the higher incidence of toxicity associated with large doses of this antibiotic.

Absorption. The amount of absorption and the rapidity of effect will depend on how drugs are administered, the total amount of the drug, the condition of the absorptive surface, the solubility of the drug in water and tissue fluids, and the adequacy of the circulation of the blood. Obviously the drugs that can be injected will be absorbed more rapidly than the ones that must be given orally. An extensive surface from which the drug is absorbed will permit faster absorption than a smaller surface. Volatile anesthetics act rapidly because of the extensive pulmonary epithelium from which they are absorbed during anesthesia. Patients in shock may not respond to drugs even when the drug is injected, if the circulation is sluggish. Absorption tends to be rapid where the supply of blood and lymph capillaries is large.

Distribution. The extent to which a drug is spread through the tissues and fluids of the body varies greatly from drug to drug. Some are evenly distributed and can be found in all cells of the body, e.g., ethyl alcohol. Others are found only in the extracellular fluids or chiefly in the cells of certain organs or tissues. Iodine is found principally in the cells of the thyroid gland. Some antibiotics pass from the blood stream and are found in therapeutic amounts in the cerebrospinal fluid or in the intrapleural and peritoneal fluids, and other antibiotics diffuse poorly into these spaces. When drugs are excreted from the body they tend to concentrate in the organs of excretion.

Fate of drugs. Drugs may be chemically inactivated (detoxified) or excreted from the body unchanged. Detoxication may be accomplished by hydrolysis, oxidation, reduction, or conjugation (some of the various chemical processes which alter the chemical structure of the drug). The products of detoxication are not always less potent or less toxic than the original substance; sometimes they are more toxic. For this reason the term "drug detoxication" can perhaps be better replaced by "drug metabolism" to indicate the mechanical reactions by which drugs are altered in the body. Ethyl alcohol is oxidized in the liver to acetaldehyde, and if this is not itself rapidly consumed, serious toxic symptoms can result from the ingestion of alcohol. Since the liver is often the chief organ of detoxication, hepatic damage may slow drug metabolism to such an extent that the effect of the drug is unduly prolonged.

The extent to which a drug is converted to a pharmacologically inactive substance and the time required for this process are very significant in drug therapy. Drugs that are changed or excreted slowly exert a prolonged effect, whereas those that are eliminated rapidly may not stay in the tissues long enough to produce more than a transitory effect.

Elimination of drugs from the body either in an active or inactive form occurs by way of all the usual channels of excretion. The kidney is an important organ of excretion. Urine, bile, sweat, saliva, milk, tears, and expired air have been found to contain drugs or the degradation products of drugs. Some are excreted directly into the intestine.

Questions
for study and review

1 What term could be used to describe the use of infusion of Peruvian bark in the early treatment of patients who suffered from a fever?

2 How does the systemic action of drugs differ from the local action?

3 What are some of the reasons why knowledge of the chemical structure of drugs has become important?

4 What are some of the ways drugs are known to bring about effects, and what are some of the theories about how drugs act?

5 What terms could be used to describe the following effects? Fill in the blanks with the appropriate term.

A. A general anesthetic brings about decreased activity in many of the cells of the brain. This action would be called _____

B. Epinephrine brings about increased activity in the muscle cells of the heart. Epinephrine might be called a myocardial _____

C. Thyroid extract when given to a patient with a certain disorder of the thyroid gland relieves the patient's symptoms. _____

D. When administered to a normal person having no need for it, thyroid extract can cause nervousness, irritability, and rapid pulse. _____

E. Certain cathartics produce a slight damage to the intestinal mucosa, resulting in an increase of peristalsis. This action is known as _____

F. When morphine is given to a patient following surgery it is likely to be given to prevent or relieve pain, but it is also likely to produce some constriction of the pupil, and in certain individuals it may cause restlessness and excitement.

a. The action of morphine which results in the relief of pain is known as _____

b. The production of restlessness and excitement would be called _____

c. The action resulting in constriction of the pupil is _____

d. The capacity of certain cells to react to morphine while other cells do not react to it is known as

_____

e. If promethazine hydrochloride is administered with morphine to prolong and intensify the effect of the morphine, the resulting effect could be said to be _____

f. Atropine brings about decreased activity of certain muscle and gland cells, whereas eserine brings about increased activity of these same cells.

_____

g. Mrs. Smith took cathartics for a long time. She found it necessary to increase the dosage from time to time to secure a satisfactory effect. This is known as _____

h. A patient tells you that she gets a skin rash, breaks out with hives, and has considerable itching every time she takes a dose of aspirin.

_____

i. A patient has taken a drug for chronic pain over a long period of time. Now he becomes "upset," restless, perspires, and exhibits a number of symptoms when he does not get his hypodermic as usual. This is likely to mean that _____

G. Name four factors that could influence the action of drugs in the body. Can you think of other factors that could also effect drug action?

References

Beckman, H.: Drugs, Their Nature and Use, Philadelphia, 1958, W. B. Saunders Co.

Bovert, D.: Isoterism and Competitive Phenomena in Drugs, Science **129**: 1255, 1959.

Drill, V. A. (editor): Pharmacology in Medicine, ed. 2, New York, 1958, Blakiston Division, McGraw-Hill Book Co., Inc.

Goodman, L., and Gilman, A.: The Pharmacological Basis of Therapeutics, New York, 1955, The Macmillan Co.

Kleiner, I. S., and Orten, J. M.: Human Biochemistry, St. Louis, 1958, The C. V. Mosby Co.

Modell, W. (editor): Drugs of Choice, St. Louis, 1960, The C. V. Mosby Co.

Woods, D. D.: Relations of p-Aminobenzoic acid to Mechanism of Action of Sulphanilamide, Brit. J. Exper. Path. **31**: 74. 1940.

Chapter 8

Anti-infectives—antibiotics

An antibiotic is a chemical substance, produced by microorganisms, which prevents the growth of or destroys other microorganisms. Antibiosis, a condition in which one microorganism injures or is antagonistic to another microorganism, has been known since the days of Pasteur. Antagonism occurs between many living organisms—plants, animals, and bacteria—and in nature this force keeps a state of relative equilibrium between species. Man ordinarily lives in equilibrium with normal intestinal microorganisms, but when the typhoid bacillus enters and causes disease, man fights the disease by antibodies, fever, etc. Few pathogens survive in the soil because nonpathogens in the soil are antagonistic to them. For this reason soil microorganisms have been an excellent source of antibiotics useful to man.

In 1928 Alexander Fleming observed that a mold contaminating a culture of *Staphylococcus aureus* inhibited the growth of the bacteria. He extracted the substance produced by the mold (genus, Penicillium) and called it penicillin. Florey, Chain, and their group at Oxford became interested in the chemistry of penicillin and in 1940 isolated small amounts of impure penicillin. They used penicillin in man and achieved striking results, although these were only temporary because their supply soon became exhausted. In 1941, under the stimulus of wartime need, manufacture of penicillin was started in the United States. The work in the United States was largely a search for improved methods of growing the mold, for strains of the mold which would produce the highest yield of penicillin, and for methods of purifying penicillin. Since the discovery of penicillin, many new antibiotics have come into use. Hope and enthusiasm are aroused whenever a new one is discovered.

How do antibiotics act?

The ability of antibiotics to inhibit or kill microorganisms without seriously damaging human cells depends upon the interference with metabolic functions essential to the microorganism and not present in man. For example, an antibiotic may interfere with a particular enzyme system necessary for the nutrition of a microorganism. Antibiotics are bacteriostatic or bactericidal, depending on the concentration and the nature of the antibiotic. In using an antibiotic as a bacteriostatic agent, the normal body defenses, such as the white blood cells and the immune bodies, are depended upon to kill the inhibited microorganism. It is believed that when an antibiotic is used as a bactericide little immunologic resistance will be built up to succeeding infections.

Current status of antibiotics

The penicillins, streptomycin, the tetracyclines, and erythromycin are among the most effective and the most widely used of the antibiotics at the present time. Certain infections can be effectively treated with the use of only one of the antibiotics. In other infections any one of several agents may be effective. When a choice can be made, ease of administration, toxicity, and cost of the drug must be considered.

The initial and maintenance doses must be adequate to bring about recovery from illness as soon as possible and to discourage the development of drug resistance by the microorganism. Excessive dosage, however, increases the likelihood of toxic reactions and adds to the patient's expense.

Resistance is the ability of a microorganism to withstand an antibiotic. Some microorganisms have never been susceptible to the action of a particular antibiotic, whereas others which were once susceptible have become resistant. Resistance appears either because resistant strains (not at first very apparent) may flourish when susceptible strains are killed or because resistant mutants occur. Much scientific work has demonstrated that usually the drug does not produce resistant mutants but that the mutations occur at random and that the resistant mutants are selectively favored by the presence of the drug and hence tend to overgrow the susceptible strain. The introduction of antibiotics and the clinical problems of drug-resistant mutations in microbes is one of many examples of the increasing importance in medicine of the science of genetics.

There are factors within antibiotics and within microorganisms related to resistance which are not well understood. Staphylococci are adept at developing resistance to many antibiotics and their increased resistance to a growing number of antibiotics is one of the most serious problems to be solved in the field of hospital infections.

Superinfections may occur when the normal flora of the body, which prevents other microorganisms from getting a foothold, is disturbed. Microorganisms not ordinarily pathogenic may then cause disease. For example, *Candida albicans* has caused monilial vaginitis when antibiotics killed the bacteria normally found in the vagina. Staphylococcic enteritis (pseudomembranous enterocolitis) has occurred when the intestinal flora has been disturbed. When superinfection develops, the use of the antibiotic is usually stopped or another antibiotic is used to destroy the microorganisms causing the superinfection.

A combination of two antibiotics may be *synergistic* (helpful to each other), *antagonistic*, or merely *additive* in action. More study is needed to understand the results of combining the various antibiotics.

Although most pathogenic bacteria are susceptible to one or another of the antibiotics, the search still goes on for antibiotics that will be more effective against tuberculosis, viruses, protozoa, and some of the gram-negative bacilli such as Proteus and Pseudomonas.

Indiscriminate use of antibiotics for trivial ailments is not considered good medical practice. Overuse of an antibiotic may result in many persons becoming hypersensitive to it so that when a serious ailment arises the drug cannot be used or must be used with caution. It is also considered wise to reserve certain new antibiotics for use in treating serious infection due to organisms such as the staphylococci, which are known to develop resistance to antibiotics in common use.

In considering antibiosis it should be remembered that in dealing with living organisms we deal with constant change. Man adapts to his environment which includes the microorganisms with which he must live. The microorganisms, in turn, represent populations of billions of cells which can divide as often as every twenty minutes. Many random mutational changes may occur from which the environment will rapidly select the most favorable, permitting mobile adaptation to new conditions. Thus the status and usefulness of antibiotics change as man and microorganisms adapt to their changing environment.

What constitutes a good antibiotic?

A good antimicrobial drug for clinical use should be harmless to human tissues, especially those of the blood and the blood-forming organs, the liver, and the kidney. For an antibiotic to be effective it must remain in the body tissues for a relatively long period of time, and if the infection is a severe one, the dosage, as well as the length of time during which it is administered, may have to be increased; hence, low toxicity is a primary qualification. There are other characteristics of a good antibiotic: It should preferably be a stable substance, not destroyed by tissue enzymes, not inhibited by the presence of serum, pus, or blood, and not eliminated too rapidly by the kidney; the infecting microorganisms should not develop resistance to it, and it should be powerful in its action against at least some microorganisms. It should be soluble in water and salt solutions. It should diffuse readily through the body tissues, and it should not sensitize the patient. It should not alter the normal flora of the body so that superinfections will not occur. It should be well absorbed from the intestinal tract and be tolerated when given by other routes of administration. It should not be antagonistic to other antibiotics. No antibiotic, however, meets all of these requirements.

Systemic antibiotics generally used

Penicilllin

Penicillin is an antibiotic derived from a number of strains of *Penicillium notatum* and *Penicillium chrysogenum,* common molds often seen on bread or fruit. Commercially the mold is grown in corn-steep liquor and to this medium may be added sugar, inorganic salts, and pre-formed chemical radicals; these radicals are incorporated by the mold into the penicillin molecule and help to form the type of penicillin desired. The various penicillins are known as penicillin F, G, K, O, V, and X. Penicillin G has been synthesized chemically, but the synthetic preparation is not practical because of increased cost and difficulties encountered.* The most commonly used penicillin is penicillin G; it is easy to manufacture and is widely used at present in the form of its sodium or potassium salt. Penicillin O and penicillin V are also used therapeutically. The other penicillins are not used therapeutically because of various disadvantages. The penicillins differ from each other in that different side chains are attached to the basic nucleus of the molecule. The basic formula for the penicillins is shown below, the R standing for the different side chains attached to the group common to all penicillins.

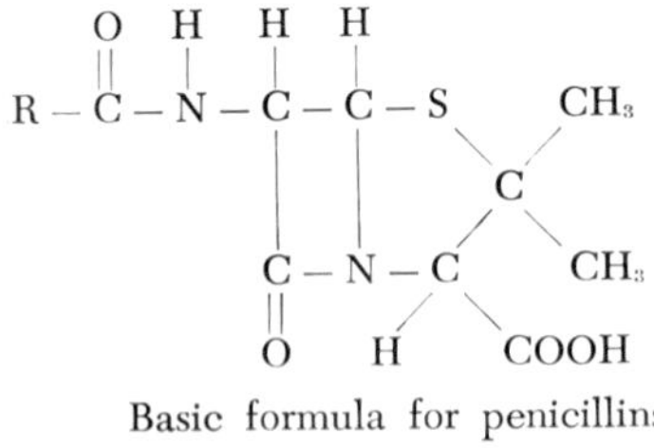

Basic formula for penicillins

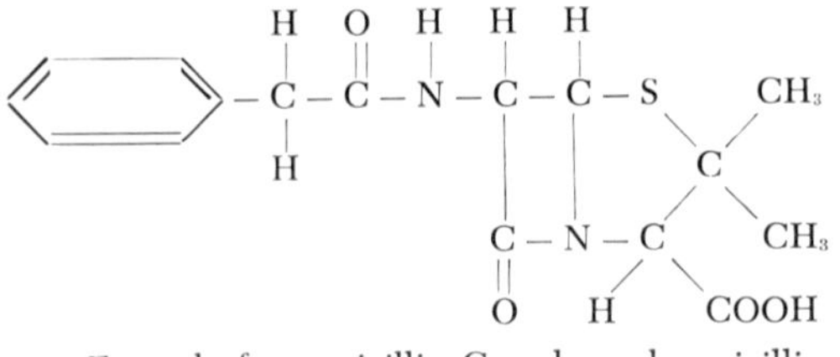

Formula for penicillin G or benzyl penicillin

*Recently a new synthetic penicillin, potassium phenoxyethyl penicillin (Syncillin), has been marketed.

140

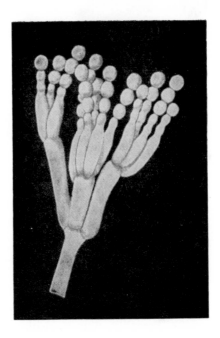

Fig. 22 Typical penicillus of *Penicillium notatum;* Fleming's strain. (From Raper, K. B., and Alexander, D. F.: J. Elisha Mitchell Sc. Soc. **61:** 74, 1945.)

For the other two commonly used penicillins the R in the formula is as follows:

Allylmercaptomethyl penicillin	(O)	$CH_2{=}CH-CH_2-\overset{\underset{\textstyle|}{SH}}{CH}-$
Phenoxymethyl penicillin	(V)	$\langle\underline{\hspace{1cm}}\rangle-O-CH_2-$

The penicillins are organic acids which are white or slightly yellow in color. The dry preparations are stable; however, in solution the penicillins are relatively unstable so that the expiration date should be noted when a nurse prepares the solution.

Standardization. Penicillin is standardized by comparing the effect of the penicillin to be assayed with the growth of a test organism (Staphylococcus, Streptococcus, or *Bacillus subtilis*) with the effect of a standard penicillin preparation. The U.S.P. unit is the antibiotic activity of 0.6 mcg. of U.S.P. Penicillin G Sodium Reference Standard, 1 mg. being equal to 1,667 units.* The term reference standard means a specific lot of penicillin G which serves as the standard of comparison in determining potency.

Penicillin dosage is still expressed in units, but the use of doses measured according to weight is increasing.

*The U.S.P. states that 1 mg. of other kinds of penicillin contains different numbers of units. For example, 1 mg. of potassium phenoxymethyl penicillin represents 1,530 U.S.P. units and 1 mg. of benzathine penicillin G represents 1,211 U.S.P. penicillin units.

Action and result. Penicillin is thought to interfere with the synthesis of cell walls by bacteria. Animal cells do not have the rigid chemically complex cell walls that give most bacteria their shape, which accounts for the high selectivity of penicillin, i.e., its virtual lack of direct toxicity for man or other mammalian hosts. Penicillin slows the growth of susceptible microorganisms and frequently kills them. The nurse is often in a position to observe the end results of the action of penicillin in the sick person. There is often a reduction of fever, improved appetite, and a general increased sense of well-being.

Absorption, distribution, and excretion. Penicillin G and penicillin O are partially inactivated by the gastric juice and by the enzyme penicillinase formed by bacteria in the intestine; therefore their absorption from the intestine is uncertain unless they are buffered by an antacid such as calcium carbonate. The benzathine or aluminum salts of penicillin G are only slightly soluble and so can withstand the action of gastric juice. Penicillin V (phenoxymethyl penicillin) is acid-insoluble and so passes through the stomach unchanged.

Penicillin diffuses readily into most body tissues, with the exception of the brain, spinal fluid, bone marrow, and fluids of the eye; in these, the levels of penicillin are considerably lower than the levels of the blood. Penicillin passes easily from the maternal blood into the blood of the fetus.

Most of the penicillin absorbed is excreted quickly by the kidneys because, like certain other drugs, penicillin is not only filtered through the glomeruli but is also secreted directly across the epithelium of the kidney tubules. A small amount appears in the bile, saliva, and serous sacs. After an intramuscular injection of an aqueous solution of penicillin, the drug appears in the urine in ten minutes and most of it is excreted within two hours. Because penicillin is absorbed so quickly from the muscles, ways have been devised to slow the passage from the muscle into the blood stream. Relatively insoluble salts such as procaine and benzathine penicillin pass slowly into the blood stream; placing penicillin in vehicles such as insoluble oils also slows its absorption.

To decrease the rate of excretion of penicillin, it is possible to give a drug which inhibits its excretion from the kidney. Probenecid (Benemid) is a drug that can be used for this purpose; however, penicillin is now relatively inexpensive, and it is usually simpler to give large doses to make up for urinary losses.

Uses. Penicillin should be used for any patient who is not allergic to it and who has an infection caused by a penicillin-sensitive organism. These include the following:

1. Gram-positive bacteria—all sensitive strains of staphylococci, *Streptococcus pyogenes, Streptococcus viridans, Diplococcus pneumoniae,*

Bacillus anthracis, Actinomyces bovis, Clostridium tetani, the clostridia of gas gangrene, and *Corynebacterium diphtheriae*.

2. Gram-negative bacteria—*Neisseria gonorrhoeae, Neisseria meningitidis*, and Vincent's organisms.

3. Others—*Treponema pallidum* and *Treponema pertenue*.

Penicillin is not effective against infections caused by (1) protozoa, such as those causing malaria and amebiasis, (2) the gram-negative bacilli, such as colon-typhoid dysentery group of organisms, (3) the tubercle bacillus, (4) the rickettsias, (5) the true viruses, and (6) fungi. It is somewhat effective against the larger viruses of psittacosis and lymphogranuloma venereum.*

In deciding on the use of penicillin against the organisms listed, the doctor's decision depends on a number of factors related to the microorganism, the patient, and the disease. For example: The microorganism may prove to be resistant to penicillin; the patient may be sensitive to penicillin; past experience with the disease may indicate that penicillin should be combined with another agent in this particular disease, as in diphtheria where penicillin is used with antitoxin and in meningococcic infections where a sulfonamide may be given simultaneously.

Penicillin-resistant organisms. Most of the organisms originally susceptible to the action of penicillin have remained sensitive. However, the staphylococci have become increasingly resistant to penicillin. The appearance of resistant staphylococci has been due to the suppression of sensitive strains which has permitted resistant strains to emerge from the occurrence of resistant mutants. When staphylococcal infections are acquired in hospitals today, the infective organisms are nearly all penicillin-resistant.

It has recently been reported that it is not uncommon for gonococci to fail to respond to an adequate course of penicillin therapy.† Up to the present it had been thought that the gonococcus has not developed resistance to penicillin. The evidence that a penicillin-resistant strain of *Neisseria gonorrhoeae* has emerged means that a re-evaluation of penicillin in the treatment of gonorrhea will need to be made.

Preparation and dosage of crystalline penicillin for parenteral use.

Buffered Penicillin G for Injection, U.S.P.; *Benzylpenicillin Injection*, B.P. This is potassium penicillin G or sodium penicillin G buffered with sodium citrate.

Potassium Penicillin G (Benzyl Penicillin Potassium), U.S.P.; *Benzylpenicillin*, B.P.

---

*These larger viruses are classified as Rickettsiales in the seventh edition of *Bergey's Manual of Determinative Bacteriology*.

†Epstein, E.: Failure of Pencillin in Treatment of Acute Gonorrhea in American Troops in Korea, J. A. M. A. **169:** 1055, 1959.

Sodium Penicillin G (Benzyl Penicillin Sodium), U.S.P.; *Benzylpenicillin*, B.P.

The usual intramuscular dose of the preceding preparations is 400,000 U.S.P. units four times a day, whereas the usual intravenous dose is 10,000,000 units daily.

*Sodium Penicillin O** (Cer-O-Cillin Sodium). This is allylmercaptomethyl penicillin, produced by growing the mold in a medium containing allylmercaptoacetic acid. It has the same dosage, action, and effects as penicillin G except that it is less likely to cause sensitivity or allergic reactions. In patients sensitive to penicillin G, penicillin O may be tried; however, of patients who are sensitive to penicillin G, an appreciable proportion will also be sensitive to penicillin O. The dosage of penicillin O is the same as that for potassium penicillin G.

Crystalline preparations may be dissolved in sterile distilled water, isotonic solution of sodium chloride, or 5 per cent dextrose solutions. They diffuse quickly and are excreted rapidly. They are usually administered by the intramuscular route, although the intravenous method is also used. They are used for severe infections or infections in which the organism is only moderately or fairly susceptible to penicillin. They are also used when the organism is not very accessible, as in subacute bacterial endocarditis in which the infecting organism is protected by vegetative lesions. In these cases the dose may total many millions of units per day. When given intramuscularly they are given at frequent intervals. A continuous intravenous drip may be employed in treatment of severe infections.

Preparation and dosage of penicillin for intramuscular administration and prolonged action.

Benzathine Penicillin G, U.S.P., B.P. The usual intramuscular dose is 600,000 U.S.P. units, repeated as necessary. The usual dose range is 300,000 to 3,000,000 units.

Sterile Benzathine Penicillin G Suspension, U.S.P. The dose is the same as that for benzathine penicillin G.

Procaine Penicillin G, U.S.P., B.P. The usual intramuscular dose is 300,000 U.S.P. units once or twice a day. The usual dosage range is 300,000 to 1,200,000 units.

Sterile Procaine Penicillin G Suspension, U.S.P.; *Procaine Penicillin Injection*, B.P. The dose is the same as that for procaine penicillin G.

Sterile Procaine Penicillin G with Aluminum Stearate Suspension, U.S.P. The intramuscular dose is 300,000 U.S.P. units on alternate days. The usual dosage range is 300,000 to 1,200,000 units.

Fortified Procaine Penicillin Injection, B.P. This is a sterile suspension of procaine penicillin in water for injection containing benzylpenicillin

*Described in annual publication of A. M. A. Council on Drugs, N.N.D., 1960.

in solution. The dose is determined by the physician in accordance with the needs of the patient.

Penicillin-Streptomycin for Suspension, Sterile, N.F.

Penicillin G, Procaine, and Buffered Crystalline Penicillin G for Suspension, Sterile, N.F.

Penicillin, Procaine, in Oil Injection, N.F.

The above preparations are examples of relatively insoluble penicillin G preparations which are called "depot" preparations because they remain in the muscle a long time. Since they are slowly absorbed, their action lasts a longer time than the crystalline preparations and permits them to be given less often. They are administered intramuscularly only.

Procaine penicillin is usually given once or twice a day, and the procaine penicillin in oil with aluminum monostearate needs to be given only every 24 to 48 hours. The amount of procaine in these preparations is small, but if a patient is allergic to procaine he may have a reaction to it and these preparations should not be used. Some preparations of procaine penicillin have crystalline penicillin G in them; this would provide both a rapid and a slow action in cases of severe infection.

Benzathine penicillin G is very slowly absorbed. Depending on the size of the dose, a single intramuscular injection produces an effective blood level for 1 to 4 weeks or longer. It may be used when prolonged action at low levels is desirable, as for example, to prevent streptococcic infections in patients who have had rheumatic fever. For primary and secondary syphilis a single dose of 2,400,000 units is considered effective.

Preparation and dosage of penicillin for oral administration.

*Aluminum Penicillin.** This preparation is available in tablets containing 50,000 units of the drug and is given orally or sublingually. Dosage is similar to that of potassium penicillin G.

Phenoxymethyl Penicillin (Penicillin V), U.S.P., B.P. (Pen-Vee, V-Cillin). Official preparations of phenoxymethyl penicillin include capsules, oral suspension, and tablets. The usual dose is 125 mg. (approximately 200,000 U.S.P. units) four times a day. The usual dosage range is 500 mg. to 2 Gm. (approximately 800,000 to 3,200,000 units) daily.

Potassium Phenoxymethyl Penicillin (Penicillin V Potassium), U.S.P. (Compocillin-VK, Pen-Vee K, V-Cillin K). The dose is the same as that for phenoxymethyl penicillin. The official preparations include tablets.

Potassium Phenoxyethyl Penicillin. This is a synthetic penicillin which is water soluble and relatively resistant to the destructive action of acids. It is given orally in doses of 125 or 250 mg. three times daily. Larger doses may be used if indicated. It is available in the form of tablets and a solution for pediatric use. The brand names include Syncillin and Darcil.

*Described in annual publication of A. M. A. Council on Drugs, N.N.D., 1960.

Penicillin G Tablets, U.S.P.; *Benzylpenicillin Tablets*, B.P. These contain potassium penicillin G or sodium penicillin G with one or more suitable buffers. The usual dose is 400,000 U.S.P. units four times a day. The usual dose range is 200,000 to 1,000,000 units.

Benzathine Penicillin Tablets, B.P. The dose is 300,000 to 600,000 units every 6 hours.

Potassium penicillins G and O may be administered orally, but because they are, to a great extent, inactivated by the gastric juice and by the intestinal bacteria, doses approximately five times greater than the parenteral doses must be given. The preparations are usually buffered with an antacid, such a sodium citrate or aluminum hydroxide, to protect them from the acid of the gastric juice. Their use has largely been replaced by the preparations that resist destruction.

Relatively insoluble preparations such as benzathine and aluminum penicillin resist the destructive action to some degree. The newer penicillin V is acid insoluble and is currently popular as an oral preparation of penicillin.

Administration. Crystalline penicillin is very soluble in water and can be given by almost any method of administration. When it was first used, it was commonly given by intramuscular injection; because it was excreted quickly it was administered at intervals of every 3 hours. With further study it was found that maintenance of high blood levels was not essential in many patients and this, added to the fact that frequent injections are inconvenient and uncomfortable, has led to the use of preparations of penicillin which are absorbed more slowly after intramuscular injection and to the use of oral preparations. Although these preparations do not lend themselves to the maintenance of high blood levels, in most cases they have been therapeutically satisfactory.

Intramuscular. Intramuscular administration is the most common parenteral method of administration. The slowly absorbed, insoluble depot preparations are those used most; procaine penicillin G and benzathine penicillin G are the most popular preparations at present.

Intravenous. Water-soluble salts of penicillin such as penicillin G sodium and penicillin G potassium are given intravenously when treatment of severe infections requires fast action and high blood levels. Continuous intravenous drip is employed for infections in which a large dose of penicillin is needed to conquer the infection.

Oral. Oral administration is highly desirable because it eliminates the need for injections and because anaphylactic reactions to orally administered penicillin are infrequent. It is not as effective are parenteral administration, for high blood levels are not attained since it is excreted almost as fast as it is absorbed. However, it is satisfactory for most infections except those that are very severe.

Aerosol. When penicillin is administered by inhalation as a fog or fine dust, the local concentration is high in the respiratory tract and absorption is such that satisfactory blood levels are reached. However, administration is cumbersome, sensitization is more likely to occur, and the effects on respiratory infections are satisfactory by other means of administration. Therefore, aerosol administration has limited usefulness.

Intrathecal. Penicillin administered orally or parenterally normally does not diffuse into the spinal fluid in large amounts. When the meninges are irritated, the diffusion is increased but high levels in the spinal fluid are not reached. Penicillin is toxic to the central nervous system so that the amount and concentration of solutions of penicillin injected intrathecally must be carefully regulated. For this reason, intrathecal administration of penicillin has limited usefulness.

Topical. Topical administration of penicillin is associated with a higher incidence of allergic reactions than any other route of administration and hence it is given this way less and less. Other safer antimicrobial agents should probably be used.

Subcutaneous. Subcutaneous injection is seldom used because the blood levels attained tend to be unpredictable.

Side effects and toxic effects. Penicillin is remarkably low in toxicity. The only tissue injured by penicillin is that of the central nervous system when penicillin is placed in direct contact with it; headache, tenseness, muscular twitching, convulsions, and cyanosis may occur when it is applied to the brain during surgical operations.

Superinfections may occur as a result of insensitive or resistant organisms. These include staphylococcic enterocolitis and monilial infections. Blacktongue is due to an overgrowth of fungi, usually Candida. Nausea, vomiting, and diarrhea may also occur.

Allergic reactions to penicillin are not uncommon. These constitute by far the most important type of untoward effect to penicillin and include contact dermatitis, urticaria, asthma, pruritus, local reaction at the site of injection, fever, erythema, polyarthritis, and exfoliative dermatitis. Anaphylactic shock is rare, but it is increasing in frequency; death has followed in some instances.

Patients known to be sensitive to penicillin G may be able to tolerate penicillin O; if this does not prove feasible another antibiotic should be used. To treat minor allergic reactions one of the antihistaminic drugs such as diphenhydramine hydrochloride (Benadryl Hydrochloride) or tripelennamine hydrochloride (Pyribenzamine Hydrochloride) may be prescribed. For acute reactions, such as anaphylactic shock, epinephrine should be available. For severe reactions, one of the adrenocorticosteroids may be helpful. It is of interest that some persons highly sensitive to penicillin may react to it even when they encounter it on a

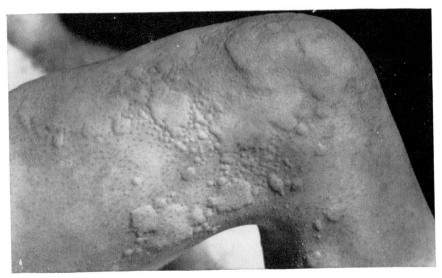

Fig. 23 Urticaria such as may be seen in patients who are sensitive to penicillin.

nontherapeutic basis, e.g., in poliomyelitis vaccine, in milk from penicillin-treated cows, or even from contact with penicillin designed for another patient.

Superinfections can sometimes be successfully treated with a different antibiotic; e.g., nystatin may be used for moniliasis. In other cases of superinfection the use of penicillin must be stopped.

Penicillinase (Neutrapen)

Penicillinase is an enzyme produced by *Bacillus cereus, Escherichia coli,* and many strains of staphylococci. It hydrolyzes penicillin to penicilloic acid. Penicillinase has been recommended for the treatment of allergic reactions to penicillin. The drug is usually given intramuscularly in doses of 800,000 units,* after which penicillin reactions generally subside in 24 to 48 hours. A second and a third dose may be needed. In case of anyphylactic shock it can be given intravenously, followed by an intramuscular injection. The commercial preparation Neutrapen is marketed in the form of a vial of dry powder containing 800,000 units. This is dissolved in 2 ml. of sterile distilled water for injection. Although penicillinase was at first thought to be nontoxic, reports of reactions, including anaphylactic shock, are presently being reported.† Its place in drug therapy will need to be determined by further study.

*One unit is the amount of penicillinase that will inactivate 1 unit of penicillin per minute or 60 units of penicillin per hour at a temperature of 25° C. and a pH of 7.
†Hyman, A. L.: Anaphylactic Shock After Therapy With Penicillinase, J. A. M. A. **169:** 593, 1959; Reisch, M.: Penicillinase Therapy—Clinical Reports of Severe Reactions, J. A. M. A. **169:** 594, 1959.

The tetracyclines

The tetracycline family consists of chlortetracycline (Aureomycin), oxytetracycline (Terramycin), and tetracycline (Achromycin). Chlortetracycline, the first to be discovered, was isolated from *Streptomyces aureofaciens*. Oxytetracycline was isolated from *Streptomyces rimosus*, and tetracycline, which was obtained from another streptomyces, has also been prepared chemically by removing chlorine from chlortetracycline.

Formulas for the tetracyclines

As can be noted from the formulas, the tetracyclines are similar to each other. They form salts which are soluble in water. In crystalline form the salts are stable, whereas in aqueous solution there is progressive loss of antibacterial activity; the acid solutions are generally more stable and are used for parenteral administration.

The three compounds can be considered together because their action against bacteria is the same. Cross resistance between them is common. Tetracycline has largely supplanted the use of the other two. It is the most stable and the least likely to produce gastrointestinal symptoms, and it passes more easily into the cerebrospinal fluid than do the other two members of the family.

Action. The tetracyclines are said to be bacteriostatic when used in therapeutic doses against susceptible microorganisms. However, the precise mechanism of their action is not known.

Absorption, distribution, and excretion. The tetracyclines are readily absorbed when administered orally. They are widely distributed through the body, except in the cerebrospinal fluid where levels are much lower than in the plasma. The tetracyclines are excreted chiefly by the kidneys.

Uses. The tetracyclines are so-called broad-spectrum antibiotics which are extremely useful against a wide variety of gram-negative and gram-positive bacteria, including the brucella, the larger viruses of the psittacosis-lymphogranuloma group, rickettsias (Rocky Mountain spotted fever and typhus fever), *actinomycetes* (actinomycosis), and *Entamoeba his-*

tolytica (amebiasis). They are particularly useful against infections caused by gram-negative bacilli since penicillin and many of the other antibiotics do not have much action on this group. The tetracyclines are said to be effective in certain stages of syphilis, but its value as compared to penicillin must be determined by further study. They seem to be as effective for yaws, as is penicillin.

Preparations.

Chlortetracycline Hydrochloride, N.F., B.P. (Aureomycin Hydrochloride). The B.P. lists *Chlortetracycline Capsules* and *Chlortetracycline Injection,* whereas N.F. lists these two preparations and also *Chlortetracycline Hydrochloride, Ophthalmic.* Other preparations are topical ointment, ophthalmic ointment, powder for injection, nasal powder, ophthalmic powder, optic powder, tablets, and troches.

Oxytetracycline, N.F.

Oxytetracycline for Suspension, Oral, N.F.

Oxytetracycline Dihydrate Tablets, B.P.

Oxytetracycline Hydrochloride, N.F., B.P. The N.F. preparations include capsules and *Oxytetracycline Hydrochloride, Ophthalmic,* whereas both N.F. and B.P. list *Oxytetracycline Hydrochloride for Injection.*

Oxytetracycline and Procaine Injection, B.P.

Tetracycline, U.S.P.

Tetracycline Oral Suspension, U.S.P.

Tetracycline Hydrochloride, U.S.P., B.P.

Tetracycline Hydrochloride Capsules, U.S.P., B.P.

Tetracycline Hydrochloride for Injection, U.S.P., B.P.

Tetracycline Hydrochloride for Ophthalmic Solution, U.S.P.

Tetracycline Hydrochloride Solution, U.S.P.

Tetracycline and Procaine Injection, B.P.

Tetracycline Tablets, B.P.

Tetracycline Phosphate Complex* (Panmycin Phosphate, Sumycin, Tetrex).

Tetracycline phosphate complex has the same actions and uses as the parent antibiotic tetracycline or its hydrochloride. However, the phosphate complex is more rapidly and completely absorbed from the digestive tract and therefore produces higher blood levels. In other respects it does not differ from other preparations of tetracycline. It is administered orally.

Dosage and administration. The tetracyclines are usually given orally in doses of 250 to 500 mg. every 6 hours. Solutions buffered with a suitable agent may be given intravenously in emergencies or when patients cannot tolerate the drug by mouth. For intravenous administration, 500 mg. is given every 6 to 12 hours. Phlebitis after intravenous administra-

---

*Described in annual publication of A. M. A. Council on Drugs, N.N.D., 1960.

tion is not uncommon. The drugs may be administered topically in suitable preparations. Intramuscular absorption is fairly satisfactory, except with chlortetracycline. The intramuscular doses range from 100 to 200 mg. every 6 to 8 hours.

Side effects and toxic effects. The tetracyclines are relatively nontoxic. They do not injure the kidneys, liver, or the eighth cranial nerve. The chief reactions occur in the gastrointestinal tract and include nausea, vomiting, and diarrhea. This type of reaction occurs more often with the tetracyclines than with any of the other commonly used antibiotics. Tetracycline is the least likely of the three drugs to cause these symptoms. Part of the gastrointestinal reaction is due to local irritation; this irritation may occur at the site of injection when tetracyclines are given intramuscularly or intravenously. The incidence of nausea and vomiting can be reduced if the drug is given with milk or sodium bicarbonate or calcium carbonate in amounts of 0.3 Gm. with each 250 mg. of the antibiotic.*

In addition to the local irritation, gastrointestinal symptoms may be caused by the suppression of the normal intestinal flora, which allows resistant or insensitive organisms to become established.

Staphylococcal enterocolitis is one of the most serious of these superinfections and requires that administration of the drug be discontinued immediately. Antibiotics such as novobiocin and erythromycin may be employed against the staphylococci if the organisms are sensitive to these antibiotics.

Superinfections with fungi such as *Candida albicans* may also occur. Nystatin is sometimes used to treat monilial infections.

Symptoms of stomatitis, gastrointestinal irritation, or vaginitis, which indicate that superinfections have developed, should be promptly reported when a patient is receiving antibiotics.

Streptomycin and dihydrostreptomycin

Streptomycin is an antibiotic obtained from certain strains of *Streptomyces griseus*. Dihydrostreptomycin is produced by the hydrogenation of streptomycin. The dry powders of these drugs are stable; the solutions are stable for 7 to 10 days under refrigeration. These antibiotics inhibit the growth of, and in sufficient concentrations, destroy, susceptible pathogens.

Absorption, distribution, and excretion. The streptomycins are poorly absorbed from the intestinal tract. When given parenterally they are distributed to all parts of the body, although they pass poorly into the cerebrospinal fluid. Excretion by the kidneys is slow.

*Shirger, A., Martin, W. J., and Nichols, D. R.: Antibiotic Therapy; Clinical Application of Available Agents, GP **19:** 102, 1959.

Uses. The main use of streptomycin is in the treatment of tuberculosis. It is also effective against a wide variety of gram-negative organisms, such as the gram-negative intestinal bacilli, and the pasteurella, hemophilus, and brucella organisms. It is used occasionally against gram-positive organisms that are penicillin resistant.

In tuberculosis the drugs of greatest value are streptomycin, dihydro-streptomycin, PAS, and isonicotinic acid hydrazide (isoniazid or INH). The latter two are discussed in Chapter 21. The streptomycins exert a marked suppressive action in tuberculosis. Because the treatment of tuberculosis is prolonged, resistance in the organisms may develop and toxicity may occur. To delay the appearance of resistance, PAS is given with the streptomycins. Some believe that it is best not to give streptomycin and isoniazid together except in extreme need, so that resistance to both drugs at the same time will not deprive the patient of the two most powerful antituberculosis drugs. To prevent toxicitiy in tuberculosis, the dosage of streptomycin is carefully regulated. In all types of tuberculosis, except the miliary and meningeal forms, doses of streptomycin 1 Gm. are given intramuscularly two or three times a week along with PAS for 120 days. In tuberculous meningitis, intrathecal administration of 50 mg. of streptomycin every day or two may be given along with the streptomycin intramuscularly. In acute miliary tuberculosis, 2 Gm. or more of streptomycin are given daily.

Originally a number of gram-negative and gram-positive bacteria were susceptible to the streptomycins. However, these drugs have a great tendency to induce resistance in bacteria, and the majority of strains of certain gram-negative pathogens such as *Proteus vulgaris, Pseudomonas aeruginosa,* and *Aerobacter aerogenes* now being isolated in infections are resistant. In addition, many organisms, with the exception of the tubercle bacillus, that are sensitive to streptomycin are sensitive to the tetracyclines; the latter are safer to use and organisms usually do not acquire resistance to the tetracyclines as rapidly as to streptomycin. Therefore, it is recommended by many authorities that streptomycin be limited to the treatment of tuberculosis and to infections in which the bacteria are resistant to other safer antibiotics but susceptible to streptomycin.

Preparation, dosage and administration.

Streptomycin Sulfate, U.S.P., B.P. The commercial preparations of streptomycin sulfate are powders for injection and solutions for injection containing 500 mg. in 1 ml., 1 Gm. in 2 ml., or 5 Gm. in 10 and 20 ml.

Dihydrostreptomycin Sulfate, U.S.P., B.P. The commercial preparations are similar to those for streptomycin.

Streptoduocin for Injection, U.S.P. (Dihydrostreptomycin-Streptomycin for Injection).

The dose stated in the U.S.P. for the above preparations of streptomycin and streptoduocin is the equivalent of 1 Gm. of the base daily, intramuscularly. The dose stated in the U.S.P. for dihydrostreptomycin is the equivalent of 500 mg. of the base every 6 hours intramuscularly. For systemic effects these antibiotics are usually given intramuscularly. Other methods of administration for streptomycin include intravenous drip, oral, intrathecal, topical, and nebulization. When given orally it is used as an intestinal antiseptic.

Dihydrostreptomycin must not be given intravenously; ordinarily it should not be given intrathecally because administration by this route increases the likelihood of loss of hearing; dihydrostreptomycin is not recommended for tuberculous meningitis.

Side effects and toxic effects. Both streptomycins may produce toxic effects such as kidney and liver damage. Allergic reactions include erythema, rashes, urticaria, fall in blood pressure, headache, nausea, vomiting, and drug fever. Contact dermatitis may develop in persons who handle these drugs, so protective measures such as the use of rubber gloves are advised.

Damage to the eighth cranial nerve, resulting in deafness and severe vertigo, is one of the most serious toxic effects of the streptomycins. Streptomycin causes more vertigo but less deafness than dihydrostreptomycin. The peculiar specificity of these toxic reactions is not understood. At one time it was believed that a half-and-half mixture of streptomycin and dihydrostreptomycin would result in less damage to the eighth cranial nerve. Recent evidence shows that loss of hearing occurs more often with the mixture than with streptomycin alone. Because the therapeutic results of the two drugs are similar and the toxicity of streptomycin is less distressing than the irreversible deafness which may result from dihydrostreptomycin, streptomycin is the drug of choice except in cases of seriously ill patients who are sensitive to streptomycin, at which time the use of dihydrostreptomycin may be justified. Dihydrostreptomycin also has the disadvantage that the deafness produced may have a latent period, that is, the deafness may appear after the drug has been discontinued.

Erythromycin (Ilotycin)

Erythromycin is an antibiotic obtained from *Streptomyces erythreus.*

Absorption, distribution, and excretion. It is readily absorbed from the gastrointestinal tract. Because it has a bitter taste and is destroyed by the gastric acid, it is administered in enteric-coated tablets or in the form of insoluble preparations which are slowly hydrolyzed. It diffuses through most of the body but is not found in appreciable amounts in the cerebrospinal fluid. It passes from the maternal blood to the fetus in amounts sufficient to be antibacterial. It is excreted by the kidneys and the liver.

Uses. Erythromycin is similar to penicillin in its range of antibacterial activity. It is more effective against gram-positive than gram-negative bacteria. However, it does inhibit *Neisseria gonorrhoeae*, *Bordetella pertussis*, rickettsias, the larger viruses, and to some extent the spirochetes. It is also useful for the treatment of amebiasis. Penicillin is chosen in most cases in preference to erythromycin; the latter is used when organisms are penicillin-resistant or when the patient is allergic to penicillin. Unfortunately, the staphylococci develop resistance to erythromycin quite rapidly. In hospital infections due to staphylococci, penicillin-resistant strains are often erythromycin-resistant.

Preparation, administration, and dosage.

Erythromycin, U.S.P., B.P. (Ilotycin, Erythrocin). The official preparations include tablets, sterile solutions for injection, and an oral suspension. Orally, as the base or in the form of a suitable derivative, the dose is the equivalent of 250 mg. of erythromycin base every 6 hours. Intravenously, it is given in the form of a suitable derivative, in the dosage of the equivalent of 250 mg. of erythromycin base, as a 0.1 per cent solution, every 6 hours. The usual dosage range is 1 to 2 Gm. daily.

Erythromycin Ethylcarbonate, U.S.P. This is an oral preparation. The dose is the same as that for erythromycin.

Erythromycin Glucoheptonate, U.S.P. This intravenous preparation has the same dose as erythromycin.

Erythromycin Lactobionate, U.S.P. (Erythrocin Lactobionate). This water-soluble salt is suitable for intravenous and intramuscular injection and for ophthalmic use in the form of an ophthalmic ointment, 1 per cent.

*Erythromycin Propionate*** (Ilosone). This is an oral preparation administered in the same doses as erythromycin.

Erythromycin Stearate, U.S.P. This is prepared in a suspension and tablet form for oral administration. The dose is the same as that for erythromcyin.

Side effects and toxic effects. Erythromycin is relatively nontoxic. Mild gastrointestinal symptoms may be produced. Large doses cause nausea, vomiting, diarrhea, and prostration. It rarely causes superinfection due to suppression of the intestinal flora.

Chloramphenicol (Chloromycetin)

Chloramphenicol is an antibiotic originally derived from *Streptomyces venezuelae*, but it is now produced synthetically. Chloramphenicol is a bitter substance, whereas chloramphenicol palmitate is a tasteless deriva-

---

*Described in annual publication of A. M. A. Council on Drugs, N.N.D., 1960.

tive which is therapeutically effective. Crystalline chloramphenicol is stable, as are neutral and acid solutions.

Absorption, distribution, and excretion. Chloramphenicol is absorbed from the gastrointestinal tract. It is widely distributed throughout the body. It is excreted by the kidney and liver; that excreted in the bile is again absorbed, so that the kidney is the eventual place of excretion.

Uses. Chloramphenicol is a broad-spectrum antibiotic which is effective against a wide range of gram-positive and gram-negative bacteria, the rickettsiae, and certain of the large viruses (psittacosis and lymphogranuloma group). It is the antibiotic of choice in typhoid fever. It should not be used indiscriminately because it depresses the bone marrow. However, under adequate supervision chloramphenicol can be used and is especially important when bacteria become resistant to less toxic antibiotics; for example, it has been used against penicillin-resistant staphylococci.

Preparation, dosage, and administration.

Chloramphenicol, U.S.P., B.P. (Chloromycetin). The U.S.P. lists as official preparations *Chloramphenicol Capsules, Chloramphenicol Ophthalmic Ointment, Chloramphenicol for Ophthalmic Solution,* and *Sterile Chloramphenicol for Suspension.* The usual dose is 500 mg. every 6 hours orally or 1 Gm. every 8 hours intramuscularly. The usual dosage range is 1 to 4 Gm. daily, orally and intramuscularly. For external use, topically as a 0.5 to 1 per cent ointment or solution.

Chloramphenicol Capsules, B.P.

Chloramphenicol Palmitate, U.S.P. The U.S.P. lists *Chloramphenicol Palmitate Oral Suspension* as an official preparation. The usual dose is 865 mg., the equivalent of 500 mg. of chloramphenicol base, four times a day. The usual dosage range is 1.7 to 6.9 Gm., the equivalent of 1 to 4 Gm. of chloramphenicol base, daily.

Side effects and toxic effects. Nausea, vomiting, and diarrhea may occur, although these occur less often with chloramphenicol than with other broad-spectrum antibiotics. The diarrhea is partly due to irritation, but most often it is the result of a change in intestinal flora.

The most serious toxic effect is depression of the bone marrow, resulting in blood dyscrasias such as aplastic anemia and agranulocytosis. Although the incidence of this toxicity is low, it has limited the use of chloramphenicol. Careful selection of cases and frequent blood studies to detect early signs of toxicity should reduce the hazards of its use.

Systemic antibiotics occasionally used

The systemic antibiotics previously discussed are among the most effective and widely used or are ones that have a special use in certain diseases. Those that follow are used less often but are very valuable in certain cases. They are listed alphabetically, not in the order of frequency of use.

Amphotericin B (Fungizone)

Amphotericin B is a new antibiotic agent that gives evidence of usefulness as an effective antifungal drug. It is derived from an unidentified species of Streptomyces found in a South American soil sample. It is intended for use in the treatment of disseminated mycotic infections, including coccidioidomycosis, cryptococcosis, disseminated moniliasis, histoplasmosis, and North American blastomycosis.

Preparation, dosage, and administration.

Amphotericin B, U.S.P.* (Fungizone). The commercial preparation is called Fungizone and contains 50 mg. of dry powder per vial. The powder should be stored in the refrigerator and protected from light. Solutions should be protected from light, and any unused material should be discarded after 24 hours.

Because only a minimal amount of absorption occurs on oral administration, it is administered parenterally for systemic infections. It is recommended that it be given by slow intravenous infusion over a period of approximately 6 hours. The recommended concentration is 0.1 mg. per milliliter of 5 per cent dextrose in water, for intravenous administration.† Dosage varies with the tolerance of each patient. An initial daily dose of 0.25 mg. per kilogram of body weight is recommended. This can gradually be increased until an optimum level is reached. Generally the daily dose may range up to 1.0 mg. per kilogram of body weight. Within this range the dosage should be maintained at the highest level not accompanied by toxic manifestations. Intrathecal injection of the drug dissolved in sterile water may be given in coccidioidal meningitis.

Side effects and toxic effects. Phlebitis at the site of injection, chills, fever, vomiting, diarrhea, respiratory distress, and azotemia (presence of nitrogenous bodies in the blood) may result from the administration of amphotericin B. Blood urea nitrogen and nonprotein nitrogen levels should be checked routinely during therapy. If therapy is prolonged, liver, kidney, and bone marrow studies should be done at appropriate intervals.

Bacitracin (Baciguent)

Bacitracin is an antibiotic obtained from *Bacillus subtilis*.

Action and uses. Bacitracin is bactericidal. It is effective against a wide variety of gram-positive bacteria (streptococci, staphylococci,

---

*U.S.P. Interim Admission.
†N.N.D., 1960, p. 76.

pneumococci, clostridia of the gas gangrene group, and corynebacteria), and the spirochete of syphilis. It has little effect against most gram-negative bacteria, except the neisseria.

Because it is toxic to the kidneys and its antibacterial spectrum is similar to penicillin and other antibiotics, the use of bacitracin has been limited. However, bacitracin is now being used for infections in which the organisms are resistant to the more commonly used antibiotics but sensitive to bacitracin. Fortunately, patients rarely become sensitive to it and bacteria are slow in developing resistance to it.

Preparation, dosage, and administration.

Bacitracin, U.S.P., B.P. (Baciguent). The commercial preparations are marketed as ophthalmic and topical ointments, as powder for injection and topical use (2,000 and 10,000 units in 20 ml. vials; 50,000 units in a 50 ml. vial), and soluble tablets containing 2,500 units.

For systemic action bacitracin is administered intramuscularly in doses of 20,000 units every 8 hours. It can be administered by local injection into circumscribed areas of infections, such as abscesses. It is also used as an intrathecal or intraventricular injection, as an aerosol mist, and as a topical application. Because little is absorbed from the intestines when given orally, it is used as an intestinal antiseptic; it has been found useful against staphylococcic enterocolitis.

Side effects and toxic effects. Pain at the site of intramuscular injection may occur. Damage to the kidney may occur; albuminuria and an increase in the concentration of urea in the blood are indications that renal injury is occurring. The fluid intake should always be adequate (2,500 ml. per day) for patients receiving bacitracin intramuscularly. If the urine output remains above 1,000 ml. and there is no undue retention of urea, nephrotoxicity is evidently not occurring.

Carbomycin (Magnamycin)

Carbomycin is an antibiotic derived from *Streptomyces halstedii*.

Absorption, distribution, and excretion. It is well absorbed after oral administration and seems to diffuse well throughout bodily tissues. An appreciable amount is excreted unchanged by way of the kidney.

Action and uses. Carbomycin appears to exert a strong inhibitory action against a number of gram-positive bacteria. For the present, it is recommended only for the treatment of infections due to staphylococci, pneumococci, and hemolytic streptococci. It is useful therefore in the treatment of pneumonia and infections of soft tissue or of the urinary tract, abscesses, or tonsillitis, caused by the organisms named. Some strains of staphylococci readily develop resistance to carbomycin, and there is a high degree of cross resistance between carbomycin and erythromycin.

Preparation, dosage, and administration.

Carbomycin* (Magnamycin). The commercial name of carbomycin is Magnamycin; it is available in tablets of 100 and 250 mg.

Carbomycin is given orally. For adults the usual daily dose is 2 Gm. given in four equal doses. This may need to be increased in severe infections and decreased for infections of the urinary tract. Carbomycin is recommended for those patients who are sensitive to penicillin or the tetracyclines or in cases where the infecting organisms have developed resistance to these antibiotics.

Side effects and toxic effects. Nausea, vomiting, and diarrhea are the side effects that have been reported. No serious toxic effects on the blood, liver, or kidneys have been noted. Its use may result in superinfections by nonsensitive organisms, particularly monilia.

Cycloserine (Seromycin)

Cycloserine is an antibiotic obtained from strains of *Streptomyces orchidaceus* or *Streptomyces garyphalus*. It exhibits a wide range of antibacterial activity, inhibiting both gram-positive and gram-negative organisms. However, its antimicrobial activity is said to be less than that of many antibiotics in general use. It is being used along with other tuberculostatic drugs in the treatment of tuberculosis, although its effectiveness is not as pronounced as that of streptomycin, isoniazid, and probably aminosalicylic acid (PAS).

Absorption, distribution, and excretion. Cycloserine is rapidly absorbed from the gastrointestinal tract, and effective blood levels are reached in 4 to 8 hours after administration, depending on the size of the dose. Significant concentrations in the cerebrospinal fluid are said to be reached after oral administration. It is excreted in the urine and feces.

Uses. It is indicated in the treatment of severe pulmonary tuberculosis in patients who do not respond to other tuberculostatic drugs or whose organisms have developed resistance to the older drugs (named above). It is not recommended as the initial form of chemotherapy for tuberculosis. It is also used in the treatment of stubborn urinary tract infections which do not respond to other forms of therapy because of bacterial resistance or drug sensitivity. It is ineffective against *Proteus vulgaris*, pseudomonas, and *Neisseria gonorrhoeae*. Bacterial resistance to cycloserine develops, although the rate of development is uncertain.

Preparation, dosage, and administration.

Cycloserine* (Seromycin). The commercial name of cycloserine is Seromycin; it is available in 250 mg. capsules.

Cycloserine is administered orally. The patient receiving cycloserine should preferably be hospitalized, where close observation can be pro-

---

*Described in annual publication of A. M. A. Council on Drugs, N.N.D., 1960.

vided and accurate blood level determinations can be made. It is said that the incidence of toxic side effects can be minimized by restricting the dosage to 250 to 500 mg. daily and by not allowing the blood level to exceed 30 mcg. per milliliter.

Side effects and toxic effects. Incidence of toxic effects from cycloserine seems to exceed that of other drugs commonly used for the treatment of tuberculosis. Reported side effects have been of a neurologic nature and include dizziness, lethargy, headache, psychotic reactions, and convulsive seizures.

Cycloserine should not be given to patients who have a history of mental disturbance or epilepsy. Renal insufficiency is also a reason for withholding the drug or for giving it with caution.

Kanamycin (Kantrex)

Kanamycin is a new antibiotic derived from *Streptomyces kanamyceticus*. Chemically, it is closely related in structure to neomycin and it has some features in common with streptomycin, but it is clearly distinct from both.

Uses. Kanamycin appears to be active against many strains of staphylococci, Neisseria, mycobacteria, salmonella, shigella, Klebsiella, Aerobacter, *Escherichia coli*, and some strains of proteus. In the treatment of tuberculosis, experience suggests that kanamycin exerts some favorable effects on the disease; further experience will reveal its place in tuberculosis. It appears to be relatively inactive against the majority of strains of streptococci, pneumococci, clostridia, pseudomonas, enterococci, Brucella, and some strains of proteus. Resistance of staphylococci and *Escherichia coli* to kanamycin has been induced in vitro. Apparently there is almost complete cross resistance between organisms able to resist neomycin and kanamycin and one-way cross resistance between organisms that can resist streptomycin and kanamycin; i.e., organisms made resistant to kanamycin are resistant to streptomycin, but organisms made resistant to streptomycin are sensitive to kanamycin.

Preparation, dosage, and administration.

Kanamycin Sulfate, U.S.P.* (Kantrex). The official preparations include *Kanamycin Sulfate Capsules* and *Kanamycin Sulfate Injection.*

Kanamycin sulfate is usually given intramuscularly for systemic effect. The daily intramuscular dose for adults and children should not exceed 15 mg. per kilogram of body weight given in two or three divided doses.† Intravenous administration is recommended only for very ill patients with overwhelming infections or with impending vascular collapse; a 0.25 per cent solution is administered by slow intravenous in-

*U.S.P. Interim Admission.
†Council on Drugs, J. A. M. A. 172: 699, 1960.

fusion at a rate of 3 to 4 ml. per minute, the daily dose being 15 to 30 mg. per kilogram of body weight given in two or three divided doses. For local effect the drug may be administered orally, intraperitoneally, by inhalation as an aerosol, or by instillation into cavities. The drug is only slightly absorbed when given orally. For preoperative preparation of the large intestine, it is given orally in doses of 1 Gm. every hour for 4 hours, then 1 Gm. every 6 hours for 36 to 72 hours before surgery. It has also been used orally for antibacterial effects within the intestines in infections caused by organisms susceptible to it.

Commercial preparations include 500 mg. capsules and solutions for injection containing 500 mg. in 2 ml. and 1 Gm. in 3 ml.

Side effects and toxic effects. Toxic effects include impaired renal function, damage to the eighth cranial nerve, abnormal sensations such as numbness and tingling, dermal reactions, and pain on injection. The drug should be given with caution to patients with renal damage; it is excreted by the kidneys and if it is not excreted adequately, damage to the eighth cranial nerve is more likely to occur. Patients should be well hydrated, and ear symptoms such as tinnitus should be reported immediately. Deafness can be partial or complete and, in most cases, has been irreversible.

Neomycin Sulfate

Neomycin is an antibiotic obtained from *Streptomyces fradiae.*

Uses. Neomycin is effective against a variety of gram-positive and gram-negative bacteria. Its antibacterial spectrum is broader than that of bacitracin, penicillin, or streptomycin. It is sometimes effective in the treatment of strains of pseudomonas and proteus, which are resistant to most antibiotics.

Unfortunately it is toxic to the kidneys and to the eighth cranial nerve when given parenterally. Its use systemically is reserved for infections that are sufficiently serious to warrant its use and in cases in which safer antibiotics are not successful.

It is not absorbed from the intestinal tract and thus is useful as an intestinal antiseptic when given orally, because bactericidal concentrations are achieved in the intestines. Topically it is effective and nonirritating. It appears to have a low degree of sensitization.

Preparation, dosage, and administration.

Neomycin Sulfate, U.S.P., B.P. Neomycin sulfate is administered topically in the form of a 0.5 per cent ointment or solution. Intramuscularly the dose is 10 to 15 mg. per kilogram of body weight per day, not to exceed a total of 1 Gm. daily, and it is injected at 6-hour intervals. Orally the dose is 1 Gm. every 4 hours for 24 to 72 hours prior to surgery.

Side effects and toxic effects. In addition to kidney damage and injury to the eighth cranial nerve, fever, tingling and numbness of the hands and feet, tinnitus, and dizziness occur. A mild laxative effect occurs when it is given orally. Superinfection by resistant organisms such as *Candida albicans* may occur.

Novobiocin

The calcium and sodium salts of the antibiotic novobiocin, derived from *Streptomyces niveus* or *Streptomyces spheroides,* are used mainly for the treatment of staphylococcic infections. The antibiotic has a moderate antimicrobial spectrum, the scope of which has not been completely determined. It inhibits the growth of many gram-positive organisms and a few gram-negative organisms. Novobiocin is indicated for the treatment of staphylococcic infections. Because of its side effects and the ease with which resistance may develop, it is best reserved for serious infections in which the patient is allergic to other drugs or in which the staphylococci are resistant to other commonly used antibiotics. It has also been used for proteus infections, especially urinary infections that are resistant to other drugs. There is no cross resistance with older antibiotics.

Absorption, distribution, and excretion. Novobiocin is rapidly absorbed from the intestinal tract. It is well distributed in the body but not into the cerebrospinal fluid. It is excreted in the feces and urine.

Preparation, dosage, and administration.

Novobiocin Sodium, U.S.P. (Albamycin, Cathomycin). The commercial preparations are marketed as 250 mg. capsules and 500 mg. of powder for injection.

Novobiocin Calcium, U.S.P. (Albamycin Calcium, Cathomycin Calcium).

Novobiocin Calcium Oral Suspension, U.S.P.

Novobiocin sodium is usually administered orally. The dosage commonly used is 250 mg. every 6 hours or 500 mg. every 12 hours. In more severe infections, 500 mg. every 6 to 8 hours may be necessary. It may be administered intravenously when oral administration is not advisable; the intravenous injection should be given slowly to avoid venous irritation. The drug can be given intramuscularly, if necessary, though this usually causes pain and irritation at the site of injection.

The novobiocin calcium preparation has the same actions and uses as the sodium salt but is more stable in aqueous suspension; thus it is better suited for oral administration in liquid form.

Side effects and toxic effects. Novobiocin has a relatively high index of sensitization. Skin rashes, urticaria, and fever have occurred. Transient leukopenia, which so far has not progressed into true agranulocytosis, has been observed; therefore, frequent examinations of the peripheral blood should be made. Yellowing of the sclerae, due to a pigment produced in the metabolism of the drug, may occur.

Oleandomycin Phosphate (Matromycin)

Oleandomycin is an antibiotic produced by species of *Streptomyces antibioticus.*

It is most active in vitro against gram-positive organisms such as staphylococci, streptococci, and pneumococci. It also inhibits a few gram-negative organisms, notably *Hemophilus influenzae,* gonococci, and meningococci.

Uses. The main use of oleandomycin has been in the treatment of staphylococcic infections in which the organisms are resistant to penicillin, erythromycin, streptomycin, and the tetracyclines. For beta hemolytic streptococcic and pneumococcic infections, penicillin and the tetracyclines are considered to be the drugs of choice. Oleandomycin has been tried against a variety of other organisms such as gonococci and meningococci, and as clinical evidence accumulates, it may be that other uses will become prominent.

Prolonged therapy with oleandomycin has produced resistant strains of staphylococci. Organisms have shown cross resistance between oleandomycin and other antibiotics such as erythromycin and carbomycin. By preventing indiscriminate use of oleandomycin, its valuable antistaphylococcic properties can best be preserved.

Preparation, dosage, and administration.

Oleandomycin Phosphate* (Matromycin). The commercial preparation is called Matromycin and is available in capsules of 250 mg. and in 500 mg. of powder for injection.

The preferred route of administration is oral administration; for adults the dose ranges from 250 to 500 mg. every 6 hours.

For intravenous administration, 1 to 2 Gm. daily in divided doses every 6 to 12 hours should be sufficient for most acute infections. The intravenous solution should be made so that there is at least 250 ml. of solution, in a proportion not to exceed 2 mg. per ml. This is infused slowly at a rate not to exceed 20 mg. (10 ml.) per minute. Care should be taken to avoid extravasation into the soft tissues.

Occasionally oleandomycin may be administered intramuscularly. Because it is irritating, 7:5 ml. of a 1 to 2 per cent solution of procaine hydrochloride are added to 500 mg. of oleandomycin phosphate powder so that each 1.5 ml. of solution contains 100 mg. of the antibiotic. The usual intramuscular dose for adults is 200 mg. every 6 to 8 hours by deep intragluteal injection, using alternating sites and buttocks. Extreme care

*Described in annual publication of A. M. A. Council on Drugs, N.N.D., 1960.

should be taken to avoid injection of the procaine solution into a vein, subcutaneously, or into the fat layer.

Side effects and toxic effects. These effects have been few and mild. They include anorexia, nausea, loose stools, and occasional skin reactions.

Triacetyloleandomycin (Cyclamycin)

Triacetyloleandomycin* has the same actions and uses as oleandomycin phosphate, but it is more rapidly and completely absorbed from the gastrointestinal tract and thus less frequent doses are necessary. It is administered orally and the dose is the same as that for the phosphate. The commercial product is called Cyclamycin. The preparations consist of capsules containing 125 and 250 mg.; a suspension containing 25 mg. per milliliter; and drops (oral), 100 mg. per milliliter.

Polymyxin (Aerosporin)

Polymyxin is a name used to designate several related antibiotics derived from different strains of *Bacillus polymyxa*. Polymyxin B is the least toxic of the polymyxins which have been studied.

Uses. Polymyxin B is effective against many gram-negative organisms, including the coliform bacteria. Because of its toxicity, polymyxin B is usually reserved for infections that do not respond to other safer agents. It is employed mainly against infections caused by *Pseudomonas aeruginosa*, which are resistant to most antibiotics. Polymyxin B and oxytetracycline act synergistically against most strains of pseudomonas, permitting lower doses of polymyxin B to be given. Infections by pseudomonas have become more common, apparently because the use of antibiotics eliminates many other bacteria and, lacking competition, *Pseudomonas aeruginosa* becomes dominant.

Preparation, dosage, and administration.

Polymyxin B Sulfate, U.S.P., B.P. (Aerosporin Sulfate). The commercial preparations are marketed in the form of an ophthalmic ointment, powder for injection, topical powder, otic solution, and tablets.

Polymyxin B sulfate is administered orally, topically, or parenterally. Intramuscularly the usual daily dose is 10,000 to 20,000 units per kilogram of body weight. The total daily dose is given in divided portions every 6 hours. The drug may be given intrathecally and topically. Because it is not absorbed from the intestinal tract, oral doses, when used, are given to combat intestinal infections due to susceptible organisms. The usual oral dose is 750,000 units four times a day.

Side effects and toxic effects. When given parenterally polymyxin B may produce nephrotoxic and neurotoxic effects. The nephrotoxic effects are manifested by albuminuria and increases in the blood urea. The

*Described in annual publication of A. M. A. Council on Drugs, N.N.D., 1960.

injury to the nervous system may lead to dizziness, mild weakness, and numbness and tingling of the face and extremities. Fever and pain at the site of injection also occur.

Ristocetin (Spontin)

Ristocetin is an antibiotic produced by *Nocardia lurida*, a species of actinomycetes. The commercial product contains two components, ristocetin A and ristocetin B, the chemistry of which is not completely known.

Uses. Ristocetin is active in vitro against the following gram-positive organisms: streptococci, enterococci, pneumococci, and staphylococci. It is also active in vitro against mycobacteria, but it is not recommended for tuberculosis at present because studies showing its efficacy are lacking.

It is not as active, as a rule, as other antibiotics, such as penicillin, and is not absorbed orally. For these reasons, penicillin and certain oral antibiotics such as the tetracyclines are usually used as first choice for various infections. However, for staphylococci and enterococci, both of which tend to become resistant to other antibiotics, ristocetin may be the drug of choice. Sensitivity tests should be done to show that the organisms are resistant to other antibiotics but susceptible to ristocetin. For pneumococci and beta hemolytic streptococci, which rarely, if ever, develop resistance to other antibiotics, ristocetin is not usually indicated. Bacterial resistance to ristocetin has not developed to the same degree as with certain other antibiotics; this may change with increasing use of the drug.

Preparation, dosage, and administration.

*Ristocetin** (Spontin). The commercial preparation of ristocetin is called Spontin and is available in the form of 500 mg. of powder for injection.

It is administered intravenously only because it is inadequately absorbed orally and is too irritating to the tissues to be given extravascularly. It irritates the veins and should not be given in too high a concentration. The drip technic is preferred, the drug to be given over a period of 35 to 45 minutes every 8 to 12 hours; the powder is dissolved to make a 0.2 per cent solution using 5 per cent dextrose solution. Occasionally more concentrated solutions have been given by direct intravenous injection. For staphylococcic infections the usual total daily dose is 25 to 50 mg. per kilogram of body weight. In certain serious infections, doses as high as 75 mg. per kilogram may be used. Doses in excess of 2 or 3 Gm. per day are seldom required and at this dosage level side effects are relatively uncommon.

*Described in annual publication of A. M. A. Council on Drugs, N.N.D., 1960.

Side effects and toxic effects. Side effects of ristocetin include depression in white blood cell counts, with relative neutropenia, drug fever, skin rash, and diarrhea. Therefore, blood counts including a differential leukocyte count should be done at frequent intervals. Occasional allergic reactions consisting of skin rashes, either at the site of the injection or all over the body, have occurred. To date, anaphylactic reactions have not been reported. Thrombocytopenia and toxic effects on the eighth cranial nerve have been reported. Because of its irritating effect, thrombophlebitis has occurred; extravasation of the drug into the tissues should be avoided.

Vancomycin (Vancocin)

Vancomycin, an antibiotic introduced in 1958, is derived from strains of *Streptomyces orientalis*. It is highly active against gram-positive cocci, including streptococci, pneumococci, and staphylococci.

Uses. Vancomycin should be reserved for critically ill patients with life-endangering infections caused by staphylococci which are resistant to the commonly used antibiotics. The drug is not intended for routine use nor for mild infections. To date, no staphylococcic resistance to vancomycin has been reported. Cross resistance to other antibiotics has not been observed. If staphylococci continue to be susceptible to vancomycin, it may become the drug of choice for severe staphylococcic infections that fail to respond to other antibiotics. Because it must be administered intravenously, the indiscriminate use of vancomycin will, in large measure, be discouraged.

Vancomycin has been used to treat severe infections caused by penicillin-resistant strains of alpha or nonhemolytic streptococci. Because beta hemolytic streptococcic or pneumococcic infections respond well to penicillin, its use for these infections is not recommended.

Preparation, dosage, and administration.

Vancomycin* (Vancocin). The commercial preparation is called Vancocin, intravenous; 500 mg. of the dry sterile powder are supplied in 10 ml. rubber-stoppered ampules.

The drug is administered intravenously only. For adults, the usual dose is 2 Gm. in 24 hours. Generally this is administered in amounts of 500 mg. every 6 hours; some investigators have used two infusions of 1 Gm. each at a 12-hour interval. Doses of 3 to 4 Gm. should be used only in desperately ill patients who have normal renal function. For children, the daily dose is 20 mg. per kilogram of body weight.

Side effects and toxic effects. Toxic symptoms include impairment of auditory acuity, thrombophlebitis because it is irritating, macular skin rashes, and febrile reactions. Toxicity is minimal for most short-term

*Described in annual publication of A. M. A. Council on Drugs, N.N.D., 1960.

therapy. The drug should be used with caution in patients with renal damage because it may accumulate in the blood and the chance of ototoxicity is increased. If doses of more than 2 Gm. per day are used, periodic determinations of the blood urea nitrogen level are suggested.

Viomycin Sulfate (Vinactane Sulfate, Viocin Sulfate)

Viomycin sulfate is the salt of an antibiotic obtained from *Streptomyces puniceus*. It is an antituberculosis agent which is less active than streptomycin but more active than aminosalicylic acid.

Uses. Because of its potential toxicity, its use should be restricted to the treatment of patients who are unable to tolerate other antituberculosis drugs or in patients with tuberculosis caused by organisms resistant to them. Apparently cross resistance does not develop between viomycin and streptomycin or isoniazid.

Absorption, distribution, and excretion. When given orally, effective blood levels of viomycin sulfate are not achieved. When given parenterally, the drug is absorbed and well distributed except to the spinal fluid or pleural and peritoneal cavities. It is excreted largely by the kidneys.

Preparation, dosage, and administration.

Viomycin Sulfate* (Vinactane Sulfate, Viocin Sulfate). Viomycin sulfate should be administered by slow intramuscular injection. Intravenous injection should be avoided because it results in greater danger of toxic reactions. More investigation of the intrathecal route for tuberculous meningitis is needed.

When administered intramuscularly in tuberculosis, the usual dose is 2 Gm., given in two doses of 1 Gm. each, 12 hours apart, every third day. It can be given alone or with aminosalicylic acid orally. This dosage can be continued at least four to six months. In special instances, dosage might be increased (for not more than one month), but the patient must be carefully watched for toxic symptoms.

Side effects and toxic effects. Viomycin sulfate is a potentially toxic drug. Toxic symptoms include allergic reactions, renal irritation, eosinophilia, edema, electrolyte disturbance, abnormal renal function, dizziness, electrocardiographic abnormalities, and partial loss of hearing.

Nonsystemic antibiotics

Fumagillin (Fumidil)

Fumagillin is an antibiotic derived from strains of *Aspergillus fumigatus*.

Action and uses. Fumagillin is used clinically for intestinal infection with *Entamoeba histolytica*. Because it has no effect on fungi or bac-

*Described in annual publication of A. M. A. Council on Drugs, N.N.D., 1960.

teria, oral therapy is not accompanied by changes in the normal flora of the intestinal tract. The excretion and fate of fumagillin in the body are not completely known; because systemic side effects occur, partial absorption of the drug is indicated. Fumagillin has no effect on extraintestinal amebiasis.

Preparation, dosage, and administration.

Fumagillin* (Fumidil). The commercial preparation is called Fumidil and is available in 10 mg. tablets.

The usual daily dose is 40 mg. given in four divided doses; therapy is continued for 10 to 14 days. Doses up to 60 mg. may be tried in resistant cases. It is given orally.

Side effects and toxic effects. Side effects are frequent, especially at high dosage levels. They are seldom serious and usually reversible. They include abdominal cramping, a sensation of epigastric burning, anorexia, nausea, vomiting, diarrhea, headache, dizziness, and vesicular skin eruptions. It is believed that fumagillin may have caused a few cases of neutropenia; therefore, peripheral blood cell counts are advised during prolonged therapy.

Nystatin (Mycostatin)

Nystatin is an antibiotic obtained from *Streptomyces noursei.*

Absorption and excretion. Nystatin is poorly absorbed from the intestinal tract. It is excreted almost entirely in the feces after oral administration. The parenteral administration of nystatin is not feasible at present because of local irritation and questionable absorption. Apparently it is not absorbed through the skin and mucous membrane when applied topically.

Action and uses. Nystatin is useful in treating infections caused by the monilial organism *Candida albicans.* In vitro, nystatin is effective against many yeasts and molds. However, its clinical effectiveness against mycotic infections other than those caused by *Candida albicans* has not been established.

Preparation, dosage, and administration.

Nystatin, U.S.P. (Mycostatin). Nystatin is available in the following official preparations: oral suspension, ointment, and tablets.

For gastrointestinal moniliasis, the proposed dose is 500,000 to 1,000,-000 units, given orally three times a day. The oral route may be used concurrently with local application in resistant anal or vaginal moniliasis to decrease the possibility of reinfection from the intestines.

For monilial lesions of the mouth (thrush), suspensions of nystatin in water, honey, or other vehicles, containing 100,000 units per milliliter, may be dropped into the mouth or applied locally by applicator. Vaginal

*Described in annual publication of A. M. A. Council on Drugs, N.N.D., 1960.

tablets or suppositories containing 100,000 units are inserted once or twice a day for vaginal moniliasis. A concentration containing 100,000 units of nystatin per gram may be applied to mycotic lesions of the skin or mucous membranes once to several times a day.

To prevent intestinal moniliasis, patients undergoing oral therapy with broad-spectrum antibiotics may be given nystatin concurrently.

Side effects and toxic effects. Nystatin has few side effects, and these are mild and transitory. They include nausea, vomiting, and diarrhea after oral administration.

Tyrothricin (Soluthricin)

Tyrothricin is an antibacterial substance produced by *Bacillus brevis*. It consists of two substances called gramicidin and tyrocidine. Gramicidin is more active than tyrocidine and probably accounts for the action of tyrothricin. It is active against many gram-positive bacteria. However, it is rapidly inactivated in the body and has so many toxic reactions that it cannot be used systemically. It causes hemolysis, injury to the spleen, kidneys, and liver, and irritation of the meninges.

Its usefulness is limited to topical applications for the treatment of local infections. With caution, it may be used in body cavities if there is no direct connection with the blood stream.

Preparation, dosage, and administration.

Tyrothricin, N.F. (Soluthricin). For local application, a solution containing 500 mcg. per milliliter is used. The N.F. lists tyrothricin spray and troches in addition to the solution.

Questions
for review and study

Single choice
Encircle the answer of your choice.

1 Which of the following has constituted the richest source of antibiotic substances?
  a. molds
  b. bacteria
  c. Streptomyces
  d. chemical synthesis
2 For which of the following pairs of diseases is the administration of penicillin considered ineffective?
  a. syphilis and gonorrhea
  b. pneumococcic pneumonia and anthrax
  c. malaria and tuberculosis
  d. actinomycosis and Vincent's infection
3 Which of the following methods of administration is used most frequently to give penicillin for systemic effects?
  a. by inhalation
  b. oral

  c. intravenous
  d. intramuscular
4 Which of the following constitute side effects to be watched for in a patient getting tetracycline?
  a. nausea, vomiting, loose stools
  b. dizziness, incoordination, deafness
  c. urticaria, dermatitis, pruritus
  d. leukopenia, anemia
5 The official name for Achromycin is:
  a. chlortetracycline
  b. oxytetracycline
  c. tetracycline
  d. Tetracyn
6 From which of the following sources is streptomycin obtained?
  a. *Streptomyces erythreus*
  b. *Streptomyces fradiae*
  c. *Streptomyces rimosus*
  d. *Streptomyces griseus*
7 Which of the following antibiotics is effective only against gram-negative organisms?

a. neomycin
b. bacitracin
c. polymyxin
d. erythromycin

8 Which of the following antibiotics, when given for systemic effects, may cause kidney damage?
a. carbomycin and erythromycin
b. polymyxin, neomycin, and bacitracin
c. penicillin, Aureomycin, and Terramycin
d. novobiocin and oleandomycin

9 Which of the following constitutes the most distinct advantage of Aureomycin over penicillin?
a. wider range of antibacterial activity
b. no side effects
c. satisfactory blood levels result from the usual oral dosage
d. less expensive

10 Which of the following pairs of antibiotics have been found effective in the treatment of certain viral and rickettsial infections?
a. streptomycin and neomycin
b. oxytetracycline and tetracycline
c. bacitracin and tyrothricin
d. penicillin and dihydrostreptomycin

11 If a patient is getting chloramphenicol, which of the following laboratory tests would you expect the doctor to order?
a. stool examination
b. audiometric and vestibular function tests
c. blood cell counts
d. urinalysis

12 If a patient becomes sensitive to penicillin, which of the following statements best explains the situation?
a. The infecting organisms are more affected by penicillin than usual.
b. The patient will not react to penicillin one way or the other.
c. The patient will show allergic symptoms when given penicillin.
d. The infecting organisms will be able to grow in spite of the presence of penicillin.

13 When in the course of treatment with an antibiotic, resistance is said to have developed, which of the following will have developed the resistance?
a. the antibiotic
b. the patient's body cells
c. the infecting organisms
d. immune bodies in the patient's blood

14 Which of the following reasons *best* explains why penicillin is not prescribed for an ordinary cold (no complications)?
a. The cold virus develops resistance easily.
b. The patient may be sensitized.
c. Penicillin has no effect on the virus causing a cold.
d. Penicillin is very expensive.

References

General references

A. M. A. Council on Drugs: New and Nonofficial Drugs, Philadelphia, 1960, J. B. Lippincott Co.

Antibiotics Today (editorial), Bull. Am. Soc. Hosp. Pharmacists 11: 449, 1954.

Beckman, H.: Drugs, Their Nature, Action, and Use, Philadelphia and London, 1958, W. B. Saunders Co.

Drill, V. A.: Pharmacology in Medicine, New York, 1958, McGraw-Hill Book Co., Inc.

Dubos, R.: Mirage of Health, New York, 1959, Harper & Brothers.

Editorial Staff: Antibiotics Symposium, Am. Prof. Pharmacist 20: 51, 1954.

Heilman, F. R.: Antibiotics, Ann. Rev. Microbiol. 7: 219, 1953.

Jager, B. V.: Untoward Reactions to Antibiotics, Am. J. Nursing 54: 966, 1954.

Martin, W. J.: Some Notes on Antibiotics and Chemotherapy in Infectious Diseases, M. Ann. District of Columbia 22: 283, 1953.

Martin, W. J., Nichols, D. R., and Geraci, J. E.: General Principles and Use of Antibiotics, Am. Pract. & Digest Treat. 10: 813, 1954.

Modell, W. (editor): Drugs of Choice, 1960-1961, St. Louis, 1960, The C. V. Mosby Co.

Nichols, D. R., and Andersen, H. A.: Treatment of Pneumonia, M. Clin. North America 38: 981, 1954.

Shirger, A., Martin, W. J., and Nichols, D. R.: Antibiotic Therapy: Clinical Applications of Available Agents, GP 19: 102, 1959.

Spink, W. W.: Clinical Problems Relating to the Management of Infections With Antibiotics, J. A. M. A. 152: 585, 1953.

Chlortetracycline

Dearing, W. H., and Heilman, F. R.: The Effect of Aureomycin on the Bacterial

Flora of the Intestinal Tract of Man, Proc. Staff Meet. Mayo Clin. **25:** 87, 1950.

Hargraves, M. M., Mills, S. D., and Heck, F. J.: Aplastic Anemia Associated With Administration of Chloramphenicol, J. A. M. A. **149:** 1293, 1952.

Herrell, W. E., and Heilman, F. R.: Aureomycin: Studies on Absorption, Diffusion and Excretion, Proc. Staff Meet. Mayo Clin. **24:** 157, 1950.

Chloramphenicol

Altemeier, W. A., and Giuseffi, J.: Chloromycetin in Surgical Infections, Surg. Gynec. & Obst. **90:** 583, 1950.

Friedman, A.: An Evaluation of Chloramphenicol Therapy in Typhoid Fever in Children, Pediatrics **14:** 28, 1954.

Ley, H. L., Woodward, T. E., and Smadel, J. E.: Chloramphenicol in the Treatment of Murine Typhus, J. A. M. A. **143:** 217, 1950.

Erythromycin

Dearing, W. H., and Heilman, F. R.: Micrococcic (Staphylococcic) Enteritis as a Complication of Antibiotic Therapy; Its Response to Erythromycin, Proc. Staff Meet. Mayo Clin. **28:** 121, 1953.

Heilman, F. R., Herrell, W. E., Wellman, W. E., and Geraci, J. E.: Some Laboratory and Clinical Observations on a New Antibiotic, Erythromycin (Ilotycin), Proc. Staff Meet. Mayo Clin. **27:** 285, 1952.

Martin, W. J., Nichols, D. R., and Geraci, J. E.: The Present Status of Erythromycin, Proc. Staff Meet. Mayo Clin. **28:** 609, 1953.

Penicillin

Epstein, E.: Failure of Penicillin in Treatment of Acute Gonorrhea in American Troops in Korea, J. A. M. A. **169:** 1055, 1959.

Fleming, Sir Alexander: Penicillin, Its Practical Application, St. Louis, 1950, The C. V. Mosby Co. (Butterworth & Co., Ltd., London).

Ford, J. H., Churchill, B. W., and Colingsworth, D. R.: Penicillin O, Antibiotics & Chemother. **4:** 1149, 1953.

Geraci, J. E., and Manning, P. R.: Antibiotic Therapy in Bacterial Endocarditis. III. Penicillin O and Hypoallergic Penicillins in the Treatment of Subacute Bacterial Endocarditis, Minnesota Med. **38:** 466, 1953.

Hyman, A. L.: Anaphylactic Shock After Therapy With Penicillinase, J. A. M. A. **169:** 593, 1959.

Reisch, M.: Penicillinase Therapy—Clinical Report of Severe Reactions, J. A. M. A. **169:** 594, 1959.

Streptomycin and dihydrostreptomycin

Carr, D. T., Brown, H. A., Hodgson, C. H., and Heilman, F. R.: Neurotoxic Reactions to Dihydrostreptomycin, J. A. M. A. **143:** 1223, 1950.

Council on Pharmacy and Chemistry: Chemotherapy of Tuberculosis in Man Present Status, J. A. M. A. **154:** 52, 1954.

Waksman, Selman A.: Tenth Anniversary of the Discovery of Streptomycin, the First Chemotherapeutic Agent Found to Be Effective Against Tuberculosis in Humans, Am. Rev. Tuberc. **70:** 1, 1954.

Oxytetracycline (Terramycin)

Herrell, W. E.: Newer Antibiotics, Ann. Rev. Microb., Jan., 1949, through Feb., 1950.

Herrell, W. E., Heilman, F. R., Wellman, W. E., and Bartholomew, L. G.: Terramycin, Some Pharmacologic and Clinical Observations, Proc. Staff. Meet. Mayo Clin. **25:** 183, 1950.

Melcher, G. W., Gibson, C. D., Rose, H. M., and Kneeland, Y.: Terramycin in Pneumonia, J. A. M. A. **143:** 1303, 1950.

Tetracycline

Cunningham, R. W., and others: Pharmacology of Tetracycline, Antibiotics Ann., pp. 63-69, 1953-1954.

Finland, M., and others: Clinical and Laboratory Observations of a New Antibiotic, Tetracycline, J. A. M. A. **154:** 561, 1954.

Putnam, L. E., Hendricks, F. D., and Welch, H.: Tetracycline, a New Antibiotic, Antibiotics Ann., pp. 88-91, 1953-1954.

Welch, Henry: An Appraisal of Tetracycline (editorial), Antibiotics & Chemother. **4:** 375, 1954.

Kanamycin

Finland, M.: Summary of the Monograph on the Basic and Clinical Research of the New Antibiotic, Kanamycin, Annals of the New York Academy of Sciences, **76:** 391, 1958.

170

Chapter 9

Drugs that affect
the central
nervous system

The central and peripheral nervous systems of the body constitute the mechanism by which the body makes rapid adjustments to its environment. Not all adjustments are rapid, but when rapid reactions are needed, the nervous system makes them possible.

Action of drugs on the central nervous system

Drugs act to increase or decrease the activity of nerve centers and conducting pathways. Stimulants and depressants of the brain, the spinal cord, or specific centers of each have been developed, and their effects, on the whole, are highly predictable.

The *cerebral cortex* is the site of consciousness. Drugs depressing cortical activity cause effects which range from decreased acuity of sensation to drowsiness and sleep. When the sensory areas of the cortex are stimulated, more numerous and more vivid impulses are received and the patient is more alert, responsive, and more aware of his surroundings. When the motor centers are stimulated the patient is likely to be more active and restless, but when overstimulated, coordination may be lost and convulsions may result. When the speech center is stimulated the patient becomes more talkative, and if the stimulation is excessive, speech becomes incessant and incoherent and the patient may become delirious. Such effects can also be due to depression of higher centers of control, as can be seen in acute alcoholism.

The association areas of the cerebral cortex are concerned with memory, perception, and the integration of various sensory experiences, and they function in what is spoken of as *higher mental activity*. This means thinking, reasoning, the exercise of judgment, will, imagination, and attention. Drugs that stimulate these centers enable the individual to think faster (not necessarily better) and form judgments more quickly. In some instances flights of imagination are produced. Cortical depressants bring about loss of interest in the surroundings and decreased ability to concentrate. The specific response brought forth by a drug depends to a large extent also on the personality of the individual and a number of other factors as well as on the nature of the drug itself.

The *thalamus* is composed of sensory nuclei and serves as a relay center for impulses to and from the cerebral cortex. It also serves as a center of unlocalized sensations; e.g., it enables us to have impressions of agreeableness or disagreeableness about a sensation. Drugs that depress cells in the various portions of the thalamus may interrupt the free flow of impulses to the cerebral cortex. This is one way pain is relieved.

The *hypothalamus* lies below the thalamus and contains centers which regulate body temperature, carbohydrate and fat metabolism, and water balance. There is evidence that there is also a center for sleep and wakefulness here. Some of the sleep-producing drugs are thought to depress centers in the hypothalamus; others are known to affect the heat-regulating center, e.g., aspirin. The thalamus and the hypothalamus constitute important regions of the brain known as the diencephalon.

The *medulla oblongata* contains the so-called vital centers, the respiratory, vasomotor, and cardiac centers. If the respiratory center is stimulated it will discharge an increased number of nerve impulses over nerve pathways to the muscles of respiration. If it is depressed it will discharge fewer impulses, and respiration will be correspondingly affected. Other centers in the medulla that respond to certain drugs are the cough center and the vomiting center. The medulla, pons, and the midbrain constitute the *brain stem* and contain many important correlation centers (gray matter) as well as ascending and descending pathways (white matter).

The *reticular formation* is a part of the central nervous system that has been studied increasingly in recent years and its importance is only beginning to be appreciated. It is made up of cells and fine bundles of nerve fibers which extend in many directions. The formation extends from the upper part of the spinal cord forward through the brain stem to the diencephalon.* It exhibits both inhibitory as well as excitatory functions in relation to other parts of the nervous system. It receives afferent impulses from all parts of the body and relays impulses to the cortex to promote wakefulness and alertness, thus affecting many cerebral functions, e.g., consciousness and learning. It also inhibits or excites activity in motor neurons, promoting both reflex and voluntary movements. Its over-all function is thought to be that of an integrating system which influences activities of other parts of the nervous system.

*Greisheimer, E. M.: Physiology and Anatomy, Philadelphia, 1955, J. B. Lippincott Co., p. 305.

Depression of the reticular formation produces sedation and loss of consciousness. Many drugs are now believed to exert an effect on the reticular formation.

The *cerebellum* contains centers for muscle coordination, equilibrium, and muscle tone. It receives afferent impulses from the vestibular nuclei as well as the cerebrum and plays an important role in the maintenance of posture. Drugs that disturb the cerebellum or vestibular branch of the eighth cranial nerve cause loss of equilibrium and dizziness.

The *spinal cord*, a center for reflex activity, also functions in the transmission of impulses to and from the higher centers in the brain and may be affected by the action of drugs. Large doses of spinal stimulants may cause convulsions; smaller doses may increase reflex excitability.

When a drug is described as having a *central action* it means that it has an action on the brain or the spinal cord.

Stimulants

The drugs included under this heading will be limited, for the most part, to those whose major effect is on the central nervous system. There are other drugs such as atropine, cocaine, and ephedrine whose action as central nervous system stimulants is secondary to their other effects; that is, these latter drugs do act on the central nervous system but, medically, have even more important actions on other systems of the body.

The central nervous system stimulants may at times produce dramatic effects, but their therapeutic usefulness is limited because of the multiplicity of their actions and the nature of their side effects and because repeated administration and large doses are prone to precipitate convulsive seizures, often alternating with periods of coma and exhaustion. The number of drugs that stimulate the central nervous system is large, but the number actually employed for this purpose is limited. Those having particular therapeutic value are the respiratory stimulants and the analeptics.

Classification

These drugs are classified on the basis of where in the nervous system they exert their major effects, i.e., on the cerebrum, the medulla and brain stem, or on the spinal cord. Amphetamine is mainly a stimulant of the cerebral cortex, nikethamide acts mainly on the centers in the medulla and the brain stem, and strychnine is a spinal stimulant. These drugs may also affect other parts of the nervous system.

The xanthines

Caffeine, theobromine, and theophylline are known as methylated xanthines. Their actions are similar, although their effect on specific structures varies in intensity.

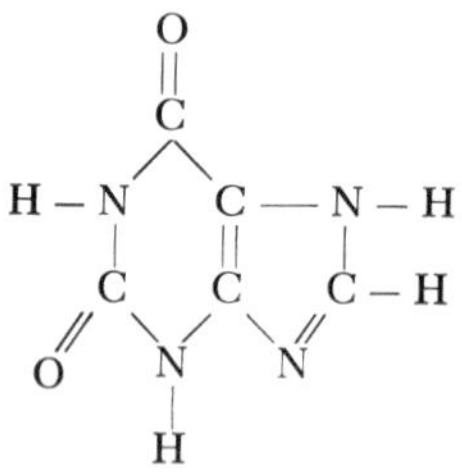

Xanthine

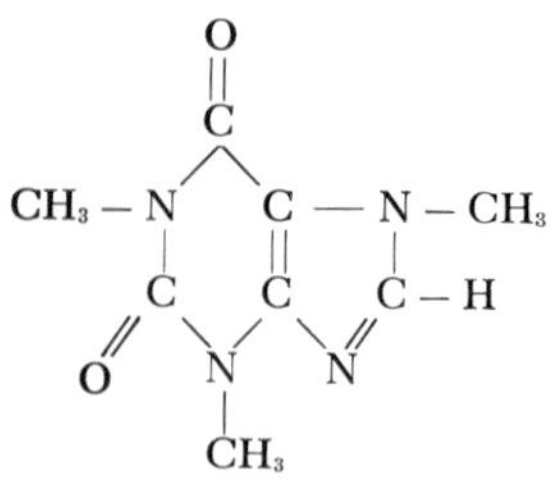

Caffeine
(1,3,7-trimethyl-
xanthine)

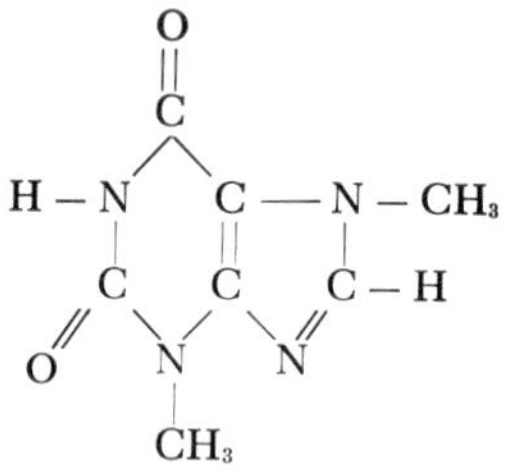

Theobromine
(3,7-dimethyl-
xanthine)

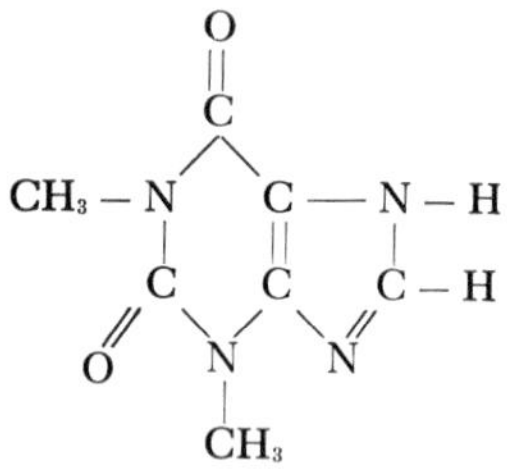

Theophylline
(1,3-dimethyl-
xanthine)

Note that caffeine is a trimethylxanthine (three methyl groups) and theobromine and theophylline are dimethylxanthines (two methyl groups). Caffeine, theophylline, and theobromine are alkaloids which all act on the central nervous system, the kidney, the heart, the skeletal muscle, and the smooth muscle, but the degree of their action on these structures varies considerably. For example, of the three xanthines, caffeine is the most effective stimulant of the central nervous system, theophylline is less effective, and theobromine has little effect. On the kidney, theophylline ranks first in effectiveness, theobromine second, and caffeine third. Aminophylline (a theophylline compound) is the xanthine preparation of choice to produce relaxation of the smooth muscle of the coronary vessels and the bronchial tubes and to produce diuresis. Theobromine and theophylline will be discussed further in later chapters (see Index).

Caffeine

Source. Caffeine, U.S.P., is a white crystalline powder commercially obtained from tea leaves. It is the active alkaloid occurring in a number of plants used as beverages: e.g., coffee, the seed of the *Coffea arabica;*

174

Caffeine—Descending Stimulant of the Central Nervous System

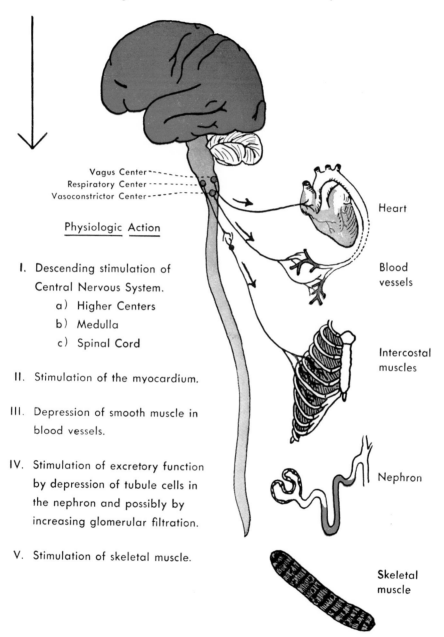

Vagus Center
Respiratory Center
Vasoconstrictor Center

Heart

Blood vessels

Intercostal muscles

Nephron

Skeletal muscle

Physiologic Action

I. Descending stimulation of
   Central Nervous System.
   a) Higher Centers
   b) Medulla
   c) Spinal Cord

II. Stimulation of the myocardium.

III. Depression of smooth muscle in
   blood vessels.

IV. Stimulation of excretory function
   by depression of tubule cells in
   the nephron and possibly by
   increasing glomerular filtration.

V. Stimulation of skeletal muscle.

Plate 1

Areas shaded in red represent degrees of stimulation. Areas shaded in
blue represent depression.

tea, the leaves of *Thea sinensis;* the kola nut of Central America; gua-
rana, derived from the seeds of a Brazilian plant and from yerba maté
or Paraguay tea. Tea contains from 1 to 5 per cent of caffeine; coffee,
from 1 to 2 per cent. Tea contains 10 to 24 per cent of tannin. Coffee
contains a variable amount of caffeo-tannic acid (av., about 12 per cent)
which is not very astringent.

Action and result. Caffeine stimulates the central nervous system,
especially the cerebral cortex. Its action is a descending one, i.e., small
doses (100 to 150 mg.) stimulate the cerebrum, and larger doses stimulate the medullary centers and the spinal cord. Doses large enough to
stimulate the spinal cord are never ordered. As a result of the cortical
stimulation the individual is more alert, thinks faster, has a better memory, forms judgments more quickly, learns faster (temporarily), and has
a decreased reaction time. Drowsiness and fatigue disappear. The sense
of touch may be more discriminating and the sense of pain more keen.
The latter effect may not be desirable in the sick person when it brings
about greater realization of the gravity of an illness. Stimulation is not
necessarily followed by depression except as it brings about exhaustion
of natural reserves.

Caffeine, when taken orally in ordinary therapeutic doses, has little
or no effect on medullary centers. Large doses given parenterally will
stimulate the respiratory center, especially if it is moderately depressed.
There is some stimulation of the vagus and vasoconstrictor centers of
the medulla, although this is partially masked by the peripheral action
on the heart and blood vessels.

Large doses of caffeine stimulate the entire central nervous system,
including the spinal cord. There is first an increased reflex excitability
which may with increasing dosage result in muscle twitching, especially
in the limbs and face.

Caffeine stimulates the myocardium, bringing about both an increased
cardiac rate and an increased cardiac output. This effect is antagonistic
to that produced on the vagus center; consequently a slight slowing of
the heart may be observed in some individuals and an increased rate in
others. The latter effect usually predominates after large doses. Overstimulation may cause a harmful tachycardia and cardiac irregularities.

Peripherally, caffeine depresses the smooth muscle of the blood vessels, thus causing vasodilation in contrast to the vasoconstriction produced by its central action. However, after therapeutic doses the peripheral action predominates and results in increased flow of blood and improved circulation. A slight and somewhat transitory elevation of blood
pressure is sometimes noted. Some investigators are of the opinion that
caffeine constricts the intracranial blood vessels and brings about some
lowering of intracranial pressure.

Improved muscle tone and lessened susceptibility to fatigue have also been observed, but whether the action is a direct one on the striated muscle cells or whether the effect is produced by masking the sense of fatigue through cerebral stimulation is not fully understood.

Like the other xanthines, caffeine increases the flow of urine, but its action is relatively weak. The mode of action seems to be that of depressing the tubule cells and preventing reabsorption of fluid.

The metabolic rate is slightly increased after caffeine. An appreciable tolerance to certain effects of caffeine is readily established, although apparently not to the cerebral effects. Caffeine is also used to relieve fatigue, depression, and headache.

Caffeine stimulates the output of pepsin as well as hydrochloric acid in the gastric juice.* Coffee therefore is usually contraindicated in the diet of patients with gastric or duodenal ulcer.

Uses. Caffeine is used as a mild cerebral stimulant. It is used also occasionally as a respiratory stimulant, provided the depression of the medullary center is not severe. In cases of severe respiratory depression there are better respiratory stimulants. Caffeine is no longer used for the relief of narcotic depression unless more effective drugs are not available.

Caffeine is used with one or more analgesic drugs or with ergotamine tartrate for the relief of headache. Its effect in such cases is thought to be due to its effect on the cerebral blood vessels.†

Preparation, dosage, and administration.

Caffeine, U.S.P., B.P. Usual dose is 0.2 Gm. (3 gr.).

Caffeine and Sodium Benzoate Injection, U.S.P. It is available in 2 ml. ampules. Usual dose is 0.5 Gm. (7½ gr.).

Citrated Caffeine, N.F. Usual dose is 0.3 Gm. (5 gr.).

Ergotamine with Caffeine (Cafergot). Each tablet contains 1 mg. of ergotamine tartrate and 100 mg. of caffeine. The drug is given orally for migraine headache (1 to 2 tablets).

Caffeine is usually prescribed as Citrated Caffeine or Caffeine and Sodium Benzoate because they are more soluble than caffeine itself. Caffeine and Sodium Benzoate is usually given intramuscularly, whereas the citrated form is given orally. Caffeine may also be given in the form of a beverage either orally or by rectum. The caffeine content of an average cup of coffee "as made in the United States" is from 2 to 3 gr.‡ Caffeine sometimes exhibits a local irritant action on the gastric mucosa, resulting in nausea and vomiting or gastric distress. Sick persons often

*Roth, J. A., and Ivy, A. C.: Am. J. Physiol. 141: 461, 1944.

†Horton, B. T., and others: Clinical Observations on the Use of E. C. 110, A New Agent for the Treatment of Headache, Proc. Staff Meet. Mayo Clin. 23: 105, 1948.

‡Cooper, L. F., Barber, E. M., Mitchell, H. S., and Rynbergen, H. J.: Nutrition in Health and Disease, Philadelphia, 1958, J. B. Lippincott Co., p. 410.

do not tolerate coffee well as a beverage, especially if they are slightly nauseated. Weak tea is often much better tolerated by the patient who is resuming oral fluids after anesthesia.

Side effects and toxic effects. Fatal poisoning by caffeine is rare, partly due to the fact that it is readily excreted. The fatal dose is presumably about 10 Gm. Toxic doses produce excessive irritability, restlessness, insomnia, nervousness, profuse flow of urine, nausea and vomiting, headache, and heart palpitation, particularly in susceptible individuals. The more chronic symptoms of poisoning include insomnia, anxiety, and functional cardiac symptoms. The signs of chronic caffeine poisoning are more commonly seen among workers such as night nurses, who use coffee to keep awake and continue work when physically tired. The symptoms of nervousness disappear when the overuse of coffee is remedied. The use of coffee to combat fatigue is like a whip to a tired horse, and it would be better to get needed rest than to continue using coffee to "keep going."

The question is sometimes raised as to whether or not caffeine causes habituation and addiction. Many persons note that if they do not have their usual cup or two of coffee in the morning, they feel irritable and nervous and develop a headache. This probably indicates habituation rather than true addiction.* Both tea and coffee should be omitted from the diets of children, partly because they have no need for stimulants and partly because they need food such as milk instead.

Treatment. Stopping the intake of caffeine and providing rest and quiet are sufficient. In certain individuals a short-acting sedative may be indicated.

The amphetamines

The amphetamines are a group of drugs known as the sympathomimetic amines. They exert a stimulating action on the cerebral cortex and, in addition, exert an effect similar to that obtained when the sympathetic nervous system is stimulated. The latter action of these drugs will be presented in Chapter 10, Autonomic Drugs. The amphetamines are synthetic preparations.

Amphetamine

Source. Amphetamine is prepared synthetically from ephedrine. The following formulas indicate points of similarity and difference.

Ephedrine   Amphetamine

*See discussion of addiction and habituation, p. 129.

Action and result. Amphetamine stimulates the central nervous system, particularly the cerebral cortex. The effects depend upon the personality of the individual, the mental state, and the amount of drug administered. The results of action seen after oral administration usually include an elevation of mood which may become a true euphoric exhilaration, decreased feeling of fatigue, increased willingness to work, increased confidence, alertness, power of concentration, and sometimes talkativeness. Continued use may cause irritability, sleeplessness, dizziness, anorexia. Large doses tend to be followed by fatigue and mental depression. Amphetamine may fortify a person for prolonged physical and mental exertion, but the end result in terms of fatigue is correspondingly greater and requires a longer period for rest than usual. When the respiratory center is depressed amphetamine exerts a stimulating effect upon it; this is significant in treatment of poisoning from depressant drugs.

Uses. Amphetamine is used to bring about symptomatic treatment of narcolepsy. Many patients can be relieved of overpowering attacks of sleep.

For various manifestations of postencephalitic parkinsonism the drug is given to bring about improvement in muscle strength, decreased rigidity, and a sense of increased energy. Subjective improvement may be more marked, however, than objective decrease in tremor and rigidity.

In the total treatment of alcoholism, amphetamine may play a part because of its favorable effect on mental depression.

This drug is useful in the treatment of certain patients with mental disease in which depression is a prominent symptom. It is also used to treat many mild psychogenic states, particularly those attending childbirth, menopause, old age, chronic fatigue, etc. Its use, however, is subordinate to treatment that will bring about removal of the underlying causes of the disorder.

Amphetamine may be useful to depress the appetite of the patient who is dieting to overcome obesity. Many physicians, however, do not recommend its use for this purpose because as soon as the drug is withdrawn the former appetite returns, and unless the patient has established a new food pattern he or she usually returns to the old habit of overeating. Furthermore, obese persons may have disturbances of the cardiovascular system which contraindicate the use of the amphetamines.

Amphetamine may be used as an analeptic in certain cases of poisoning from depressant drugs. "Analeptic" is a general name for drugs that restore consciousness and mental alertness, as from a state of anesthesia or hypnosis. Other uses for amphetamine and related compounds are mentioned in Chapter 10.

Preparation, dosage, and administration.

Amphetamine Sulfate, U.S.P., B.P. This drug is marketed in tablets of

5 and 10 mg. each, in an elixir (0.5 mg. per milliliter), in solution for injection (20 mg. per milliliter), and in 15 mg. sustained release capsules (Spansules). It is marketed under the trade name of Benzedrine. Amphetamine sulfate is usually administered orally and given in divided doses; i.e., the total daily dose is divided into several smaller doses and distributed through the day. To prevent interference with sleep the final dose of the day preferably should not be given after 4 P.M. When injected it is given intramuscularly or by slow intravenous drip.

Amphetamine Phosphate, N.F. (Raphetamine Phosphate). This form is available in 5 mg. tablets and as an elixir (1.25 mg. per milliliter) for oral administration and in solution for injection (100 mg. per 10 ml.). Small initial doses, 5 mg. or less, are recommended, to be followed if necessary with gradually increased amounts. Amphetamine phosphate has the same effects and uses as amphetamine sulfate, but its physical property of increased solubility in water makes it better suited for parenteral administration, although it may also be given orally.

Side effects and contraindications. There is danger in using amphetamine promiscuously to overcome sleepiness and lack of alertness because the natural warning signs associated with fatigue may be eliminated. Furthermore, amphetamine is a habit-forming drug. It is to be avoided by persons with hypertension and cardiovascular disease and by persons who are unduly restless, anxious, agitated, and excited. Side effects include dryness of the mouth, headache, insomnia, irritability, a sense of intoxication, and possibly constipation.

Benzedrex

Benzedrex is the trade name for propylhexedrine and serves as a substitute for the previously used Benzedrine Inhaler. Benzedrex has a minimal of central effects, although it is useful to relieve nasal congestion.

Dextro Amphetamine Sulfate (Dexedrine Sulfate)

Action and uses. Dextro amphetamine sulfate, for the most part, has the same action and uses as amphetamine sulfate, although it exhibits a greater stimulating effect on the central nervous system. It is considered to be less toxic than the previously mentioned amphetamine because of its diminished sympathomimetic activity; i.e., it seldom causes rapid pulse, changes in blood pressure, tremor, etc. However, the same dangers attend its indiscriminate use as is true of the other amphetamines.

The racemic compound, amphetamine sulfate, contains two optical isomers which behave differently in relation to polarized light. The one, when in solution, will cause a beam of polarized light to be bent to the left and the other will cause it to be bent to the right. They are spoken of, respectively, as the levo (l), or levorotatory, and the dextro (d), or dextrorotatory, parts of the parent substance. In the racemic compound both forms are present, i.e., dl-amphetamine. In the case of amphetamine sulfate, as for other asymmetric compounds, the physiologic activity of the two forms is different. The levo component has more effect on the cardiovascular system, and the dextro component is more active as a stimulant of the central nervous system. Dextro amphetamine is chemically separated from the parent substance dl-amphetamine or amphetamine sulfate.

Preparation, dosage, and administration.

Dextro Amphetamine Sulfate, U.S.P. (Dexedrine Sulfate); *Dexamphetamine Sulfate*, B.P. It is available in 5 and 10 mg. tablets, as an elixir (5 mg. per 5 ml.), and in sustained release capsules (Spansules) containing 5, 10, or 15 mg. of drug. It is also marketed in combination with analgesics such as aspirin or phenacetin or with one of the barbiturates such as amobarbital. The latter combination is sometimes used when elevation of blood pressure and insomnia constitute problems. The usual dose of dextro amphetamine is 5 mg. twice daily, and it is given orally.

Methamphetamine Hydrochloride (Desoxyephedrine Hydrochloride)

Methamphetamine hydrochloride greatly resembles amphetamine sulfate, the two drugs differing in their action only in degree. The central stimulant action of this drug is slightly greater and the cardiovascular action is slightly less than that of amphetamine. Like amphetamine, it is used in the treatment of narcolepsy, to relieve symptoms of postencephalitic parkinsonism, as part of the treatment for alcoholism, and in various types of depressed states. Because it allays hunger and depresses motility in the gastrointestinal tract, it has been used in the treatment of obesity. It has the same disadvantages as a form of treatment for obesity as was mentioned under amphetamine sulfate.

It is contraindicated for patients with hypertension, cardiovascular disease, hyperthyroidism, anxiety states, or undue restlessness.

Preparation, dosage, and administration.

Methamphetamine Hydrochloride, N.F. (Desoxyephedrine Hydrochloride); *Methylamphetamine Hydrochloride*, B.P. It is marketed in 5 and 10 mg. capsules, 2.5, 5, 7.5, and 10 mg. tablets, as an elixir (0.667 and 1 mg. per milliliter), and in solution for injection (20 mg. per milliliter). Methamphetamine is given parenterally as well as orally. The beginning oral dose is 2.5 mg. daily; this is increased to 2.5 to 5 mg. two or three times a day until the desired response is obtained. In case of emergency, 10 to 15 mg. may be given slowly by intravenous injection.* In emergency, usual dose is 15 to 30 mg. when the drug is given intramuscularly.

*Council on Drugs, N.N.D., 1960, p. 225.

180

Phenmetrazine Hydrochloride (Preludin)

Phenmetrazine hydrochloride* is a relatively new preparation which resembles amphetamine pharmacologically, especially in its ability to depress appetite. It is a mild stimulant of the central nervous system, and it rarely causes changes in pulse rate and blood pressure. It is administered orally in 25 mg. doses two or three times a day, an hour before meals.

Other stimulants

The amphetamines have effects on the cardiovascular and other systems besides the central nervous system; hence these effects become unwanted side effects when the drugs are used primarily for their stimulating effects on the central nervous system. This has led to a search for compounds with similar central effects but fewer side effects; two new analeptic compounds have resulted, pipradrol and methylphenidate.

Pipradrol Hydrochloride (Meratran Hydrochloride)

Both pipradrol and methylphenidate are derivatives of piperidine, and the two compounds exhibit pharmacologic similarities.

Pipradrol   Methylphenidate

Action and result. Pipradrol is said to resemble amphetamine, although it produces less anorexia, insomnia, and euphoria. It seems to have little effect on pulse, blood pressure, and respiration when dosage is kept within therapeutic range. It is a mild cerebral stimulant producing elevation of mood, increased ability to work, heightened confidence, and increased ability to concentrate.

Uses. Pipradrol has been used to produce an increased sense of well-being, especially in elderly patients who feel that life no longer holds anything for them, in persons ill with chronic disease and in cases in which depressed states are not associated with compulsive behavior or pronounced anxiety. It has also been used in treatment of narcolepsy and for depression caused by oversedation.

*Described in annual publication of A. M. A. Council on Drugs, N.N.D., 1960.

Preparation, dosage, and administration.

Pipradrol Hydrochloride* (Meratran Hydrochloride). It is available in 1 and 2.5 mg. tablets. It is usually given orally in doses of 1 to 2 mg. several times a day. Dosage must be carefully geared to needs and responses of individual patients.

Side effects and toxic effects. Pipradrol hydrochloride seems to have a wide margin of safety and is relatively low in toxicity when therapeutic limits of dosage are maintained. Side effects may include mild insomnia, excitability, and anorexia. It is contraindicated in agitated patients, paranoid and prepsychotic persons, and those suffering from chorea, anxiety, or hyperexcitability.

Methylphenidate Hydrochloride (Ritalin Hydrochloride)

Action and result. Methylphenidate is a central nervous system stimulant the potency of which is said to be somewhere between that of caffeine and amphetamine. Its effect on the heart and blood vessels is less than that of the latter two drugs. It does not ordinarily elevate the blood pressure and it does not affect appetite as readily as do the amphetamines. It is also claimed that it does not as readily interfere with sleep at night. When given intravenously it will terminate within a minute or two the respiratory depression produced by medication given prior to a general anesthetic or that caused by fairly large doses of thiopental sodium given intravenously.†

Uses. Methylphenidate is used as a mild cortical stimulant in the treatment of various kinds of depression. It improves the mood and behavior of depressed patients who are neurotic or psychotic, and it increases their motor and mental activity. It counteracts lethargy, lassitude, depression, and oversedation associated with the side effects of tranquilizing agents, barbiturates, anticonvulsants, antihistamines, and, in some instances, anesthetics. It appears to be effective in relieving symptoms of narcolepsy.

Preparation, dosage, and administration.

Methylphenidate Hydrochloride* (Ritalin Hydrochloride). It is available in 5, 10, and 20 mg. tablets and in multiple-dose vials for parenteral use. The usual oral dose is 10 mg. two or three times a day. Methylphenidate is administered orally and parenterally (subcutaneously, intramuscularly, and intravenously).

Side effects and toxic effects. Methylphenidate exhibits a relatively low level of toxicity. Occasionally, patients experience nervousness, insomnia, dizziness, loss of appetite, nausea, headache, and palpitation.

---

*Described in annual publication of A. M. A. Council on Drugs, N.N.D., 1960.

†Lundy, J. S.: Available New Drugs for Systemic Control of Previously Difficult Pain Problems, J. A. M. A. **163:** 1456, 1957.

Tolerance may develop after long-term administration, but this does not seem to constitute a serious problem. It is recommended that this drug be used cautiously for patients with epilepsy and hypertension, and it should be avoided for hyperexcitable and agitated patients. The ultimate status of this drug as a safe agent for prolonged administration is uncertain.

Nikethamide (Coramine)

Nikethamide is a synthetic compound chemically related to nicotinamide, the vitamin that prevents pellagra.

Action and result. It acts mainly as a stimulant on the medullary centers of the nervous system, producing increased rate and depth of respiration and peripheral vasoconstriction. Its action on a depressed respiratory center is more effective than on a normal one. Blood pressure is sometimes raised, but this effect may be secondary to improved respiration and to stimulation of reflex centers. It also stimulates the cerebral cortex acting as an analeptic. Claims have been made that nikethamide increases the flow of blood in the coronary vessels, but evidence is said to be inconclusive. Although it has been tried as a cardiac stimulant, it has not proved to be especially efficient and seems to be of benefit only when circulatory depression is of central origin. Toxic doses produce convulsions from stimulation of motor centers in the cerebrum. Death results from respiratory paralysis.

Uses. The main therapeutic use of nikethamide is as a respiratory stimulant when excessive depression has resulted from the use of central depressant drugs.

Preparation, dosage, and administration.

Nikethamide Injection, N.F., B.P. (Coramine). It is available in 1.5 ml. ampules containing 0.4 Gm. of drug and 5 ml. ampules containing 1.25 Gm. The usual dose is 1 ml. The preferred route of administration is by intravenous injection, especially in situations of an emergency nature. However, the drug may also be given intramuscularly, orally, and subcutaneously.

Pentylenetetrazol (Metrazol)

Pentylenetetrazol is a central nervous system stimulant which is chemically related to camphor but is said to be more stable and dependable than camphor.

Action and result. Pentylenetetrazol stimulates the higher centers of the cerebrum as well as other parts of the central nervous system. It will awaken lightly anesthetized persons in a few seconds when injected intravenously. It stimulates the respiratory and vasomotor centers of the medulla, and reflex activity in the spinal cord appears to be increased, particularly when the drug is given after this part of the nervous system has been depressed. It does not seem to have any direct effect on the myocardium or on the blood vessels.

Uses. Pentylenetetrazol has been used to induce convulsive seizures in patients with mental illness, but electric shock is more convenient, more reliable, and more acceptable to the patient. It has been recommended for long-range treatment of elderly patients suffering from arteriosclerosis who are troubled and disabled by changes of an organic as well as emotional nature. Differences of opinion are expressed about its value for this group of patients. Pentylenetetrazol speeds recovery from narcotic depression, especially that produced by the barbiturate group of drugs. It is rapidly detoxified; hence its action can be reasonably well controlled.

Preparation, dosage, and administration.

Pentylenetetrazol Injection, N.F. (Metrazol); *Leptazol Injection,* B.P. It is available as a 10 per cent aqueous solution in 1 and 3 ml. ampules and in 30 ml. bottles (100 mg. per milliliter). Available preparations also include 0.1 Gm. tablets. Usual dosage is 100 to 500 mg., as necessary. Administration is usually by the intravenous route, although it can be given orally, intramuscularly, and subcutaneously. It is well absorbed from the gastrointestinal tract.

Side effects. Pentylenetetrazol is a relatively nontoxic drug in that large doses are necessary to produce serious poisoning. The major untoward effect is the production of convulsive seizures which is followed by deep depression. Death results from lack of oxygen and respiratory failure.

Picrotoxin

Source. Picrotoxin is a drug obtained from a climbing shrub, *Anamirta cocculus,* indigenous to Malabar and the East Indies. The drug is present in the berries of the shrub, commonly called fishberries because of a native custom of throwing the berries onto the water to catch fish. The fish are stupefied by the berries and float on the surface of the water. The chemical structure of picrotoxin is still unknown.

Action and result. Picrotoxin is a powerful central nervous system stimulant and convulsant. Its most prominent action is apparently on the midbrain and medulla. It stimulates the respiratory, vasomotor, vomiting, and vagus centers in the medulla, producing increased respiration, elevation of blood pressure, emesis, and slowing of the heart. These effects are seen particularly in the anesthetized or narcotized individual. It is a dangerous stimulant because the range of safety between the therapeutic dose and the toxic dose is a narrow one. Large doses produce convulsions.

Uses. Although highly toxic to normal persons, this drug is less toxic to individuals who have taken an overdose of barbiturates. It has, in fact, a special analeptic action against the narcosis produced by a large dose of barbiturates. It is also useful in combating depression caused by paraldehyde and Avertin, but it is not useful in overcoming depression of the nervous system caused by alcohol or morphine. It is used chiefly in treatment of serious barbiturate poisoning. The drug is rapidly destroyed in the body.

Preparation, dosage, and administration.

Picrotoxin Injection, N.F., B.P. This is available as a 3 per cent solution in isotonic saline (3 mg. per milliliter). Total dosage is determined on an individual basis according to the needs of the patient. Picrotoxin is administered intravenously. In cases of barbiturate poisoning it is recommended by some that 6 mg. of picrotoxin be given initially and an additional 3 mg. at 15-minute intervals until 15 mg. have been injected or until the desired response has been obtained. Other restorative measures should accompany the administration of picrotoxin, e.g., oxygen administration, intravenous fluids, artificial respiration, etc. It is worth noting here, however, that there is considerable difference of opinion among physicians about the optimal treatment for barbiturate poisoning, and many hospitals avoid the use of analeptics entirely on the basis that their hazards do not justify their beneficial effects.

Strychnine

Source. Strychnine is an alkaloid derived from the seeds of the *Strychnos nux vomica*, a tree grown in the East Indies. The seeds are large, grayish, disk-shaped seeds which are very poisonous and are known by such terms as *poison nut, dog button,* and *Quaker button.* Strychnine is an alkaloid found in nux vomica.

Action and result. Strychnine belongs to the "spinal cord group" of central nervous system stimulants. Small doses increase the reflex excitability of the spinal cord and larger doses affect the higher centers. However, the margin of safety between the dose that will stimulate medullary centers and the one that will precipitate convulsive seizures is narrow. Its actions are pharmacologically interesting, but its ancient reputation as a therapeutic agent is undeserved and furthermore it is a potent poison.

Uses and preparation. Today strychnine is believed to have no uses for which we do not have a better therapeutic agent. The present U.S.P. lists no preparations of strychnine, although Strychnine Hydrochloride is official in the B.P., and Iron, Quinine, and Strychnine Elixir and several preparations of Nux Vomica are listed in the *National Formulary.* There are no official laxative pills containing strychnine, but some are still ob-

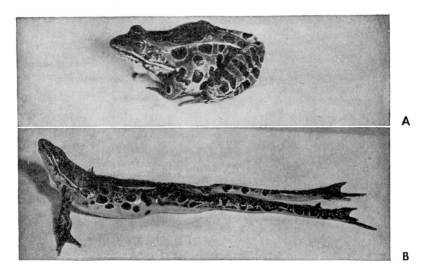

Fig. 24 Strychnine convulsion. **A,** Normal frog. **B,** Same frog in convulsion five minutes after the injection of 0.5 mg. of strychnine sulfate hypodermically. Note marked extension of back and hind legs. All the muscles in the body are contracting, but the extensor muscles are stronger than the flexors. (From Gilbert, A. J., and Moody, S.: Essentials of Pharmacology and Materia Medica for Nurses, St. Louis, The C. V. Mosby Co.)

tainable in drugstores. These constitute a grave hazard around a household where young children can get them, thinking they are candy. They are medications without justification, for their cathartic action offers no particular advantage and their toxicity, when many pills are swallowed, can be grave. Some rat poisons also contain strychnine, although other forms of poison have replaced strychnine to a great extent. The only reasons for continuing to include something about strychnine in this book is because strychnine poisoning continues to occur (although fortunately the incidence is low) and because strychnine has an important place in the early history of pharmacology.

Poisoning. Acute strychnine poisoning results from an overdose of the drug, taken by mistake or with suicidal intent. Strychnine poisoning in children occurs occasionally due to their accidentally gaining access to some preparation containing strychnine. The symptoms occur within fifteen or twenty minutes after the drug has been taken and begin with a feeling of stiffness in the muscles of the face and neck, followed by twitchings of the face and limbs, and presently violent convulsions of the whole body, which occur at intervals varying from a few minutes to an hour. Between the attacks there is usually complete relaxation of muscles. Death may result during a convulsion from asphyxia due to spasm of the respiratory muscles or during the period of relaxation from respiratory paralysis. The convulsions are due to excessive stimulation of nuclei in the spinal cord. The patient is usually conscious to the end and suffers intensely.

Treatment. The main object of treatment is to control and prevent convulsive seizures. Anesthetic agents or barbiturates may be used to control them. It is advisable to postpone evacuation of the stomach and give a moderately fast-acting barbiturate such as the sodium salt of amobarbital or pentobarbital intravenously. Other central depressants such as chloroform, paraldehyde, or tribromethanol are recommended if barbiturates are not available. If there is reason to believe that some of the poison is still in the stomach, gastric lavage may be done. Lavage may be done with solutions of potassium permanganate 1:1,000 or 2 per cent tannic acid. When the stomach has been emptied and the convulsions have been checked, chloral hydrate or phenobarbital may be needed to keep the convulsions from returning. If respiration fails at any time, artificial respiration and oxygen should be administered.

During treatment the patient should be in a cool, quiet room and protected from sudden noise, jar, or change of any kind which might precipitate another seizure.

Depressants

Mild drug-induced depression of the central nervous system is frequently characterized by lack of interest in surroundings, inability to focus attention on a subject, and lack of inclination to move or talk. The pulse and respiration may become slower than usual, and as the depression deepens acuity of all sensations such as touch, vision, hearing, heat, cold, and pain diminish progressively. Psychic and motor activities decrease, reflexes become sluggish and finally are abolished. If the depression is not checked it progresses to unconsciousness, stupor, coma, respiratory failure, and death. Some depressant drugs such as the general anesthetics act upon the entire central nervous system, but others such as the anticonvulsant drugs are more selective in their action. The nonselective depressants include the following: (1) analgesics, which are drugs that relieve pain, (2) hypnotics and sedatives, which produce sleep and rest, and (3) general anesthetics, which produce loss of sensation and loss of consciousness.

Nonselective depressants
Analgesics

Analgesics are drugs that relieve pain without producing loss of consciousness. Opium and its derivatives, related synthetic compounds, and the analgesic antipyretics, such as acetylsalicylic acid (aspirin) and acetophenetidin (phenacetin), belong to the analgesic group of drugs.

The search for an ideal analgesic continues, but it is difficult to find one that does all we desire of it. It should (1) be potent so that it will afford maximum relief of pain, (2) be nonaddicting, (3) exhibit a minimum of side effects such as constipation, respiratory depression, nausea, and vomiting, (4) not cause tolerance to develop, (5) act promptly and over a long period of time with a minimum amount of sedation so that the patient is able to remain awake and be responsive, and (6) be relatively nonexpensive. Needless to say, no present-day analgesic has all of these qualifications and so the search for one continues. Opium is one of the oldest analgesics about which we have any record.

Narcotic analgesics

Opium and its derivatives

Opium is described in Chinese literature written long before the time of Christ. The name comes from the Greek *opos*, meaning juice.

Source. Opium is the hardened dried juice of the unripe seed capsules of the *Papaver somniferum*, a species of poppy grown largely in China, India, Iran, and Asia Minor. The poppy plant is indigenous to Asia Minor, and from there knowledge of opium spread to Greece and Arabia where physicians became well versed in its use. Arabian traders were responsible for its introduction into the Orient where it was known as "smoking dirt." The Chinese used it chiefly to control some of the symptoms of dysentery until its cultivation was exploited for commercial reasons by European powers, and the opium habit spread through many parts of the Orient.

Paracelsus is credited with compounding the preparation "laudanum." Paregoric was first used as an elixir for asthma, and was prepared by a chemistry professor at Leyden. Thomas Dover, an English physician, used the powder as a sweating agent for gout in 1732.*

Opium in the crude form was used until well into the nineteenth century, before the chief alkaloid, morphine, was isolated. The discovery of other alkaloids soon followed and their use came to be preferred to that of the crude preparations.

Composition. The active principles of opium are alkaloids, of which there are some twenty in number although but three are used widely in the practice of medicine, namely, morphine, codeine, and papaverine.

The alkaloids of opium belong to two distinct classes. Morphine and codeine belong to the phenanthrene group and papaverine is known as

*Goodman, L., and Gilman, A.: The Pharmacological Basis of Therapeutics, New York, 1955, The Macmillan Co., p. 217.

188

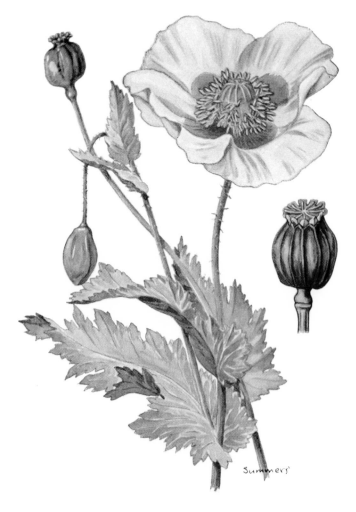

Plate 2

Papaver somniferum (opium poppy). (From Jackson, D. E.: Experimental Pharmacology and Materia Medica, St. Louis, The C. V. Mosby Co.)

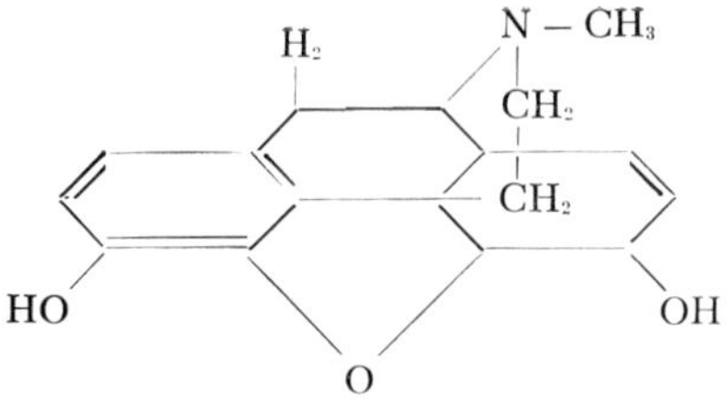

Morphine

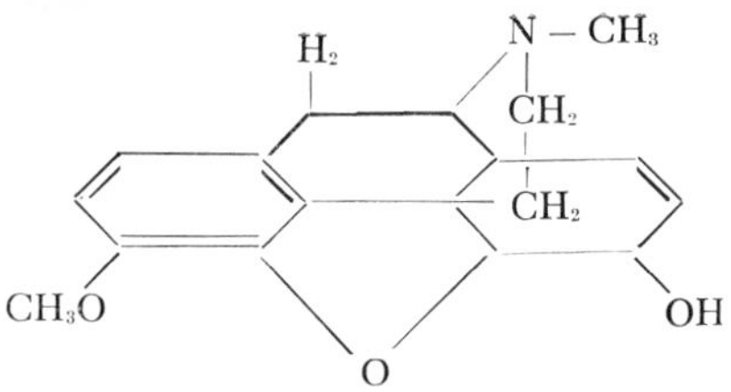

Codeine

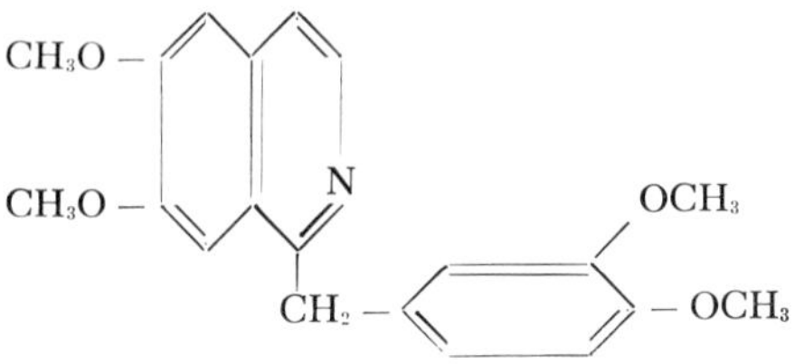

Papaverine

a benzylisoquinoline derivative. This helps to explain why papaverine has a much different effect in the body from the other alkaloids. Papaverine has little effect on the nervous system but produces relaxation of certain smooth muscles in the body. Morphine and codeine act mainly on the central nervous system where they produce a combination of depressing and stimulating effects. Both promote contraction of the smooth muscle, especially muscle in organs of the gastrointestinal tract.

The alkaloids form 25 per cent of the active constituents of opium, the rest being made up of such substances as gums, oils, resins, proteins, etc.

Action and result. The effects of opium are due chiefly to the morphine which it contains; hence the two preparations will be considered together.

On cerebrum. Morphine exerts a narcotic* action on the cerebrum which results in analgesia and sleep. The site of its depressant action is thought to be the sensory cortex, psychic or higher centers, and the thalami. Morphine elevates the mood, causing euphoria in many patients, relieves fear and apprehension, and produces feelings of peace and tranquility. Prolonged concentration becomes difficult, and the patient becomes apathetic, with a slowing of both mental and physical activities. The exact mode of action is still not known. The most outstanding effect of morphine is the *relief of pain*. This is highly specific because pain may be effectively relieved without affecting other sensations appre-

---

*The word "narcotic" can be confusing because it is used in at least three different ways: (1) a central nervous system depressant, (2) an addicting drug, and (3) a drug that may be neither of these but may be like papaverine, which comes under the restrictions of the federal narcotic law (Harrison Narcotic Act).

ciably. Continuous dull pain is more effectively relieved than sharp intermittent pain. It is especially effective for visceral pain, although when used in large enough doses it will abolish almost all forms of pain.

Morphine continues to be the most valuable analgesic in medicine, and ordinarily a nurse does not need to fear habit formation in a patient who is receiving the drug, over a short period, for severe pain.

In small doses at least, morphine seems to have little or no effect on the motor areas of the brain. The diminished restlessness is probably due to the drowsiness and sleep that is produced.

On brain stem and hypothalamus. Morphine has a highly selective action on the respiratory center. Doses that have little or no effect on other parts of the brain will depress respiration. The respiratory center is made less sensitive to the stimulating effect of carbon dioxide. The rate and minute volume are decreased and toxic doses cause slow shallow respiration. Death from poisoning is due to respiratory failure. Codeine is less potent as a depressant of the respiratory center than morphine.

Therapeutic doses of morphine and related alkaloids have little or no effect on the medullary centers concerned with blood pressure, heart rate, or rhythm.

Morphine acts as a miotic, i.e., it constricts the pupil of the eye. The exact mechanism or site of action is not clear. Some authorities say it is probably due to stimulation of a pupil-constricting center in the brain. There seems to be agreement that the action is central. Instillation of morphine in the eye does not cause miosis. Tolerance to this effect of morphine does not develop. In poisoning, pupils become pinpoint in size.

After administration of morphine the cough center is depressed and coughing is relieved. Morphine and related compounds will abolish the cough reflex but codeine is the drug of choice for this effect since it is less likely to cause respiratory depression and addiction.

The heat-regulating center is slightly depressed after therapeutic doses of morphine. Reduction of body temperature may be due in part to this effect, but it is also due to increased perspiration, decreased physical activity, and increased loss of heat because of peripheral vasodilation.

Nausea and vomiting may occur after the administration of morphine and related alkaloids. This is thought to be due to stimulation of a chemoreceptor trigger zone of the medulla.* Patients who remain in a recumbent position have nausea and vomiting less often than patients who are ambulatory.

On spinal cord. There is evidence that in laboratory animals morphine may stimulate the cord to the extent that convulsive seizures result. In

*Goodman, L., and Gilman, A.: The Pharmacological Basis of Therapeutics, New York, 1955, The Macmillan Co., p. 225.

man reflex centers of the spinal cord are stimulated but the depressant action of morphine on higher centers prevents a convulsive reaction at the cord level.

On cardiovascular system. Toxic amounts of morphine or related alkaloids are required to produce significant changes in heart rate and blood pressure. Changes that occur after therapeutic doses are believed to be due to decreased physical activity and sleep. Toxic amounts will stimulate the vagal center and depress the vasomotor center, causing a lowering of blood pressure and a slowing of the heart rate. Diminished oxygen to the brain greatly contributes to the hypotension which develops in morphine intoxication. Therapeutic doses of morphine will produce relaxation of small blood vessels in the face, neck, and upper chest, making the patient feel flushed and warm. Sweating is common. Itching of the nose is frequently observed and is thought to be due to altered circulation in the skin.

On gastrointestinal tract (smooth muscle and glands). In general, glandular activity throughout the length of the alimentary tract is diminished. Gastric, biliary, and pancreatic secretions are decreased and the digestion of food in the small intestine is hindered. The tone of smooth muscle in the sphincters is increased, and this delays the emptying of the stomach and small intestine. Although the nonpropulsive type of rhythmic contractions in the intestine are increased, propulsive peristalsis is decreased and a type of spasm has frequently been observed. The tendency to increased tone extends also to the biliary ducts and the sphincter of Oddi.* The defecation reflex is depressed due to diminished sensitivity of the bowel and rectum and the increased tone and spasticity of the muscle of the large bowel. The papaverine group of alkaloids differ in their effect on the muscle of the gastrointestinal tract in that they produce relaxation.

Many of the actions mentioned explain why patients receiving opiates and especially morphine are prone to develop "gas pains," constipation, and sometimes abdominal distention. The stomach empties more slowly, peristalsis fails to keep the intestinal contents moving, water continues to be absorbed from the intestinal content, and the feces gradually become hardened. When the rectum does fill, there is little or no inclination to empty it. Decreased peristaltic activity may give rise to local accumulations of gas which causes a painful stretching of the intestine. These effects are observed particularly in the postoperative patient who has had not only several doses of morphine but also an anesthetic and one or more doses of a sedative.

The effect of morphine on the smooth muscle of the gastrointestinal

---

*Woods, L.: Narcotic Analgesics, Opium Alkaloids. In Drill, V. A. (editor): Pharmacology in Medicine, New York, 1958, McGraw-Hill Book Co., Inc., p. 221.

organs also explains why morphine does not always alleviate the pain and distress in these organs when, for some reason, the muscle already has become hypertonic. For example, the presence of a stone in the common bile duct may cause the muscle of the duct to contract painfully and this may be intensified by the effect of morphine rather than be relieved, unless the dose of morphine is large enough to make the analgesic effect more pronounced than the effect on the smooth muscle.

These effects also help to explain the kind of diet that should be given to a patient who has had morphine. It is obvious that the patient is not likely to have either the inclination or ability to enjoy or digest a full meal. Tolerance to the effects of morphine on the gastrointestinal muscle develop slowly if at all.

On other smooth muscle. The tone of the muscle in the ureters and the detrusor muscle of the urinary bladder is said to be affected much the same as the tone of the muscle in the gastrointestinal organs. Increased tone in the sphincter muscle of the bladder may contribute to difficulty in urination. This sometimes explains a patient's inability to void and the need for catheterization.

Morphine promotes contraction of the bronchial musculature, but this effect is significant only in persons subject to allergic reactions and asthma. Allergic reactions to morphine and related alkaloids are said to be rather common.

Although there seems to be no direct action of morphine on uterine muscle, normal labor may be delayed because of central depression, and the respiration of both the mother and the child will be depressed.

Therapeutic uses of opium and the natural alkaloids of opium. Morphine especially is used primarily as an analegesic for the control of severe pain. It should not be used if other analgesics will suffice, but when pain is severe the narcotic analgesics probably have no rival. When morphine is given to a patient who is already in severe pain, the chief effect seems to be that the patient's emotional reaction to the pain is altered. He is no longer afraid of the pain or thrown into a panic because of it. If the nurse asks such a patient about his condition half an hour or so after she has given him a hypodermic of morphine, he is likely to say, "I still have pain, but I can stand it."

If the morphine is given before the patient begins to experience pain, its effect seems to be somewhat different; a better blocking of the pain impulses occurs and the patient may experience no pain. This explains why, on the first or possibly the second postoperative day, a patient should not be allowed to wait until he is "full of pain" if the fullest analgesic effect of morphine is to be achieved.

In surgical conditions in which the alleviation of severe pain may make diagnosis more difficult and lead to undue delay in operating, morphine should not be used or it should be employed only in very small doses and with great caution. It should not be used in chronic conditions in which there is pain, as prolonged administration is almost certain to result in habit formation. Exceptions to this rule are to be found in such conditions as inoperable cancer, in which the patient cannot recover and may be spared much unnecessary suffering by their use. The administration of a drug such as chlorpromazine or promethazine can be used to potentiate the action of morphine and reduce the amount of morphine needed by such patients. Morphine should not be used for the relief of pain in persons of neurotic or hysteric temperaments, unless its use is absolutely necessary.

Ordinarily morphine or related alkaloids are not given to produce sleep unless sleeplessness is due to pain or dyspnea. There are occasionally conditions in which the relief of restlessness and apprehension are essential, such as for the patient who is threatened with abortion or the patient who has had a severe pulmonary hemorrhage; in such cases morphine may be used advantageously.

Morphine is used to check peristalsis in conditions such as peritonitis, hemorrhage, severe diarrhea, and after surgery on the stomach and bowel. Preparations of opium are prescribed more often than morphine to check diarrhea because of opium's slow absorption and effect on smooth muscle.

Morphine is frequently used as premedication prior to the administration of a general anesthetic to relieve apprehension and decrease resistance to the anesthetic. Atropine (or scopolamine) is frequently given with the morphine to decrease secretions of the respiratory tract and to prevent spasm of muscle in the larynx (laryngospasm).

Codeine is opiate of choice in relieving a cough because it effectively depresses the cough center and is less habit-forming than morphine.

Papaverine is sometimes used to relieve the reflexly constricted blood vessels in pulmonary embolism, peripheral arterial embolism, or in the treatment of coronary occlusion. These are instances in which the antispasmodic effects of papaverine may be beneficial.

Opium—preparation, dosage, and administration.

Opium Tincture, U.S.P., B.P. (Laudanum). Usual dose is 0.6 ml. (10 minims); range of dosage, 0.3 to 1 ml. It is used to check intestinal peristalsis. It contains approximately 10 mg. of morphine per milliliter.

Camphorated Opium Tincture, U.S.P., B.P. (Paregoric). Usual dose is 5 ml.; range of dosage, 5 to 10 ml. This is a 1:250 solution of opium together with benzoic acid, camphor, oil of anise, glycerine, and diluted alcohol. Paregoric is given to check intestinal peristalsis, e.g., for diarrhea. It contains approximately 0.4 mg. of morphine per milliliter.

Preparations of whole opium must be given by mouth and are not suited to parenteral injection. This is partly because the two tinctures contain alcohol and because preparations of whole opium contain resins and other substances that are not readily soluble in water and tissue fluids.

Alkaloids of opium and derivatives—preparation, dosage, and administration.

Morphine Sulfate, U.S.P., B.P. Morphine sulfate tablets are official in the U.S.P. Usual dose is 10 mg. (gr. $\frac{1}{6}$); range of dosage, 5 to 20 mg. (gr. $\frac{1}{12}$ to $\frac{1}{3}$).

Although the dosage (15 mg.) for both morphine sulfate and morphine hydrochloride is sometimes ordered, investigators are of the opinion that 10 mg. (gr. $\frac{1}{6}$) per 70 kilograms of body weight comes closer to being an optimal dose than 15 mg. Larger doses may sometimes be needed but they are associated with a higher incidence of untoward (side) effects.

Morphine Hydrochloride, B.P. Usual dose is 15 mg. (gr. $\frac{1}{4}$); range of dosage, 8 to 20 mg. (gr. $\frac{1}{8}$ to $\frac{1}{3}$).

The action and uses of these two salts are the same. They may be given by mouth but more frequently are given by hypodermic injection. When given by mouth they act in from 10 to 15 minutes; when given by hypodermic, in 5 to 10 minutes. Peak analgesia after subcutaneous administration is said to be achieved in 60 to 90 minutes.[*] Actual increase in the pain threshold may last only a few hours, but the decreased emotional reaction to the pain may make the patient able to endure the pain for six hours or more.

Morphine Injection, U.S.P. This is a sterile solution of a suitable salt of morphine in water for injection.

Codeine Phosphate, U.S.P., B.P.; *Codeine Phosphate Tablets,* U.S.P., B.P. Usual dose is 30 mg. (gr. $\frac{1}{2}$); range of dosage, 15 to 60 mg. (gr. $\frac{1}{4}$ to 1). Codeine is a natural alkaloid of opium but it is made from morphine. Codeine Sulfate, N.F., is like the phosphate except that it is less soluble in water. Codeine is about one sixth as analgesic as morphine. It is also less constipating (although it does cause constipation), less depressing to respiration, and less habit-forming than morphine, although tolerance and addiction do occur. It is a preparation of choice in cough mixtures for the treatment of a dry, unproductive cough. Doses beyond 60 mg. are thought to be inadvisable because if effect is not secured with 60 mg. it will not be accomplished with a higher dosage. Large doses of codeine tends to stimulate the brain stem; codeine has a greater tendency to excite nerve centers than is true of morphine.

Terpin Hydrate and Codeine Elixir, N.F. Usual dose is 4 ml. which contains 8 mg. of codeine (gr. $\frac{1}{8}$).

[*]Goodman, L., and Gilman, A.: The Pharmacological Basis of Therapeutics, New York, 1955, The Macmillan Co., p. 226.

Dihydrocodeinone Bitartrate, N.F. (Hycodan Bitartrate). This is similar in action to codeine sulfate (or phosphate) but more active and more addicting. It is used to relieve cough. The dose is 5 to 15 mg. (gr. $\frac{1}{12}$ to $\frac{1}{4}$). It is marketed in oral tablets and a syrup.

Pantopon. This is an artificial mixture, composed of the purified alkaloids of opium in the same proportion as they are found in opium but in about five times the concentration. It is free from gums, resins, etc. Some think it is more valuable than opium itself. This is questionable. Pantopon has an advantage in that it can be injected and opium cannot. Patients who are sensitive to morphine can sometimes tolerate pantopon satisfactorily. The dosage is twice that of morphine. It may be administered orally or subcutaneously. The usual therapeutic dose is 20 mg. (gr. $\frac{1}{3}$).

Papaverine Hydrochloride, U.S.P., B.P.; *Papaverine Hydrochloride Injection*, U.S.P. Usual intramuscular dose is 30 mg. (gr. $\frac{1}{2}$); the range of dosage is 30 to 60 mg. (gr. $\frac{1}{2}$ to 1), although larger doses are sometimes given. The usual oral dose is 100 mg. (gr. $1\frac{1}{2}$). It can be administered orally, intramuscularly, or intravenously. In emergencies it is usually given slowly by intravenous injection. It has been known to cause cardiac arrhythmias when given intravenously. The depressant effects on the brain are much less than those of morphine. Papaverine has an antispasmodic action on smooth muscle of the body. The muscle that responds most to this alkaloid is that of the heart, coronary, and pulmonary blood vessels. It has a weakly antispasmodic action on gastrointestinal musculature.* Since papaverine is one of the alkaloids of opium it comes under the federal narcotic law, although practically devoid of narcotic action. *Copavin* contains 15 mg. each of codeine sulfate and papaverine hydrochloride. It is a cough depressant.

Dihydromorphinone Hydrochloride, U.S.P. (Dilaudid Hydrochloride). This is prepared from morphine. The usual dose is 2 mg., and it is about one fifth as potent as morphine. It may be given orally, subcutaneously, or by suppository. The latter preparation allows for slower absorption and more prolonged effect, which is an advantage because the duration of analgesic effect is shorter than that of morphine. Its analgesic effect is accompanied by minimal hypnotic effect which is desirable when the drug is given for pain to patients in whom it is important to relieve pain without producing a stupifying effect. It depresses respiration, but side actions such as euphoria, nausea, vomiting, and constipation seem to be less marked than with morphine. Both addiction and tolerance occur. Federal narcotic regulations apply to this drug.

Tolerance. Different individuals require varying periods of time be-

---

*Goodman, L., and Gilman, A.: The Pharmacological Basis of Therapeutics, New York, 1955, The Macmillan Co., pp. 251-252.

fore the repeated administration of opium derivatives fails to have the effect which it originally produced. This condition is known as tolerance. A patient who suffers considerable pain may be relieved at first by ¼ gr. of morphine, but if the painful condition persists, the time will come when he requires an ever-increasing dose to experience the same relief which he received in the beginning. The person who has developed tolerance may eventually take doses that would have caused death if given as an initial dose. Tolerance does not develop uniformly, i.e., tolerance is developed to the hypnotic, analgesic, and respiratory depressant effects of opiates but not to their effects on the pupil of the eye and on the gastrointestinal muscle. Tolerance develops faster when the dosage is administered regularly and is large. The exact mechanism of action whereby tolerance develops is not known.

Idiosyncrasy. Any unusual effect of opium or its derivatives other than the expected one is an idiosyncrasy. There may be idiosyncrasy of effect or idiosyncrasy of dosage.

Idiosyncrasy of effect is an effect such as nausea and vomiting, excitement and restlessness, tremors, delirium, and insomnia instead of relaxation and sleep. In some persons the nausea and vomiting are pronounced aftereffects which may last for hours. Urticaria, skin rash, itching, and sneezing are allergic manifestations which may be caused by morphine and its derivatives. Infants are believed to be less sensitive to morphine than was formerly thought to be true, provided dosage for them is calculated on the basis of their body weight. Aged, debilitated, or weakened individuals are likely to be more sensitive to the effects of morphine and need to have correspondingly smaller doses when it is given.

Idiosyncrasy of dosage is noted when a pronounced depression is observed following moderate or small doses or, on the other hand, little or no effect is secured when moderate or larger doses are given.

Contraindications. Because of its depressant effect on respiration and its tendency to increase intracranial pressure and because it is likely to make the patient less responsive, morphine is contraindicated or used cautiously for patients with head injuries and for patients who have had a craniotomy performed. Other persons for whom it may not be indicated are those with bronchial asthma, hypertrophy of the prostate gland, or stricture of the urethra (because of the effect on the smooth muscle involved). Morphine is also contraindicated in acute alcoholism and in convulsive disorders, and it must be used with caution for patients who, for some reason, have difficulty in getting sufficient oxygen, e.g., anemic and cyanotic individuals.

Side effects and toxic effects.

Acute poisoning. Poisoning with opium or morphine occurs from over-

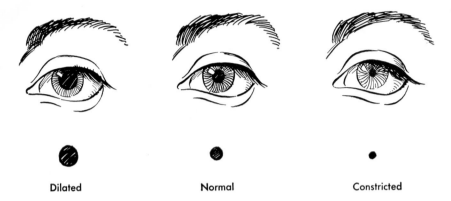

Dilated   Normal   Constricted

Fig. 25 Salts of morphine produce constriction of the pupil. Pinpoint pupils occur only in advanced states of poisoning.

doses taken as a medicine or with suicidal intent. As a rule, the toxic dose of morphine for the adult who is not in pain is about 60 mg. (1 gr.), and the lethal dose is approximately 250 mg. (4 gr.).* Death may come within the hour after the ingestion of a fatal dose, or the patient may linger for six to twelve hours. The longer the patient lives, the better are his chances for recovery, because the drug is being destroyed and excreted and restorative measures can be instituted. The nurse is often in a position to detect the early symptoms of poisoning, and, if she is alert to her responsibilities, she will not allow the poisoning to reach an advanced stage.

The symptoms begin with depression which progresses into a deep sleep from which the patient at first is easily aroused; then it becomes increasingly difficult to arouse him (stupor), and finally he cannot be aroused at all (coma). A significant early symptom of overdosage is slow and somewhat shallow respirations (10 or 12 per minute). In advanced poisoning the respirations may be 2 to 4 per minute, and Cheyne-Stokes breathing may be observed. Death usually results from asphyxia brought on by a developing respiratory failure; hence this condition becomes a focal point toward which therapy must be directed. The pupils of the eyes are at first constricted, later they become pinpoint sized, and, as the asphyxia deepens, the pupils dilate. The patient, as a rule, perspires freely and increasingly so as poisoning advances. In early stages the skin is warm, as well as moist, and the color fairly normal, but later the body temperature falls and the skin feels cold and clammy and appears cyanotic or gray. The heart action is not much affected at first, but

*Goodman, L., and Gilman, A.: The Pharmacological Basis of Therapeutics, New York, 1955, The Macmillan Co., p. 239.

later the pulse becomes weak and irregular. The blood pressure is usually maintained near normal until the lack of oxygen becomes pronounced and shock develops.

The early symptoms of poisoning which the nurse should regard as particularly significant are *slow respirations (less than 12 per minute), deep sleep, and constricted pupils.* Further doses of morphine should be withheld when these symptoms appear and the patient carefully watched to prevent the development of more serious symptoms. If a toxic dose has already been taken, however, prompt treatment is necessary to save the patient's life. Attention must be focused especially on the respiration. Respiratory stimulants such as nikethamide, caffeine and sodium benzoate, or ephedrine sulfate may be prescribed to be given parenterally. Analeptics such as amphetamine and ephedrine stimulate respiration and increase blood pressure. Artificial respiration should be given without delay if breathing has become dangerously slow, and it should be continued until a supply of oxygen can be fed directly into the trachea.

Treatment is also directed toward elimination of the poison from the body. If the drug has been taken orally, the stomach should be emptied. Repeated lavage, however, is not recommended. Tannic acid or dilute potassium permanganate solution (1:2,000) may be used to wash out the stomach, since these agents attack alkaloids chemically and thereby inactivate them. Strong black coffee as hot as may be given with safety may be administered by tube, by mouth, and also by rectum. Additional measures consist largely of keeping the patient warm and dry as possible and changing the patient's position frequently to prevent the development of hypostatic pneumonia. Prolonged stupor also requires that attention be given to food intake, fluids, and distention of the bladder. Measures should be avoided which uselessly exhaust the patient.

Two morphine antagonists have been used for morphine poisoning with seemingly good results. See *Nalorphine Hydrochloride,* p. 205, and *Levallorphan Hydrochloride,* p. 206.

Chronic poisoning. Addiction to opiates as well as other true forms of addiction is characterized by *tolerance, physical dependence,* and *habituation.* Frequent repeated doses of these drugs lead not only to marked tolerance but also to a strong desire for the drug which the victim seems powerless to resist. Results vary in different persons, but, in general, long-continued use leads to depression and weakness, not only of the body but also of the mind and morals. The patient suffers loss of appetite and various other digestive disturbances and may become thin and anemic.

Later, he grows nervous and irritable, is unable to work except under the influence of the drug, and may engage in low moral practices. He seems particularly incapable of telling the truth and will resort to any method of obtaining the drug. Ill health, crime, degeneracy, and low standards of living are the result, not of the effects of morphine itself but of the sacrifice of money, social position, food, and self-respect in order to get the daily dose of the drug.

Symptoms of addiction may be difficult to identify unless the addict is deprived of his drug. Constricted pupils, constipation (or diarrhea), skin infections, scars, abscesses, especially on the anterior surfaces of the body where the addict is able to inject his own drug, all may cause an observer to be suspicious of addiction. The truly identifying symptoms occur when the drug is withheld four to twelve hours and the patient exhibits a variety of withdrawal symptoms such as marked craving for the drug, insomnia, yawning, sneezing, vomiting, diarrhea, tremor, sweating, mental depression, muscular aches and pains, chilliness, and numerous other symptoms of both organic and psychogenic origin. Euphoria tends to disappear unless the dosage is consistently increased. After administration of the drug to which the victim is addicted, withdrawal symptoms disappear.

The cause of addiction varies. A defective personality seems to be the greatest underlying cause. Contributing factors may be the prolonged use of an opiate for the relief of pain, easy access to drugs and curiosity about their effects, inability to deal with frustrations such as are encountered in an unfavorable home environment, etc.

The number of addicts in the United States is unknown, but all strata of society are represented among them. The increased incidence of addiction among children and juveniles is cause for grave concern in all socially responsible persons.

Morphine and heroin are the opiates that are most desired by the addict. Codeine has less tendency to cause addiction, although it does occur. Addicts frequently use other drugs as well as opiates, e.g., cocaine, one of the barbiturates, or alcohol.

Treatment is best carried on in a hospital or sanitarium where the patient has the benefit of care from specially trained personnel and can be given a combination of medical, nursing, and psychiatric therapy. The federal government maintains two hospitals for the study and management of narcotic addicts under the United States Public Health Service. One is at Lexington, Kentucky, and the other is at Fort Worth, Texas. It is generally agreed that the longer a patient has been addicted, the longer and more difficult will be the treatment and the less is the likelihood of permanent cure.

Role and responsibility of the nurse. Because addiction may have its origin in the use of opiates for the pain associated with disease processes, the nurse is a factor in the cause and prevention of drug addiction. She is protected by hospital rules and regulations, because of the necessity of following written orders which must be rewritten at frequent intervals if the drug is to be continued. But even within such restrictions she should be alert to the possibilities of a growing dependence on a drug. On the other hand, she must not withhold opiates when their need is indicated. The situation of a postoperative patient with extensive surgery going through the first twenty-four hours after operation and that same patient five days later is quite different. Although p.r.n. orders may be left in both instances, the interpretation of the opiate needs for the patient should be quite different and requires the exercise of discriminating judgment on the part of the nurse. In the first situation there may be a need not only to control pain and general restlessness but also to prevent hemorrhage, stress and strain on sutures, etc. The physician has a right to expect that sufficient opiate be given to keep such conditions under control. In the second situation if the patient is convalescing satisfactorily, the free use of opiates instead of more mild sedatives or hypnotics may be laying an early basis for habit formation. It often means more work for the nurse to help a patient through a day or night without narcotics, but no nurse worthy of the name would hesitate at the course to be followed. The young or inexperienced student, who is puzzled about the best way to interpret orders, should never hesitate to consult her head nurse or supervisor.

Another point to be remembered about the judicious use of opiates is that addiction is much less likely to occur if the drug can be given orally rather than subcutaneously. Many times the nurse can help a doctor to decide whether or not the patient can get along on an oral medication.

Furthermore, morphine and the related compounds should not be given if another analgesic, which is not habit-forming, will suffice. Addiction sometimes can be prevented by using the analgesic that is least habit-forming, or which is not habit-forming, but will at the same time relieve distress adequately.

Every nurse in the course of her life is likely to come in contact with one or more persons addicted to the use of drugs in some form. While a nurse needs to know what to look for and what to avoid doing, she should remember that the addict is only another sick individual, worthy of everything she can do to help him recover. Kindness, sympathy, gentleness, and firmness are essential attributes of a nurse, no matter what a patient's psychologic or sociologic deficiencies may happen to be. The addict has learned to use a drug to help him bear things in his life which have become intolerable to him, therefore the treatment must go further and deeper than just breaking the physical dependence on the drug. There is usually, if not always, need for psychiatric treatment.

Unfortunately, addiction to drugs occurs among doctors and nurses in spite of their opportunity to become aware of the results of drug addiction. Everything possible should be done to prevent the likelihood of people being tempted to use drugs inadvisedly. Once a nurse forms this habit she automatically puts herself out of her profession sooner or later, for no one can assume the responsibility of allowing her to care for helpless patients.

Synthetic narcotic analgesics

Mention has been made that morphine falls short of being an ideal analgesic not because it is not sufficiently potent but because it depresses respiration, produces constipation, and may produce addiction. Consequently there has been an almost continuous search for an analgesic with fewer of the disadvantages of morphine. Some new agents have been found which exhibit some advantages over morphine.

Meperidine Hydrochloride (Demerol Hydrochloride)

Meperidine hydrochloride is a synthetic substitute for morphine discovered by two German scientists who were searching for a substitute for atropine. It is a stable, white crystalline powder soluble in alcohol and very soluble in water.

Action and result. Meperidine depresses the central nervous system probably at both the cortical and subcortical levels. The exact mechanism of action is unknown. Its most outstanding effect is to produce analgesia. It is especially effective for visceral pain, although it also relieves pain in structures of the body wall. Its analgesic potency is said to be slightly greater than codeine and lasts two to six hours, depending on the dosage. It is about one tenth as analgesic as morphine; hence severe pain is not well controlled by meperidine. Euphoria is produced in some patients and lasts for an hour or so. Compared to morphine it is less likely to cause sleep and sedation unless large doses are given. There is little depression of the respiratory center with the usual therapeutic doses; however, toxic doses can produce marked depression. Compared to morphine it is less likely to cause nausea and vomiting and it does not produce pupillary constriction. It does not depress the cough center.

Meperidine in therapeutic doses has little or no effect on the cardiovascular system, particularly if the patient is in a recumbent position. When given to patients who are up and about or when given by rapid intravenous injection, postural hypotension and fainting may result. Like morphine it is prone to cause an elevation of intracranial pressure and must be used cautiously in patients with head injuries or conditions in which there is an elevation of cerebrospinal pressure.

Meperidine was formerly thought to be a useful agent to relieve the spasm of smooth muscle, but it has been found that it resembles morphine in some of its effects on smooth muscle; e.g., it has been found to promote spasm of muscle in the biliary tract. It exerts a rather weak antispasmodic effect on the bronchial musculature and can more safely be used than morphine for the asthmatic patient who has need for an analgesic. On the gastrointestinal tract the tendency to produce spasm in the smooth muscle is said to be somewhere between that of morphine and codeine.* It is rather mildly spasmogenic and does not produce constipation; hence it is of no value in the therapy of severe diarrhea. It has more effect on the small intestine than on the colon. The emptying of the stomach is somewhat retarded.

Uses. Meperidine is used primarily as a substitute for morphine to produce analgesia. When so used it has the advantage of producing much less respiratory depression, sedation, and constipation. However, it does not take the place of morphine for the relief of severe pain.

Meperidine is widely used as a preanesthetic agent.

In obstetrics it is frequently combined with scopolamine, promethazine, or one of the short-acting barbiturates to produce obstetric amnesia.

Preparation, dosage, and administration.

Meperidine Hydrochloride, U.S.P. (Demerol Hydrochloride); *Pethidine Hydrochloride*, B.P. This drug is available for oral use in 50 and 100 mg. tablets and in ampules for parenteral administration as well as in powder form for prescription purposes. The single oral or parenteral dose usually varies from 50 to 100 mg. For severe pain doses up to 150 mg. may be given. Meperidine may be given orally, but better effects seem to be obtained when it is given intramuscularly. Occasionally it is given rectally. It is rarely administered intravenously. It may be given orally for relief of chronic pain. It is irritating to subcutaneous tissue.

Side effects and toxic effects. Side effects include dizziness, nausea and vomiting, dry mouth, sweating, headache, fainting, and drop in blood pressure. Toxic effects include dilated pupils, mental confusion, tremor, incoordination, convulsions, respiratory depression, and death.

Meperidine has a distinct capacity to produce habituation and addiction. Some physicians are of the opinion that addiction develops more rapidly than with morphine. Withdrawal symptoms develop more rapidly but are thought to be less severe. Tolerance develops less rapidly than with morphine. It is subject to provisions of the Harrison Narcotic Law.

Treatment. Treatment of acute intoxication depends upon the severity of the symptoms. Cautious use of barbiturates may be indicated. If respiratory depression becomes severe it can be antagonized by the administration of nalorphine.

Contraindications. Meperidine is contraindicated in severe dysfunc-

---

*Goodman, L., and Gilman, L.: The Pharmacological Basis of Therapeutics, New York, 1955, The Macmillan Co., p. 263.

tion of the liver, in certain conditions involving the gallbladder and the bile ducts, and in cases in which there is increased intracranial pressure.

Methadone Hydrochloride

Methadone was synthesized during World War II by German chemists. It occurs as a white crystalline substance which has a bitter taste and is soluble in both alcohol and water.

Action and result. Methadone resembles morphine in a number of respects. It also depresses the central nervous system and acts as a potent analgesic, although it has a weaker sedative effect than morphine. Only in minimal doses does it cause less respiratory depression than morphine. Euphoria is less intense than that which is produced by morphine. The effects of methadone on smooth muscle are somewhat more variable than morphine, but, on the whole, the results are similar.

Uses. Methadone is used primarily as an analgesic. The duration of its effect is about the same as for morphine. It is somewhat more satisfactory for the relief of chronic pain than morphine, but it is not as useful as a preanesthetic medication.

It is given to relieve cough, because of its depressant effect on the cough center. This type of drug is called an antitussive.

Methadone is sometimes substituted for morphine in the treatment of morphine addiction. This can be done because addiction develops more slowly and the withdrawal symptoms are less severe than those associated with morphine.

Preparation, dosage, and administration.

Methadone Hydrochloride, U.S.P., B.P. This is available in 2.5, 5, 7.5, and 10 mg. tablets and in solutions dispensed in ampules or multiple-dose vials containing 10 mg. per milliliter. It is also available as an elixir (1 mg. per milliliter) and as a syrup (0.33 mg. per milliliter). The usual oral or subcutaneous dose is 7.5 mg. every 4 hours as necessary; range of dosage, 2.5 to 10 mg. To relieve cough 1.5 to 2 mg. are given. Methadone is sometimes administered orally but more often parenterally. It is more effective than morphine when given orally. Subcutaneous injections sometimes cause local irritation, in which case intramuscular injection is preferred. If it is given intravenously the patient should be in recumbent position.

Side effects and toxic effects. Methadone exhibits some of the same disadvantages as morphine. It causes nausea and vomiting, itching of the skin, constipation, light-headedness, and respiratory depression. Death is due to respiratory failure.

Both tolerance and addiction occur following repeated doses of methadone. The same precautions need to be observed in the administration of methadone as for morphine. Nalorphine acts as an antagonist to methadone as it does for morphine and meperidine. The use and administration of methadone is subject to restrictions of the federal narcotic laws.

Metopon Hydrochloride

Metopon hydrochloride was a morphine derivative which was used for relief of severe and persistent pain. It could be given orally but it was expensive and at present is not commercially available in the United States.

Alphaprodine Hydrochloride (Nisentil Hydrochloride)

Alphaprodine hydrochloride is a white crystalline powder with a bitter taste and a fishy odor. It is a synthetic narcotic analgesic which is chemically related to meperidine.

Action and result. Its analgesic potency is said to be between that of meperidine and morphine. It resembles morphine in that it produces euphoria, mild sedation, slight dizziness, itching, and sweating. It is less likely to cause depression of respiration, nausea, and vomiting than morphine. Its analgesic and general depressant actions are less intense than those of morphine, but it acts more quickly and over a shorter time (about two hours). It passes the placental barrier easily, especially if given in conjunction with a barbiturate, and can depress respiration in the fetus unless it is given long enough before the time of delivery. Its effect on smooth muscle is similar to that of morphine. It has little or no cumulative action.

Uses. Alphaprodine is suited for the temporary relief of pain in obstetrics, for urologic examinations, and as a preoperative narcotic for minor surgical procedures involving the musculoskeletal system, the eye, the nose, or the throat.

Preparation, dosage, and administration.

Alphaprodine Hydrochloride[*] (Nisentil Hydrochloride). It is available in 1 ml. ampules containing 40 or 60 mg. and 10 ml. vials of solution containing 60 mg. per milliliter. The usual dose is 40 to 60 mg., depending on the size of the patient. The dose may be repeated after 2-hour intervals. Alphaprodine hydrochloride is usually administered subcutaneously. When very rapid and brief analgesia is desired, it is given intravenously.

Side effects and toxic effects. The undesirable effects are similar to those of morphine. Death can result from respiratory failure. Nalorphine is an effective antidote. Tolerance and addiction may develop, although the establishment of addiction is thought to be unlikely under conditions in which this drug is used.

[*]Described in annual publication of A. M. A. Council on Drugs, N.N.D., 1960.

204

Levorphanol Tartrate (Levo-Dromoran Tartrate)

Levorphanol tartrate is a white, odorless crystalline powder. It has a bitter taste and is sparingly soluble in water. It is a synthetic analgesic pharmacologically and chemically related to morphine.

Action and result. Its analgesic potency is comparable to that of morphine. The analgesic effect is said to last somewhat longer than in the case of morphine, but authorities do not agree on this point. Maximum analgesic effects are obtained in 60 to 90 minutes after subcutaneous injection. In man, 2 to 3 mg. of levorphanol tartrate are said to relieve pain as effectively as 10 to 15 mg. of morphine.* It has less effect than morphine on the smooth muscle of the gastrointestinal tract.

Uses. This drug is useful to relieve severe visceral pain such as that associated with terminal carcinoma, renal and biliary colic, myocardial infarction, and gangrene. It is also used as a preanesthetic narcotic as well as for the relief of postoperative pain. It can be used for practically all the same conditions for which morphine is employed.

Preparation, dosage, and administration.

Levorphanol Tartrate† (Levo-Dromoran Tartrate). It is available in solution, dispensed in 1 ml. ampules and 10 ml. vials of solution containing 2 mg. per milliliter. It is also available in scored 2 mg. tablets for oral administration. Recommended average dose for adults is 2 to 3 mg. Initial dose should be as small as possible to delay the development of tolerance. This drug is usually given subcutaneously, but, unlike morphine, it is almost as effective after oral administration as when given subcutaneously. This constitutes a possible advantage over morphine.

Side effects and toxic effects. The side effects are the same as those for morphine except for a lower incidence of constipation. As is true of most narcotics, dizziness and emesis are observed more in ambulatory patients than in bed patients. The drug is capable of causing tolerance and addiction and must be used with the same precautions that are observed in the use of other addicting drugs. It is subject to the restrictions of the federal narcotic law.

Narcotic antagonists

Nalorphine Hydrochloride (Nalline Hydrochloride)

Nalorphine, a synthetic congener of morphine, acts as an antagonist of morphine, meperidine, and methadone in the event of narcotic poisoning. There is evidence that it also reverses the respiratory depression caused by overdoses of dihydromorphinone (Dilaudid), levorphanol (Levo-Dromoran), and alphaprodine (Nisentil). It does not reverse the respiratory depression caused by barbiturates or some general anesthetics.

*Goodman, L., and Gilman, A.: The Pharmacological Basis of Therapeutics, New York, 1955, The Macmillan Co., p. 274.
†Described in annual publication of A. M. A. Council on Drugs, N.N.D., 1960.

Uses. Nalorphine is of value in the treatment of acute poisoning from morphine and related analgesics, but its use should not exclude the use of other supportive measures for the patient. It is not recommended for the treatment of the addict. It can be used to prevent respiratory depression in the newborn when given to mothers shortly before delivery, provided they have been given morphine or one of the related analgesics.

Large doses of nalorphine hydrochloride are said to cause feelings of drowsiness, lethargy, sweating, and dysphoria (misery). In morphine addicts it produces rapid onset of withdrawal symptoms and can therefore be used in diagnosing cases of addiction. Doses beyond 40 mg. are not recommended.

Preparation, dosage, and administration.

Nalorphine Hydrochloride, U.S.P., B.P. (Nalline Hydrochloride). This is a white powder and *Nalorphine Injection,* U.S.P., B.P., is a solution suited for parenteral administration. It is available in 1 and 2 ml. ampules and in 10 ml. vials. The concentration of the solutions vary from 0.2 mg. to 5 mg. per milliliter. It can be given subcutaneously, intramuscularly, or intravenously. The usual adult dose is 5 to 10 mg., which can be repeated if the respirations are not adequate. Since it is a derivative of morphine it is subject to the restrictions of the federal narcotic law.

Levallorphan Tartrate (Lorfan Tartrate)

This drug is a narcotic antagonist which is said to bear the same structural relationship to levorphanol as nalorphine bears to morphine.° It relieves the respiratory depression due to the action of narcotics but not the depression that may result from the action of anesthetics, barbiturates, or pathologic conditions. It is said to abolish the respiratory depression without affecting the state of analgesia. When given alone, however, it acts as a respiratory depressant and produces slight analgesia.

Uses. The uses for levallorphan are much the same as those for nalorphine. When given after or together with narcotics it relieves or prevents respiratory depression. It is fully as effective as nalorphine to antagonize the respiratory depression of morphine, some physicians considering it more effective. It is less expensive than nalorphine.

Preparation, dosage, and administration.

Levallorphan Tartrate, U.S.P. (Lorfan Tartrate). It is available for adults as a solution in which 1 mg. is contained in each milliliter; for children, it is available in concentration of 0.05 mg. per milliliter. Total dosage varies with the patient and the degree of depression. One or more doses of 0.4 to 0.6 mg. may be given as is deemed necessary. In acute poisoning with morphine, 1 mg. may be the initial dose. Levallor-

°Bonica, J. J.: The Choice of Drugs for the Relief of Pain. In Modell, W. (editor): Drugs of Choice 1960-1961, St. Louis, The C. V. Mosby Co., p. 226.

phan is administered intravenously, as a rule, although it may be given subcutaneously and intramuscularly. This drug is not a narcotic.

Synthetic nonnarcotic analgesics

Dextro Propoxyphene Hydrochloride (Darvon)

Dextro propoxyphene hydrochloride is a synthetic analgesic compound.

Pharmacologically it is related to codeine in analgesic potency and both can be used for the relief of the same kind of pain. Like codeine, it does not depress respiration when given in ordinary therapeutic amounts, but unlike codeine, it produces little or no relief of cough. It relieves mild to moderate pain better than severe pain. The onset of its action and the duration of its effects are similar to codeine. It does not act as an antipyretic.

Uses. It is used alone or along with certain other analgesics such as aspirin for the relief of pain associated with chronic or recurring diseases like rheumatoid arthritis and migraine headache.

Preparation and dosage.

Dextro Propoxyphene Hydrochloride* (Darvon). It is available in 32 and 65 mg. capsules. The usual dose for adults is 65 mg. four times a day with or without other medication for the relief of pain.

Darvon Compound contains the following: Dextro propoxyphene hydrochloride 32 mg., acetophenetidin (phenacetin) 162 mg., acetylsalicylic acid (aspirin) 227 mg., and caffeine 32.4 mg. Dosage 1 to 2 capsules three or four times a day. Darvon and Darvon Compound are given orally. Dextro propoxyphene hydrochloride is not suited to parenteral administration because of a local irritating action.

Side effects and toxic effects. Therapeutic doses do not produce euphoria, tolerance, or physical dependence. Sudden cessation of administration has not been known to produce withdrawal symptoms. While it does seem to be able to suppress withdrawal symptoms in cases of morphine addiction, its action is weak and not considered to be of sufficient significance to establish the drug as an addicting agent. It appears to have a low level of toxicity. Side effects of nausea, vomiting, and constipation are considered minimal. Large doses may cause drowsiness and dizziness. Patients are occasionally sensitive to this drug. There are no known contraindications except sensitivity. It is not subject to the restrictions of the federal narcotic law.

Nonnarcotic analgesics that are also antipyretics

During the latter part of the nineteenth century when chemists were trying to find a cheaper source of quinine than the natural source, they

---

*Described in annual publication of A. M. A. Council on Drugs, N.N.D., 1960.

discovered a number of compounds which differed in some respects from quinine but resembled it in their ability to reduce fever and relieve pain. Several of these compounds have survived chiefly because of their analgesic properties.

The salicylates

Source. The natural source of salicylic acid is willow bark, although it is now made synthetically from phenol. The cheaper synthetic product is identical with and therefore as effective as the natural product. Salicylic acid itself is irritating and can be used only externally, necessitating the synthesis of derivatives for systemic uses. All of these compounds will be referred to as "salicylates" and will be discussed as a group. Usefulness of the various members of the group depends upon their solubility, their salicylic acid content, and their tendency to cause local irritation. A chemical relationship among several members of the group can be seen in the following formulas.

| Salicylic acid | Acetylsalicylic acid | Sodium salicylate | Methyl salicylate |

Action and result. Both local and systemic effects may occur.

Local action. Salicylic acid is irritating to both skin and mucous membrane. It softens epidermis without producing inflammation. The salts of salicylic acid have no effect on the skin, but when salicylic acid is released, after their oral ingestion, it is likely to cause gastric irritation, nausea, and vomiting. Methyl salicylate produces irritation of both skin and mucous membranes and at one time was used for its counterirritant effects, i.e., it was rubbed on sore and painful parts to produce some degree of redness and improved circulation. It now is rarely prescribed for this purpose but is more of a home remedy. In solution the salicylates are weakly bacteriostatic and are capable of inhibiting certain fermentative and putrefactive processes.

Systemic action. The systemic action may, in turn, be either analgesic or antipyretic.

ANALGESIC ACTION. The salicylates demonstrate a selective type of depression of the central nervous system. Some authorities are of the opinion that the site of action is in or near the hypothalamus, but definite proof has not been found. Since analgesic doses do not produce dulling of consciousness, mental sluggishness, or disturbance of memory, the site of action is apparently not in the cortex. The analgesia produced by this group of drugs differs from the opiates in that it is not accompanied by euphoria and sedation. The salicylates do not cause addiction and they relieve pain associated with the musculoskeletal system better than pain in the visceral organs. Their analgesic potency is less than that of codeine.

There is reason to believe that the salicylates exert other actions in the relief of symptoms associated with rheumatic conditions but just what they are is not clear. Aspirin seems to have an effect on inflamed tissues which brings about reduction of edema, and there apparently is a relationship between edema and pain in conditions of muscle and joint pathology. It has also been suggested that salicylates may bring about relief of painful symptoms through promoting the release of adrenal hormones.

ANTIPYRETIC ACTION. Little or no effect is observed in persons with a normal body temperature, but in the febrile patient, a marked fall in temperature may be brought about. The salicylates seem to reduce fever by increasing the elimination of heat. It is believed that they act upon the heat-regulating center in the hypothalamus and reset the human thermostat for a normal or more nearly normal body temperature. As a result of this action, water is drawn from the tissues into the blood, peripheral blood vessels dilate, and heat is lost from the body by radiation and by evaporation of increased perspiration. There is evidently no effect on heat production.

On respiration. Therapeutic doses of acetylsalicylic acid (aspirin) and sodium salicylate do not affect respiration. Large or toxic doses stimulate the respiratory center, producing increased depth and rate of respiration.

On cardiovascular system. Therapeutic and even large doses of the salicylates have no harmful effect on the heart. In patients receiving large doses, the plasma volume of the blood increases somewhat and this may be significant if the patient has cardiac insufficiency. The patient's heart will have an extra load to pump.

On gastrointestinal organs. Salicylates in large doses are prone to produce gastrointestinal irritation (gastric distress, nausea, and vomiting). This effect is attributed to both a local and a central action, i.e., the gastric mucosa may be affected and also the vomiting center in the brain. The administration of sodium bicarbonate with the oral doses of salicylates helps to prevent irritation, but it also promotes excretion via the kidney and this is not an advantage when the maintenance of a definite blood level is desirable. It has been suggested that gastric irritation is decreased appreciably when aspirin is buffered with aluminum glycinate and magnesium carbonate and that it is also absorbed more rapidly.* Unlike sodium bicarbonate, these substances do not increase the sodium intake which is an advantage in certain instances.

Liver damage from salicylates seldom occurs, although massive doses may lower the prothrombin content of the blood.

Absorption and excretion. Salicylates are rapidly absorbed from the stomach and duodenum and are rapidly excreted from the kidney, giving the urine a greenish brown color. Rapid excretion explains the need for large and frequent dosage. Salicylic acid, as well as methyl salicylate, to some extent, is absorbed from the skin.

Uses based on local effects. *Salicylic acid* is a constituent of some corn and callus removers, and it is used to remove warts and upper layers of the skin in the treatment of certain diseases of the skin. It is also used for the treatment of some fungous infections. Whitfield's ointment contains benzoic acid and salicylic acid. This type of preparation loosens the outer horny layers of the skin and is known as a *keratolytic*.

Methyl salicylate is used as a flavoring agent. It was formerly used as a counterirritant but this type of therapy for painful muscles and joints is considered more or less obsolete. Methyl salicylate is absorbed from the skin and poisoning in children has resulted from application to large areas of skin surface.

Sodium salicylate is sometimes used as a sclerosing agent in the treatment of varicose veins.

Uses based on systemic effects. The major use of salicylates (aspirin and sodium salicylate) is for the relief of pain (analgesia). When compared on the basis of weight, the former compound is said to be the more potent analgesic. These preparations are especially effective for headache, neuralgia, dysmenorrhea, myalgia, fibrositis, neuritis, rheumatoid arthritis, and rheumatic fever. Aspirin is probably more widely used than any other single therapeutic agent. Feldman,† in quoting from a report of the United States Tariff Commission, states that 13,481,000 pounds were produced in 1951. A more recent figure of the estimated amount used yearly in the United States is approximately 8,000 tons.‡

Salicylates are also used to produce antipyresis when reduction of fever is beneficial to the patient. Care must be exercised to avoid giving any of these preparations if the patient is benefiting from the fever or if the cause of the illness is obscured by the reduction of the temperature.

The preparations are helpful in the symptomatic treatment of gout. They are less valuable for this purpose than certain other agents, but

*However, careful objective studies have failed to verify either advantage from the addition of a buffer.

†Feldman, W. H.: Modern Chemotherapy of Infectious Diseases, Dis. Chest **26:** 5, 1954.

‡Smith, P.: Nonnarcotic Analgesics: Salicylates. In Drill, V. A. (editor): Pharmacology in Medicine, New York, 1958, McGraw-Hill Book Co., Inc., chap. 20.

they are also less toxic. They decrease the renal threshold of uric acid and promote its excretion.

Unpleasant symptoms associated with a cold or attack of influenza may be relieved by one or more of the salicylates since they relieve muscular aching, headache, and fever, but their use should be accompanied by rest in bed. They exert no effect on the progress of the infection. In other words, it is impossible to "break up" a cold with aspirin as is commonly believed.

Preparation, dosage, and administration.

Acetylsalicylic Acid, U.S.P., B.P. (Aspirin). This is a white, crystalline, odorless powder. It has a bitter taste and is poorly soluble in water. In the presence of moisture it hydrolyzes to acetic acid and salicylic acid. It is available in capsule and tablet form. Enteric-coated tablets are available for those who do not tolerate well the plain tablets, e.g., patients with gastric or duodenal ulcers. The usual dose is 0.6 Gm. (10 gr.) every 3 to 4 hours as necessary. It is available in 150, 300, and 600 mg. tablets (2½, 5, and 10 gr.) for adults and 65 mg. (1 gr.) tablets for children. The latter are coated with a sweet-tasting material which may lead the child to think of aspirin as candy. Aspirin is also available in suppository form.

Sodium Salicylate, U.S.P., B.P. This preparation is a white or pinkish powder which has a sweetish saline taste. The usual dose is 0.6 Gm. (10 gr.) every 2 to 4 hours as needed. It is relatively soluble in water and is absorbed more rapidly than aspirin. It is available in 300 mg. and 600 mg. tablets (5 and 10 gr.) plain or enteric coated. It is also available in ampules of sterile solution for injection.

Both aspirin and sodium salicylate may be given in large doses to patients having acute rheumatic conditions, as much as 1 Gm. every hour until untoward symptoms appear, e.g., ringing in the ears. The route of administration is usually oral, and both preparations should be accompanied by ample amounts of water. Sodium salicylate is occasionally given intravenously when high concentrations in the blood are desired and it is difficult to attain them with oral administration.

Salicylic Acid, U.S.P., B.P. This form is too irritating for oral administration, but it is a component of many ointments and preparations for external use.

Methyl Salicylate, U.S.P., B.P. (Wintergreen Oil). This preparation is too irritating to be used internally except in low concentrations as a flavoring agent.

Phenyl Salicylate, N.F. This salicylate was used at one time as a mild intestinal antiseptic but is now used mainly as material with which to coat tablets to prevent them from dissolving in the stomach 'enteric coating).

Side effects and toxic effects. The safety range of the salicylates is wide and most cases of poisoning are mild. However, the indiscriminate use of these drugs by lay persons for every kind of ache or pain has resulted in numerous instances of toxic reactions. Mild poisoning is called salicylism and consists of ringing in the ears, dizziness, disturbances of hearing and vision, sweating, nausea, vomiting, and diarrhea. The so-called "salicylic jag" results from stimulation of the central nervous system and may progress to a state of delirium. Skin eruption and other allergic manifestations as well as deaths from salicylate poisoning have been reported. Intensive therapy with salicylates and massive doses can produce a decreased prothrombin level in the blood and hemorrhagic manifestations. This appears to accompany a deficiency or diminished intake of vitamin K.* There is little likelihood of hemorrhage if the dosage is kept at 1 Gm. or less, a day.† Methyl salicylate in doses as small as 6 ml. has caused death in children. Other dangerous symptoms include depression, coma, inconstant pulse, first a rise and then a fall in blood pressure, and deep labored respirations which became slower and slower until respiratory failure results. Poisoning and untoward reactions to the salicylates are frequently a matter of personal idiosyncrasy.

Treatment. There is no specific antidote for salicylate poisoning; hence treatment is largely symptomatic. All that is usually necessary in mild cases of poisoning is to stop the administration of the drug and give plenty of fluids. If massive doses have been taken, it may be necessary and desirable to empty the stomach, preferably with gastric lavage, and then instill a saline evacuant. If the symptoms are those of depression, stimulants may be ordered; if the symptoms are those of overstimulation, mild sedatives may be prescribed.

Overdosage in children. Although aspirin and aspirin compounds are among the safest analgesics known, the ease with which they can be purchased has contributed to carelessness in their use. The so-called "Baby Aspirin," which is available in 1 grain flavored tablets or dulcets, has been responsible for a high incidence of poisoning in young children. Children eat it thinking it is candy. Then, too, the usual form of aspirin is left about the house within easy reach of children, who may swallow many tablets before detection. This has produced severe and sometimes fatal poisoning. The younger the child the more dangerous overdosage is likely to be. Methyl salicylate should not be left where children can obtain it. The fact that it is used as a flavoring agent suggests to the child that it is good to eat.

All salicylates should be kept out of the hands of children and mothers should be helped to understand that indiscriminate administra-

*Sollmann, T.: A Manual of Pharmacology, Philadelphia, 1957, W. B. Saunders Co., p. 738.
†Queries and Minor Notes, J. A. M. A. 145: 1306, 1951.

tion of these drugs to children and particularly to young children can be dangerous.

Drugs that may be combined with salicylates. Codeine and aspirin are frequently given together, and aspirin is also combined with other analgesics and sedatives. Such combinations are believed to bring more effective relief of pain than any one of the drugs given alone.

Para-aminobenzoic acid (PABA), when administered with sodium salicylate, was found to raise the level of salicylate in the blood plasma. It acts by inhibiting the metabolism of the salicylates as well as their excretion from the kidney. Para-aminobenzoic acid can be given orally for this purpose.

Salicylamide (Salamide, Salicylamide)

Salicylamide, the amide of salicylic acid, shares the actions and uses of aspirin. It has no advantage over aspirin with the exception that it can be used effectively for patients who are allergic to aspirin. Administration, dosage, etc. are essentially the same as for aspirin.

Other analgesics and antipyretics

Acetanilid, acetophenetidin, aminopyrine, and antipyrine are synthetic derivatives of products of coal tar and have been often referred to as "coal tar analgesics." Acetanilid and acetophenetidin (phenacetin) are known as para-aminophenol derivatives or aniline derivatives. Antipyrine and aminopyrine belong to a different chemical family and are called phenyl-pyrazolone derivatives. Since their actions and uses are much the same they will be discussed together. They differ mainly in their toxic qualities. Phenylbutazone, a compound related to aminopyrine, also has been introduced into therapy.

Action and result. The two chief effects of these drugs is to produce analgesia and to reduce fever. In this respect they are similar to the salicylates. It is thought that they exert their depressant action in the thalamus and hypothalamus and interrupt the passage of nerve impulses which would ordinarily result in pain and that they affect the heat-regulating center in such manner as to bring about an increased elimination of heat through mobilization of body fluid, vasodilation, and sweating.

There is little or no effect on normal temperature, but in febrile patients they cause a definite drop in temperature. The depressant action in the brain is thought to be subcortical since there is no decrease in intellectual activities. Acetanilid and acetophenetidin are said to be converted in the body to N-acetyl-p-aminophenol, to which they are believed to owe their analgesic and antipyretic effects. Therapeutic doses of these drugs seem to have no effect on the cardiovascular and respiratory systems.

Drugs that affect central nervous system   213

Uses. Members of this group of drugs have been used as analgesics, especially for the relief of headache, and one or more of them have been the active ingredient of many headache remedies. They also have been used to relieve muscular aches and pains of various kinds. Acetophenetidin (phenacetin) is probably used more than any other member of this group at the present time. It is often combined with aspirin and caffeine. Acetanilid and particularly aminopyrine are prone to cause toxic effects in susceptible individuals. The presence of aminopyrine in proprietary preparations is now prohibited by law.

Antipyretics were more in demand when effort was made to cure fevers by antipyresis. Today many physicians look upon fever as a reaction of the body which helps the individual to combat infection, and therefore reduction of the fever is not always desirable. Antipyretic drugs are still used, however, for the relief of high fever, especially in children. Aspirin is probably used more than any other single agent for this purpose.

Preparation, dosage, and administration.

Acetanilid. Available in 0.2 Gm. and 0.3 Gm. tablets. Usual dose is 0.2 Gm. (3 gr.). This preparation is no longer included in U.S.P. or N.F.

Acetophenetidin, U.S.P., B.P. (Phenacetin). Available in powder, capsule, and tablet form. Usual dose is 0.3 Gm. (5 gr.).

Aminopyrine, N.F. (Pyramidon). Available as a powder or as tablets containing 0.3 Gm. (5 gr.) per tablet and as an elixir (4 Gm. per 100 ml.). This drug is seldom prescribed because of its tendency to destroy white blood cells in susceptible persons.

Antipyrine, N.F. Usual dose is 0.3 Gm. (5 gr.).

Acetylsalicylic Acid, Acetophenetidin, and *Caffeine Capsules,* N.F. Each capsule contains 0.3 Gm. acetylsalicylic acid (aspirin), 0.3 Gm. acetophenetidin, and 0.2 Gm. caffeine. These same drugs are found in combination and marketed as *Empirin Compound, Anacin, Aspirin Compound, APC Capsules,* and a number of others. These three drugs are also combined with codeine or with one of the barbiturates.

The above preparations are best given orally.

Side effects and toxic effects. Poisoning may occur from a single dose or overdose, but it is usually the result of the prolonged use of some proprietary headache remedy. The symptoms include profuse sweating, nausea and vomiting, skin eruption, weakness, cyanosis, slow weak pulse, and slow respirations. Most severe cases of poisoning show subnormal temperature, leukopenia, and collapse. Aminopyrine seems to be a particularly bad offender and should be used with caution, if at all. It can cause agranulocytosis, although the incidence of this reaction fortunately is low. It is seldom prescribed in the United States.

Acetanilid is likely to cause cyanosis, due to the formation of methemoglobin. It may also cause hemolytic anemia. Acetophenetidin produces allergic reactions, but neither acetanilid nor acetophenetidin is likely to cause agranulocytosis. Considerable individual susceptibility to these drugs seems to exist; some persons are unharmed by them whereas others develop severe reactions.

Nurses should remember that fever, malaise, sore throat, and ulcerated mucous membranes may be symptoms of a developing agranulocytosis. If a patient develops such symptoms the physician should be informed immediately. Not only members of this group of drugs but also a number of other medicines can damage the blood and bone marrow if the patient is susceptible to the drug. This constitutes a strong point against self-medication.

Although the coal tar analgesics are not considered to be truly addicting, they are habit-forming in the sense that the patient can become habituated. Prolonged administration is discouraged.

Treatment. In cases of mild poisoning, it is usually sufficient simply to discontinue the drug and wait for its elimination from the body. In more severe cases gastric lavage may be indicated if there is reason to think that some of the drug remains in the stomach. Provision should be made for rest and warmth. Oxygen is sometimes indicated if the patient is cyanotic. Treatment of agranulocytosis is supportive and it also is directed toward prevention of infection. The death rate is high.

Phenylbutazone (Butazolidin)

Phenylbutazone is a white or light yellow powder with a slightly bitter taste and a slight aromatic odor. It is a synthetic preparation which is chemically related to aminopyrine and antipyrine and exhibits similar analgesic and antipyretic actions. It is absorbed rapidly and completely from the digestive tract and more slowly from intramuscular sites of injection. It is likely to cause some irritation regardless of the channel of administration. *Renal excretion of sodium and chloride is reduced, causing temporary retention of fluid.* In patients with gout the drug brings about a reduction of uric acid in the blood.

Uses. Phenylbutazone is regarded as a potent analgesic to relieve the pain of rheumatoid arthritis and associated conditions (bursitis, peritendinitis, painful shoulder, etc.). It is said to suppress inflammation, to relieve stiffness and swelling, and to shorten the period of disability. However, because of the high incidence of toxic effects, its use is recommended only for those patients who do not respond to older, less toxic drugs. It is used particularly to relieve symptoms of gout when the patient has an acute episode of this disease and does not respond well to conservative measures.

Drugs that affect central nervous system 215

Preparation, dosage, and administration.

*Phenylbutazone** (Butazolidin). This preparation is available in 100 mg. enteric-coated tablets. The initial daily dose for adults is 300 to 600 mg., given in divided portions. The minimal effective dose is then determined and may be as low as 100 to 200 mg. Phenylbutazone is usually administered orally. To avoid gastric irritation it should be given at mealtime or just after a meal or with a glass of milk. Nonsodium antacids also help to minimize irritation without increasing the ingestion of sodium. A diet that is restricted in sodium chloride is recommended while the patient is receiving this drug.

Side effects and toxic effects. The administration of phenylbutazone is accompanied by a rather high incidence of side effects (approximately 40 per cent of the patients). Side effects include edema, nausea, gastric distress, stomatitis, rash, and dizziness. Severe reactions include hepatitis, hypertension, temporary psychosis, leukopenia, thrombocytopenia, and agranulocytosis. Some patients experience a reactivation of peptic ulcers with bleeding, and others complain of nervousness, confusion, visual disturbances, and fever and may develop disturbances of the rhythmn of the heart.

Contraindications. Phenylbutazone is contraindicated for patients with edema, those threatened with cardiac insufficiency, those who have a history of peptic ulcer or blood dyscrasia, and those with hepatic or renal dysfunction. Patients receiving this drug should be under close medical supervision, and periodic examination of their blood is recommended to detect early indications of toxic effects.

Drugs used in the treatment of gout

Gout is a metabolic disease of unknown origin. Heredity is thought to have a bearing on the incidence of the disease since it occurs more often in relatives of persons with gout than in the general population. It is seen mostly in males. It is characterized by defective purine metabolism and manifests itself by attacks of acute pain, swelling, and tenderness of joints such as those of the great toe, ankle, instep, knee, and elbow. The amount of uric acid in the blood becomes elevated, and tophi, which are deposits of uric acid or urates, form in the cartilage of various parts of the body. These deposits tend to increase in size. They are seen most often along the edge of the ear. Chronic arthritis, nephritis, and premature sclerosis of blood vessels may develop if the disease is uncontrolled.

Drugs given to relieve gout are those given to relieve pain and increase elimination of uric acid. The latter are called *uricosuric agents*. Salicylates, probenecid, and colchicine are drugs of choice at the present

*Described in annual publication of A. M. A. Council on Drugs, N.N.D., 1960.

time. Other drugs that are occasionally used are cinchophen, neocincho-phen, and phenylbutazone; ACTH, cortisone, and related compounds are also effective in relieving attacks of acute gouty arthritis and may be used when the administration of colchicine is not feasible.

The *salicylates* increase urinary output of uric acid and, in milder cases of gout, may afford considerable relief. The dosage must be large to accomplish this effect. The recommended dose is 5 or 6 Gm. a day in divided portions for three to five consecutive days of the week and omissions of the drug for the remainder of the week. Dosage must be determined according to the needs of the patient. The effect and dosage of acetylsalicylic acid and sodium salicylate in the treatment of gout are the same. The former preparation is preferable for patients who must have a diet restricted in sodium. The salicylates should not be administered with probenecid, since each is said to counteract the uricosuric effect of the other.

Since uric acid is not very soluble in acid urine but is readily soluble in alkaline urine, the use of an alkalinizing agent is indicated in conjunction with uricosuric agents. The maintenance of an alkaline medium in the kidney prevents the deposit of uric acid and the formation of renal stones and gravel. The amount needed differs with individual patients.

Colchicine

Source. Colchicine is an alkaloid obtained from the seeds and corm (bulbous root) of the *Colchicum autumnale* (meadow saffron), which belongs to the lily family of plants. Extracts of this plant have been used for hundreds of years in the treatment of gout.

Action and result. Locally, colchicine is an irritant. The mechanism of its systemic action remains unknown. It does not affect the amount of uric acid in the blood or in the urine, and it has no effect on the size of the tophi. It does not effectively relieve pain other than that of acute gouty arthritis. It is an interesting drug not only because of its potent analgesic effect in gout but also because of its ability to arrest mitotic division of cells when they are in metaphase. During this phase it prevents the development of the spindle. This occurs in both normal and cancer cells. The formation of new cells requires an extra amount of activity in the synthesis of nucleic acids and their breakdown into uric acid. It has been suggested that colchicine may relieve gout by arresting the formation of nucleic acids.* There is also a possibility that some intermediate metabolic product other than uric acid is formed in gout and is the cause of the pain and inflammation.*

Uses. Colchicine is used to prevent or relieve acute attacks of gout. The response is often dramatic and pain may be relieved within a few

*Stetten, DeWitt, Jr.: Gout and Metabolism, Scient. Am. 198: 80, June, 1958.

hours, the fever and swelling diminishing sometime after the relief of pain. It frequently must be used in doses large enough to cause some gastrointestinal irritation. Tolerance does not seem to develop. It is sometimes given every night or every other night to prevent the development of an acute attack.

Preparation, dosage, and administration.

Colchicine, U.S.P., B.P. This drug is available in 0.5 mg. and 0.6 mg. tablets. The initial dose of 1 mg. is usually followed by 0.5 mg. every hour or every two hours until the pain is relieved or the patient begins to have diarrhea, nausea and vomiting, or abdominal pain. Camphorated opium tincture or bismuth subcarbonate may be required to control the diarrhea. A preparation of colchicine has been prepared for intravenous injection. An ampule contains 1 mg. in 2 ml. of solution. Colchicine is usually administered orally. Occasionally it is given by intravenous injection when rapid relief is important or when oral administration is not feasible. It is very irritating if injected outside a vein and therefore cannot be given subcutaneously or intramuscularly.

To be effective, colchicine must be given promptly at the first indication of an oncoming attack and dosage must be adequate. Once the dose that will cause diarrhea has been determined, it is often possible to reduce subsequent doses to prevent the diarrhea and still achieve satisfactory relief of pain.

Side effects and toxic effects. In acute poisoning the patient complains of abdominal pain, nausea and vomiting, and diarrhea which may become bloody as poisoning advances. Excessive loss of fluid and electrolytes and the dilatation of capillaries result in shock. Scanty urine and blood in the urine indicate damage to the kidney. The pulse becomes rapid and weak, and the patient becomes exhausted. Death results from respiratory failure. Prolonged use can cause agranulocytosis, peripheral neuritis, and aplastic anemia.

Treatment. The main measures used in the treatment of poisoning depend upon the patient and the symptoms that are presented. Treatment is directed toward removal of the poison if possible (gastric lavage) and the prevention of shock. Atropine and morphine will relieve abdominal pain. Artificial respiration and the administration of oxygen are indicated should there be symptoms of respiratory involvement.

Probenecid (Benemid)

Probenecid is a white crystalline powder which is soluble in alcohol but relatively insoluble in water. Chemically it is related to the sulfonamides and was first introduced into medicine as an agent to inhibit the excretion of penicillin by the kidney.

Action and result. It has been found to affect renal excretion of a number of other substances including para-aminosalicylic acid and uric acid. It inhibits the reabsorption of urate in the kidney, and this results in reduction of uric acid in the blood. It is not an analgesic.

Uses. Probenecid is especially useful for the treatment of chronic gout and gouty arthritis. It is not effective in acute attacks of gout. Precipitation of urates in the kidney can be prevented by keeping the urine alkaline. It is also used in connection with therapy with penicillin when it is desirable to maintain high levels of the antibiotic in the blood plasma.

Preparation and dosage.

Probenecid, U.S.P. (Benemid). This is available in 500 mg. tablets. The usual dose is 1 to 2 Gm. daily in divided portions. The daily dose must be increased for some patients.

Administration. Probenecid is administered orally and frequently with sodium bicarbonate (2 to 5 Gm. daily) to maintain alkalinity of the urine. In gout, probenecid should not be given with salicylates because their effects are said to be antagonistic.*

Side effects and toxic effects. Probenecid is well tolerated by most patients. A few persons may experience nausea, constipation, or skin rash.

Cinchophen and Neocinchophen

Cinchophen was introduced into medicine under the name of Atophan. Its systemic action is similar to that of sodium salicylate, although its effect may sometimes be more potent and also more prompt. It has been used as an analgesic in gout and chronic arthritic conditions. Its tendency to cause gastrointestinal irritation and toxic effects in the liver has resulted in its being replaced by drugs less likely to produce harmful effects. *Cinchophen* (Atophan) may be given in doses which vary from 0.5 to 1 Gm. three times a day. *Neocinchophen,* N.F. (Novatophan), greatly resembles cinchophen except that it is less effective in promoting elimination of urates and it is less irritating. This may be due to the fact that it is less soluble than cinchophen and is less well absorbed from the intestine. The dosage is the same as that for cinchophen.

New drugs for gout

A number of new drugs are being investigated as to their usefulness in the treatment of gout. *Zoxazolamine* (Flexin) has been used as a muscle relaxant and has been found to be significantly effective as a uricosuric agent. It is available in 250 mg. tablets. *Sulfinpyrazone* is another drug whose effectiveness in gout is being studied.†

---

*Council on Drugs, N.N.D., 1960, p. 674.

†United States Department of Health, Education, and Welfare: Trial of Drugs for Gout, Pub. Health Rep. 74: 315, 1959.

Hypnotics and sedatives

A hypnotic is a drug that produces sleep, and as a group of drugs they have been widely used both for hospitalized patients and by the public at large. Since most of them can be secured only on a prescription basis, the possibility of self-medication is somewhat reduced.

Hospitalized patients often find it difficult to obtain rest and sleep for a variety of reasons. The surroundings are unfamiliar; there may be more noise or a different kind of noise than what they are accustomed to hear; they may have reason to be worried about many things; and they may have sufficient pain or discomfort to prevent them from sleeping. Equally important as a deterrent to sleep are the minor discomforts such as cold feet, an aching back, a wrinkled bed, lack of sufficient ventilation, too few or too many blankets, a full bladder, or a distended rectum. Occasionally a patient cannot sleep because he is hungry. It would be a poor nurse who would rely entirely on the effects of a hypnotic or sedative to remedy such discomforts.

The only difference between a hypnotic and a sedative action is one of degree. When a drug is given around the hour of retirement and is given in full dosage, producing sleep soon after administration, it is known as a hypnotic. When it is given in reduced dosage and given several times during the day and perhaps again at bedtime, it is called a sedative. Sedation is a calming, quieting effect, and, of course, the patient who is calm and relaxed during the day usually sleeps better at night. The terms soporific and somnifacient are synonymous with hypnotic. Many of the drugs known as tranquilizers are used for some of the same effects as the sedatives.

The mechanism of action which produces sleep is not well understood. It is believed that at least some of these drugs affect the reticular formation of the brain which is concerned with states of wakefulness and sleep.

Hypnotics act much like general anesthetics if large enough doses are given. They characteristically spare the medullary centers until large doses have been given.

Characteristics of a satisfactory hypnotic

Since rest and sleep are so important to relieve the effects of fatigue, stress, and strain in everyday life, it is equally if not more important that the sick individual have adequate help in securing the benefits of sleep and relaxation. A hypnotic should produce sleep that is refreshing and as much like natural sleep as possible. In addition, the hypnotic should act within a reasonable length of time after administration and allow the patient to awaken somewhere near his usual time of awakening with no "hang-over" effects. The hypnotic should not be habit-forming and should produce no adverse effects on body organs.

The barbiturates

The barbiturates were among the first drugs to be synthesized. The first one was introduced into medicine by Emil Fischer and Joseph von Mehring in 1903 under the name of Veronal. Phenobarbital is the second oldest of the barbiturates and is known also as Luminal. Since the time of their introduction hundreds of similar compounds have been synthesized, but only a limited number have proved clinically useful. New compounds have resulted from slight changes in the basic barbiturate molecule, and these changes have resulted in compounds which vary from the earlier compounds mostly in speed and duration of action. The accompanying formulas show the relationship of certain present-day compounds with the basic structure of barbituric acid and barbital. Various members of this family of drugs are made by substituting other substances for hydrogen atoms, at position 5.

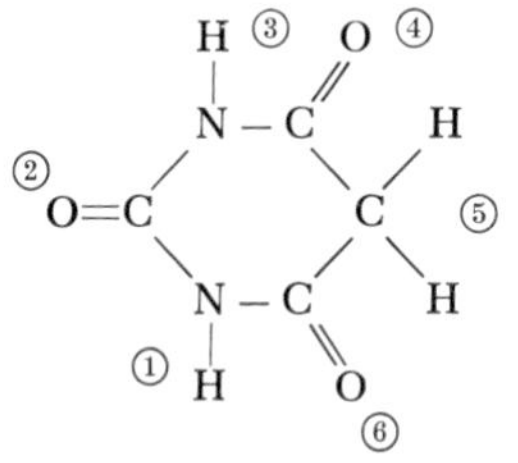

Barbituric acid (contains no carboxyl group but is capable of forming a salt)

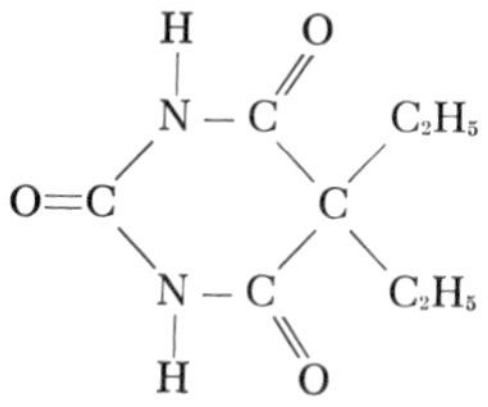

Barbital (diethyl barbituric acid)

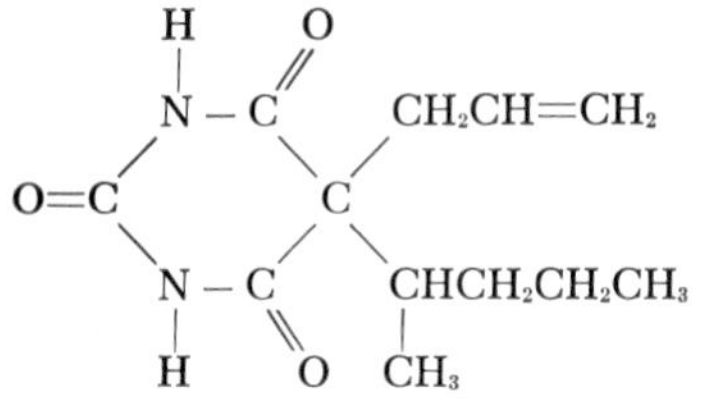

Secobarbital (Seconal)

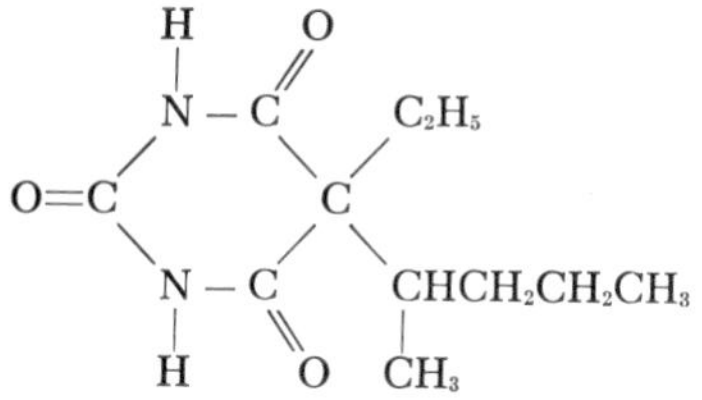

Pentobarbital (Nembutal)

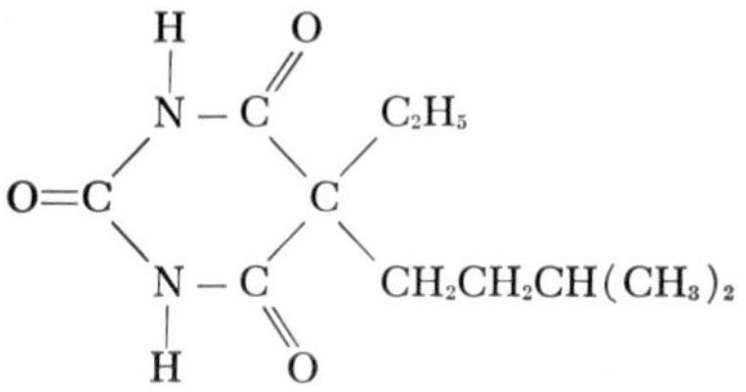

Amobarbital (Amytal)

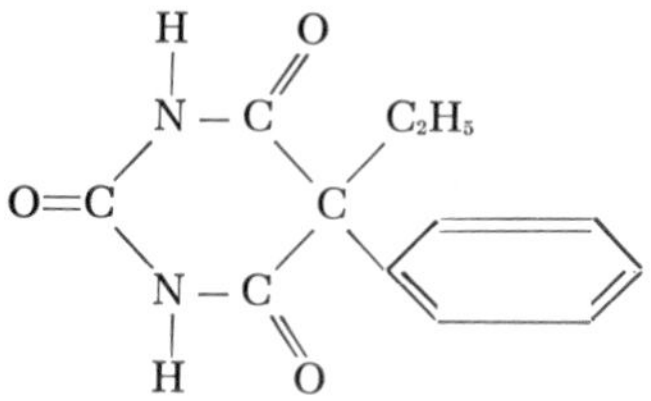

Phenobarbital (Luminal)

Some of the barbiturates have stood the test of time very well. Large amounts of these drugs are prescribed and used, as is evident from the fact that 864,000 pounds were produced in 1955.*

The barbiturates are all colorless, white crystalline powders which have a more or less bitter taste. They are sparingly soluble in water but freely soluble in alcohol. The sodium salts of these compounds are freely soluble in water.

Action and result. An important action appears to be that of depression of cells of the diencephalon, which contains the fundamental vegetative and sleep centers.† However there is evidence that the barbiturates act at all levels of the central nervous system. The extent of effect varies from mild sedation to deep anesthesia, depending upon the drug selected, the method of administration, the dosage, and also the reaction of the individual's nervous system. The barbiturates are not regarded as analgesics and cannot be depended upon to produce restful sleep when insomnia is due to pain.‡ However, when combined with an analgesic the sedative action seems to re-enforce the action of the analgesic. Therapeutic doses of the longer-acting barbiturates may result in depression of spirits and lowered vitality on the following day. On the other hand, many of the barbiturates produce a dreamless sleep from which the patient awakes refreshed.

All of the barbiturates, used clinically, depress the motor cortex of the brain when given in large doses, but phenobarbital, mephobarbital, and metharbital exert a selective action on the motor cortex, even in small doses. This explains their use as anticonvulsants.

Ordinary therapeutic doses have little or no effect on medullary centers, but large doses, especially when administered intravenously, depress the respiratory and vasomotor centers. Death from overdosage is due, as a rule, to respiratory failure accompanied by hypotension.

Smooth muscles of blood vessels and of the gastrointestinal organs are depressed after large amounts of barbiturates, but clinical doses, as a rule, do not produce untoward effects. The motility of the gastrointestinal organs may be reduced and the emptying of the stomach delayed slightly, but there is apparently little interference with the ability to respond to normal stimuli. Uterine muscle is affected little by hypnotic doses of barbiturates and the force of uterine contractions at the time of childbirth is not diminished, unless anesthesia has been produced.

Uses. The barbiturates have many uses.

As hypnotics. For best effects the barbiturates should be administered

*Adams, Elijah: Barbiturates, Scient. Am. 198: 60, Jan., 1958.
†Salter, W. T.: Textbook of Pharmacology, Philadelphia, 1952, W. B. Saunders Co., p. 99.
‡Goodman, L., and Gilman, A.: The Pharmacological Basis of Therapeutics, New York, 1955, The Macmillan Co., p. 127.

at such times as will coincide with the usual hour of retirement. Long-, short-, or intermediate-acting barbiturates are chosen to meet the needs of individual patients.

As sedatives. The barbiturates have, for purposes of sedation, a wide range of therapeutic uses. Although the tranquilizing drugs have come into a position of great prominence, the barbiturates are still used to calm and sedate the nervous patient, and they are also used for patients who have physical illness in which there is usually an emotional factor, as in the case of hypertension, chronic ulcerative colitis, and gastric ulcer.

As anticonvulsants. Barbiturates are used to prevent or control convulsive seizures associated with tetanus, strychnine poisoning, cerebral pathology, and epilepsy. Phenobarbital has been especially valuable in the prevention and control of grand mal epilepsy. It may be prescribed alone or in conjunction with other anticonvulsant drugs. Mephobarbital and metharbital are also effective in the symptomatic treatment of certain types of epilepsy.

As anesthetics. For selected forms of surgical procedures and especially for surgery of short duration, the rapid-acting barbiturates are employed. Thiopental Sodium is the preparation most widely used in the United States. These barbiturates are further discussed under *Basal Anesthetics* (see Index).

As preanesthetic medications. The short-acting barbiturates such as pentobarbital sodium are selected for this effect. They are often ordered to be given the night before surgery to enable the patient to have a restful sleep, and they may also be ordered to be given the morning of the day of operation. They are frequently supplemented by other medications just before the patient is called to the operating room. Other medications may be morphine, meperidine (Demerol), atropine, scopolamine, or one of a number of others, depending on the surgeon and on what he thinks the patient needs.

For obstetric sedation and amnesia. For obstetric sedation and amnesia the barbiturates are used either alone or in combination with other drugs such as scopolamine or meperidine (Demerol). Drugs that cause respiratory depression of the mother are likely to cause respiratory depression in the infant as well.

In psychiatry. Barbiturates are sometimes used in psychiatry to temporarily release a patient from strong inhibitions and enable him to cooperate more effectively with his therapist. Amobarbital, pentobarbital, and thiopental are the barbiturates likely to be chosen for this purpose.

Absorption, fate, and excretion. Barbiturates are readily absorbed after both oral and parenteral administration. The sodium salts being more soluble are more rapidly absorbed than the free acids. Most of the barbiturates, with the exception of barbital, undergo change in the liver before they are excreted by the kidney. Some are excreted partly in an altered form and partly unchanged, and others are excreted in a completely altered form. The longer-acting barbiturates are said to be metabolized or chemically altered more slowly than the rapidly acting members.[*] The more slowly a barbiturate is altered or excreted, the more prolonged is its action. If excretion is slow and administration prolonged, cumulative effects will result.

Preparation and dosage. The barbiturates are classified according to the duration of their action as long, intermediate, short, and ultrashort acting. This means that the short-acting drugs produce an effect in a relatively short time (10 to 15 minutes) and also act over a relatively short period (3 hours or less). Long-acting barbiturates require 30 to 60 minutes to become effective and act over a period of 6 hours or more. The others act in a correspondingly shorter or longer time. Thiopental sodium, which belongs to the ultrashort-acting group of barbiturates, acts rapidly and can produce a state of anesthesia in a few seconds. See Table 12 for dosage, methods of administration, and length of action and page 229 for further discussion on the choice of a barbiturate.

Administration. The oral channel of administration is preferred and should be used whenever possible. Certain preparations may be given subcutaneously, intramuscularly, intravenously, or rectally, depending on the purpose to be achieved and the general condition of the patient. The intravenous route is the most dangerous one and is used only for the production of anesthesia or in emergencies. Parenteral administration is also used when a patient is too ill to take the drug orally or suffers from nausea and vomiting or when for some reason it is important to have a rapid depressant action.

Contraindications. Barbiturates should be avoided for patients who manifest a sensitivity toward them or have been previously addicted to them. If a patient tells the nurse that he is sensitive to this group of drugs she should record the statement and make the information known to the physician. The patient usually knows and perhaps has had previous experience to justify his comments. Seriously impaired hepatic or renal function may also constitute a contraindication for the use of these drugs, although only the physician can decide whether the degree of damage warrants the use of a different type of drug.

Side effects and toxic effects. Unusual effects or reactions may be exhibited as one or more of the following: (1) marked symptoms of "hang-over"—listlessness, prolonged depression, nausea, and emotional

*Shideman, F. E.: Sedatives and Hypnotics. II. Barbiturates. In Drill, V. A. (editor): Pharmacology in Medicine, New York, 1958, McGraw-Hill Book Co., Inc., p. 169.

Table 12

Preparation	Usual adult dose	Usual method of administration	Length of action
*Barbital, N.F. (Veronal); Barbitone Sodium B.P.	300 mg. (5 gr.)	Orally	Long acting
*Phenobarbital, U.S.P. (Luminal); Phenobarbitone, B.P.	30-100 mg. (½ to 1½ gr.)	Orally	Long acting
Mephobarbital (Mebaral)	400-600 mg. (6 to 10 gr.)	Orally	Long acting
Metharbital† (Gemonil)	100 mg. (1½ gr.)	Orally	Long acting
*Amobarbital, U.S.P. (Amytal)	100 mg. (1½ gr.)	Orally	Intermediate
Aprobarbital, N.F. (Alurate)	60-120 mg. (1 to 2 gr.)	Orally	Intermediate
Probarbital Sodium (Ipral Sodium)	120-250 mg. (2 to 4 gr.)	Orally	Intermediate
Butethal (Neonal)	100 mg. (1½ gr.)	Orally	Intermediate
Butabarbital Sodium† (Butisol)	8-60 mg. (⅛ to 1 gr.)	Orally	Intermediate
Pentobarbital Sodium, U.S.P. (Nembutal Sodium); Pentobarbitone Sodium, B.P.	100 mg. (1½ gr.)	Orally; rectally	Short acting
Secobarbital Sodium, U.S.P. (Seconal Sodium); Quinalbarbitone Sodium, B. P.	100-200 mg. (1½ to 3 gr.)	Orally; rectally	Short acting
Cyclobarbital Calcium, N.F. (Phanodorn); Cyclobarbitone, B.P.	200 mg. (3 gr.)	Orally	Short acting
Butallylonal (Pernoston)	200 mg. (3 gr.)	Orally	Short acting
Hexobarbital Sodium, N.F. (Evipal Sodium)	2-4 ml. 10%	Intravenously	Ultrashort acting
Thiopental Sodium, U.S.P. (Pentothal Sodium); Thiopentone Sodium, B.P.	2-3 ml. 2.5% in 10 to 15 sec. repeated in 30 sec. as required	Intravenously	Ultrashort acting

°Sodium salts are available.
†Described in annual publication of A. M. A. Council on Drugs, N.N.D., 1960.

Drugs that affect central nervous system

disturbances; (2) skin rash, urticaria, swelling of the face, and asthmatic attack; (3) bad dreams, restlessness, and delirium.

Bad dreams, restlessness, and delirium may be experienced especially by elderly or debilitated patients. Night nurses find that they need to watch older patients carefully when they have been given a hypnotic dose of a barbiturate. Such patients naturally go to the bathroom more frequently than younger adults and under the influence of a barbiturate may become confused and have difficulty in orienting themselves. Barbital, amobarbital, and pentobarbital are said to exert this effect more often than phenobarbital.

Restlessness is also produced when barbiturates are administered to patients in severe pain. The drug, in this instance, does not relieve the pain but depresses the higher centers which normally serve as control centers. Mental confusion and delirium may result. An analgesic should accompany a barbiturate if the patient has pain.

Acute poisoning. Because barbiturates are widely known and are obtained with comparative ease, they have been one of the agents of choice for suicide. Poisoning also occurs accidentally and can occur when these drugs are given intravenously by persons insufficiently experienced in giving anesthetics. The fatal dose varies, but when fifteen to twenty times the usual therapeutic dose is absorbed, severe poisoning and possibly death will result. The lethal dose is said to be 1 to 1.5 Gm. or more.[*] When seen in the earlier stages of poisoning the patient is usually in a deep sleep or stupor. Occasionally confusion and excitement precede heavy sleep. When poisoning is fully advanced the patient is comatose and many of his reflexes are sluggish or absent. Respiration is either slow or rapid and shallow. Lack of oxygen affects the cardiovascular system and results in shock. The blood pressure drops, the pupils may become pinpoint in size, and the pulse is rapid and weak. Death is usually the result of respiratory failure, especially if one of the more rapidly acting barbiturates has been taken. If death is delayed it is more likely to be due to hypostatic pneumonia or pulmonary edema.

TREATMENT. The treatment prescribed by the physician will vary with the condition and needs of the patient. Sometimes little more than general supportive measures are required (keeping the patient warm and turned periodically, providing for adequate fluids and nutrition, etc.). If the patient is deeply comatose and unresponsive and is having serious difficulty with respiration, great effort may be required to save his life.

If the drug has been swallowed and there is reason to think that part or most of it remains in the stomach, prompt gastric lavage may be done. A saline cathartic is sometimes instilled, after lavage, to hasten elimination of the drug. The danger of aspiration of gastric content at the time

[*] Adams, Elijah: Barbiturates, Scient. Am. 198: 62, Jan., 1958.

of lavage is always a calculated risk. Only the physician can decide whether or not that risk should be taken. The nurse frequently is expected to arrange to have some of the gastric washings saved in the event that a toxicologic examination is to be made. At all times the maintenance of an open airway is of primary importance. In severe depression the physician may plan to use an endotracheal tube or a respirator and administer oxygen or oxygen and carbon dioxide. The nurse will be expected to keep a careful check and to make repeated observations of the respirations, pulse, blood pressure, and degree of responsiveness, especially if circumstances are such that the physician cannot be with the patient continuously.

Extensive use of analeptic drugs is looked upon with disfavor by some clinicians because many of these drugs are themselves capable of producing toxic symptoms. Picrotoxin and pentylenetetrazol (Metrazol) are analeptics which may be prescribed for certain patients to overcome severe general depression as well as respiratory depression. Amphetamines, ephedrine, and nikethamide are examples of central nervous system stimulants which are advocated for the less severe types of depression associated with poisoning from barbiturate drugs. Levarterenol, amphetamines, and phenylephrine may be used to combat circulatory collapse. A relatively new drug which was introduced under the name of bemegride (Megimide) is under investigation as a barbiturate antagonist. The exact mode of its action is unknown, but it appears to be of value in the treatment of patients who are comatose from overdosage with a barbiturate as well as the central nervous system depressants. This drug can cause convulsive seizures, but it is effective for the depressed patient in doses below that which will cause convulsions. It is administered in 50 mg. doses every 3 or 4 minutes, until the laryngeal and pharyngeal reflexes are restored. Total dosage depends on the individual patient.

Chronic poisoning. Both addiction and habituation to the barbiturates can develop. Tolerance is said to develop slowly and to a lesser degree than it does to morphine and related drugs. Occasional doses of barbiturates in doses of 0.1 Gm. (1½ gr.) causes neither addiction nor habituation. In fact, it takes an appreciably larger daily dose such as 0.8 Gm. (12 gr.) or more over a period of time to establish addiction.

In recent years the abuse of barbiturates has become a problem of increasing concern. The seriousness of the situation is reflected in the large number of state laws that have been passed to regulate the sale of barbiturates and in the continued effort to get some kind of federal control of them.

Symptoms of chronic intoxication include slowness of thought, mental depression, incoherent speech, failing memory, skin rash, weight loss, gastrointestinal upsets, and anemia. There is frequently an ataxic gait, coarse tremor of the lips, fingers, and tongue, increased emotional instability, and some mental confusion. The clinical manifestations are similar to those of chronic alcoholism. Because of the poor motor coordination, patients may fall and be injured. They are likely to fall asleep while smoking and set the bed or room furnishings on fire. They are unable to work, and they constitute a real hazard if they attempt to drive power machinery, e.g., an automobile. Their judgment may be so impaired that they take additional doses of their drug when they are already seriously intoxicated. It is thought that some instances of reported suicide with barbiturates are explained on this basis. Long-continued use of particularly the short-acting barbiturates in large doses results in withdrawal symptoms characterized by great weakness, tremor, anxiety, nausea, and vomiting and by a series of grand mal convulsions or psychosis or both. Withdrawal symptoms are precipitated when the drug is appreciably reduced or stopped altogether.

Many opium addicts are also barbiturate addicts. They resort to barbiturates when they have difficulty getting their supply of opiates. The barbiturates most commonly selected by them seem to be pentobarbital, secobarbital, and amobarbital or the sodium salts of these compounds. Some authorities feel that the addiction resulting from the overuse of the barbiturates is, in some respects, more dangerous and undesirable than the addiction resulting from the misuse of opiates.*

TREATMENT. The best results in the way of treatment are probably obtained in an institution with well-prepared personnel, and even then there is a rather high percentage of discouraging results. Abrupt withdrawal of the drug is not recommended.

Advantages and disadvantages encountered in the use of barbiturates. Barbiturates lend themselves to a variety of uses. They are anticonvulsants, anesthetics, hypnotics, and sedatives, although no one of them excels in all of these types of action. They are easily administered in tablets or capsules, for the most part, although they may be given in other ways, e.g., rectally or parenterally. They have a reasonably wide margin of safety, especially those which the nurse is likely to give.

The main disadvantages are that in large doses they all depress the respiratory center; and they are often used for suicide. In addition, they are habit-forming. These are drugs which should never be left at the bedside for the patient to take at will. Patients have been known to hoard barbiturates until they had enough to commit suicide.

*Harris, Isbell, and others: Chronic Barbiturate Intoxication, An Experimental Study, Arch. Neurol. & Psychiat. 64: 1, 1950.

Legislation. These drugs in the past have had a wide use and have been easy to get, which resulted in indiscriminate use and use for suicidal purposes. At present many states have passed legislation patterned after the Harrison Narcotic Act which restricts the sale of hypnotic drugs and prohibits the sale or possession of barbiturates except under proper licensure. Barbiturates may not be purchased or dispensed without a physician's prescription and the prescription may not be refilled without the physician's personal sanction.

Choice of barbiturate

In choosing barbiturate preparations, consideration is given primarily to the duration of effect produced by the drug and to individual needs of patients. Phenobarbital is an outstanding member of the group of barbiturates because of its anticonvulsant action and will be described in greater detail. Secobarbital and pentobarbital are good examples of short-acting barbiturates, and the ultra short-acting ones will be described under anesthetics.

Barbiturates may be combined in the same capsule so that a long-acting and a short-acting or moderately long-acting preparation can be used to advantage in overcoming the type of insomnia in which the patient has difficulty both in getting to sleep and remaining asleep for the desired number of hours. *Tuinal* is an unofficial combination of secobarbital sodium and amobarbital sodium. It is available in capsules containing ¾ gr. (0.05 Gm.) of each barbiturate (total 0.1 Gm., 1½ gr.) or 1½ gr. of each (total 0.2 Gm., 3 gr.)

Phenobarbital (Luminal)

Phenobarbital not only requires a relatively long time to take effect but it also exerts an effect over a long period (six or more hours) and is used when prolonged sedation is required. It is used as a hypnotic as well as a sedative for a variety of nervous conditions such as chorea, gastrointestinal neuroses, disturbances of menopause, and preoperative and postoperative states of tension. It is also proposed as a sedative in certain circulatory and cardiac disorders. Because its action is rather slow, it is not the best drug for certain kinds of insomnia or for use as a preanesthetic medication.

Phenobarbital has a selective depressant action on the motor cortex of the brain *when given in sedative doses* to epileptic patients. It is the best-known member of the group about which this can be said, although many, if not all, depress the motor cortex in large or anesthetic doses. When effective anticonvulsant doses are given, unfortunately some degree of central depression also results. (The patient feels tired, relaxed, and perhaps dull and sleepy.) In this respect phenobarbital is inferior to

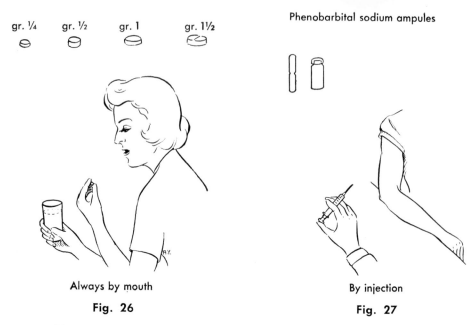

Phenobarbital tablets

gr. ¼ gr. ½ gr. 1 gr. 1½

Phenobarbital sodium ampules

Always by mouth

Fig. 26

By injection

Fig. 27

Figs. 26 and 27 These illustrations emphasize the point that phenobarbital and phenobarbital sodium are not one and the same drug. Phenobarbital sodium is suitable for parenteral administration, whereas the plain phenobarbital is not.

the anticonvulsant drug Dilantin. On the other hand, phenobarbital is regarded as one of the least, if not *the* least, toxic of the antiepileptic drugs.* The adult dose varies between 0.1 and 0.13 Gm. (1½ and 2 gr.). This may be given in one dose at the time the patient retires, or it may be given in divided doses and spread throughout the day. Should it be necessary to discontinue the drug for an epileptic patient, it should be done gradually and never stopped suddenly or severe epileptic seizures may be precipitated. Phenobarbital is often given to patients following surgical operation on the brain, to minimize the irritating effect of the procedure. Patients may continue to take the drug for a year or more under medical supervision.

The action and uses of phenobarbital sodium are the same as those of phenobarbital except that it can be injected when phenobarbital either cannot be given by mouth or the desired effects are not being secured by oral administration.

CAUTION: Errors sometimes occur if the nurse forgets, or does not un-

---

*Goodman, L., and Gilman, A.: The Pharmacological Basis of Therapeutics, New York, 1955, The Macmillan Co., p. 142.

derstand, that phenobarbital (Luminal) and phenobarbital sodium (Sodium Luminal) are not one and the same drug. The latter, the sodium salt, can be given parenterally but the former cannot.

Preparation, dosage, and administration.

Phenobarbital Tablets, U.S.P.; *Phenobarbitone Tablets,* B.P. Usual dose is 30 mg. (½ gr.) orally.

Phenobarbital Elixir, U.S.P. Usual dose is 4 ml. (1 fluidram) orally.

Phenobarbital Sodium, U.S.P.; *Phenobarbitone Sodium,* B.P. Usual dose is 30 mg. (½ gr.). This is a powder dispensed in ampules for parenteral or oral administration.

Phenobarbital Sodium Injection, N.F. Usual dose is 30 mg. (½ gr.). A sterile solution of phenobarbital sodium in a suitable solvent is used intramuscularly or subcutaneously. Aqueous solutions of phenobarbital sodium decompose upon standing.

Phenobarbital Sodium Tablets, N.F.; *Phenobarbitone Sodium Tablets,* B.P. Usual dose is 30 mg. (½ gr.) orally.

Phenobarbital is also available in 60 mg. and 100 mg. Spansules.

Secobarbital Sodium (Seconal Sodium)

Although similar in its actions to that of barbital, secobarbital is a short-acting barbiturate, more active than barbital, and given in correspondingly smaller doses. Small doses produce a sedative effect and larger doses, a hypnotic effect.

Preparation, dosage, and administration.

Secobarbital Sodium, U.S.P. (Seconal Sodium); *Quinalbarbitone Sodium,* B.P. Dosage is 0.1 to 0.2 Gm. (1½ to 3 gr.) for adults. As a pre-anesthetic agent, 0.2 to 0.3 Gm. is given one-half to one hour before the patient goes to the operating room. It is available in 30, 50, and 100 mg. capsules and in 30, 60, 120, and 200 mg. rectal suppositories. Secobarbital is usually given by mouth, although it may be given rectally, in which case the drug should be dissolved in about an ounce of tepid water and given with a small rectal tube. Rectal suppositories are also available.

Pentobarbital Sodium (Nembutal Sodium) and related compounds

Pentobarbital sodium is similar in its actions to barbital, but it is effective in smaller doses. It acts over a rather brief period of time (three to six hours) which is sometimes an advantage, particularly if large doses have been given. It is used as a hypnotic and as a sedative prior to anesthesia.

Pentobarbital is one of the short-acting derivatives of barbituric acid, and both pentobarbital and pentobarbital calcium share in the action and uses of pentobarbital sodium. Pentobarbital calcium has no advantage except that it is better suited for making compressed tablets than pentobarbital sodium.

Preparation, dosage, and administration.

Pentobarbital Sodium Elixir, U.S.P. (Nembutal Sodium Elixir). Usual dose is 4 ml. (1 fluidram). It is marketed in the form of an elixir for preoperative sedation of children or for elderly patients.

Pentobarbital Sodium, U.S.P., B.P. (Nembutal Sodium); *Pentobarbitone Sodium,* B.P. Usual dose is 0.1 Gm. (1½ gr.). Range of dosage may vary from 0.1 to 0.5 Gm. for oral hypnotic or sedative use. The preparation is available in capsules, ampules containing the drug in powder form or in solution for injection, as suppositories for rectal administration, and in Spansules for slow, continuous absorption. *Pentobarbital Sodium Injection,* U.S.P., may be given intravenously if prompt action is essential, e.g., to control convulsive seizures associated with some types of drug poisoning, rabies, tetanus, chorea, eclampsia. Aqueous solutions of pentobarbital are not stable and decompose on standing or after boiling.

*Pentobarbital Calcium** (Nembutal Calcium). Dosage is 0.1 Gm. (1½ gr.). It is available in tablet form rather than capsules for oral administration. It is usually administered orally or rectally.

Thiopental will be discussed under anesthetics.

Nonbarbiturate sedatives and hypnotics

Ethchlorvynol (Placidyl)

Ethchlorvynol is a colorless to yellow liquid with a pungent odor. It is a mild hypnotic somewhat less predictable than the barbiturates. An advantage over the barbiturates which is claimed for this drug is that it has not been known to cause addiction and the incidence of "hangover" effects has been less. It acts within 15 to 30 minutes after administration, and the duration of its effects is about 5 hours.

Uses. Ethchlorvynol is said to be useful in the treatment of insomnia if pain and anxiety are not complicating factors. It is also useful for patients who are unable to take barbiturates. It may also be used as a daytime sedative. Careful observation of patients who receive this drug over long periods of time is thought advisable since clinical experience with it has been limited.

Preparation, dosage, and administration.

*Ethchlorvynol** (Placidyl). This drug is available in 100, 200, and 500 mg. capsules. The usual adult hypnotic dose is 500 mg.; sedative doses are correspondingly smaller. It is administered orally.

Side effects. This drug seems to have a wide margin of safety. Side effects include headache, fatigue, ataxia, dizziness, mental confusion, nightmares, nausea, and vomiting.

*Described in annual publication of A. M. A. Council on Drugs, N.N.D., 1960.

Ethinamate (Valmid)

Ethinamate exerts a mild sedative effect upon the central nervous system. The duration of its effects is shorter than that produced by the barbiturates. It is effective within 15 to 25 minutes, and the duration of its effects is about 4 hours. It has not been known to cause habituation or addiction, and tolerance does not seem to develop. It is readily absorbed from the gastrointestinal tract and rapidly destroyed or excreted from the body.

Uses. It is used chiefly as a rapidly acting hypnotic for the treatment of simple insomnia. It can be used for patients with impaired function of the liver and kidney. It is not a hypnotic of choice for patients requiring heavy or continuous sedation.

Preparation, dosage, and administration.

Ethinamate (Valmid). This preparation is available in 500 mg. tablets. The minimal effective hypnotic dose for adults is 500 mg. Larger and repeated doses may be required to produce a full night's sleep. It is administered orally.

Side effects. Toxic effects have not been reported, but careful observation of patients who receive the drug over long periods of time is recommended.

Glutethimide (Doriden)

Glutethimide is a hypnotic and sedative that depresses the central nervous system and produces effects similar to those produced by the short-acting barbiturates. The main advantage claimed for it is that it can be used for patients who do not tolerate the barbiturates. It is effective in 15 to 30 minutes, and its effects last 4 to 8 hours. "Hang-over effects" do not seem to be noticeable unless the drug is administered late at night or unless the dose is repeated in the course of the night. It is not considered to be an addicting agent.

Uses. At present the greatest use for glutethimide seems to be for relief of simple or nervous insomnia, provided it is uncomplicated by pain or severe agitation. It can be used both as a preoperative and as a daytime sedative.

Preparation, dosage, and administration.

Glutethimide (Doriden). This drug is marketed in 125, 250, and 500 mg. tablets. The usual hypnotic dose for adults is 500 mg. given orally at bedtime. For daytime sedation, 250 mg. may be given orally three times daily after meals.

Side effects. The principal side effects seem to be nausea and occasionally rash on the skin. Toxic effects and the treatment are much the same as those for poisoning with the barbiturates.

*Described in annual publication of A. M. A. Council on Drugs, N.N.D., 1960.

Methyprylon (Noludar)

Methyprylon depresses the central nervous system in a manner similar to the barbiturates except that it has less tendency to depress the respiratory center. The onset and duration of its action are said to be similar to those of the short-acting barbiturates. Its capacity to cause addiction is thought to be less than that of the barbiturates, although further study of this property may prove otherwise.

Uses. Methyprylon is used in the treatment of simple and nervous insomnia. It acts rapidly and produces several hours of sleep.

Preparation, dosage, and administration.

Methyprylon* (Noludar). It is marketed in 50 and 200 mg. tablets and as an elixir containing 10 mg. per milliliter. Doses of 50 to 100 mg. three or four times daily are prescribed to produce sedation, and 200 to 400 mg. is the usual adult hypnotic dose given at bedtime.

Side effects. The incidence of side effects is thought to be low, although the following have been observed: nausea, vomiting, constipation, diarrhea, headache, itching, and rash on the skin.† No serious toxic effects on the kidney, liver, or bone marrow have been reported.

There are a number of hypnotics which were almost abandoned when the barbiturates became popular. They seem to be gradually regaining some of their lost popularity. They include chloral hydrate and paraldehyde as well as a number of others.

Chloral Hydrate

Source. Chloral hydrate was first synthesized in 1862. It is the oldest of the hypnotics and is still used. It is a chlorinated derivative of acetaldehyde, or it may be described as a hydrate of trichloracetaldehyde. It is a crystalline substance that has a bitter taste and a penetrating odor. It is readily soluble in water, alcohols, and oils, e.g., olive oil.

Action and result. Locally, chloral hydrate is an irritant. Systemically, it depresses the central nervous system and decreases awareness of external stimuli. It acts promptly (10 to 15 minutes) and produces sleep which lasts 5 hours or more. The sleep greatly resembles natural sleep; the patient can be awakened without difficulty. It produces little or no analgesic effect, and it is neither an anesthetic nor an anticonvulsant.

In therapeutic doses there is little or no effect on the heart and respiratory center. The pulse and blood pressure are not lowered more than can be observed in ordinary sleep. In large doses chloral hydrate depresses the respiratory and vasomotor centers, resulting in slowed res-

---

*Described in annual publication of A. M. A. Council on Drugs, N.N.D., 1960.

†Lasagna, L.: The Newer Hypnotics, M. Clin. North America, p. 361, 1957.

234

piration and dilatation of cutaneous blood vessels. The effect on the heart is said to be similar to that of chloroform. Overdoses will cause cardiac depression, especially in patients with heart disease.

Uses. Chloral hydrate is used as a sedative. It produces sedation similar to paraldehyde and the barbiturates. It is sometimes used to relieve symptoms during the withdrawal phase of drug addiction (alcoholism, opiate, or barbiturate).

Chloral hydrate is used as a hypnotic when insomnia is not due to pain. It is one of the cheapest and best hypnotics. Its chief disadvantage is that it can produce gastric irritation. It also has an unpleasant taste, but this problem is remedied by administering the drug in capsule form.

Preparation and dosage.

Chloral Hydrate, U.S.P., B.P. This is a crystalline substance. The usual adult dose is 500 mg. given up to 3 times a day. Larger doses may also be prescribed (250 mg. to 1 Gm.). It is marketed in soft gelatin capsules containing 250 and 500 mg. and in suppository form. It can be prepared as an aqueous solution or a syrup (dissolved in a syrup).

Administration. If the liquid solution is administered it should be well diluted with water or given in a syrup or milk to disguise the taste. It is sometimes given to children in the form of a retention enema (dissolved in oil). It is too irritating to be given parenterally. It should not be given with alcohol to avoid the additive effects of two depressant drugs. Such a combination is sometimes referred to as a "Mickey Finn" or "knock-out drops."

Side effects and toxic effects. Symptoms of both acute and chronic toxicity are sometimes observed.

Acute poisoning. Although chloral hydrate has a wide safety range, acute poisoning can occur. Symptoms are similar to those of any central depressant and include the following: deep sleep, stupor, coma, lowered blood pressure, slow weak pulse, slow respiration, and cyanosis. The local effects of the drug may cause nausea and vomiting when it is taken orally. Death is usually caused by respiratory depression or it may result from sudden heart failure in patients who have cardiac damage. If the patient survives, there is a possibility that damage may have been done to the liver and kidneys.

Treatment is essentially the same as that for acute poisoning with barbiturates.

Chronic poisoning. Chloral hydrate habitues develop some tolerance to the drug, but habituation is rare. It results in degenerative changes in the liver and kidneys, nervous disturbances, weakness, skin manifestations, and gastrointestinal disturbances. Treatment consists in gradual withdrawal of the drug and rehabilitative measures similar to those used in the treatment of the chronic alcoholic.

Contraindications. Chloral hydrate is contraindicated for patients with serious heart disease or impaired function of the liver and kidney and sometimes for patients with gastric or duodenal ulcer.

Petrichloral (Periclor)

Petrichloral is a derivative of chloral which exhibits a hypnotic and sedative action similar to chloral hydrate. It is better tolerated than the latter drug because it has no odor or aftertaste, and it does not produce gastric irritation. It has a wide margin of safety.

Preparation, dosage, and administration.

Petrichloral° (Periclor). This drug is available in 300 mg. gelatin capsules. The usual hypnotic dose is 600 mg., and the sedative dose for daytime effect is 300 mg. every 6 hours.

Chlorbutanol (Chloretone)

Chlorbutanol is similar to chloral hydrate both chemically and pharmacologically. It does not cause gastric irritation but produces a local anesthetic action on mucous membranes. It is used as a hypnotic and as a preservative in sera, solutions of epinephrine hydrochloride, etc. As a hypnotic, the same precautions should be observed for its use as given for chloral hydrate.

Preparation, dosage, and administration.

Chlorbutanol, B.P. (Chloretone). It is available in 300 mg. capsules for oral administration. The usual adult dose is 0.3 to 1 Gm.

Paraldehyde

Paraldehyde has been used as a hypnotic since 1882, when it was introduced into medicine. It is a polymer of acetaldehyde, i.e., it is formed from three molecules of acetaldehyde which join together when in the presence of an acid. It is a colorless, transparent liquid with a strong odor and a disagreeable taste. It is only slightly soluble in water but freely soluble in oils and in alcohol.

Action and result. Paraldehyde depresses the central nervous system, producing drowsiness and sleep in 10 to 15 minutes after a hypnotic dose. The sleep closely resembles a natural sleep and lasts for 4 to 8 hours. Therapeutic doses do not depress the medullary centers and do not affect the heart and respiration. It is less potent than chloral hydrate but also less toxic. It is not an analgesic, and it may compel sleep in spite of pain.

Absorption and excretion. Paraldehyde is rapidly absorbed from the mucosa of the gastrointestinal tract and also from intramuscular sites of injection, although it may cause some irritation when given parenterally.

°Described in annual publication of A. M. A. Council on Drugs, N.N.D., 1960.

The fate of paraldehyde in the body is not known, but a large part of it is thought to be destroyed in the liver. It is therefore contraindicated for patients who have serious impairment of liver function. It is not contraindicated for patients with renal disease. A part of the drug is excreted by the lungs, where it tends to increase bronchial secretions, and for this reason it is avoided for patients with bronchitis and pneumonia.

Uses. Paraldehyde is employed for its hypnotic and sedative effects in treatment of conditions in which there is a threat of convulsive seizures or nervous hyperexcitability. It is used therefore in delirium tremens, tetanus, strychnine poisoning, and mania. It is sometimes used as a basal anesthetic, particularly for children; when so used it is given rectally.

Preparation, dosage, and administration.

Paraldehyde, U.S.P., B.P. This drug is available as a plain liquid for oral administration or as a sterile solution dispensed in ampules (2 ml. and 10 ml.) for parenteral use. Usual adult oral dose is 8 ml. (2 fluidrams) but may be increased to 10 or 15 ml. in some instances. When paraldehyde is given orally it should be disguised in a suitable medium such as a flavored syrup, fruit juice, wine, or milk, and it should be given very cold to minimize the odor and taste. It can also be given as a retention enema (mixed with a thin oil). When given intramuscularly a pure sterile preparation should be used. The usual intramuscular dose is 5 ml. It is rarely given intravenously.

Side effects and toxic effects. The chief disadvantages of paraldehyde are its obnoxious odor, disagreeable taste, and irritating effect on the throat and stomach if the drug is not well diluted in a suitable medium. Because of the odor it is not suitable for patients who are up and about, for they will reek with the odor of the drug. Fortunately, if the patient is capable of noticing the odor, his sense of smell becomes dulled after a time. Paraldehyde has a wide safety range. Symptoms of overdosage resemble those of alcohol in that mild poisoning can usually be "slept off." The incidence of acute toxicity is low, although deaths from paraldehyde depression have been reported. The symptoms of poisoning and treatment are essentially the same as those for chloral hydrate.

The bromides

Bromide was discovered in the waters of the Mediterranean in 1826 by Balard. In 1864 potassium bromide was used by Behrend in certain cases of sleeplessness and a little later by Vigouroux and Voisin in epilepsy. It was assumed that its action was similar to that of potassium iodide, and it was given in large doses (30 Gm. per day) for glandular swellings of syphilis and tuberculosis. These large doses revealed its peculiar narcotic or sedative action which at present is the most important effect.

The bromides are white crystalline substances which are odorless and have a pungent saline taste. They are readily soluble in water.

Action and result. The main therapeutic action of the bromide ion is on the central nervous system.

Nervous system. Bromides are given mainly for their depressant action on the central nervous system. The depression may vary from a mild sedation to a deep coma, depending upon dosage given. Bromides are not directly hypnotic in the same way that morphine and chloral hydrate are but favor sleep by depressing the centers, which prevent orderly impressions from exerting a disturbing influence. The entire cerebrospinal axis, with the exception of the medulla, is readily affected. Large therapeutic doses depress the psychic centers, motor areas, and many of the reflexes of the brain and spinal cord. The sensory areas concerned with pain, as well as the respiratory center, are not much affected except by large doses. The irritability of the cough center is lessened, and coughing may be allayed. After the bromides have been given long enough to build up the level in the blood, the mind becomes less alert, special senses are less keen, and the patient becomes apathetic, relaxed, indifferent, and more or less drowsy. Nervous excitement, worry, and anxiety are relieved. Sleep, however, after large doses is not necessarily refreshing but may be followed by a drowsy hang-over and a sense of weariness. Reflexes are diminished, and example of which is the disappearance of the gagging reflex when the fauces is irritated.

Circulatory system. Ordinary doses of the bromides have little effect on circulation. They sometimes favorably influence cardiac disturbances due to an abnormal irritability of the central nervous system. Large doses depress the heart and vasoconstrictor center.

Gastrointestinal system. Although bromides are given to allay vomiting of central origin, they have no effect on the alimentary canal, with the possible exception of producing nausea and vomiting when large doses are given. This is attributed to irritation by their saline action.

The bromides of potassium, ammonium, and sodium have identical actions, but the ammonium ion is somewhat stimulating and the potassium ion depressing, whereas the sodium ion is neutral in effect.

Absorption, distribution, and excretion. Bromides are rapidly absorbed and are excreted almost entirely in the urine. There is a tendency to accumulation since they are not excreted as rapidly as absorbed.

Bromides when absorbed occur in all the secretions and fluids of the body. Traces are found in sweat, in the milk, in the hair, and in other places where chlorides occur naturally. The brain and spinal cord do

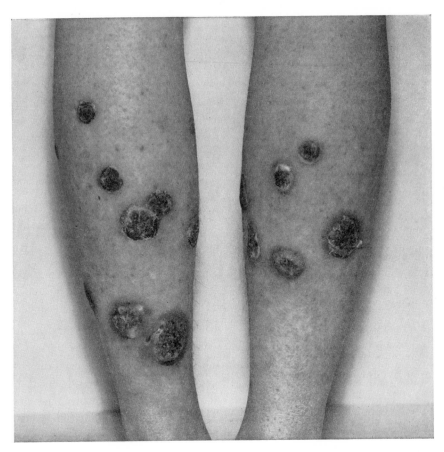

Fig. 28 Skin eruption which followed prolonged administration of a medicine that contained a bromide. The medicine had been administered for insomnia.

not contain any more than other organs and never approach the concentration found in the blood plasma.

Uses. Bromides are given primarily as anticonvulsants and as sedatives. They are not, however, preparations of choice if a rapid action is desired. Sedation is not obtained by a single dose but rather by consecutive doses in order to obtain the desired level of the bromide in the blood. They are less effective as anticonvulsants than phenobarbital and Dilantin.

Preparation, dosage, and administration.

Potassium Bromide, N.F. Usual dose is 1 Gm. (15 gr.).

Sodium Bromide, N.F. Usual dose is 0.3 Gm. (5 gr.) three times a day; range of dosage, 0.3 Gm. to 1 Gm. Sodium bromide is said to be the least irritating to gastric mucosa and it is the least expensive.

Sodium Bromide Elixir, N.F. Usual dose is 4 ml. (1 fluidram).

Drugs that affect central nervous system 239

Sodium Bromide Tablets, N.F. Usual dose is 1 Gm. (15 gr.).

Three Bromides Elixir, N.F. Usual dose is 4 ml. (1 fluidram). This is a mixture of sodium, potassium, and ammonium bromide.

Bromides are always given by mouth in the form of capsules, tablets, or in specially flavored vehicles to disguise the disagreeable salty taste. Effervescent preparations are not unpleasant to take. They should be given after meals and with plenty of fluid to minimize the gastric irritation and the dehydrating effect of the medication. Administration is usually three to five times a day.

Side effects and toxic effects. Poisoning may be acute or chronic.

Acute poisoning. Acute poisoning is comparatively rare. Large doses, however, may produce deep stupor, ataxia, extreme muscular weakness, and collapse. Treatment consists of stopping the drug and giving large quantities of physiologic salt solution to hasten the excretion of the drug.

Chronic poisoning. Repeated administration of bromides often leads to a condition known as *bromism.* This condition varies according to individual susceptibility. The first symptom may be a bromide acne, which is seen on the face, chest, and back. The cause of the skin disturbance is not definitely known but is probably due to a peculiar sensitization of the skin by the bromide ion. Other poisonous symptoms from long-continued use are salty taste in the mouth, foul breath, gastrointestinal disturbance, mental depression, faulty memory, pronounced apathy, ataxia, slurred speech, muscular weakness, malnutrition, and anemia. As a rule, the symptoms of bromism rapidly abate if the drug is withdrawn.

Contraindications. Bromides should be given with caution to patients with advanced arteriosclerosis, debilitation, and dehydration. A state of delirium can be rather easily produced in the patient with cerebral arteriosclerosis. Poor renal function, chronic alcoholism, malnutrition, and mental depression are all conditions in which bromide therapy is not indicated. Since bromides are not good analgesics, their use when the patient is in pain may cause delirium. Bromides are contraindicated for patients who are to receive the drug for long periods of time unless they can be kept under close medical observation.

Nonselective depressants
Anesthetics

Anesthetics are drugs that produce loss of sensation. General anesthetics produce loss of sensation accompanied by loss of consciousness. They produce analgesia before they produce loss of consciousness. The anesthetic state is accompanied by varying degrees of muscular relaxation. In recent years there has been a renewal of interest in drugs that

240

produce analgesia without loss of consciousness. Local anesthetics abolish sensation in regions of application or injection or in the part supplied by nerves that have been blocked by the anesthetic agent.

Historical points of interest

It is more than a hundred years since the first volatile anesthetics were used to produce relief of pain and unconsciousness during a surgical operation. Prior to that, agents to relieve pain were limited to alcoholic beverages, belladonna preparations, and opium. The psychic as well as physical trauma associated with surgery without a good anesthetic definitely limited what the surgeon could do for a patient. An English physician, Sir Clifford Allbutt, is quoted as follows: "When I was a boy, surgeons operating upon the quick were pitted one against the other like runners on time. He was the best surgeon both for the patient and the onlooker, who broke the three minute record in an amputation or a lithotomy."[*]

Nitrous oxide was discovered in 1772 by Joseph Priestley, who did not realize that the gas had anesthetic properties. Sir Humphrey Davy in 1799 suggested that because of its pain-relieving property, it might be tried in connection with surgery, but his suggestion passed unheeded for many years. Three hundred years elapsed from the time of the discovery of ether until it began to be used for the relief of pain during surgery. Dr. Crawford Long, of Georgia, in 1842 had a patient inhale ether while he removed a tumor from the neck. Dr. Long failed to publish a report of this administration in the medical literature and therefore failed to receive full credit for being the first to discover the value of ether as an anesthetic agent.

Horace Wells, a dentist, observed some of the properties of nitrous oxide and began to use it in connection with his dental practice. In 1845 he attempted to demonstrate its capacity to relieve pain during a surgical operation. The demonstration failed and his efforts were ridiculed, with the result that this useful agent received little attention for some time thereafter. It was not appreciated in that day how difficult it is to produce a good level of anesthesia with nitrous oxide alone and over the period of time required for a surgical operation.

In 1846 William Morton, another dentist, who later studied medicine, successfully anesthetized a patient with ether at the Massachusetts General Hospital in Boston. The success of this undertaking launched a new era in surgery.

Chloroform was discovered in 1831, and in 1847 James Simpson of England successfully demonstrated its usefulness. Queen Victoria knighted him for his contribution to the relief of pain.

[*]Beecher, H. K.: Anesthesia, Scient. Am. 196: 70, Jan., 1957.

The action of general anesthetics

It is known that general anesthetics depress the central nervous system, but relatively little is known of how these chemical agents bring about the depression. There are a number of interesting theories, one of which is that anesthetics depress the function of the cellular enzymes controlling oxidation.[*] A great deal of investigational work is being done, but regardless of the ultimate explanation, anesthesia is produced by progressively increasing the amount of the anesthetic agent, first in the blood and subsequently in the nervous system.

Unlike many other drugs, the anesthetics that can be given by inhalation are absorbed, transported, and excreted by the body without undergoing chemical change.[†]

For the most part, they are exhaled and excreted by way of the lungs, except for small amounts lost by way of the kidneys, skin, etc. They are therefore relatively safe agents since their anesthetic effect can be reversed by elimination from the lungs, provided respiration is maintained satisfactorily.

The pattern of depression is similar for all anesthetics, *irregular descending depression*. The cerebral cortex is depressed first, then structures of the diencephalon, midbrain, spinal cord, and lastly, the medullary centers. It is fortunate that the medulla is spared temporarily, since it contains the vital centers concerned with heart action, blood pressure, and respiration.

In recent years the concept of "balanced anesthesia" has become increasingly well known. This means the use of a combination of agents and methods so that part of the burden of pain relief is borne by the preanesthetic drugs, part by local anesthetics, and part by one or more of the general anesthetics.[‡] It has been found that by combining several drugs, each in small amounts, the desired state of anesthesia can be produced with slight disturbance of physiologic functions and at the same time place a minimal burden on each of the organs of detoxication and excretion. Many new and important measures are utilized in the field of supportive therapy to prevent and control shock, hypoxia, disturbance of electrolyte balance, as well as circulatory and respiratory depression. An effort is made to avoid saturating the tissues of the patient with any one agent. Many times the patient is now kept in a state of analgesia and unconsciousness and does not need to be in a deep state of anesthesia,

[*]McCarthy, K. C.: Nitrous Oxide. In Hale, D. E. (editor): Anesthesiology, Philadelphia, 1955, F. A. Davis Co., p. 274.

[†]Vandam, L. D.: Transport of Anesthetics and Stages of Anesthesia. In Drill, V. A. (editor): Pharmacology in Medicine, New York, 1958, McGraw-Hill Book Co., Inc. p. 45.

[‡]Lundy, J. S., and Courtin, R. F.: The Present Status of Balanced Anesthesia and Supportive Therapy, Collected Papers at the Mayo Clinic and the Mayo Foundation, Philadelphia, 1949, W. B. Saunders Co., p. 653.

since muscle relaxants can be made to do what the anesthetic agent once had to do, i.e., produce muscular relaxation necessary for the surgical procedure. Considerable emphasis is placed on adequate oxygenation throughout the period of anesthesia and also in the immediate post-anesthetic recovery period.

More recently Dr. John Lundy had this to say about balanced anesthesia:

"It is interesting at this particular time that 'balanced anesthesia' has arrived at an unforeseen goal, and I now speak of it as 'precision balanced anesthesia.' This fortunate circumstance has gradually developed since more and more drugs that antagonize the deliberate effects of anesthetics and analgesics have been developed. An example is the advent of phenazocine (Prinadol) which can be administered intravenously or orally, and when either a local anesthetic or nitrous oxide and oxygen is used with it, anesthesia becomes under almost perfect control. Five milligrams of Prinadol plus 1 mg. of Lorfan are administered. Good analgesia develops with little respiratory depression. The important point in this 'precision balanced anesthesia' is that it is not drug against drug but rather dose of drug against dose of drug. If the approved proportions between Prinadol and Lorfan are used, good respiration results with good analgesia. If two to four times as much Lorfan is used, then the desirable drug effect of Prinadol is eliminated. We are able to antagonize muscle relaxants with Tensilon; we are able to antagonize the effect of Pentothal with Megimide so that we have almost perfect control of the situation if only a plan is made prior to beginning the use of the drugs and then one uses oxygen and nitrous oxide rather than to say 'nitrous oxide and oxygen' so that the emphasis is on ample oxygen."*

Preanesthetic medications

Satisfactory anesthesia is partly dependent on the preparation of the patient. Several hours of restful sleep and relief from worry and anxiety help the patient to tolerate the stress of anesthesia and the operation. Sedative and hypnotic drugs are usually administered the night before as well as the morning of the operation. This type of medication decreases apprehension and worry, tends to produce serenity and amnesia, and decreases reflex excitability. The latter brings about a lowered metabolic rate which in turn decreases the amount of anesthetic required.† Preanesthetic medications, given properly, promote a smooth, even, and comfortable induction period of the anesthesia.

One of the barbiturates such as pentobarbital sodium (Nembutal Sodium) is often administered the night before the operation to ensure a sound and restful sleep, and it may be repeated the morning of the day of surgery.

Narcotics, such as morphine sulfate, meperidine hydrochloride (Demerol Hydrochloride), alphaprodine hydrochloride (Nisentil Hydrochloride), methadone hydrochloride (Dolophine Hydrochloride), and levor-

*From Lundy, J. S.: Personal communication.
†Faulconer, A., and Lundy, J. S.: Selection of the Anesthetic. In Hale, D. E. (editor): Anesthesiology, Philadelphia, 1955, F. A. Davis Co., p. 219.

phanol tartrate (Levo-Dromoran Tartrate), with or without atropine or scopolamine, may be prescribed for the patient prior to the time that he is taken to the operating room. It is important that the nurse administer the medications at the time they are ordered to be given, because a narcotic like morphine, if given too close to the time of the administration of the general anesthetic, may achieve its full effect after the administration of the general anesthetic has begun and cause severe respiratory depression.

Some physicians prefer to use a drug such as promethazine (Phenergan) or chlorpromazine (Thorazine) in combination with one of the following—ethchlorvynol (Placidyl), methprylon (Noludar), glutethimide (Doriden), or pentobarbital—to produce a sound sleep the night before operation, and they may prescribe promethazine again in the morning, along with morphine or atropine.

Atropine is effective in reducing bronchial and salivary secretions and in preventing spasm of the vocal cords (laryngospasm). It is also a mild respiratory stimulant. Scopolamine augments the action of narcotics and is an exceptionally effective drug to produce amnesia. Dosage of any of the preanesthetic drugs will depend upon the weight, age, and general condition of the patient.

Requirements of an ideal general anesthetic

It is highly desirable that the anesthetic agent have a wide safety range; considerable difference should exist between the therapeutic and the toxic dose.

The anesthetic should produce anesthesia rapidly and not be unpleasant to take.

The recovery should be rapid and free from discomfort.

The anesthetic should be readily excreted from the body without damage to body tissues.

The anesthetic should produce maximum muscular relaxation and should not increase capillary bleeding.

The anesthetic should be of such potency that the levels of anesthesia are easily controlled and that oxygen may be administered freely with it.

The anesthetic should be a stable substance and not explosive.

There is no known anesthetic that fulfills all of the above requirements, but these criteria may be used to evaluate the properties of the various anesthetic agents.

Stages of anesthesia

Anesthetists have learned to observe a patient's reactions while under anesthesia and have come to know when conditions are satisfactory for surgical procedure and when a reaction constitutes a danger signal.

244

The stages of anesthesia vary with the choice of anesthetic, the speed of induction, and the skill of the anesthetist. It is possible to administer some anesthetics so that the first two stages are scarcely discernible. However, if the drug is given slowly enough, usually all stages can be observed. It has become traditional to outline the stages of anesthesia. They are most easily seen when ether is used as the only anesthetic. In present-day practice, ether may be used along with a number of other agents, in which case the patient may not go beyond the first stage, or some other anesthetic is used for induction and then a switch is made to ether.

Stage of analgesia or stage of local irritation and diminished sensation

This stage begins with the first inhalation and lasts until consciousness is lost. The difficulty of getting air through a mask and the irritating effects of anesthetics such as ether may cause choking, coughing, and increased secretion of tears and saliva (unless atropine was administered). The breathing may be rapid and irregular. These reactions can be avoided to some extent by gradual induction and by the skill of the anesthetist in gaining the cooperation of the patient. The pulse and blood pressure may be somewhat elevated because of the excitement, unless the patient has been well sedated by the preliminary medication. Senses become less acute, and numbness and loss of sensation gradually spread over the body. Pain is abolished before consciousness is lost. Speech becomes difficult and indistinct. The pupils are normal and react to light but dilate as the patient passes into the second stage. The body feels stiff and unmanageable.

Stage of excitement

The second stage varies greatly in different individuals. It is not always seen in the adult, and it is frequently absent in children. In some persons there is merely a tremor, stretching of the extremities, or irregularity in respirations, but in others, especially in habitual users of alcohol, there is great excitement and violent movements. This stage begins with movements of the arms, designed to push the mask away or to enable the patient to rise. Then other muscles are used and the patient may struggle, sing, shout, laugh, swear or talk. The patient must be fastened securely to the table at the beginning of this stage. Excitement and involuntary motor activity are said to be due to depression of the higher centers of the brain. The pulse is usually faster than usual, and the blood pressure is elevated. Muscular tone is increased, and all reflexes are present. Exaggerated respiratory reflexes are responsible for irregular respiration and may be the cause of uneven absorption of the anesthetic into the blood. The irritant effect of the anesthetic may cause the patient to hold his

Drugs that affect central nervous system 245

breath temporarily and then inspire deeply. This constitutes one of the dangers in this stage of anesthesia. The pupils are dilated but continue to react to light. There is an exaggerated response to painful stimuli; hence premature surgery and painful stimuli are avoided. Correct use of preanesthetic medication is said to do much to prevent accident in this stage. The first two stages constitute the *period of induction*.

Stage of surgical anesthesia

The third stage is divided into four planes. Whether a patient is in one or the other of these four planes is determined by the character of the respirations, the nature and movement of the eyeballs, the size of the pupils, and the degree to which reflexes are present or absent. Most operations are done in plane 2 or in the upper part of plane 3. As the patient moves into plane 1 the respiratory irregularities of the second stage have usually disappeared and respiration becomes full and regular. As anesthesia deepens, respiration becomes more shallow and also more rapid. Paralysis of the intercostal muscles is followed by increased abdominal breathing; finally only the diaphragm is active. Preliminary medications affect the respiratory rate and volume during all stages of anesthesia. The eyeballs, which exhibit a rolling type of movement at first, gradually move less and then cease to move at all. The size of the pupils depends in part on the amount and kind of preliminary medication. Normally, if the pupils were reflexly dilated in the second stage, they now constrict to about the size they are in natural sleep. The reaction to light becomes sluggish. The pupils dilate as plane 4 is approached.

The face is calm and expressionless and may be flushed or even cyanotic. The musculature becomes increasingly relaxed as reflexes are progressively abolished. Most abdominal operations cannot be done until the abdominal reflexes are absent and the abdominal wall is soft. The body temperature is lowered as the anesthetic state continues. The pulse remains full and strong. Blood pressure may be slightly elevated, but in plane 4 the blood pressure drops and the pulse becomes weak. The skin, which was warm, now becomes cold, wet, and pale.

With an anesthetic such as ether the third stage (upper planes) may be maintained for hours, with little change by the repeated administration of small amounts of the drug.

Stage of medullary paralysis (toxic stage)

The fourth stage is characterized by respiratory arrest and vasomotor collapse. Respiration ceases before the heart action so that artificial respiration may lighten the anesthetic state (if a gaseous agent has been used) and save the patient's life.

Methods of administering anesthetics by inhalation

Open method

Liquid anesthetics such as ether are frequently given by dropping the anesthetic on gauze or cotton placed on a wire mask which fits over the patient's nose and mouth. This is called the open drop method. There is free access to air. No attempt is made to confine the vapor, and there is no rebreathing of the anesthetic mixture. Another form of the open method is seen when a gaseous agent such as nitrous oxide merely flows over the patient's face.

Semi-open

This refers to the use of some means to decrease the escape of the anesthetic vapor. A towel may be placed around the base of the mask. There is some rebreathing of the anesthetic mixture and a greater retention of carbon dioxide than with the open method, but a higher concentration of anesthetic vapor is provided.

Closed

This method can be used for both gases and volatile liquids. An anesthetic machine is used and an apparatus fits over the nose and face of the patient, or a tube, i.e., an endotracheal tube, connects the respiratory tract of the patient with the anesthetic machine, thus forming a closed system. Provision is made for removal of carbon dioxide, absorption of moisture, and regulation of the intake of the anesthetic agent or agents, as well as oxygen. Regulation of respiration by the anesthetist is made possible by the periodic and rhythmic compression of the breathing bag. The closed method affords better control of the anesthetic state, as well as greater economy of the anesthetic since rebreathing of the mixture occurs. The anesthetist must be an expert to use this method safely and advantageously.

General anesthetics

Ether (Diethyl Ether)

$$\begin{matrix} C_2H_5 \\ \diagdown \\ \diagup \\ C_2H_5 \end{matrix} O$$

Ether is a clear, colorless liquid with a pungent odor and a bitter, burning taste. It is formed by the action of sulfuric acid on ethyl alcohol. It is highly volatile and very flammable. Mixtures of ether and air or ether and oxygen are explosive. It is decomposed by light and air and should therefore be kept in sealed metal containers. Ether is a good solvent for fats, oils, resins, and adhesive plaster.

Action and result. Ether may have either a local or systemic reaction.

Drugs that affect central nervous system 247

Local. When applied to the skin and allowed to evaporate, ether cools the skin. If it is not allowed to evaporate, it reddens the skin and acts as a rubefacient. Ether irritates mucous membranes and causes increased secretion of mucus, saliva, and tears. When moderately dilute, it acts as a carminative in the digestive tract. Nausea and vomiting may result from gastric irritation or from central stimulation of the vomiting center.

Systemic. The systemic action of ether has been described in the presentation of the stages of anesthesia. Ether progressively depresses the central nervous system, beginning with the highest intellectual centers and then affecting the sensory and motor centers, basal nuclei, cerebellum, spinal cord, and finally the medullary centers. Learned reactions are lost first, and sensory functions are lost before motor functions. Consciousness gradually recedes. Muscles gradually relax and voluntary movement becomes impossible. Ether has an action similar to that of curare at the myoneural junctions. It is said to be the only anesthetic to possess this action. When ether and a member of the curariform drugs are used together, the dose of the latter must be reduced. The induction period is comparatively slow and the period of recovery is longer than for a number of the other general anesthetics.

For a time, ether makes the heart beat faster and stronger; then, as the vagus nerve is blocked, the heart is reflexly accelerated for a time. In the deeper planes of surgical anesthesia the myocardium is directly depressed. Ether produces peripheral vasodilatation by slight depression of the vasomotor center and also by direct depression of the smooth muscle of the blood vessels, particularly the peripheral blood vessels in the skin. Blood pressure is lowered as anesthesia deepens. The skin feels warm, and the face is frequently flushed. Loss of considerable heat from the body is thus explained. The temperature of the body may be reduced several degrees during a long operation.

The respiratory center is stimulated during induction, and this can result in uneven breathing and sudden changes in the rate of absorption of the ether. Respirations are usually full and even during surgical anesthesia. As anesthesia deepens, respiration is depressed and finally ceases.

The pupils of the eye are dilated somewhat, as a rule, during the first and second stages and appear more like they do in normal sleep in the third stage. As the patient regains consciousness slight dilatation recurs. Sudden, marked dilatation is regarded as a danger signal, as it may mean the beginning of respiratory failure. Of course, the size of the pupil may be modified by the action of the preanesthetic drugs such as morphine and atropine.

Some degree of irritation in the kidney is indicated by the presence of albumin in the urine and scanty urine formation for several hours following surgery. Postoperative retention may be due to poor tone in the urinary bladder. There is no evidence that ether causes any damage to the liver.

Contractions of the uterus are not much affected by moderate degrees of anesthesia, but they are slowed and decreased by deep anesthesia. Ether is not an entirely satisfactory anesthetic to relieve the pain of childbirth because its analgesic effect cannot be obtained fast enough unless the pains are coming regularly and each pain is carefully anticipated. There are better analgesics for this purpose.

In the early stages of anesthesia there may be sufficient stimulation of smooth muscle of the gastrointestinal tract to cause nausea and vomiting. During moderate or deep surgical anesthesia, ether produces diminished peristalsis and tone of smooth muscle of the gastrointestinal organs. This is sometimes responsible for the development of distention. Early ambulation is believed to be helpful in prevention of local accumulations of gas.

Recovery from ether anesthesia proceeds in reverse order, i.e., the patient goes from the stage of surgical anesthesia through the stage of excitement and on through the stage of analgesia before becoming fully conscious. The nurse must make sure that the patient's face is turned to the side to prevent aspiration of mucus or vomitus. No patient should ever be left alone until he is fully conscious. The present-day use of postanesthetic recovery rooms, in which the patient is under constant observation, may be indirectly responsible for a nursing student forgetting this precaution should some patient be sent directly to his room from the operating suite.

The sense of hearing returns comparatively early. This is a fact worth noting. Postanesthetic doses of morphine or similar narcotics should be withheld until the gagging, swallowing, and coughing reflexes have returned fully. Return of function of these reflexes coincides with the return of consciousness.

Uses. Ether continues to be used widely as a general anesthetic. A combination of nitrous oxide gas, oxygen, and ether (G-O-E) is commonly used also. Nitrous oxide may be used for induction, and thus the unpleasant suffocating effects of ether, as well as much of the excitement of the second stage, are avoided. Ether can be used to check convulsive seizures associated with tetanus and strychnine poisoning. It is used as a fat solvent to cleanse the skin prior to surgical procedures.

Preparation, dosage, and administration.

Ether, U.S.P., B.P. The dose depends upon the patient, the length of operation, and the depth of anesthesia maintained.

Ethyl Oxide, N.F.; *Solvent Ether,* B.P. This is not used for anesthesia. Ether is administered in any of the ways mentioned under administration on p. 247. It is often given by the open drop method, although the closed system is also employed, especially if it is combined with a number of other agents.

Side effects and toxic effects. Acute toxicity due to overdosage may occur during administration. If induction is pushed too rapidly there may be a temporary respiratory arrest. Removal of the mask or facepiece is usually all that needs to be done. Respiration is usually resumed at the normal rate. Prolonged administration of ether may result in respiratory depression and respiratory failure. The pulse becomes feeble and irregular, and the blood pressure drops. The skin becomes cold, clammy, and gray. The pupils dilate widely and do not react to light. Other dangers associated with ether anesthesia are those that arise from aspiration of mucus or vomitus or from some other form of obstruction of the airway.

Treatment of overdosage is prevented by keeping the patient in the lighter planes of surgical anesthesia. Oxygen and artificial respiration will hasten the elimination of the ether and lighten the anesthesia.

Advantages. Ether is considered to be a relatively safe anesthetic. There is a wide margin of safety between the anesthetic dose and the toxic dose. Ether is a potent chemical, so that adequate amounts of oxygen can be given with it. It brings about excellent muscular relaxation. It is said that if anesthetists could have but one anesthetic agent they would probably choose ether.

Disadvantages. Ether is flammable and potentially explosive. It is irritating to mucous membranes and unpleasant to inhale. The recovery period from ether anesthesia may be unpleasant because of nausea and vomiting.

Contraindications. Although ether has long been thought to be contra-indicated in pulmonary disease, this opinion has, to some extent, been reversed. Ether depresses activity of the vagus nerve, which is desirable in thoracic surgery. When ether is administered in a closed system with adequate amounts of oxygen and continual removal of carbon dioxide and when steps are taken to prevent accumulations of secretions in the bronchial tubes and trachea, this anesthetic seems to serve satisfactorily for thoracic surgery even when pulmonary disease is present. Its use is not recommended for patients in acidosis or for those who have advanced renal disease. Unless special precautions are taken it should not be administered when an open flame or cautery must be used.

Vinyl Ether (Divinyl Ether, Vinethene)

$$H - C = C - O - C = C - H$$
$$\begin{array}{cccc} | & | & & | & | \\ H & H & & H & H \end{array}$$

Vinyl ether is a clear, colorless fluid which greatly resembles ether. It is more volatile but about as flammable and explosive as diethyl ether. Partial decomposition may occur when it is exposed to light and air.

Action and result. Vinyl ether depresses the central nervous system but it acts more rapidly, which means that the toxic stage is also reached more rapidly. To prevent overdosage the patient must be watched with more than the usual care. Induction is rapid and smooth and surgical anesthesia is produced two or three times more quickly than with ordinary ether.* Continuous administration is necessary to maintain anesthesia; otherwise the patient promptly recovers consciousness. The effects on respiration and circulation are similar to those produced by diethyl ether. It produces satisfactory muscular relaxation with minimal respiratory irritation.

Uses. Vinyl ether is used especially for minor operations or surgical procedures of short duration. It is sometimes used as an induction agent prior to the administration of another anesthetic. It is a useful anesthetic in dentistry, for post-partum repair work, and in surgery of the ear, eye, nose, and throat.

Preparation and administration.

Vinyl ether, U.S.P., B.P. It is available in 10, 25, 50, and 75 ml. bottles with droppers. It can be administered by the open drop method and also by the semi-closed and the closed methods.

Side effects and toxic effects. This drug has a narrow safety range and can cause damage of the liver and kidney. It may cause increased flow of saliva, even after the administration of atropine. It is contraindicated in the aged and for patients with hepatic and renal insufficiency. It is particularly important to prevent hypoxia during its administration since lack of oxygen is believed to be the cause of the hepatic damage. Repeated administration of vinyl ether after short intervals or prolonged administration at any time is not recommended. Nausea and vomiting seldom occur.

Chloroform

$$H - \overset{\displaystyle Cl}{\underset{\displaystyle Cl}{\overset{|}{\underset{|}{C}}}} - Cl$$

Chloroform is a heavy, clear, colorless liquid. It has a characteristic odor and a sweet taste. It is prepared by the action of the chlorine on alcohol or by the direct chlorination of methane. It should be protected from bright light when stored. It is not flammable, and when mixed with oxygen it does not form an explosive mixture.

Action and result. Chlorofrom, like ether, progressively depresses the central nervous system. It resembles ether in that all degrees of surgical anesthesia may be obtained along with adequate oxygenation of the

---

*Goodman, L., and Gilman, A.: The Pharmacological Basis of Therapeutics, New York, 1955, The Macmillan Co.

patient. Chloroform is more pleasant to inhale than ether. It provides a faster induction and is not as irritating to mucous membranes, since a lower concentration can be used. It provides excellent muscular relaxation. It is excreted mainly from the lungs much the same as ether.

Uses. Chloroform is little used in the United States. It is used more often in tropical countries where it is difficult to give ether by the drop method because of its high volatility. In this country it has, to a great extent, been replaced by agents that are considered safer anesthetics. It is now used chiefly as an emergency anesthetic and for surgical or obstetrical patients in a home.

Preparation and dosage.

Chloroform, U.S.P., B.P. Dosage is determined for patients on an individual basis.

Side effects and toxic effects. Chloroform is said to have caused five times as many deaths as ether. It may disturb the rhythm of the heart and cause it to slow or to stop beating. This is thought to be preventable by the proper use of atropine. Chloroform has also been blamed for damage of the liver and the kidney. Some authorities are of the opinion that the dangers of chloroform have been exaggerated and believe that, because of its advantages, its status should be re-evaluated. They maintain that with present-day facilities for supplying adequate oxygen and removing carbon dioxide, chloroform is not necessarily more toxic than a number of other anesthetics.

Nitrous Oxide (Nitrous Monoxide)

Nitrous oxide is a colorless gas somewhat heavier than air, with a slight odor and a sweetish taste. It long has been known as "laughing gas." It is unique in that it is an inorganic compound (contains no carbon atoms). It is made from ammonium nitrate. It is nonflammable and nonexplosive, but at sufficiently high temperatures it will dissociate, release oxygen, and support combustion. It will therefore increase explosiveness of certain other anesthetics, such as ethylene and ether.

Action and result. The central nervous system is the only part of the body that seems to react to nitrous oxide. When the gas is mixed with air and inhaled it produces an effect similar to that of a mild intoxicant. The patient feels merry, laughs, and talks, but he does not go to sleep.

When the pure gas is inhaled, the patient first feels warm, numb, dizzy, and confused. Vivid dreams and hallucinations may be experienced. After a few deep inspirations the patient becomes pale and soon loses consciousness. If administration is continued the patient becomes cyanosed and death results from asphyxia. The upper planes of surgical anesthesia are reached in one or two minutes, but by this time the patient is already becoming seriously depleted of oxygen. Respirations are deep and rapid, later becoming irregular and shallow. If administration is stopped before cyanosis is marked, consciousness is regained rapidly. Because many untoward effects are associated with anoxia, administration of undiluted nitrous oxide is not recommended. Anesthesia can be safely prolonged when a mixture of 20 per cent oxygen and 80 per cent nitrous oxide is used, but this combination is insufficiently potent to produce satisfactory surgical anesthesia without premedication. Nitrous oxide has no untoward effects on circulation, respiration, and the liver or kidneys unless oxygen deficiency is allowed to develop and persist. Nitrous oxide does not irritate the respiratory mucous membrane. Muscular relaxation is not as complete as it is with ether or cyclopropane.

Uses. If nitrous oxide were more potent it would probably be regarded as an ideal anesthetic. As it is, it is an excellent analgesic and can be given with oxygen to produce this effect, especially in certain dental procedures and in obstetrics. It is also used as an agent for induction prior to the use of other anesthetics. G-O-E refers to the use of gas (nitrous oxide), oxygen, and ether in that sequence.

When preceded by a suitable preanesthetic medication, nitrous oxide and oxygen can be combined with a drug such as thiopental sodium and a muscle relaxant. This makes it possible to maintain the patient satisfactorily in a light anesthetic state and still have sleep, satisfactory relief of pain, and the muscular relaxation needed for many operations.

The use of oxygen and nitrous oxide without other agents is limited to those surgical procedures that are brief and do not require muscular relaxation.

Preparation and administration.

Nitrous Oxide, U.S.P., B.P. This anesthetic is available in the compressed state in steel cylinders. The closed system is usually employed for administration.

Side effects and toxic effects. Nitrous oxide itself is considered a very innocuous substance. However, probably no more serious danger in anesthesia exists than that of anoxia. The chief disadvantage of nitrous oxide is its low anesthetic potency, although this can be remedied by proper use of supplemental agents. Satisfactory administration requires an experienced anesthetist and a special apparatus (machine).

Ethylene

$$H_2C=CH_2$$

Ethylene is a colorless, highly volatile gas with a slightly sweet taste and an unpleasant but not intolerable odor. When mixed with a certain amount of oxygen it is highly explosive and flammable. However, it is believed to be no more explosive than ether-oxygen or ether-oxygen-nitrous oxide mixtures when comparable precautions are taken. Ethylene was first used for clinical surgery in 1923.

Action and result. Ethylene has a direct depressant action on the central nervous system. Induction is smooth and rapid, but ethylene is less powerful as an anesthetic than either ether or cyclopropane. It is difficult to reach more than plane 1 or possibly plane 2 of surgical anesthesia. This, of course, is not a serious disadvantage if the patient has received adequate preliminary medication and/or if supplemental agents, such as ether or a muscle relaxant, are used. Analgesia definitely precedes anesthesia. Ethylene does not irritate the respiratory mucosa, and it does not increase salivary secretion. The patient awakens readily when administration of ethylene is stopped. Respiratory depression and vasomotor depression are uncommon, and postoperative complications are rare.

Uses. Ethylene is used in obstetrics to produce analgesia. It does not interfere with uterine contractions in labor. It is also used for certain surgical operations with or without supplemental agents. It is sometimes preferred for the patient who is considered a poor surgical risk.

Preparation and administration.

Ethylene, N.F. It is available in steel tanks in which the gas is kept under considerable pressure. It is administered with oxygen in a closed system technic with a gas machine. It is important for the patient to receive a preliminary medication so that adequate amounts of oxygen may be given during anesthesia to prevent hypoxia.

Disadvantages. The chief disadvantage associated with the use of ethylene is the hazard of fire and explosion. As is true of certain other anesthetics, the time of greatest danger is at the end of the operation, when the mask is lifted from the patient's face. For this reason no one should touch the anesthetist or the anesthetic machine other than those more or less constantly working with the patient or with the machine. A small spark of static electricity may set off an explosion. This precaution applies to all explosive mixtures. In other respects ethylene is considered one of the least disturbing of the general anesthetics.

Cyclopropane

$$CH_2$$
$$H_2 - C - C - H_2$$

Cyclopropane is a colorless gas, heavier than air, flammable, and explosive in most anesthetic concentrations when mixed with air or oxygen. It has a mildly pungent but not unpleasant odor. It is stable and is stored in metal cylinders where under pressure it liquefies easily.

Action and result. Cyclopropane is a potent anesthetic. Adequate amounts of oxygen can be given with it, to the extent of 20 per cent or more, and it will still produce satisfactory anesthesia. A wide margin of safety exists between the anesthetic and the toxic dose. Induction is pleasant and reasonably rapid. It does not irritate the respiratory mucous membrane and hence it is unlikely to cause respiratory irregularities. In low concentrations analgesia precedes loss of consciousness. There is little change in respiration until deep depression is produced. Laryngospasm occasionally develops; therefore atropine or scopolamine is likely to be prescribed as a preliminary medication. The insertion of an artificial airway along with the use of a muscle relaxant usually prevents further difficulty with laryngospasm. Cyclopropane produces a fair amount of muscle relaxation, although the supplemental effect of muscle relaxant may be required to obtain the amount desired. Uterine and intestinal muscle is not affected unless the patient is in the lower planes of surgical anesthesia.

Uses. Cyclopropane has been used successfully as a general anesthetic for all kinds of operations. It has been approved as an anesthetic for chest surgery, in which quiet respirations and absence of bronchial irritation are important. It is also used in obstetrics since it can be administered in amounts that do not affect uterine activity or the respirations of the child.

Preparation and administration.

Cyclopropane, U.S.P., B.P. Stored in steel cylinders, cyclopropane is administered by inhalation, preferably with the use of the closed system because it is both expensive and explosive.

Side effects and toxic effects. As anesthesia with cyclopropane deepens, disturbance of cardiac rhythm may occur. Sudden death has been known to result. This effect seems to be related to the development of hypoxia and the retention of carbon dioxide. The anesthetist often manually assists the patient to breathe by rhythmically squeezing and releasing the breathing bag on the anesthetic machine. Some anesthetists are using a device to monitor the pulse in order to pick up early changes in the action of the heart. This may be done during the administration of all anesthetics, not only during administration of cyclopropane.

The incidence of nausea, vomiting, and postoperative distention is said to be less than that after ether anesthesia but more than that seen after anesthesia with nitrous oxide or ethylene.

Ethyl Chloride

$$C_2H_5Cl$$

Ethyl chloride is a colorless, highly volatile liquid with an agreeable odor and a sweetish, burning taste. It is flammable and explosive and should be kept from any contact with fire.

Ethyl chloride is a powerful, rapidly acting general anesthetic. It closely resembles chloroform in its effects, but it acts more rapidly than chloroform. It does not provide complete muscular relaxation. Because of the ease with which the anesthesia progresses beyond the surgical stage and because of the danger of cardiac arrest associated with its administration, it is rarely used except for short and minor procedures, e.g., opening a boil. It is occasionally used as an agent for induction prior to the administration of ether. For this purpose it is given by the open drop method, although the closed technic can also be used.

Ethyl chloride also acts as a local anesthetic. After it is sprayed on the area to be anesthetized, it evaporates so rapidly it freezes the underlying tissues and produces insensibility to pain. It thus permits incision and drainage of boils, carbuncles, etc. The edema and erythema which result from the thawing of the tissues can be rather painful.

Preparation.

Ethyl Chloride, N.F., B.P. This anesthetic is marketed in sealed glass tubes or small metal cylinders.

Basal anesthetics

Basal anesthesia means the induction of unconsciousness by a non-volatile anesthetic or soporific before the production of surgical anesthesia. Basal anesthetics are usually given rectally or intravenously. They are valuable to allay emotional distress since many patients dread having a tight mask placed over their face while they are fully conscious. Basal anesthetics reduce the amount of general anesthetic required. The two principal drugs used for this purpose are tribromoethanol (Avertin) and thiopental sodium (Pentothal Sodium).

Tribromoethanol (Avertin)

$$Br - \underset{\underset{Br}{|}}{\overset{\overset{Br}{|}}{C}} - \underset{\underset{H}{|}}{\overset{\overset{H}{|}}{C}} - OH$$

Tribromoethanol is a white, crystalline powder with a slightly aromatic taste and odor. Chemically it is related to ethyl alcohol and chloral. It is unstable in light and air; it is sparingly soluble in water but very soluble in amylene hydrate. Amylene hydrate is flammable.

Action and result. Tribromoethanol depresses the central nervous system. In basal anesthetic amounts it produces drowsiness, amnesia, and sleep in about 15 minutes, reaching its maximal effect in about 30 minutes. It materially decreases the amount of inhalation anesthetic required, and, in addition, it provides a pleasant induction and state of sedation which lasts well into the postanesthetic period. There is often

256

a temporary drop in blood pressure. It is also a powerful respiratory depressant. Overdosage can produce respiratory failure. Careful attention must be given to the patient during both the anesthesia and the post-anesthetic sleep to make certain that the airway is open. An artificial airway is often inserted to prevent obstruction. Because of its effects on respiration and blood pressure and because it is difficult to regulate the depth of anesthesia, it is not considered safe to use it alone for surgical anesthesia. Since the drug is given rectally, there is no easy way of lowering the concentration in the body.

Uses. Tribromoethanol is of value as a basal anesthetic for patients who are unusually nervous and apprehensive because it can be given to the patient in his own room. He is spared the stress and anxiety as well as the respiratory irritation associated with induction with some of the general anesthetics. The drug may also be employed to control or prevent convulsive seizures associated with eclampsia, tetanus, or status epilepticus (continuous epileptic seizures). It is not extensively used.

Preparation, dosage, and administration.

Tribromoethanol, U.S.P. (Avertin with Amylene Hydrate). This contains in each milliliter 1 Gm. of tribromoethanol and 0.5 Gm. of amylene hydrate. Dosage is usually calculated on the basis of body weight, but dosage should not exceed 8 ml. for women and 10 ml. for men. It is administered rectally in 2.5 per cent solution in warm distilled water at a temperature not to exceed 40° C. or 104° F.

Side effects and toxic effects. Prolonged postanesthetic sleep complicates the nursing problems in care of patients receiving this drug since they cannot be left alone. There is difficulty in controlling the level of depression once the dose has been given and therefore tribromoethanol is contraindicated in a number of conditions. Patients should not receive this drug if they are chronic alcoholics or if they have impaired function of the liver or kidney or disease of the colon, rectum, or heart. It is thought to be inadvisable to use it for patients of advanced years.

Thiopental Sodium (Pentothal Sodium)

Barbiturates are used both as general anesthetics and as basal anesthetics. Thiopental sodium is an ultrashort-acting barbiturate and seems to be the most popular. Its use has steadily increased since it was first introduced by Dr. John S. Lundy in 1934.

Action and result. Thiopental sodium depresses the central nervous system and produces rapid loss of consciousness. The usual early stages of anesthesia are rarely seen because the drug acts so rapidly. The patient may go to sleep in the middle of a sentence. Induction is smooth, easy, and pleasant for the patient. Recovery is uneventful and rapid, and complications are rare. Its use is not accompanied by the hazard of fire or explosion. Opinion has been expressed that the experienced, skillful anesthetist finds the control of anesthesia with this agent as easy or easier than with many of the anesthetics given by inhalation. Abdominal relaxation is likely to be inadequate even with deep anesthesia, and if used as a general anesthetic its effects are frequently supplemented with those of one of the curariform drugs. Due attention must be given to the possible dangers of hypoxia, obstruction of the air passages, and respiratory depression.

Uses. Thiopental sodium is used as a basal anesthetic to carry the patient through the period of induction prior to the use of an anesthetic given by inhalation or prior to the use of a spinal anesthetic or some other form of local anesthetic. It is also used in combination with a number of other drugs for many kinds of minor and major types of surgery; e.g., it may be given by intermittent intravenous injection along with a muscle relaxant and nitrous oxide and oxygen. The nitrous oxide and oxygen may be given by inhalation through an endotracheal tube.

Preparation, dosage, and administration.

Thiopental Sodium, U.S.P. (Pentothal Sodium); *Thiopentone,* B.P. This drug marketed in glass ampules containing 0.5, 1, 5, and 10 Gm. of the powder with anhydrous sodium carbonate which acts as a buffer and makes the resulting solution less irritating to tissues. Thiopental sodium is unstable when in solution and must be freshly made. The usual dose is 2 to 3 ml. of a 2.5 per cent solution; it is given intravenously in about 10 or 15 seconds and is repeated in 30 seconds as required. A 10 per cent solution is sometimes given rectally as a basal anesthetic for children (0.2 ml. per pound of body weight).

Side effects and toxic effects. The rapid onset of action of this barbiturate is both a desirable effect and a potential danger. Medullary paralysis may develop rapidly when an overdose is given. It also has a tendency to produce laryngospasm. This can be prevented or handled successfully with the use of a drug such as atropine or a curariform drug such as succinylcholine (Anectine), or by the use of endotracheal intubation. Although some difference of opinion seems to exist as to how thiopental is metabolized, there seems to be agreement that it is detoxified chiefly in the liver and the metabolic products are excreted by the kidney. Its use is not recommended for patients with severe heart disease, hepatic disease, anemia, or respiratory difficulties.

Hexobarbital Sodium and Thiamylal Sodium

Hexobarbital Sodium, N.F. (Evipal Sodium) and *thiamylal sodium* (Surital Sodium) are both ultrashort-acting barbiturates with properties similar to those of thiopental sodium.

Local anesthetics

Although local anesthetics do not rightfully belong with the central nervous system depressants, for convenience of study they will be presented here.

Local anesthetics are drugs that, in sufficient concentration, are capable of blocking the conduction of nerve impulses along both sensory and motor nerve fibers. When concentration is carefully controlled it is possible to produce loss of sensation without producing motor paralysis because sensory fibers are affected before motor fibers. The concentration of the local anesthetic needed to block conduction of nerve impulses in a nerve is much less than the concentration of a general anesthetic found in the blood of a patient in surgical anesthesia. A similar amount of a local anesthetic in the blood would cause death. For this reason, effort is made to confine the local anesthetic to a limited region or small area near a nerve or among nerve endings. Rapid absorption of a local anesthetic is impeded by the addition of epinephrine or similar drugs which are vasoconstrictors. The action of the local anesthetic is reversible, i.e., it is followed by complete recovery and, as a rule, produces no damage to the nerve cells.

Reactions to local anesthetics

All local anesthetics are potentially toxic drugs. Most reactions to them are believed to be due to overdosage and rapid absorption into the systemic circulation. Occasionally a local anesthetic may be accidentally injected into a blood vessel; hence the use of low concentrations is considered less hazardous. Reactions to local anesthetics are usually reactions of the central nervous system, the cardiovascular system, and the skin, i.e., an allergic reaction.

Reactions of the central nervous system. The patient may exhibit nervousness, apprehension, and confusion and may complain of dizziness. He may also have muscular twitching and go on to unconsciousness and convulsions. The physician is likely to want a short-acting barbiturate such as thiopental sodium for intravenous therapy in case of convulsive seizures. Some patients have a low level of tolerance and react to a very small dose of the drug.

Reaction of the cardiovascular system. The patient suddenly becomes pale, feels faint, and has a drop in blood pressure. If the patient is sitting up it is important to have him lie down flat. This will help to restore blood pressure in the brain and may prevent the development of convulsive seizures. Cardiac arrest can be the end result of a cardiovascular reaction.

Allergic reaction. True allergic reactions are said to be uncommon. Sometimes a reaction is thought to be allergic when it is really caused by overdosage. However, allergic reactions can occur. They may be relatively mild (hives, itching, skin rash) or they may be of an acute anaphylactic nature. Small test doses are frequently given by the physician to gauge the extent of the patient's sensitivity to the anesthetic agent. Dosage and administration must be decided on an individual basis for each patient.

———

Preliminary medication is frequently prescribed prior to the use of a local anesthetic much the same as before a general anesthetic. The use of a barbiturate is believed to prevent or decrease toxic reactions. Some anesthesiologists recommend the administration of a systemic analgesic and a tranquilizing agent, e.g., levorphan tartrate (Levo-Dromoran Tartrate) and promethazine hydrochloride (Phenergan Hydrochloride), prior to the administration of a local anesthetic. The anesthetic agent chosen, its concentration, the rate of injection, and physical and emotional factors in the patient, all influence reactions to local anesthetics.

Methods of administration

Some local anesthetics are suited only for surface anesthesia, some must be injected, and some are suitable for both topical administration and injection.

Surface anesthesia. Surface anesthesia is accomplished by painting or swabbing the mucous membrane with a preparation of the local anesthetic or by the use of a pack soaked with an anesthetic solution. This method is used in connection with surgery of the eye, nose, or throat. Cocaine continues to be one of the most widely used agents for topical administration. Local anesthetics do not penetrate the unbroken skin, but preparations containing a local anesthetic are applied to mucous membranes, wounds, ulcers, etc. in the form of solutions, ointments, or powders.

Anesthesia by injection. Anesthesia by injection is accomplished by infiltration, conduction, spinal, caudal, and saddle block.

Infiltration anesthesia is produced by injecting dilute solutions of the agent into the skin and then subcutaneously into the region to be anesthetized. Epinephrine is often added to the solution of the anesthetic to intensify the anesthesia in a limited region and to prevent excessive bleeding and systemic effects. Repeated injection will prolong the anesthesia as long as it may be needed. The sensory nerve endings are anesthetized.

Conduction or block anesthesia means that the anesthetic is injected into the vicinity of a nerve trunk which supplies the region of the operative site. The injection may be made at some distance from the site of surgical procedure. A single nerve may be blocked, e.g., an ulnar nerve block, or the anesthetic may be injected in a location where several nerve trunks emerge from the spinal cord (paravertebral block).

Spinal anesthesia is a type of extensive nerve block, sometimes called a subarachnoid block. The anesthetic solution is injected into the subarachnoid space, and it affects the lower part of the spinal cord and the nerve roots. Several complications may arise with this procedure; the anesthetic may spread to upper levels of the cord and autonomic as well as sensory and motor fibers may be blocked, seriously interfering with respiration, heart action, and the maintenance of blood pressure. Spinal anesthesia is used less now than previously.

Caudal anesthesia (caudal block) is sometimes used for the obstetrical patient. The anesthetic solution is introduced into the sacral canal and affects the sacral nerves, producing anesthesia of the pelvic region.

Saddle block is sometimes used in obstetrics and for surgery involving the perineum, rectum, genitalia, and upper parts of the thighs. The patient sits upright while the anesthetic is injected, after a lumbar puncture has been done. The patient remains upright for a short time until the anesthetic has had a chance to be effective. The parts which would have been in contact with a saddle when riding become anesthetized; hence the name.

Cocaine

Cocaine is one of the oldest local anesthetics and is still an important one. It is an alkaloid derived from the leaves of the coca shrub which grows in Peru and other parts of South America. The native people of this country have been known to chew the leaves to give them added energy and ability to endure fatigue. In medicine, cocaine is used chiefly in the form of cocaine hydrochloride, which occurs as a white crystalline powder and is freely soluble in water and alcohol.

Action and result. When a moderate amount of absorption occurs, cocaine stimulates the central nervous system from above downward and produces a state of mild stimulation. The pulse is stronger and more rapid, blood pressure is elevated, respirations are faster and deeper, and the activities of the brain are increased. The patient is more talkative and active, is more alert mentally, and feels exhilarated and happy. With increasing absorption, depression rather quickly follows stimulation. The higher centers are depressed first and death is due to respiratory failure. When applied topically cocaine has no effect on unbroken skin, but it blocks the conduction of nerve impulses when in contact with mucous membranes or, abraded skin or when injected under the skin, producing insensibility to pain. Sensation is completely recovered when the drug is eliminated. Cocaine dilates the pupil of the eye and anesthetizes the cornea after topical application but only slightly affects accommodation (the ability to focus objects). It produces some vasoconstriction in the conjunctiva and sclera.

Uses. Cocaine is used chiefly for surface anesthesia of the nose, throat, and eye. It is also injected in low concentrations for the removal of tonsils and similar procedures, although some authorities do not recommend its administration by injection.

Preparation and dosage.

Cocaine Hydrochloride, U.S.P., B.P., and *Cocaine,* N.F., are official preparations. Concentrations of 1 to 4 per cent are used for surface anesthesia of the eye and 2 to 5 per cent for mucous membranes of the nose and throat. Epinephrine hydrochloride is frequently added to the cocaine solutions. Cocaine crystals may be moistened in epinephrine hydrochloride solution (1:1,000) for placement on the nasal mucosa prior to surgical operation in the nose. One fifth per cent concentration is the strength usually used for injection.

Side effects and toxic effects. Acute toxic symptoms are likely to occur if the drug is absorbed rapidly, whereas no toxic effects are likely to be noted after slow absorption because adequate time for destruction in the body is provided. Excessive absorption from overdosage may cause the following symptoms: headache, dizziness, excitement, palpitation, fainting, and sometimes convulsions and collapse. Death usually results from failure of respiration. Patients have been known to collapse and die very quickly. The most specific treatment is intravenous administration of a short-acting barbiturate. Artificial respirations may also prove helpful.

Cocaine habit. This habit is acquired either from frequent medicinal use of cocaine or deliberately for the pleasurable excitement the drug produces. Addicts usually induce others to acquire the habit and assist each other in obtaining this and other habit-forming drugs. The tolerance for cocaine is considerable and the strength of habit is such that it is doubtful whether it is ever abandoned voluntarily. Continued use of the drug results in chronic poisoning. The earliest effects may be digestive disturbances and loss of appetite and weight, but the nervous system suffers most, and gradual degeneration of mind and morals, as from the opium habit, usually results. Sleeplessness, tremors, spasm, delirium, and insanity are some of the consequences of long-continued use. To help combat the danger of habituation and addiction, cocaine and all its derivatives are under the regulations of the Harrison Narcotic Law.

Procaine Hydrochloride (Novocain)

Procaine is a synthetic local anesthetic. Many synthetic local anesthetics have points of similarity in their chemical structure, i.e., they are amino esters of aromatic acids. Procaine is a white powder which is readily soluble in water. In solution it withstands sterilization with heat, although a precipitate may form when the solution stands for a long time.

$$NH_2$$

$$O=C-O-\underset{\underset{H}{|}}{\overset{\overset{H}{|}}{C}}-\underset{\underset{H}{|}}{\overset{\overset{H}{|}}{C}}-N\overset{C_2H_5}{\underset{C_2H_5}{}}$$

Procaine is less potent than cocaine but also less toxic. It is rapidly destroyed by enzymes in the blood and other tissues. It does not constrict blood vessels and does not dilate the pupil of the eye. It produces no particular central action like cocaine, and it is not habit-forming.

Uses. Procaine is the best known of the local anesthetics and it is said to be the safest for both nerve block and infiltration.* It is probably used more than any other single local anesthetic. Reactions occur comparatively seldom, and tend to be mild; elimination is rapid and tissue damage is seldom produced. Procaine is not well absorbed from mucous membranes; hence it is not suited for topical administration. It is useful for many types of local anesthesia when given by injection. Procaine hydrochloride has been used to overcome cardiac arrhythmias, although procainamide is used more often for this purpose.

Preparation and dosage.

Procaine Hydrochloride, U.S.P., B.P. This is available as a white crystalline powder intended for parenteral solutions.

Procaine Hydrochloride Injection, U.S.P.; *Procaine and Adrenaline Injection,* B.P. The U.S.P. preparation is available in concentrations of 1 and 2 per cent procaine hydrochloride. It may or may not contain 0.002 per cent epinephrine (1 in 50,000).

The dosage of procaine used for anesthesia varies with the technic of administration employed. One or 2 per cent concentrations are adequate for most purposes, although concentrations of 0.25 to 0.5 per cent may be used for infiltration. The duration of anesthesia for a nerve block is about 45 minutes and for spinal anesthesia about 1 hour.*

*Adriani, J.: Local Anesthetics, Am. J. Nursing 59: 87, 1959.

Chlorprocaine Hydrochloride (Nesacaine Hydrochloride)

Chlorprocaine is more potent and acts more quickly than procaine.

Preparation and administration.

Chlorprocaine Hydrochloride° (Nesacaine Hydrochloride). Solutions for injection in 1, 2, and 3 per cent concentrations are available.

The drug is not a potent surface anesthetic.† It apparently can be given in all the ways that procaine can be given by injection, although its use for spinal anesthesia has not been fully evaluated.

Toxic effects. Its toxic effects are said to be similar to those produced by procaine. Since it does not produce vasoconstriction its toxicity can be decreased by giving it with epinephrine to delay absorption.

Cyclomethycaine Sulfate (Surfacaine)

Cyclomethycaine sulfate is used as a topical anesthetic for certain types of skin lesions and abrasions in which discomfort is caused from pain and itching. It is also used on vaginal and rectal mucous membranes for effect on painful fissures and ulcerations.

Preparation and administration.

Cyclomethycaine Sulfate° (Surfacaine). Available in preparations which include a topical cream and ointment, a urethral jelly, topical solutions, and suppositories. The concentration of the drug in the various preparations varies from 0.5 to 1 per cent.

Tetracaine Hydrochloride (Pontocaine Hydrochloride)

Tetracaine hydrochloride is a synthetic local anesthetic, the effects of which are said to be more potent and more prolonged than those of procaine. It is also more toxic. It can be employed in dilute concentrations and serves as a useful anesthetic for a number of purposes. It can be used to produce surface anesthesia of the eye, nose, and throat, as well as for infiltration and spinal and caudal anesthesia. Effects are believed to be more prolonged than with procaine.

Preparation and dosage.

Tetracaine Hydrochloride, U.S.P. (Pontocaine Hydrochloride); *Amethocaine Hydrochloride,* B.P. This form is available in solutions of various concentrations and also in tablets. An official ophthalmic ointment 0.5 per cent in white petrolatum is also available. The concentration used varies with the part to be anesthetized; 0.5 per cent solution is commonly employed for the eye, a 2 per cent solution for mucous membranes of the nose and throat, 0.5 per cent for spinal anesthesia, and 0.15 to 0.25 per cent for caudal anesthesia. It can be given with epinephrine.

°Described in annual publication of A. M. A. Council on Drugs, N.N.D., 1960.
†Council on Drugs, N.N.D., 1960, p. 6.

Butacaine Sulfate (Butyn Sulfate)

Butacaine sulfate acts rapidly and produces a prolonged effect. It does not produce constriction of blood vessels or dilatation of the pupil of the eye. Butacaine is used for surface anesthesia of the eye, nose, and throat and has, to some extent, replaced cocaine.

Preparation and administration.

Butacaine Sulfate (Butyn Sulfate). This drug is usually used in a 2 per cent solution. It is also available in an ointment base for local application to the eye.

Toxic effects. Its toxicity is similar to that of cocaine and its administration by injection is not recommended.

Dibucaine Hydrochloride (Nupercaine Hydrochloride)

Dibucaine hydrochloride is not only one of the more potent local anesthetics but also one of the most toxic.[*] Anesthesia is obtained within a few minutes and lasts $2\frac{1}{2}$ to 3 hours.

It is used to produce surface anesthesia and also for spinal anesthesia when prolonged effects are desired. Its use for nerve blocks is not recommended because it has been known to cause tissue damage and severe systemic effects.[†] It can be given with epinephrine.

Preparation and dosage.

Dibucaine Hydrochloride, U.S.P.; *Cinchocaine Hydrochloride,* B.P. These are marketed in ampules and vials containing various amounts of the drug. The drug is used in concentrations of 0.05 to 0.1 per cent solution for injection and topical application.[‡]

Toxic effects. Caution in its use is recommended because of its potential toxicity. It is a constituent of certain ointments used to relieve the discomfort of burns and hemorrhoids.

Hexylcaine Hydrochloride (Cyclaine Hydrochloride)

Hexylcaine hydrochloride is a relatively new local anesthetic.

Preparation, dosage, and administration.

Hexylcaine Hydrochloride.[||] This is used in concentrations up to 5 per cent for surface anesthesia, 1 per cent for infiltration and nerve block, and 2 to 2.5 per cent for spinal anesthesia. It can be administered both topically and by injection. For surface anesthesia it is said to be as effective as cocaine, and for infiltration and nerve block it is thought to be

---

[*]Goodman, L., and Gilman, A.: The Pharmacological Basis of Therapeutics, New York, 1955, The Macmillan Co., p. 367.

[†]Adriani, J.: Local Anesthetics, Am. J. Nursing 59: 88, 1959.

[‡]Robbins, B. J.: Pharmacology. In Hale, D. E. (editor): Anesthesiology, Philadelphia, 1955, F. A. Davis & Co., p .95.

[||]Described in annual publication of A. M. A. Council on Drugs, N.N.D., 1960.

faster and longer acting than equal amounts of procaine.*

Toxic effects. It exhibits toxic effects similar to other local anesthetics and must be employed with the same precautions used with similar agents.

Lidocaine Hydrochloride (Xylocaine Hydrochloride)

Lidocaine hydrochloride is another synthetic local anesthetic. It is said to produce effects more promptly and with greater intensity than those produced by an equal amount of procaine. Lidocaine is suited for surface anesthesia as well as for infiltration and block anesthesia.

Preparation and dosage.

Lidocaine Hydrochloride, U.S.P. (Xylocaine Hydrochloride). Solutions are available in 0.5 to 2 per cent concentration, with or without epinephrine hydrochloride. A 2 per cent jelly is used for mucous membranes of the urethra, and a 5 per cent ointment is available for application to burns and skin lesions.

Toxic effects. In low concentrations its toxicity is thought to be about the same as that of procaine. It has an advantage of being effective in small amounts of low concentrations. Overdosage may result in many of the toxic symptoms associated with local anesthetics, such as drop in blood pressure, nausea, vomiting, pallor, apprehension, muscular twitching and convulsions.

Piperocaine Hydrochloride (Metycaine Hydrochloride)

Piperocaine hydrochloride is chemically related to cocaine but produces effects similar to procaine. It differs from procaine in that it is suited to topical application for surface anesthesia as well as for injection. It is slightly more potent and more toxic than procaine and lasts for about the same length of time. It is compatible with epinephrine and is used for anything for which procaine can be used unless the patient is sensitive to the agent.

Preparation, dosage, and administration.

Piperocaine Hydrochloride, U.S.P. (Metycaine Hydrochloride). Solutions of various concentrations are available for injection, as well as tablets (150 mg.) and an ointment (4 or 5 per cent). The drug is used in concentrations which vary from 0.25 to 5 per cent, depending on the route of administration.

There are a number of other local anesthetics in use at the present time, some of which are described in *New and Nonofficial Drugs.*

*N.N.D., 1960, p. 11.

Local anesthetic which acts by freezing

Low temperatures in living tissues produce diminished sensation. This form of anesthesia is sometimes employed for minor operative procedures. Tissues that are frozen too intensely and over too long a period of time may be destroyed. Ethyl chloride is a local anesthetic which can be used to produce this effect. It is mentioned under general anesthetics, p. 255. It is not employed extensively.

Slightly soluble local anesthetics

A number of local anesthetic agents are only slightly soluble and hence cannot be injected. Because they are absorbed slowly they can be used safely on open wounds, ulcers, mucous surfaces, etc. They occasionally cause dermatitis, which necessitates discontinuation of their use.

Ethylaminobenzoate, N.F. (Anesthesin); *Benzocaine*, B.P. This agent acts as a local anesthetic when applied to painful wounds and ulcers of the skin and mucous membranes. It may be applied as a dusting powder or as an ointment to denuded areas of the skin and to mucous membranes. It is used to relieve itching and discomfort associated with hemorrhoids and rectal fissures. It is also available in the form of rectal and vaginal suppositories.

Ethylaminobenzoate Ointment, N.F. This is a 5 per cent preparation of the drug in white ointment.

Butyl Aminobenzoate, N.F., B.P. This preparation is used with or without a diluent as an anesthetic dusting powder. It is also marketed in the form of troches, suppositories, and ointments.

Butamben Picrate (Butesin Picrate). This agent is marketed in a 1 per cent ointment. It is used for burns, painful ulcers, and other painful lesions of the skin.

Miscellaneous local anesthetics

Eugenol, U.S.P. This anesthetic is a pale yellow liquid obtained from clove oil. It is applied topically to the skin and mucous membrane and is used especially by dentists for the relief of pain due to dental caries.

Phenolated Calamine Lotion, U.S.P. This contains 1 per cent phenol, which is included because the phenol anesthetizes the sensory nerve endings of the skin. It is used for the relief of itching caused by mild allergic reactions.

Nonselective depressants
Alcohols

Although there are many alcohols, which vary physically from liquids to solids, the alcohol usually meant, unless otherwise specified, is ethyl alcohol. Methyl alcohol, propyl alcohol, butyl alcohol, and amyl alcohol are examples of other alcohols. Chemically speaking they are hydroxy derivatives of aliphatic hydrocarbons.

Ethyl Alcohol

$$H - \underset{\underset{H}{|}}{\overset{\overset{H}{|}}{C}} - \underset{\underset{H}{|}}{\overset{\overset{H}{|}}{C}} - OH$$

Ethyl alcohol has been known in an impure form since earliest times, and it is the only alcohol used extensively in medicine. It was formerly thought to be a remedy for almost any disease or disorder. It is a colorless liquid and lighter than water, with which it mixes readily. It lowers surface tension and acts as a good solvent for a number of substances. In concentrations above 40 per cent it is flammable. Ethyl alcohol, also referred to as grain alcohol, is the product of the fermentation of a sugar by yeast. If the carbohydrate used to secure alcohol is a starch, it must first be changed to a sugar before it can be fermented.

Action and result. Ethyl alcohol may have either a local or systemic action.

Local action. Ethyl alcohol denatures proteins by precipitation and dehydration. This is said to be the basis for its germicidal, irritant, and astringent effects.[*] It irritates denuded skin, mucous membranes, and subcutaneous tissue. Considerable pain may result from a subcutaneous injection of alcohol, and slough of the tissue may result. When it is injected into or near a nerve it may produce degeneration of the nerve and anesthesia. Alcohol evaporates readily from the skin, produces a cooling effect, and reduces the temperature of the skin. When rubbed on the surface of the body it acts as a mild counterirritant. It dries and hardens the epithelial layer of the skin and helps to prevent bed sores when used externally. On the other hand, its use on skin that is already dry and irritated is usually contraindicated. Seventy per cent solutions of ethyl alcohol (by weight) seem to exert the best bactericidal effects. High concentrations have a marked dehydrating effect but do not necessarily kill bacteria. Ethyl alcohol in proper concentration is considered an effective germicide for a number of uses, but it does not kill spores.

Systemic action. According to modern scientific authorities alcohol is not considered a stimulant (popular ideas to the contrary). It is thought to interfere with the transmission of nerve impulses at synaptic connections, but how this is accomplished is not known. It exerts a progressive and continuous depression on the central nervous system (cerebrum, cerebellum, cord, and medulla). Its action is comparable to that of the

---

[*]Hulpieu, H. R., and Harger, R. N.: The Alcohols. In Drill, V. A. (editor): Pharmacology in Medicine, New York, 1958, McGraw-Hill Book Co., Inc., p. 196.

general anesthetics. The excitement stage, however, is longer, and when the anesthetic stage is reached, definite toxic symptoms are present. The margin between the anesthetic and fatal dose is a narrow one. What sometimes appears to be stimulation results from the depression of the higher faculties of man's brain and represents the loss of learned inhibitions acquired by civilization. The results of the action of alcohol vary with the individual, his tolerance, the presence or absence of extraneous stimuli, and the rate of ingestion. Small or moderate quantities produce a feeling of well-being, talkativeness, greater vivacity, and increased confidence in one's mental and physical power. The personality becomes expansive, and there is a general loss of inhibitions. The finer powers of discrimination, concentration, insight, judgment, and memory are gradually dulled and lost. Large quantities of the drug may cause excitement, impulsive speech and behavior, laughter, hilarity, and, in some cases, pugnaciousness. Others may become melancholy or unduly sentimental. The individual usually becomes ataxic, mutters incoherently, has disturbance of the special senses, is often nauseated, may vomit, and eventually lapses into stupor or coma.

The respiratory center is not depressed except by large doses.

CARDIOVASCULAR SYSTEM. Alcohol depresses the vasomotor center in the medulla and in this way brings about dilatation of the peripheral blood vessels, especially those of the skin. This causes a feeling of warmth. Because of the dilatation of the capillaries, heat is lost from the surface of the body and more must be brought from the interior. This accounts for the fact that an intoxicated person may freeze to death more quickly than a normal person. Alcohol also depresses the heat-regulating mechanism in the same manner as the antipyretics, and before the advent of the modern antipyretics it was used to reduce fever.

Small doses (10 to 25 ml.) in man produce an insignificant increase in the pulse rate, due mainly to the excitement and to the reflex effect on the gastrointestinal tract. Larger doses produce the same effect but may be followed by lowered blood pressure due to the effect on the vasoconstrictor center. Only high concentrations of alcohol depress the heart.

GASTROINTESTINAL SYSTEM. The effect of alcohol upon the function of the digestive organs depends upon the presence or absence of gastrointestinal disease, the degree of alcoholic tolerance, the concentration of the beverage used, as well as the type and amount of food present. Small doses in the patient who likes alcohol will stimulate the secretion of gastric juice rich in acid. Salivary secretion is also reflexly stimulated. Large and concentrated doses of alcohol tend to inhibit secretion and enzyme activity in the stomach, although the effect in the intestine seems to be negligible. However, when large quantities of alcohol are taken over a

Drugs that affect central nervous system 269

period of time, gastritis, nutritional deficiencies, and other untoward results have been observed.

Absorption and excretion. Since alcohol does not require digestion in the stomach or intestine, it is readily absorbed from both organs. Ninety per cent or more of the alcohol that is absorbed is metabolized, chiefly in the liver. It is oxidized first to acetaldehyde and eventually to carbon dioxide and water. It is oxidized at the rate of about 10 grams per hour which amounts to about 70 calories.* Alcohol does not form glycogen and hence it cannot be stored, so that it is a food only in the sense that it contributes calories. It supplies no minerals or vitamins.

The alcohol that escapes oxidation is excreted by way of the lungs and kidneys and some is found in a number of excretions, e.g., sweat.

Alcohol produces an increased flow of urine because of increased fluid intake which ordinarily accompanies the drinking of alcoholic beverages. Recently it has been suggested that alcohol may also act as a diuretic through central nervous system depression and inhibition of the ADH (antidiuretic hormone) release. If the patient has pre-existing renal disease, there may be further damage to the kidney. Large and concentrated doses of alcohol are thought to injure the renal epithelium.

Since alcohol, after absorption, is distributed in the tissues of the body in *approximately* the same ratio as their water content, a rough estimate of the quantity taken may be obtained from an analysis of the blood and urine. Muehlberger gives his analysis as shown in Table 13.

The National Safety Council regards concentrations of alcohol in the blood up to 0.05 per cent as evidence of unquestioned sobriety. Concentrations between 0.051 and 0.149 per cent are regarded as grounds for suspicion and for use of performance tests, and anything more than 0.15 per cent is evidence of unquestionable intoxication. The states differ as to what is accepted as a legal limit.

Effects of alcohol which may not be discernible to the casual observer become apparent when the individual who has had a number of doses of alcohol attempts to operate a piece of power machinery such as an automobile. Visual acuity (especially peripheral vision) is diminished, reaction time is slowed, judgment and self-control are impaired, and the individual tends to be complacent and pleased with himself. Many drivers will take chances when under the influence of alcohol that they would never take ordinarily. This leads to disaster, as statistics reveal.

Uses. Ethyl alcohol is used topically as an astringent and antiseptic. It is rubbed on the backs and buttocks of patients to prevent decubiti. It is used to cleanse the skin, and it is poured on dressings over wounds. It is a popular disinfectant for the skin.

*Salter, W. T.: A Textbook of Pharmacology, Philadelphia, 1952, W. B. Saunders Co.

Table 13*

Relation between clinical indications of alcoholic intoxication and concentration of alcohol of the blood and urine

Stage	% Blood alcohol	% Urine alcohol	Clinical observations
Subclinical	0-0.11	0-0.15	Normal by ordinary observation, slight changes detectable by special tests
Emotional instability	0.09-0.21	0.13-0.29	Decreased inhibitions; emotional instability; slight muscular incoordination; slowing of responses to stimuli
Confusion	0.18-0.33	0.26-0.45	Disturbance of sensation; decreased pain sense; staggering gait; slurred speech
Stupor	0.27-0.43	0.36-0.58	Marked decrease in response to stimuli; muscular incoordination approaching paralysis
Coma	0.36-0.56	0.48-0.72	Complete unconsciousness; depressed reflexes; subnormal temperature; anesthesia; impairment of circulation; possible death
Death (uncomplicated)	Over 0.44	Over 0.60	

*From Muehlberger. In McNally: Toxicology, 1937.

It is an excellent solvent and preservative for many medicines and medicinal mixtures (spirits, elixirs, fluidextracts).

It cools the skin and therefore alcohol sponges are given to lower the temperature of the patient with a high fever.

It is sometimes injected into a nerve to destroy the sensory nerve fibers and thus relieve the pain associated with a severe and protracted neuralgia, e.g., trifacial neuralgia (tic douloureux). An injection of 80 per cent ethyl alcohol is used. Effects may persist for one to three years or until regeneration of the peripheral nerve fibers takes place. Alcohol also may be injected into nerves to relieve the pain due to inoperable carcinoma.

It is used to produce vasodilation in peripheral vascular disease. Concentrated solutions often produce greater peripheral vasodilation than any other drug.* The pain associated with Buerger's disease may be relieved with the use of ethyl alcohol administered orally. It is sometimes prescribed to decrease the frequency of attacks of coronary disease, but effects are said to be unreliable. Benefits to the cardiac patient, if they occur, are believed to be due to the rest and relaxation which the alcohol produces.

*Beckman, H.: Drugs, Their Nature, Action and Use, Philadelphia, 1958, W. B. Saunders Co., p. 236.

It is occasionally used as an appetizer or food accessory for patients with poor appetite during periods of convalescence and debility. Five to 10 per cent solutions of alcohol have also been given in intravenous fluids (5 per cent dextrose and isotonic saline solution) to supplement the caloric intake.

The use of some form of alcohol has long been advocated to thwart the development of a head cold. It may be useful in so far as it makes the patient more comfortable, drowsy, and sleepy so that he will go to bed for extra sleep and rest. Increased circulation of blood through the skin will relieve feelings of chilliness. It seems to have no effect on the course of the cold itself.

It is sometimes used as a hypnotic, especially for older persons who do not tolerate other hypnotics well. It is used thus more as a home remedy or for an occasional hospitalized patient who requests it. It is occasionally given in intravenous fluids for its sedative effects, e.g., to reduce the amount of opiate or barbiturate needed to keep a patient comfortable.

Preparation and dosage.

Alcohol (Ethyl Alcohol), U.S.P., B.P. Alcohol contains not less than 92.3 per cent by weight corresponding to approximately 94.9 per cent by volume of C_2H_5OH.

Diluted Alcohol, U.S.P. The diluted form contains not less than 41 per cent and not more than 42 per cent by weight of ethyl alcohol. The B.P. lists a number of dilute alcohols.

Whisky (Spiritus Frumenti), N.F. Whisky is an alcoholic liquid which is obtained by the distillation of the fermented mash of wholly or partly malted cereal grain and which contains not less than 47 per cent and not more than 53 per cent by volume of ethyl alcohol. It must have been stored in charred wood containers for a period of not less than two years.

Brandy (Spiritus Vini Vitis), N.F. Brandy is an alcoholic liquid which is obtained by the distillation of the fermented juice of sound, ripe grapes and which contains not less than 48 per cent and not more than 54 per cent by volume of ethyl alcohol. It must have been stored in wood containers for a period of not less than two years.

Other spirits are solutions of volatile substances in alcohol. In most cases the dissolved substance has a more important action than the alcohol which is used merely as a solvent.

Wines are fermented liquors made from grapes or other fruit juices. Besides alcohol, wines may contain various acids, such as tartaric, tannic, malic, etc.

Dry wines are those that contain no added sugar. They contain about 10 per cent alcohol.

Sweet wines are those to which sugar has been added. They contain about 15 per cent alcohol.

Sparkling wines contain carbon dioxide which makes them effervescent, e.g., champagne, sparkling burgundy, etc.

Red wines are made by fermenting grapes with the skins. They contain 15 to 40 per cent alcohol.

White wines are made from grapes without the skins, or from white grapes.

Dosage varies with the purpose for which the alcohol is administered. When whisky is prescribed as a vasodilator, 30 ml. may be ordered to be given two or three times a day. When an alcoholic beverage is given for its effects as an appetizer it should be given before meals (30 to 60 ml. usually).

Acute alcoholism. In states of acute intoxication, the patient is stuporous or comatose, the skin is cold and clammy, respirations are noisy and slow, and pupils are dilated or normal. The breath is usually heavy with alcoholic fumes. Death may result if the coma is prolonged or if injury, hypostatic pneumonia, or infection complicates the picture.

Treatment. Ordinary intoxication treats itself with time and sleep. In severe intoxication the stomach should be emptied. Emetics in cases of deep narcosis are inactive and worse than useless because they add to the depression. The stomach therefore, should be emptied with a stomach tube. If one is sure that alcohol alone is causing the intoxication, emptying the stomach may be of little value, but often other intoxications are hidden by the alcohol. The patient should be kept warm. Difference of opinion exists as to the use of analeptic drugs, but if the depression is deep and the patient cannot be aroused, drugs, such as amphetamine phosphate, pentylenetetrazol (Metrazol), methylphenidate hydrochloride (Ritalin Hydrochloride), and others have been recommended. In case of threatened respiratory failure, artificial respiration and the inhalation of oxygen and carbon dioxide may be beneficial. The patient's position should be changed frequently to combat development of hypostatic pneumonia. As the patient emerges from a comatose state he may become acutely active and require the administration of a sedative. (Chlorpromazine should *not* be given; it potentiates the effects of alcohol.) Recovery is comparable to recovery from an anesthetic.

The headache, nervousness, and gastric irritability which frequently follow acute alcoholism are best relieved by antacids and demulcents, e.g., sodium bicarbonate and bismuth subcarbonate. The combined use of glucose and insulin therapy has given favorable results since it promotes the detoxication of alcohol. The administration of isotonic saline solution, intravenously, will help the dehydrated patient by re-establishing the electrolyte pattern of the blood.

Chronic alcoholism. The more common manifestations of chronic alcoholism are redness of the face, nose, and conjunctivae due to the injection of the blood vessels, gastroenteritis, cirrhotic changes in the liver, nephritis, arteriosclerosis and chronic myocardial changes, amblyopia due to orbital optical neuritis, dulling of the mental faculties, tremors due to nerve degeneration, muscular weakness, and moral deterioration. Not infrequently the prolonged use of alcohol leads to insanity, or the mental change may manifest itself in the gradual weakening of the mental powers, with hallucinations and delusions, or other forms of psychosis. To be successfully treated the chronic alcoholic must want to be treated and must want to get well. Early establishment of rapport between the patient and his physician as well as with his nurse is very important. Treatment must include rehabilitation and help in making better adjustments to the patient's living conditions. The best results are probably obtained in a hospital or sanitarium.

Careful attention should be given to the patient's physical needs, such as his diet, fluid balance, and general hygiene, since optimal physical fitness makes the patient feel better and increases his ability to deal with the problems that have contributed to his illness or have caused it to continue. Particular attention is given to supplying adequate amounts of vitamin B complex and ascorbic acid.

The use of sedatives and tranquilizing agents make the patient more comfortable, help him to sleep better, and relieve anxiety. The patient is also likely to eat better.

There is need for adequate medical supervision at all times as well as good nursing care if good results are to be attained. Relapses are frequent but are said to be fewer than those seen after the treatment for morphine addiction.

In the treatment of chronic alcoholism, two additional aspects of treatment are deserving of mention because of the success which has been attained.

1. The psychologic approach to the problem or problems of the chronic alcoholic as made by *Alcoholics Anonymous.* This is an organization composed entirely of rehabilitated former alcoholics who are therefore in a unique position to understand the problems of other alcoholics. The organization has its headquarters in New York and has many local groups in cities and towns throughout the United States. Frequent meetings, mutual assistance and understanding, and a definite program of constructive rehabilitation have resulted in the fact that approximately 50 per cent of those who enter the organization with a sincere desire to stop drinking do so. Another 25 per cent are reclaimed after one or more failures, and most of the remaining 25 per cent are for one reason or another never successfully reclaimed.

2. The development of an unpleasant conditioned reflex associated with the drinking of alcoholic beverages. The patient is given a dose of a drug which, when taken with alcohol, makes him very sick (nausea and vomiting). By repeating this procedure a few times, the patient becomes nauseated when he takes the alcohol without the drug or sometimes at the very thought of drinking. Emetine hydrochloride has been used for this purpose, or, more recently, a drug called disulfiram (Antabuse) has been reported favorably by some Danish physicians. Disulfiram is said to interfere with the metabolism of alcohol by retarding the oxidation of acetaldehyde. Increased amounts of acetaldehyde in the blood account for the unpleasant effects. The drug must be used cautiously because it has been known to cause personality changes, as well as death. Psychotherapy aimed at mental and social rehabilitation should accompany the use of such drugs if permanent effects are likely to be obtained.

Delirium tremens is a form of psychosis which sometimes develops in the chronic alcoholic. It usually follows excessive drinking over a period of weeks followed by abstinence. In the alcoholic who has been drinking for some time, it may be precipitated by exposure, surgical operation, or serious illness, especially pneumonia. There may be warning symptoms such as restlessness, insomnia, anorexia, anxiety, fear, and tremor. Chronic alcoholics refer to the first stage of delirium tremens as the "shakes." During the attack the patient continues to have tremor, insomnia, delirium, and also terrifying hallucinations of such things as snakes and small animals creeping over him. The patient may have a temperature of 102° to 103° F. Death may result from collapse, traumatism, or infection.

Many methods of treatment have been tried. Sedatives such as paraldehyde, amobarbital sodium, mephobarbital, and some of the tranquilizing agents are tried when the patient is maniacal. Symptomatic treatment of the patient includes attention to fluids, nutrition, vitamins, etc. Some physicians have found ACTH and cortisone beneficial in promoting recovery.

Contraindications. Ethyl alcohol is contraindicated for certain persons and should be avoided by others. This includes the following:

1. Patients who have some type of ulceration in organs of the gastrointestinal tract, especially patients with hyperacidity and gastric or duodenal ulcers.

2. Patients with acute infections of the genitourinary organs.

3. During pregnancy.

4. Epileptics.

5. Patients with disease of the liver or kidney.

Drugs that affect central nervous system   275

6. Persons with personality problems, those who are maladjusted, or those who have at one time been addicted.

Alcohol and life span. The effect of alcohol on resistance to infection and on the life span has been a subject of controversy for many years. It is believed that evidence is lacking to prove that moderate amounts of alcohol have much effect one way or the other. Statistics show, however, that chronic alcoholics and heavy drinkers have a shorter life span than those who abstain from alcohol. Some of the ill effects that have been attributed to alcohol have been found to be due to general impairment of health which in turn is due to malnutrition, poor hygiene, etc. Apparently it often is not so much the direct effect of alcohol that injures the person as the inability of the alcoholic to take care of himself and others.

Methyl Alcohol (Wood Alcohol)

$$H - \underset{\underset{\displaystyle H}{|}}{\overset{\overset{\displaystyle H}{|}}{C}} - OH$$

Methyl alcohol is prepared on a large scale by the destructive distillation of wood. It has also been prepared synthetically. It is important in medicine chiefly because of the cases of poisoning that have resulted from its ingestion. The main effects are on the central nervous system. However, intoxication, i.e., a state of drunkenness, does not occur as readily as with ethyl alcohol, unless large amounts are consumed. Methyl alcohol is oxidized in the tissues to formic acid, which is only poorly metabolized. This is the basis for the development of a severe acidosis. Symptoms of poisoning include nausea and vomiting, abdominal pain, headache, dyspnea, blurred vision, and cold clammy skin. Symptoms may progress to delirium, convulsions, coma, and death. In nonfatal cases the patient may become blind or suffer from impaired vision. Treatment is directed toward the relief of acidosis since this seems to be related to the severity of the visual symptoms. Large amounts of sodium bicarbonate may be needed to treat acidosis successfully. One dose of 60 ml. has been known to cause permanent blindness. Obviously methyl alcohol is much more toxic than ethyl alcohol. Fluids containing methyl alcohol usually bear a *Poison* label, although this may be disregarded or overlooked.

Isopropyl Alcohol

$$H - \underset{\underset{\displaystyle H}{|}}{\overset{\overset{\displaystyle H}{|}}{C}} - \underset{\underset{\displaystyle OH}{|}}{\overset{\overset{\displaystyle H}{|}}{C}} - \underset{\underset{\displaystyle H}{|}}{\overset{\overset{\displaystyle H}{|}}{C}} - H$$

Isopropyl alcohol is a clear, colorless liquid with a characteristic odor and a bitter taste. It is miscible with water, chloroform, and ether but insoluble in salt solutions. It is a good solvent for creosote and compares favorably with ethyl alcohol in its antiseptic action. It has been recommended for disinfection of the skin and for rubbing compounds and lotions to be used on the skin. Its bactericidal effects are said to increase as its concentration approaches 100 per cent. It differs in this respect from ethyl alcohol.

It is occasionally misused as a beverage. It can cause severe poisoning and death. The first symptoms are similar to intoxication from ethyl alcohol, but the symptoms progress to coma, from which the patient may not recover.

Butyl and Amyl Alcohols

Butyl and *amyl alcohols* are said to be several times as toxic as ethyl alcohol.

Selective depressants
Anticonvulsant drugs

In this part of the chapter dealing with depressants of the central nervous system a number of drugs used for the symptomatic treatment of various kinds of convulsive seizures will be described.

Epilepsy is regarded as a symptom of disease or disorder of the brain rather than a disease in itself. It is associated with marked changes in the electric pulsations of the cerebral cortex and these alterations are often detected in the electroencephalogram. Hence, the EEG is often a valuable aid to the physician in making a diagnosis. Sometimes the convulsive seizure is associated with a brain tumor, growth of scar tissue, or the presence of a toxin or a poison, but at other times no specific cause can be found. Epileptic seizures differ somewhat one from another and are often grouped according to the following: grand mal seizures, petit mal seizures, Jacksonian epilepsy, and psychomotor attacks. There are about 1 million epileptic persons in the United States.

Grand mal epilepsy is the type most frequently seen. Such attacks are characterized by sudden loss of consciousness; the patient falls forcefully and experiences a series of tonic and clonic muscular contractions. The eyes roll upward, the arms are flexed, and the legs are extended. The force of the muscular contractions causes air to be forced out of the lungs, and this accounts for the cry which the patient may make as he falls. Respiration is suspended temporarily, the skin becomes cyanotic, perspiration and saliva flow, and the patient may froth at the mouth and bite his tongue if it gets caught between his teeth. When the seizure subsides the patient regains partial consciousness and may complain of aching. He then tends to fall into a deep sleep.

Petit mal seizures are most often seen in childhood and consist of temporary lapses of consciousness which last for a few seconds. Patients appear to be staring into space and may exhibit a few rhythmic movements of the eyes or head. They do not convulse. They may experience many attacks in a single day. Sometimes an attack of petit mal is followed by one of grand mal.

Jacksonian epilepsy is described by some authorities as a type of focal seizure, i.e., it is associated with irritation of a specific part of the brain. A single part, such as a finger or an extremity, may jerk and such movements may end spontaneously or spread over the whole musculature. Consciousness may not be lost unless the seizure develops into a generalized convulsion.

Psychomotor attacks are characterized by brief alterations in consciousness, unusual stereotyped movements (such as chewing or swallowing movements) repeated over and over, temperamental changes, confusion, and feelings of unreality. It is often associated with grand mal seizures and is likely to be rather resistant to therapy with drugs.

Some patients have more than one type of seizure or have mixed seizures. This is significant because different types of seizures respond rather specifically to certain anticonvulsant drugs. The aim of therapy is to find the drug or drugs that will effectively control the seizures and will at the same time cause a minimum of undesirable side effects.

Mechanism of action of the anticonvulsant drugs

The effectiveness of anticonvulsant drugs is often measured by the amount of increased voltage necessary to provoke an electroconvulsion in an animal who has previously received the anticonvulsant to be tested or by the degree of their antagonism to chemical substances capable of producing convulsions. Pentylenetetrazol (Metrazol) is a drug against which anticonvulsants are often measured for effectiveness.

The mode and site of action of these drugs are still regarded as uncertain. The convulsive seizure may be effectively suppressed, but the abnormal brain waves may or may not be altered. All clinically useful drugs for epilepsy inhibit the spread of the seizure, but how this is accomplished is not clear.

Although there is no ideal anticonvulsant drug, if one could be synthesized to order, a number of characteristics would be considered highly desirable:

1. The drug should be highly effective but exhibit a low incidence of toxicity.

2. It should be effective against more than one type of seizure and for mixed seizures.

3. It should be long-acting and nonsedative so that the patient is not incapacitated with sleep or excessive drowsiness.

4. It should be well tolerated by the patient and inexpensive since the patient may have to take it for years or for the rest of his life.

5. Tolerance to the therapeutic effects of the drug should not develop.

The present-day drugs that are considered especially satisfactory and safe are *phenobarbital, diphenylhydantoin sodium,* and *trimethadione.* The bromides are among the oldest anticonvulsants known, but because they tend to cause states of chronic toxicity, they seldom are used. The barbiturates have been discussed but their use as anticonvulsants will be emphasized again. They are an important group of drugs for this purpose, especially the longer-acting members. Phenobarbital is effective against all types of epileptic seizures except certain petit mal types. It is considered one of the safest of the anticonvulsants.* Its chief disadvantage is that it must often be given in doses that produce apathy and sleepiness. Amphetamines or Ritalin may be ordered to counteract the drowsiness. Mephobarbital (Mebaral) is similar to phenobarbital, especially when given in comparable doses. The same can be said for metharbital (Gemonil).

Diphenylhydantoin Sodium (Dilantin Sodium)

$$C_6H_5 - \overset{\overset{\displaystyle C_6H_5}{|}}{\underset{\underset{\displaystyle O=C-N}{|}}{C}} - NH \diagdown \\ C-O-Na$$

Diphenylhydantoin sodium is a synthetic agent, chemically related to the barbiturates. It is an odorless, white or cream-colored powder with a bitter taste.

Action and result. Diphenylhydantoin sodium exerts a selective action on the cerebral cortex of the brain without appreciably affecting the sensory areas. It is an anticonvulsant but not a hypnotic. It is somewhat more effective in controlling grand mal seizures than phenobarbital, although patients vary in their response to these drugs. It is strongly alkaline in solution and may produce gastric irritation.

Uses. In the treatment of epilepsy it is more effective for grand mal than petit mal seizures. It may for a time increase the attacks of petit mal. Psychomotor seizures are sometimes controlled. It does not cure mental deterioration sometimes found in the epileptic. On the other hand, it does not cause mental deterioration. It is frequently prescribed in combination with phenobarbital. It may be prescribed for patients following surgical operations upon the brain, to prevent convulsive seizures.

Preparation, dosage, and administration.

Diphenylhydantoin Sodium, U.S.P. (Dilantin Sodium); *Phenytoin So-*

*Daly, D. D.: Drug Therapy in Convulsive Disorders, Proc. Staff Meet. Mayo Clin. **32:** 259, 1957.

dium, B.P. This drug is marketed in 30 mg. and 100 mg. capsules (delayed action), in 50 mg. scored tablets, and in an oral suspension (100 mg. per 4 ml.). It is also available for parenteral administration in "Steri-Vials," each containing 250 mg. of the drug. When used alone, the beginning daily dose for adults is 100 mg. orally with one-half glass of water three times a day. The dosage may be gradually increased until optimum effects are obtained. Most adults seem to tolerate 300 to 400 mg. daily without toxic effects. Children over 6 years of age may be given the adult dose. Dosage for children under 6 years should be less. Increase in dosage is made slowly and with careful observation of the patient. When the drug is combined with one or more other anticonvulsants, the dosage of individual drugs is often reduced. The transition from phenobarbital, bromides, and other hypnotics to diphenylhydantoin is made gradually, with some overlapping of drugs to prevent the precipitation of convulsive seizures.

There are a number of preparations available which are mixtures of barbiturates and one of the hydantoins. *Phelantin* contains diphenylhydantoin sodium, phenobarbital, and methamphetamine hydrochloride. *Hydantal* contains methyl-phenyl-ethyl hydantoin and phenobarbital. *Mebroin* contains diphenylhydantoin sodium and methobarbital. These preparations have the advantages of convenience (two or more drugs in one tablet) and slightly lower cost but the disadvantage of always having a fixed amount of each drug. It is advantageous for the physician to be able to make adjustments of dosage when several drugs are taken together.

Side effects and toxic effects. The incidence of toxic reactions with diphenylhydantoin sodium is greater than with phenobarbital. The less serious side effects include apathy, nervousness, dizziness, ataxia, blurred vision, hyperplasia of the gums (excessive formation of gum tissues), and hirsutism (excessive growth of hair, especially on the face). Other reactions sometimes seen are tremor, excitement, hallucinations, psychosis, nausea, and vomiting. If the patient is particularly sensitive to the drug he may develop skin rash, exfoliative dermatitis, fever, and difficult breathing.

Methyl-phenyl-ethyl Hydantoin (Mesantoin)

$$C_2H_5 - \underset{\underset{O=C-N-CH_3}{|}}{\overset{\overset{C_6H_5}{|}}{C}} - \overset{NH}{\underset{}{\diagdown}} C=O$$

Mesantoin is an anticonvulsant drug which is similar in chemical structure and activity to diphenylhydantoin sodium. It is less potent as an anticonvulsant than the latter preparation. It produces more sedation than Dilantin but less than phenobarbital.

Uses. Mesantoin seems to be more effective for grand mal and psychomotor seizures than for petit mal seizures. It sometimes provokes attacks of petit mal. Certain patients who do not respond favorably to diphenylhydantoin or to phenobarbital may be benefited by this drug.

Preparation, dosage, and administration.

Mesantoin. This drug is available in 100 mg. tablets for oral administration. The average daily dose for adults is 400 to 600 mg.; for children, 100 to 400 mg. As for all anticonvulsants, the optimum daily dosage must be calculated to meet the needs of each patient.

Side effects and toxic effects. This is a drug that can produce serious toxic effects and therefore caution in its use is recommended. In cases of sensitivity to the drug, destruction of blood cells can occur, which may vary from leukopenia to agranulocytosis and aplastic anemia. Some patients become jaundiced, indicating damage to the liver. Other symptoms of toxicity include fever and dermatitis.

Ethotoin (Peganone)

$$
\begin{array}{c}
\text{H} \\
| \\
C_6H_5 - C - N - H \\
| \qquad\qquad \diagdown \\
\qquad\qquad\quad C{=}O \\
\qquad\qquad \diagup \\
O{=}C - N - C_2H_5
\end{array}
$$

Ethotoin belongs to the hydantoin group of anticonvulsants.

Uses. It is said to be less effective than diphenylhydantoin, but it is also less toxic. It is effective in grand mal epilepsy but does not always bring about complete relief of seizures. To be satisfactory it may need to be used with other anticonvulsants. It is of limited usefulness in petit mal and psychomotor seizures. However, in certain patients, seizures may be controlled which cannot be controlled by other drugs.

Preparation, dosage, and administration.

*Ethotoin** (Peganone). The average daily dose is 2 to 3 Gm. given after meals in four to six divided portions (orally). It is available in 250 and 500 mg. tablets.

Trimethadione (Tridione)

$$
\begin{array}{c}
\text{CH}_3 \\
| \\
CH_3 - C - O \\
| \qquad\qquad \diagdown \\
\qquad\qquad\quad C{=}O \\
\qquad\qquad \diagup \\
O{=}C - N - CH_3
\end{array}
$$

*Described in annual publication of A. M. A. Council on Drugs, N.N.D., 1960.

Trimethadione belongs to a group of compounds known as the oxazolidine diones.

Action. Its primary action is on the central nervous system, although it is not restricted to the motor cortex. It exerts an analgesic effect in some instances, as well as an anticonvulsant action. It is said to surpass all other anticonvulsants in raising the threshold to pentylenetetrazol-induced seizures. The precise mechanism of action, however, is unknown.

Uses. Trimethadione is used chiefly in the treatment of petit mal epilepsy and is considered to be the drug of choice for this condition. It appears to be more effective for petit mal in children than in adults. It is not effective for grand mal seizures. It is frequently given with diphenylhydantoin or phenobarbital if the patient has attacks of both petit mal and grand mal. It rarely seems to be adequate to control psychomotor seizures.

Preparation, dosage, and administration.

Trimethadione, U.S.P. (Tridione); *Troxidone,* B.P. This drug is available in 150 mg. tablets, 300 mg. capsules, and in solution (37.5 mg. per milliliter) for oral administration. The dose for children is 300 to 900 mg. daily and for adults, 900 to 1,200 mg. daily, in divided portions. Dosage may need to be increased.

Side effects and toxic effects. Symptoms of toxicity appear infrequently, but they may be serious. Nausea and vomiting, skin eruption, blurring of vision, and sensitivity to light are considered indications for reduction of dosage or temporary withdrawal of the drug. Careful medical supervision of the patient receiving the medication is essential. Rare instances of aplastic anemia explain why it is thought advisable for the patient to have periodic examinations of the blood to detect early signs of toxic effects.

The drug is not recommended for patients with hepatic or renal disease, with disease of the optic nerve, allergic reactions to drugs, or blood dyscrasias.

Paramethadione (Paradione)

$$C_2H_5 - \underset{\underset{\displaystyle C = N - CH_3}{\overset{\displaystyle |}{\underset{\displaystyle \parallel}{}}}{\overset{\displaystyle CH_3}{\overset{\displaystyle |}{C}}} - O \diagdown C = O$$

Action and uses. The action and uses of paramethadione are similar to those of trimethadione. It belongs to the same chemical group and no significant pharmacologic difference between them is known. Some patients not benefited by trimethadione are benefited by paramethadione and vice versa.

282

Preparation, dosage, and administration.

Paramethadine* (Paradione). The initial dose for adults is 900 mg., which is given orally in divided doses. Thereafter dosage is adjusted to the minimum effective dose. Initial dosage for children varies from 300 to 600 mg., depending on age.

Side effects. Side effects are similar to those of trimethadione, except the incidence of skin rash and photophobia is said to be less with paramethadione.

Phenacemide (Phenurone)

Phenacemide bears a close chemical relationship to the hydantoin compounds as can be seen in the accompanying formulas.

```
        H                                        C6H5
        |                                         |
C6H5 — C — H    NH2              C6H5 — C———————NH
        |             \                  |           \
        |              C=O               |            C=O
        |             /                  |           /
     O=C————————N — H             O=C———————N — H
       Phenacemide                    Diphenylhydantoin
```

Uses and toxic effects. Phenacemide is a synthetic anticonvulsant which has the advantage of being effective in the treatment of grand mal, petit mal, psychomotor epilepsy, and mixed seizures. It is often effective when other anticonvulsants are not, but it is one of the more toxic agents and may cause personality changes, liver damage, and depression of bone marrow. Some physicians regard it as being too toxic for routine use.

Preparation, dosage, and administration.

Phenacemide* (Phenurone). It is available in 300 and 500 mg. tablets for oral administration. It may be prescribed alone or with other anticonvulsants. The dosage recommended is as small as will permit control of seizures.

Other anticonvulsants

There are a number of other anticonvulsants whose ultimate status will be determined after further investigation. These include *phensuximide* (Milontin) and *methsuximide* (Celontin), which are reported to be effective for petit mal seizures. *Primidone* (Mysoline) is a barbituric acid derivative whose effects are comparable to phenobarbital, although it is said to be less potent than phenobarbital. *Acetazolamide* (Diamox) is reported to be a useful drug for occasional use as a supplement to routine medication with anticonvulsants. It is primarily a diuretic and will be mentioned again in connection with the diuretics.

———————

The nurse sometimes plays an important role in helping the patient with epilepsy to learn how to live with his handicap. The patient often

*Described in annual publication of A. M. A. Council on Drugs, N.N.D., 1960.

Drugs that affect central nervous system 283

needs encouragement and help to enable him to understand why strict adherence to the routine the physician has worked out for him is so important. The patient may never be cured, but with care he may experience minimal symptoms and be able to lead a full and useful life.

Selective depressants

Ataractics (tranquilizers)

The drugs ordinarily known as tranquilizers have come into prominence in all branches of medicine. They help distraught patients secure sleep and obtain relief of tension and apprehension, as well as help promote a state of calm and relaxation. The nurse is likely to see them ordered for patients on the medical and surgical wards of the hospital almost as often as in the psychiatric unit. Anxiety in some form accompanies many, if not all, forms of illness; indeed it is encountered in everyday living. In the sick person, however, too much anxiety may have adverse effects.

The line of distinction between sedatives and ataractics is sometimes a fine one. One distinction between them is that ataractics do not produce stupor and coma even when relatively large doses are given. Sleep may occur if the patient is undisturbed after administration of an ataractic but he is easily aroused.

Ataractics have been used extensively for patients with disorders of behavior and with mental disease. Their dramatic effects on violent, overactive, psychotic patients have, in some instances, led to exaggerated expectations regarding their role in the treatment of mental illness. They do not cure mental illness but they may be invaluable in the over-all plan of the patient's therapy. Their effects have sometimes been referred to as a medical lobotomy, meaning that the effects secured are comparable to those produced by a surgical operation which severs some of the neural pathways in the brain. The drugs somehow insulate the patient from external stimuli which cause him anxiety and stress. It is quite generally accepted that this group of drugs, which decrease excessive emotional behavior, act on the brain. The exact anatomic sites of action have not been clearly identified because of the tremendously complex nature of cerebral activity. It may be that drugs affect one or more chemical transmitters which function in and around synaptic connections in the central nervous system, but to date no such definite chemical interpretation has been established, although research continues. A number of ataractics such as reserpine, chlorpromazine, and other phenothiazine derivatives are described as central sympathetic suppressants. This means that certain centers in the brain associated with the sympathetic nervous system are affected and the action of drugs on these centers accounts for some of the effects produced by this group of drugs. This concept is based largely on analogy with the many drugs that act on synapses at the peripheral (autonomic and neuromuscular) junctions.

Alkaloids of Rauwolfia

Rauwolfia serpentina is a large climbing or twining shrub which grows in India and various tropical regions of the world. The botanical name given to a whole group of these plants was *Rauwolfia,* after the German physician and botanist Leonard Rauwolf. Extracts of the root of the plant have been used for a long time (in countries where the plant is indigenous) for a variety of ills, including mental disorders. Recently the drug has aroused interest in the Western world where preparations have come to be used for their sedative and hypotensive effects. Rauwolfia is the powdered whole root of the plant.

Reserpine (Serpasil)

Source. Reserpine is an ester alkaloid obtained from the root of a certain species of Rauwolfia. It is a complex heterocyclic compound which was first synthesized in 1956, although our principal source continues to be the plant. It is a whitish crystalline powder slightly soluble in water and alcohol but soluble in organic acids such as acetic acid. It is considered the most potent of the alkaloids of Rauwolfia.

Action and result. The action of reserpine is believed to be principally a central one. The action is apparently that of depression and suppression of activity in centers at the level of the hypothalamus where autonomic functions are integrated. The precise mechanism of action of reserpine is uncertain. It is known to release a substance called 5-hydroxytryptamine (serotonin) from its bound position in tissues by interfering with the tissue-binding of this substance. What the relationship of the sedative action is to the effects of reserpine is imperfectly understood.[*]

[*]Dews, P. B.: Drugs Affecting Behavior. In Drill, V. A. (editor): Pharmacology in Medicine, New York, 1958, McGraw-Hill Book Co., Inc., p. 323.

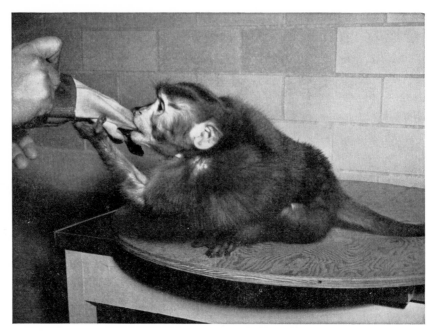

Fig. 29 A, Rhesus monkey before the administration of reserpine (Serpasil). The animal is hostile and vicious. (From the CIBA Archives.)

Reserpine produces a type of sedation different from that produced by the barbiturates. It does not alter the brain waves (EEG); it produces calm and quietude without undue drowsiness and without mental confusion or difficulty in movement. It also increases the sense of well-being. When given to animals which are hostile and vicious, they become gentle, calm, and manageable, without loss of alertness and muscle coordination. The animal may go to sleep if undisturbed, but it is easily aroused. The drug seems to reduce attention and responsiveness to outside stimuli, but it does not produce general centralized depression. Effects attributed to action on autonomic centers in the brain include the following: constriction of the pupil, slowing of the heart and increased secretion and motility of the gastrointestinal organs, and lowering of blood pressure. These effects are believed to be due to suppression of sympathetic centers which allow the activity of the parasympathetic centers to be more prominent and noticeable. Reserpine is not an analgesic and it does not potentiate the effects of analgesics.

The onset of action with reserpine is slow. In animals, a single dose, even when given intravenously, will not show maximal effects for 18 to 24 hours. Maximum therapeutic effects in man may not be obtained until the drug has been given for several weeks. When administration is stopped, effects persist and decline slowly over a period of days.

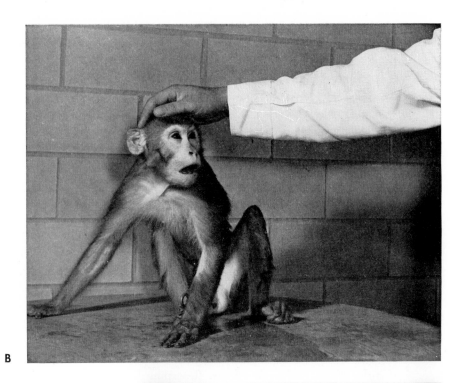

B

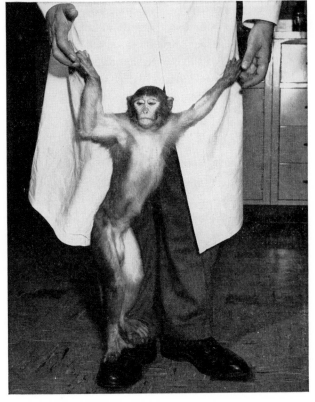

Fig. 29 (cont'd) B and **C,**
After the administration of
reserpine the animal becomes
relaxed, calm, and relatively
docile. (From the CIBA Archives.)

C

Drugs that affect central nervous system 287

Uses. Reserpine is used in the treatment of the mentally ill patient who is agitated, hyperactive, destructive, or excited. It is less useful in the treatment of the patient who is silent, withdrawn, and depressed. In fact it may make the latter type of patient worse and may provoke an increased incidence of suicide. Improvement may be noted only after weeks of administration. Effectiveness is likely to continue for a time after administration is stopped. Some patients are kept on maintenance doses indefinitely.* One of the biggest advantages is that the patient may become more accessible for psychotherapy.

Reserpine is also used in the treatment of moderate labile hypertension and will be mentioned under antihypertensive drugs, p. 438.

Preparation, dosage, and administration.

Reserpine, U.S.P., B.P. (Serpasil). It is marketed in capsules, 0.25, 0.5, 0.75 mg.; elixir, 0.05, 0.25, 0.5 mg. per milliliter; in solution for injection, 5 mg. in 2 ml.; and in tablets, 0.1, 0.2, 0.25, 0.5, 1, 2, 4, and 5 mg. Reserpine is administered orally, intramuscularly, and intravenously. For psychoneurotic patients the usual daily dose is 0.5 to 2 mg. In disturbed psychotic patients 3 to 5 mg. may be given orally along with 5 to 10 mg. intramuscularly, each day. *Reserpine Injection* and *Reserpine Tablets* are listed in the U.S.P.

Side effects and toxic effects. Reserpine is considered to have a low level of toxicity, but undesirable effects are seen as dosage levels rise. Nasal stuffiness (the patient thinks he has a head cold), gain in weight, and diarrhea are effects seen commonly. Other untoward effects include dryness of the mouth, nosebleeds, insomnia, nervousness, anxiety, fatigue, nightmares, agitated or paranoid depression, itching, and skin eruption. The drug sometimes causes gastric irritation and occasionally it brings about reactivation of an old gastric ulcer or causes a new one to form. Postural hypotension may occur after parenteral administration.

Deserpidine and Rescinnamine

Deserpidine (Harmonyl) and *rescinnamine* (Moderil) are two additional ester alkaloids of Rauwolfia. They are similar to reserpine in their pharmacologic effects. Side effects are claimed to be less marked than those seen with reserpine, but at present the drugs have not been used long enough to make possible the collection of adequate data to corroborate these claims. They are both given orally.

Phenothiazine derivatives

Chlorpromazine Hydrochloride (Thorazine Hydrochloride)

The structural formulas of phenothiazine and chlorpromazine are represented as follows.

*Bross, R. B.: The Modern Mood Changing Drugs, Am. J. Nursing **57:** 1143, 1957.

Phenothiazine   Chlorpromazine

Source. Chlorpromazine was introduced for clinical trial in 1951. It is a grayish white, crystalline powder, soluble in water. It is chemically related to the antihistamine promethazine (Phenergan), but in comparison chlorpromazine has little antihistaminic activity. It was introduced in Europe under the name of Largactil.

Action and result. Chlorpromazine was first used to relieve nausea and vomiting associated with a number of conditions. It depresses the central nervous system, its major effects seeming to be in various centers of the thalamus and hypothalamus and possibly other interconnected centers. As a result of its action, numerous and widespread effects have been observed. It does not impair intellectual functions but the patient feels less irritable, anxious, and apprehensive. He tends to feel drowsy and less active, but the drug is not considered an anticonvulsant. It lowers body temperature and may lower blood pressure. It potentiates (intensifies) the effects of opiates, sedatives, and anesthetics when administered with them or close to the same time. It acts like a local anesthetic on sensory nerve endings, and it decreases the contractions of skeletal muscles. It relieves nausea and vomiting by depressing the chemoreceptor trigger zone which activates the vomiting center.

Uses. Chlorpromazine has been found useful in alleviating the symptoms of nausea and vomiting associated with nitrogen mustard therapy, radiation sickness, action of certain drugs, carcinoma, uremia, acute infections, and recovery from an anesthetic. It is also used to relieve hiccoughs.

It is used extensively to relieve anxiety, tension, agitation, and hyperactivity in psychoneurotic and psychotic patients. This has made possible the discharge of some patients who formerly required institutional care. It has made possible a closer working relationship between the patient and his physician as well as other personnel of the hospital. As mentioned previously, it is not a cure for mental disease as we know it, but in many instances it modifies the patient's behavior and makes it more acceptable. It has greatly reduced the need for convulsive therapy.

Because it potentiates the effects of a number of drugs it permits adequate control of pain with smaller doses of analgesics such as morphine.

Drugs that affect central nervous system   289

Preparation, dosage, and administration.

Chlorpromazine Hydrochloride, U.S.P. B.P. (Thorazine Hydrochloride). It is marketed in capsules (sustained release), 30, 75, 150, 200, and 300 mg.; in solution, in ampules, and in multiple-dose vials (25 mg. per milliliter); in syrup, 2 mg. per milliliter; and in tablets, 10, 25, 50, and 200 mg. It is available also in suppository form, 25 and 100 mg.

The smallest effective dose is the one recommended. Oral dosage varies from 10 to 400 mg. or more per day. Total daily amounts are usually given in three evenly spaced doses.

Chlorpromazine is administered orally, intramuscularly, and intravenously. It usually is given orally unless for some reason the patient is unable to take the dose by mouth. It is considered too irritating to be given subcutaneously. When given intramuscularly it should be injected deeply and slowly. Massage of the site of injection helps to reduce the local irritation. There is danger of severe hypotension when the drug is given intravenously. Patients should remain in bed for an hour or two after parenteral injection. The drug is believed to be destroyed in the liver. The usual parenteral dose is 25 mg. daily.

Side effects and toxic effects. Sedation and drowsiness under some circumstances are side effects and at other times they are the effects desired. In addition, the patient may complain of dryness of the mouth, dermatitis, photosensitivity, nausea and vomiting, and nasal stuffiness. Usually these effects do not require that administration of the drug be stopped. The development of symptoms like those seen in Parkinson's disease,* as well as jaundice, leukopenia, fever, sore throat (agranulocytosis), and hypoplastic anemia, means that administration of the drug must be stopped immediately.

Contraindications. Chlorpromazine is contraindicated in all comatose patients and should be given with caution when administered with drugs that it potentiates, e.g., ethyl alcohol. Caution in its use is also recommended for patients in whom a sudden drop in blood pressure is considered dangerous. It should be avoided for patients who have hepatic disease or who have a history of disease of the liver.

A number of other phenothiazine derivatives are being used and are subject to study and investigation. They resemble chlorpromazine in that they exhibit ataractic-, antiemetic-, and narcotic-potentiating effects. Some are more potent than chlorpromazine and can therefore be prescribed in smaller doses. Patients may respond to one more than another. Which derivatives will best stand the test of time and prove to be the safest is at present difficult to predict.

*Symptoms characteristic of Parkinson's disease include tremulousness, drooling, muscular rigidity, blank expression of the face, peculiar gait, etc.

Prochlorperazine (Compazine)

Prochlorperazine is similar to chlorpromazine except that on a weight basis it is more potent than chlorpromazine.[*] It exerts a mild antihistaminic and antispasmodic effect, and its potentiating action of central depressants is said to be minimal. Its over-all toxicity is said to be less than that of chlorpromazine.

Preparation, dosage, and administration.

Prochlorperazine† (Compazine). Administered rectally, the suggested dose for adults is one 25 mg. suppository twice daily. Rectal doses for children are smaller.

Prochlorperazine Ethanedisulfonate, U.S.P. (Compazine Ethanedisulfonate). Administration can be both oral and parenteral (intramuscular). The usual oral and intramuscular dose for adults is 5 to 10 mg. This preparation is marketed in a syrup for oral administration, 1 mg. per milliliter, and in solution for injection, 5 mg. per milliliter.

Prochlorperazine Maleate, U.S.P. (Compazine Maleate). This preparation is administered orally to adults in doses ranging from 8 to 15 mg. three or four times a day. It is available in tablets and capsules.

Promazine Hydrochloride (Sparine Hydrochloride)

Promazine resembles chlorpromazine but has no chlorine in its chemical structure. Pharmacologically, however, it is similar to chlorpromazine.

Uses. It is an effective antiemetic and tranquilizing agent. It is used for many of the same conditions for which chlorpromazine is effective.

Preparation, dosage, and administration.

Promazine Hydrochloride† (Sparine Hydrochloride). The drug is administered orally, intramuscularly, and intravenously. The oral channel of administration is recommended whenever possible. The drug is mar-

[*]N.N.D., 1960, p. 396.
†Described in annual publication of A. M. A. Council on Drugs, N.N.D., 1960.

keted in solution for injection, 100 mg. per milliliter; as a syrup, 2 mg. per milliliter, and tablets, 10, 25, 50, 100, and 200 mg. for oral administration. The average daily dose for adults is 25 to 300 mg.

Side effects and toxic effects. Jaundice has not been reported, but many of the other toxic effects such as leukopenia, agranulocytosis, and convulsive seizures have been observed, as well as the milder side effects such as drowsiness, and drop in blood pressure when the patient is upright (orthostatic hypotension).

Perphenazine (Trilafon)

$$CH_2-CH_2-CH_2-N\diagdown N-CH_2-CH_2-OH$$

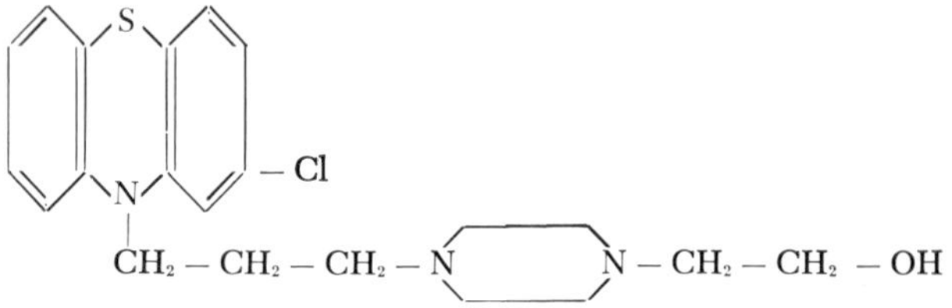

Perphenazine is similar to chlorpromazine in its depressant action and clinical uses. Milligram for milligram it is said to be more potent than prochlorperazine (Compazine).

Preparation, dosage, and administration.

*Perphenazine** (Trilafon). Administration may be orally, intramuscularly, and occasionally intravenously. The oral dosage for adults varies from 2 to 4 mg. three or four times daily to many times this amount for the seriously disturbed patient. It is marketed in solution for injection, 5 mg. per milliliter; as a syrup, 0.4 mg. per milliliter, as tablets, 2, 4, 8, and 16 mg. for oral administration, and as suppositories, 4 and 8 mg., for rectal administration.

Side effects and toxic effects. Perphenazine is also similar to chlorpromazine in its side effects. Although it is thought to be less toxic than chlorpromazine, the similarity of the chemical structure of the two chemicals suggests the possibility of similar toxic effects.

Promethazine Hydrochloride (Phenergan Hydrochloride)

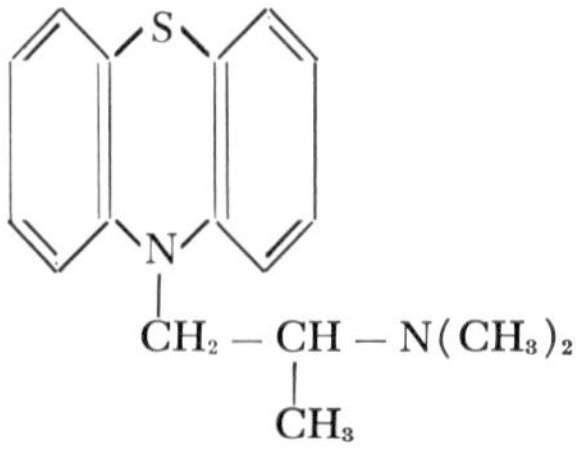

$$CH_2-CH-N(CH_3)_2$$
$$|$$
$$CH_3$$

Uses. Promethazine is a phenothiazine derivative which was introduced into medicine for its potent antihistaminic effects. It is therefore

---

*Described in annual publication of A. M. A. Council on Drugs, N.N.D., 1960.

useful in the management of certain allergic conditions. In addition, it shares the antiemetic and ataractic effects of other phenothiazine derivatives. It also potentiates the depressant effects of narcotics, barbiturates, and anesthetics. It is an effective preliminary medication prior to surgical operation and the administration of anesthetics. Unlike chlorpromazine, it is effective for motion sickness.

Preparation, dosage, and administration.

Promethazine Hydrochloride, U.S.P., B.P. (Phenergan Hydrochloride). It may be administered orally, intramuscularly, intravenously, and rectally. The average dose for adults (oral or rectal) is 25 mg. Parenteral doses vary from 12.5 to 25 mg. up to 50 or 75 mg. The oral channel of administration is preferred unless for some reason its use is not feasible. The drug is available in solution for injection (25 to 50 mg. per milliliter); as a syrup, 1.25 mg. per milliliter, and as tablets, 12.5 to 25 mg., for oral use.

Side effects. Side effects include drowsiness and dizziness, but jaundice, hypotension, and destructive effects in the blood do not seem to occur.

Mepazine (Pacatal)

Action and uses. Mepazine is a phenothiazine compound with actions and uses similar to but not identical with those of chlorpromazine. It is reported to be less potent than chlorpromazine and to produce less drowsiness and sedation. Its diminished potency makes it less effective in control of acute psychotic manifestations.

Preparation, dosage, and administration.

Mepazine Hydrochloride* (Pacatal Hydrochloride). This drug is administered orally. The initial dose for psychiatric patients varies from 25 to 100 mg. per day, depending upon the nature and severity of the symptoms. Antiemetic doses range from 50 to 100 mg. daily. The drug is marketed in 25, 50, and 100 mg. tablets.

Mepazine Acetate* (Pacatal Acetate). This form is like mepazine hydrochloride except that it is suited for parenteral administration (intramuscular or intravenous). Dosage varies from 50 to 200 mg.

Side effects. Although all of the side effects associated with this group of drugs can be expected because of its typical chemical structure, the

*Described in annual publication of A. M. A. Council on Drugs, N.N.D., 1960.

effects most frequently observed are dryness of the mouth, blurred vision, and constipation which in some instances necessitate the use of laxatives. Although the incidence of untoward effects on the blood seems to be low, granulocytopenia and agranulocytosis have been known to occur.

Other ataractics

Meprobamate (Equanil, Miltown)

$$H_2N - \overset{\displaystyle O}{\overset{\|}{C}} - O - CH_2 - \overset{\displaystyle C_3H_7}{\underset{\displaystyle CH_3}{\overset{|}{\underset{|}{C}}}} - CH_2O - \overset{\displaystyle O}{\overset{\|}{C}} - NH_2$$

Meprobamate is a synthetic drug which is chemically related to mephenesin, a skeletal muscle relaxant. As can be observed from the formula, the chemical structure differs markedly from that of reserpine or the phenothiazine derivatives. Meprobamate is a straight-chain aliphatic compound. It is a crystalline, white powder with a bitter taste.

Action and result. Meprobamate exhibits properties of an anticonvulsant, a skeletal muscle relaxant, and an ataractic. It is described as an interneuronal blocking agent; that is, it blocks the transmission of nerve impulses in spinal and bulbar reflexes (reflexes involving the brain stem) in which there are synaptic connections with connecting neurons. This action is thought to cause skeletal muscle relaxation. It also exerts a central action, probably in the thalamus, where it temporarily decreases the number of incoming stimuli, thus relieving anxiety and tension. It calms and quiets the patient without clouding consciousness. Autonomic functions such as respiration, heart action, and the secretion of gastric juice are apparently not affected.

Uses. Meprobamate has been effective in bringing about relief of anxiety and tension, abnormal fears, psychosomatic disorders, behavior disorders, and insomnia. It is not a potent hypnotic, but the relief of tension that it produces is conducive to sleep. Improvement following administration of this drug is usually characterized by decreased irritability, improved sense of well-being, and greater relaxation. However, it is not as potent a tranquilizing agent as chlorpromazine and reserpine.

Meprobamate is sometimes given to patients to relieve muscle spasm, e.g., fibrositis, wryneck, cerebral palsy, etc., and as an anticonvulsant in petit mal epilepsy. It is not beneficial for other forms of epilepsy.

It may be beneficial in the treatment of alcoholism.

Preparation, dosage, and administration.

Meprobamate, U.S.P. (Miltown, Equanil). It is marketed in sustained release capsules, 200 mg.; in an oral suspension, 40 mg. per milliliter; and in tablets, 200 and 400 mg. It is administered orally. The usual adult dose is 400 mg. three or four times daily.

294

Side effects and toxic effects. Although meprobamate is not considered a toxic drug it has been known to cause a number of side effects and untoward reactions. The more common reactions are allergic manifestations, such as skin rash, itching, and urticaria. This reaction is sometimes sufficiently severe to require the administration of a corticosteroid and cessation of administration, but the symptoms usually respond well to administration of one of the antihistaminic drugs. Drowsiness may constitute a side effect at times, but it seems to subside spontaneously. Other effects seen less frequently are chills, fever, bleeding into the skin (purpura), edema, double vision, diarrhea, and pronounced skeletal muscle relaxation. Large doses can produce coma and a sharp decline in blood pressure. Evidence exists that both habituation and physical dependence can develop.[*] Some patients seem to develop tolerance as well. Withdrawal symptoms including convulsions have been observed, although rarely. Such symptoms are seen only after prolonged administration and abrupt discontinuance of administration.

Gradual withdrawal of meprobamate therapy is recommended in the event that physical or psychic dependence develops.

Hydroxyzine Hydrochloride (Atarax Hydrochloride)

Hydroxyzine hydrochloride is chemically and pharmacologically similar to some of the antihistaminic drugs.

Action. It depresses the central nervous system and produces sedation.

Uses. It has been used for the symptomatic treatment of a great variety of emotional disorders in which anxiety, agitation, and tension are prominent symptoms. Its use for psychotic patients, however, does not appear to be promising.

Preparation, dosage, and administration.

Hydroxyzine Hydrochloride[†] (Atarax Hydrochloride). This drug is

[*]Council on Drugs: Potential Hazards of Meprobamate, J. A. M. A. **164:** 1332, 1957.
[†]Described in annual publication of A. M. A. Council on Drugs, N.N.D., 1960.

available in 10, 25, and 100 mg. tablets for oral administration. The usual adult dose is 25 mg. three times a day, although dosage varies with age, severity of symptoms, and the individual patient's response to the drug.

Side effects. Drowsiness appears to be the main side effect, and this is said to diminish after prolonged administration.

Benactyzine Hydrochloride (Suavitil, Phobex)

$$HO - C - COO - CH_2 - CH_2 - N \underset{CH_2CH_3}{\overset{CH_2CH_3}{<}}$$

Action. Benactyzine is an anticholinergic drug, the actions and effects of which are similar to those of atropine, although less potent. It also has a central action, probably in the region of the hypothalamus. The exact mechanism of action is unknown, but it is believed to somehow decrease the emotional reaction to external stimuli and thus relieve anxiety in distraught persons. More evidence is needed to establish its true status as a psychotherapeutic agent.

Preparation, dosage, and administration.

Benactyzine Hydrochloride* (Suavitil, Phobex). The drug is administered orally. The dosage for adults is 1 mg. three times a day, after meals. Dosage is gradually adjusted to a higher level as the patient may require it. The drug is marketed in 1 and 5 mg. tablets.

Side effects and toxic effects. It is believed to have a low level of toxicity. It may produce side effects similar to those of atropine, although the more commonly observed effects are those of mild confusion, dizziness, inability to concentrate, and a sense of unreality.

*Described in annual publication of A. M. A. Council on Drugs, N.N.D., 1960.

Suggestions
for review and study

1 Name the major groups of drugs that will come under the heading of central nervous system depressants. Mention several drugs that belong to each group. Indicate points of difference between one group and another.

2 What effects can you expect from drugs that act as central nervous system stimulants?

3 Explain the role of preliminary medications in the production of a satisfactory anesthetic state.

4 Discuss the advantages and disadvantages of "over-the-counter" sale of drugs without a prescription.

5 What hazards are involved in the present-day use of tranquilizing drugs? What attitude do you think should be fostered relative to their use?

6 Contrast and compare the barbiturates and the drugs known as ataractics.

7 What precautions are observed in your hospital to prevent the development of drug addiction. Name various persons with whom nurses share this responsibility.

Sample questions

Directions

Encircle number (or letter) of the part which in your judgment constitutes the best answer.

1 Drugs that produce loss of sensation and loss of consciousness are known as:
a. spinal anesthetics
b. local anesthetics
c. general anesthetics
d. basal anesthetics

2 Drugs given to produce sleep are known as:
a. sedatives
b. somnifacients
c. hypnotics
d. analgesics
   (1) a and b
   (2) b and c
   (3) c and d
   (4) c only

3 Drugs that bring about dilatation of the pupil of the eye are:
a. miotics
b. mydriatics
c. cycloplegics
d. antispasmodics

4 Opium is derived from:
a. seeds of the white poppy
b. leaves and roots of Oriental poppies
c. juice of unripened seed capsules of the white poppy
d. leaves of the *Papaver somniferum*

5 The greatest use of morphine lies in its ability to act as a (an):
a. antispasmodic
b. analgesic
c. cough remedy
d. antidiarrheic

6 The habit-forming quality of opium is explained by its effect on:
a. higher centers of the cerebral cortex
b. respiratory center

c. vasomotor center
d. smooth muscle of the bowel

7 Indicate which of the following symptoms you would consider alarming in a patient to whom you have given a dose of morphine sulfate.
a. deep sleep
b. constricted pupils
c. pulse 68 beats per minute
d. respirations 10 per minute

8 Coffee is usually withheld from the diet of the patient with gastric ulcer for which of the following reasons it:
a. tends to cause spasm of gastric muscle
b. decreases motility of the stomach
c. increases gastric acid
d. tends to irritate gastric mucosa
   (1) a and b
   (2) b and c
   (3) b and d
   (4) c and d

9 A cup of coffee before writing an examination may be considered a good use of caffeine because:
a. caffeine depresses the higher centers and thus relieves worry and tension
b. caffeine stimulates the cerebral cortex
c. caffeine stimulates the myocardium and thus improves circulation
d. caffeine stimulates fatigued muscle

10 The use of salicylic acid in corn cures and diseases of the skin is based on its ability to:
a. soften and loosen excess epithelial layers
b. deaden nerve endings in the skin
c. prevent bacterial growth in and on the skin
d. act as a mild counterirritant

11 Indicate which of the following are considered characteristics of a good hypnotic. The drug should:
a. act with reasonable promptness
b. produce a restful sleep
c. produce no undesirable hangover
d. allow a patient to awaken somewhere near his usual hour of awakening
   (1) a and b
   (2) a, b, and c
   (3) b and c
   (4) a, b, c, and d
   (5) b and d

12 Phenobarbital is one of the best of the barbiturates to prevent convulsive seizures because it:
a. depresses the motor centers in the brain stem

b. depresses the entire cerebral cortex

c. exerts a highly selective depressant action on the motor cortex

d. acts as an anticonvulsant in ordinary doses

    (1) only c

    (2) a and c

    (3) c and d

    (4) b and d

13 Indicate which of the following drugs is sometimes given with phenobarbital to control grand mal epilepsy:

a. Pentothal Sodium

b. sodium bromide

c. Dilantin Sodium

d. chloral hydrate

14 The method by which alcohol exerts a vasodilator effect is by:

a. depression of muscle in the blood vessels

b. depression of vasomotor center

c. general cerebral depression

d. depression of motor cortex

15 The anesthetic stage characterized by regular full respirations, full strong pulse, muscle relaxation, loss of consciousness, loss of reflexes, and progressive loss of body heat is known as stage of:

a. analgesia, diminished sensation

b. medullary paralysis

c. stage of excitement

d. surgical anesthesia

16 Ether has continued to be one of the widely used anesthetics because:

a. muscular relaxation can be secured

b. induction is easy and safe

c. it has a wide safety range

d. it is readily transported and used in a variety of circumstances

    (1) a and b

    (2) a and c

    (3) c and d

    (4) a and d

    (5) all are true

17 Indicate which of the following constitutes the chief disadvantage in the use of cyclopropane:

a. cost

b. availability

c. explosiveness

d. narrow safety range

18 Indicate which of the following channels of administration you would expect to use to give phenobarbital sodium:

a. oral

b. rectal

c. sublingual

d. intramuscular

19 Which of the following routes of administration would you expect to use when giving camphorated opium tincture?

a. oral

b. rectal

c. intramuscular

d. subcutaneous

20 The usual dosage of meperidine (Demerol) falls into which of the following ranges of dosage?

a. 15 to 20 mg.

b. 6 to 10 mg.

c. 50 to 100 mg.

d. 50 to 150 mg.

21 A drug that arouses a patient and makes him more alert and responsive is called a (an):

a. ataractic

b. analgesic

c. analeptic

d. antitussive

22 Which of the following groups of drugs are spoken of as tranquilizing agents?

a. Coramine, Dexedrine, Ritalin

b. Dilantin, Phenergan, Seconal

c. Promazine, Compazine, Thorazine

d. Lorfan, Nalline, Megamide

23 Another name for procaine is:

a. Phenacaine

b. Novocain

c. Butacaine

d. Dibucaine

24 Which of the following barbiturates would you expect to see ordered for a patient who has no difficulty in getting to sleep but tends to awaken about 3 A.M.?

a. Alurate Elixir

b. Seconal

c. phenobarbital

d. Nembutal

25 For the following dose of barbiturate drugs would you seek verification before administering the drug (the orders are written)?

a. Secobarbital gr. iss

b. Sodium Luminal gr. ii

c. Sodium Amytal gr. iii

d. Alurate Elixir ounce 1

26 Indicate the generic or official name for each of the following:

Nisentil   _____

Lorfan   _____

Levo-Dromoran _____

Nembutal   ———————

Aspirin   ———————

Seconal   ———————

Phenergan   ———————

Serpasil   ———————

Miltown   ———————

Darvon   ———————

27 If a patient tells you that he is taking one of the barbiturates regularly for insomnia because he has high blood pressure, and fears he may become addicted to the drug, although his doctor has reassured him regarding this danger, which of the following replies would you consider most suitable and helpful?

a. I can understand your concern and agree that such drugs do cause addiction.

b. I think you should do whatever your doctor tells you to do.

c. Your doctor no doubt feels that it is very important for you to have adequate rest and sleep but why don't you talk with him about it again?

d. Why don't you try something else for insomnia, such as a prolonged warm bath before retiring?

28 If you are approached by a relative or friend who tells you that she has headaches often and that her doctor has recommended aspirin for relief, and she asks if you know of a better remedy since you are in a position to know about new drugs, which of the following replies would you consider most suitable?

a. If your doctor has told you to take aspirin, there is probably a very good reason why he wants you to have it.

b. Why don't you try one of the other remedies which are on the market today and which you can buy without a prescription?

c. Why don't you persuade your doctor to prescribe one of the newer nonhabit-forming drugs which give relief from pain?

d. Aspirin has stood the test of time very well; it is considered one of the safest and best pain-relieving drugs on the market.

29 A doctor orders 0.5 Gm. of a drug. You find that the tablets of the drug are labeled 250 mg. How many tablets or what part of a tablet would you give?

30 A doctor's order reads: "Acetylsalicylic Acid 10 Gm. today in 6 doses q. 4 h. day and night." The stock supply of the drug is available in tablets gr. x and gr. v. How much would you give per dose from the stock supply?

References

A. M. A. Council on Drugs: New and Nonofficial Drugs, Philadelphia, 1960, J. B. Lippincott Co.

Beckman, H.: Drugs, Their Nature, Action and Use, Philadelphia, 1958, W. B. Saunders Co.

Drill, V. A. (editor): Pharmacology in Medicine, New York, 1958, McGraw-Hill Book Co., Inc.

Goodman, L., and Gilman, A.: The Pharmacological Basis of Therapeutics, New York, 1955, The Macmillan Co.

Hale, D. E. (editor): Anesthesiology, Philadelphia, 1955, F. A. Davis Co.

Henry Ford Hospital, International Symposium: Reticular Formation of the Brain, Boston, 1958, Little, Brown & Co.

Lundy, J. S.: Clinical Anesthesia, Philadelphia, 1942, W. B. Saunders Co.

Modell, W.: Drugs of Choice, 1960-1961, St. Louis, 1960, The C. V. Mosby Co.

Sollmann, T.: A Manual of Pharmacology, Philadelphia, 1957, W. B. Saunders Co.

Central nervous system stimulants

Daly, D. D., and Yoss, R. E.: The Treatment of Narcolepsy With Methyl Phenylpiperidyl Acetate: A Preliminary Report, Proc. Staff Meet. Mayo Clin. 31: 620, 1956.

French, J. D.: The Reticular Formation, Scient. Am. 196: 54, May, 1957.

Kapernick, J. S.: Metrazol for Central Nervous System Arteriosclerosis in Aging Patients, Geriatrics 12: 703, 1957.

Analgesics, hypnotics, and sedatives

Adams, E.: Barbiturates, Scient. Am. 198: 60, Jan., 1958.

Chase, H. F., Boyd, P. S., and Andrews, P. M.: (N)-Allylnormorphine in Treatment of Dihydromorphinone and Methorphinan Overdosage, J. A. M. A. 150: 1103, 1952.

Committee on Toxicology, A. M. A. Report to the Council: Precautions Regarding Salicylates Including Aspirin, J. A. M. A. 158: 831, 1955.

Eddy, N. B.: Addiction Producing Versus Habit Forming (Guest Editorial), J. A. M. A. 163: 1622, 1957.

Drugs that affect central nervous system   299

Feldman, W. H.: Chemotherapy of Infectious Diseases; Implications and Significance, Dis. Chest. **26:** 1, 1954.

Fraser, H. F.: Human Pharmacology and Clinical Uses of Nalorphine, M. Clin. North America, pp. 393-402, March, 1957.

Gross, M.: The Salicylates, Am. J. Nursing **55:** 1372, 1955.

Ingelfinger, F. J.: The Effect of Barbiturates in Patients With Liver Disease, J. Clin. Invest. **33:** 1116, 1954.

Isbell, H., and others: Chronic Barbiturate Intoxication, Arch. Neurol. & Psychiat. **64:** 1, 1950.

LaSagna, L.: The Newer Hypnotics, M. Clin. North America, pp. 359-367, March, 1957.

LaSagna, L., and Beecher, H. K.: The Optimal Dose of Morphine, J. A. M. A. **156:** 230, 1954.

Modell, W.: The Search for a Morphine Substitute, Am. J. Nursing **57:** 1565, 1957.

Prescor, M. J., and Walker, P. K.: The Treatment of Drug Addiction, Am. J. Nursing **51:** 611, 1953.

Reichard, J. D., Gupton, M. C., Buchanan, J. A., and Ingelfinger, F. J.: The Effect of Barbiturates in Patients With Liver Disease, J. Clin. Invest. **33:** 1116, 1954.

Anticonvulsants

Daly, D. D.: Drug Therapy in Convulsive Disorders, Proc. Staff Meet. Mayo Clin. **32:** 257, 1957.

Mulder, D. W., Daly, D. D., Rushton, J. G., and Yoss, R. E.: The Treatment of Epilepsy, Postgrad. Med. **25:** 404, 1959.

Unna, K. R.: Drugs in Epilepsy and Hyperkinetic States. In Drill, V. A. (editor): Pharmacology in Medicine, New York, 1958, McGraw-Hill Book Co., Inc., Chap. 15.

Gout

Hench, P. S.: Gout and Gouty Arthritis. In Cecil, R. L., and Loeb, R. F. (editors): A Textbook of Medicine, Philadelphia, 1959, W. B. Saunders Co., pp. 595-607.

Robinson, W. D.: Current Status of the Treatment of Gout, J. A. M. A. **164:** 1670, 1957.

Stetten, De Witt, Jr.: Gout and Metabolism, Scient. Am. **198:** 73, June, 1958.

United States Department of Health, Education and Welfare: Trial of Drugs for Gout, Pub. Health Rep. **74:** 315, 1959.

Anesthetics

Adriani, J.: Local Anesthetics, Am. J. Nursing **59:** 86, 1959.

Adriani, J., and Campbell, D.: Fatalities Following Topical Application of Local Anesthetics to Mucous Membranes, J. A. M. A. **162:** 1527, 1956.

Beecher, H. K.: Anesthesia, Scient. Am. **196:** 70, Jan., 1957.

Greisheimer, E. M.: The Physiological Effects of Anesthesia, Am. J. Nursing **49:** 337, 1949.

Hartridge, V. B.: Obstetric Analgesia and Anesthesia, Collected Papers of the Mayo Clinic, Philadelphia, 1958, W. B. Saunders Co., pp. 679-685.

Little, D. M., and Stephan, C. R.: Modern Balanced Anesthesia, A Concept, Anesthesiology **15:** 246, 1954.

Lundy, J. S.: Progress in Analgesia, A New Note on an Old Theme, Texas M. J. **51:** 301, 1955.

Lundy, J. S.: Contributions of Modern Anesthesia to Improvement in Surgical Technic, Collected Papers of Mayo Clinic and Mayo Foundation, Philadelphia, 1956, W. B. Saunders Co.

Lundy, J. S.: New Drugs and an Era of Analgesia and Amnesia, J. A. M. A. **162:** 97, 1956.

Ridley, R. W.: Safety in Anesthesia, Collected Papers of the Mayo Clinic and Mayo Foundation, Philadelphia, 1953, W. B. Saunders Co., pp. 779-784.

Waters, R. M., and Schmidt, E. R.: Cyclopropane Anesthesia, J. A. M. A. **103:** 975, 1934.

Alcohol

Block, M. A.: Alcoholism (Guest Editorial), J. A. M. A. **163:** 550, 1957.

Himwich, H. E. (Council on Mental Health): The Physiology of Alcohol, J. A. M. A. **163:** 545, 1957.

Jacobson, E., and Martensen, L. O.: Treatment of Alcoholism With Tetraethylthiuram disulfide (Antibus), J. A. M. A. **139:** 918, 1950.

McCarthy, R. G.: Alcoholism, Am. J. Nursing **59:** 203, 1959.

Smith, J. J.: The Treatment of Acute Alcoholic States With ACTH and Adreno-cortical Hormones, Quart. J. Stud. Alcohol. **11:** 190, 1950.

Westerfield, W. W., and Schulman, M. P.: Metabolism and Caloric Value of Alcohol, Report to the Council on Foods and Nutrition, J. A. M. A. **170:** 197, 1959.

Ataractics

Borrus, J. C.: Meprobamate in Psychiatric Disorders, M. Clin. North America, pp. 327-337, March, 1957.

Bross, R. B.: The Modern Mood-Changing Drugs, Am. J. Nursing **57:** 1142, 1957.

Council on Drugs, A. M. A.: Potential Hazards of Meprobamate, J. A. M. A. **164:** 1332, 1957.

Kierland, R. R.: Use of Sedatives and Tranquilizers, Minn. Med. **41:** 539, 1958.

Kline, N. S., and Saunders, J. C.: Reserpine in Psychiatric and Neurologic Disorders, M. Clin. North America, pp. 307-326, March, 1957.

Nance, M. R.: Chlorpromazine, Am. J. Nursing **56:** 609, 1957.

Chapter 10

Autonomic drugs

The autonomic nervous system

Autonomic (*autos*, self + *nomus*, law) means a law unto itself, or self-governing. The autonomic nervous system has been known by other names. Winslow (1732) called it sympathetic because he thought it controlled the sympathies of the body; Bichat (1800) called it vegetative to designate its control over the nutrition, as opposed to voluntary processes. Gaskell called it the involuntary nervous system to contrast it with the voluntary which controls skeletal movement. The autonomic nervous system consists of nerves, ganglia, and plexuses which regulate the heart, the smooth muscle of the body, and the glands. Thus respiration, digestion, circulation, metabolism, sweating, and the secretion of some of the endocrine glands are regulated by this system. Autonomic nerves contain cell processes known as preganglionic and postganglionic fibers. The cell bodies of origin lie within the central nervous system. The fiber which originates in the central nervous system and terminates in a ganglion is called preganglionic, and the fiber which originates in the ganglion and terminates in the organ it affects is called postganglionic. Ganglia of the sympathetic division of the autonomic nervous system lie close to the vertebrae (thoracic and lumbar regions), whereas those of the parasympathetic system lie close to the organ that is innervated.

There are a number of centers that lie in the central nervous system which are concerned with integration of all autonomic nervous system activities, i.e., activities of both the sympathetic and parasympathetic divisions. There is evidence that the hypothalamus particularly is concerned with such integrating activities. It contains centers which function in the regulation of body temperature, water balance, carbohydrate and fat metabolism, blood pressure, sleep, and emotions. There are other centers of integration, also, which are believed to be located in higher levels of the brain, but they have not been clearly identified.

Differences between the sympathetic and parasympathetic divisions

Although anatomic and physiologic differences do exist between the sympathetic and parasympathetic divisions, these differences are not as clear-cut and absolute as might be supposed. One of the differences lies in the fact that sympathetic nerve fibers ramify to a much greater extent than do the parasympathetic fibers. A preganglionic nerve fiber may not only pass through a number of ganglia in the sympathetic chain but it also frequently synapses with a large number of postganglionic fibers. In this way the sympathetic system may accomplish mass action through diffuse discharge of nerve impulses. The parasympathetic nervous system in contrast has its ganglia close to the organ which it innervates and thus is more limited in the discharge of its nerve impulses. On the other hand, the parasympathetic is more essential to life. The sympathetic is geared for mass response and the expenditure of large amounts of energy. The parasympathetic is concerned with functions of conservation and restoration. In general, if one system stimulates a function the other system inhibits that function. Viscera are usually innervated by both divisions. The action of one system may be made prominent by the blocking of effects in the opposing system.

Theories regarding transmission of nerve impulses

There is evidence to substantiate the theory that transmission of nerve impulses at synaptic connections and at myoneural junctions is brought about by the activity of chemical substances called mediators. At most autonomic junctions, i.e., synapses between preganglionic and postganglionic nerves or between postganglionic nerves and effector cells, this substance is believed to be acetylcholine, which is present in the nerve fibers and is released at the terminals (ganglia and myoneural junctions). All nerve fibers that synthesize this substance and liberate it at their terminals are known as cholinergic fibers. Acetylcholine plays an important role in transmission of nerve impulses in both the sympathetic and parasympathetic divisions of the autonomic nervous system. Acetylcholine is subject to inactivation or destruction by one or more enzymes known as cholinesterases. The most specific one to inactivate acetylcholine is said to be true acetylcholinesterase.* This enzyme hydrolyzes acetylcholine to choline and acetic acid. The enzymatic action is rapid; hence the effect of acetylcholine is brief. When the enzyme is made ineffective, as it is by certain drugs, the effect of acetylcholine is intensified and prolonged. Drugs that bring about effects in the body similar to those produced by acetylcholine are called *cholinergic drugs*. An older term used to designate this group of drugs is "parasympatho-

*Wescoe, W. C.: The Autonomic Nervous System, General Consideration. In Drill, V. A. (editor): Pharmacology in Medicine, New York, 1958, McGraw-Hill Book Co., Inc., p. 344.

mimetic," because they appeared to mimic the action produced by stimulation of the parasympathetic division of the autonomic nervous system.

The chemical mediator associated with certain nerve junctions in the sympathetic nervous system was formerly known as "sympathin." This substance greatly resembled epinephrine but differed from it in certain definite respects. Later, most investigators were led to believe that this compound, secreted at "adrenergic" nerve endings, is norepinephrine. Nerve fibers which liberate this mediator are spoken of as adrenergic fibers. In contrast to the cholinergic mediator, the adrenergic one is destroyed slowly in the body.

Drugs that produce effects like those produced by the Adrenalin-like mediator are called *adrenergic drugs*.

$$CH_3 - \overset{\overset{\displaystyle CH_3}{|+}}{\underset{\underset{\displaystyle CH_3}{|}}{N}} - CH_2 - CH_2 - O - \overset{\overset{\displaystyle O}{||}}{C} - CH_3$$

Acetylcholine

Epinephrine
(Adrenalin)

Norepinephrine
(Levarterenol)

Classification of autonomic drugs

The autonomic drugs are those drugs which either mimic or oppose the peripheral effects of nerve impulses from the autonomic nervous system. They can be grouped into *four* main classes based on the two chemical mediators within the autonomic nervous system and on the action of a given drug, that is, whether it mimics or opposes the physiologic effects of one or the other mediators.

1. Adrenergic drugs, or drugs that bring about effects similar to those produced by epinephrine and norepinephrine.

2. Cholinergic drugs, or drugs that bring about effects similar to those produced by acetylcholine.

(Since the postganglionic nerve fibers of the sympathetic nervous system are adrenergic, whereas those of the parasympathetic system are cholinergic, it has sometimes been the practice to call cholinergic drugs "parasympathomimetic" and the adrenergic drugs "sympathomimetic." However, it should be emphasized that a rational classification of the autonomic drugs must conform to the chemical substance secreted by the nerve and not to the anatomic location of the nerve; e.g., the preganglionic fibers in the sympathetic system are cholinergic and these

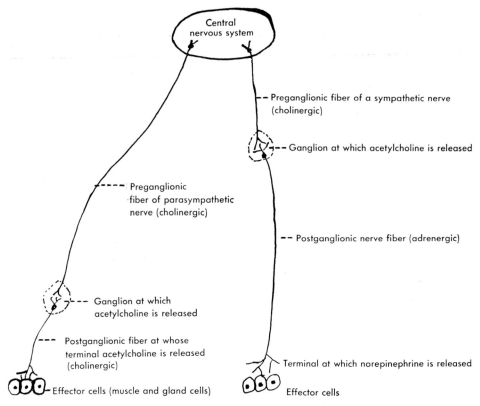

Central nervous system

—— Preganglionic fiber of a sympathetic nerve (cholinergic)

—— Ganglion at which acetylcholine is released

—— Preganglionic fiber of parasympathetic nerve (cholinergic)

—— Postganglionic nerve fiber (adrenergic)

—— Ganglion at which acetylcholine is released

—— Postganglionic fiber at whose terminal acetylcholine is released (cholinergic)

—— Terminal at which norepinephrine is released

—— Effector cells (muscle and gland cells)

Effector cells

Fig. 30 Schematic representation to show preganglionic and postganglionic fibers of the autonomic nervous system and associated chemical mediators.

junctions in the ganglia respond to cholinergic or anticholinergic drugs, not to adrenergic drugs. See Fig. 30.)

3. Adrenergic blocking agents, or drugs that block the effect of norepinephrine at the myoneural junction.

4. Cholinergic blocking agents or anticholinergic drugs, those that block the effects of acetylcholine.

In addition to the above groups of autonomic drugs there are some that produce mixed autonomic effects by partial blocking action in the ganglia of both the sympathetic and parasympathetic divisions of the autonomic nervous system. A review of the effects of stimulation of the two main subdivisions of the autonomic nervous system may be helpful in anticipating effects of autonomic drugs. See Table 14.

Site of action

Autonomic drugs act at ganglia, i.e., postganglionic nerves, and upon effector cells rather than on nerve endings. They make the cells more or less sensitive to the chemical mediator, or they may inhibit the action of the enzyme which normally destroys the mediator. For example, it is

Table 14

Effects produced by divisions of the autonomic nervous system

Sympathetic	Parasympathetic
Dilated pupils, eye adjusted to distance	Constricted pupils, eye adjusted to close vision
Increased cardiac rate	Slowed heart action
Increased cardiac output	Decreased cardiac output
Constriction of blood vessels in skin and viscera; dilated coronary blood vessels	Dilated blood vessels in nose, salivary glands, and pharynx; constricted coronary blood vessels
Elevation of blood pressure	
Relaxation of smooth muscle in bronchial tubes	Constricted bronchial tubes
Elevation of blood sugar	
Decreased activity along gastrointestinal tract (both muscular and glandular)	Increased peristalsis Increased secretions
Sphincters tightened, although this action varies	Sphincters usually relaxed
Bladder	
Detrusor muscle relaxed	Contracted
Trigone and sphincter contracted	Relaxed
Ureter tone and motility decreased	Increased
Human uterus	
Pregnant: increased contractions	Increased contractions
Nonpregnant: stimulated?	Variable

believed that physostigmine exerts its action on acetylcholinesterase to the extent that physostigmine inhibits the action of the enzyme and thus prolongs the effect of acetylcholine on the effector cells.

Adrenergic agents (sympathomimetic drugs)

Most of the agents that belong to this group of drugs have a similar chemical structure, which helps to explain similarity of effects. Their chemical structure contains a benzene ring and an amino nitrogen atom separated by a chain of two carbon atoms. For example:

$$\langle \underset{\underline{\quad\quad}}{\quad\quad} \rangle - \overset{|}{\underset{|}{C}} - \overset{|}{\underset{|}{C}} - \overset{|}{\underset{|}{N}}$$

The ring formation constitutes what is called the aromatic portion of the compound, and the two carbon atoms plus the nitrogen atom constitute the aliphatic portion of the compound. Substitutions of another atom or group of atoms for hydrogen atoms on either the aromatic or aliphatic part of the molecule account for a great number of synthetic adrenergic agents which, although exhibiting many effects characteristic of these drugs in general, also exhibit some properties that are differ-

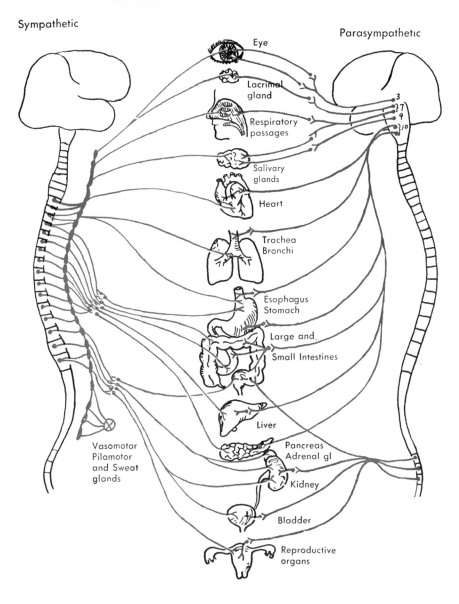

Sympathetic

Parasympathetic

Eye

Lacrimal
gland

Respiratory
passages

Salivary
glands

Heart

Trachea
Bronchi

Esophagus
Stomach

Large and

Small Intestines

Liver

Vasomotor
Pilomotor
and Sweat
glands

Pancreas
Adrenal gl

Kidney

Bladder

Reproductive
organs

3
7
9
10

Plate 3

Diagram of the autonomic nervous system. The craniosacral (parasympathetic) division is
shown in green. The thoracolumbar (sympathetic) division is shown in red.

ent, and new properties may make the compound therapeutically useful. However, it is also true that all adrenergic compounds are not chemically similar.

Epinephrine and Norepinephrine

Two physiologically important hormones are produced by the medullary portion of the adrenal gland. One is epinephrine and the other is norepinephrine (levarterenol).

Epinephrine is a hormone which exhibits a general action, whereas norepinephrine acts at or near the site of its liberation. It is now thought that norepinephrine is liberated in small amounts at all postganglionic adrenergic nerve endings and is an over-all vasoconstrictor. The activity at the sympathetic nerve endings therefore results in normal peripheral vasomotor resistance which constitutes a major factor in the maintenance of blood pressure.

Epinephrine, on the other hand, is an emergency substance liberated into the circulation under conditions of stress and causes increased cardiac output and redistribution of blood in the body. It is thought to be liberated from the gland either paroxysmally or over short periods of time to cope with stressful circumstances.

The secretion from the adrenal gland is normally a mixture of the two hormones, the amount of norepinephrine being up to 25 per cent of the total. The fundamental effect from this mixture is, however, the effect of epinephrine, since it has been shown to be the predominant hormone.

Norepinephrine is thought to be the natural synthetic intermediate substance formed by the adrenal gland. When the gland is subjected to splanchnic nerve stimulation, at first more epinephrine than norepinephrine is liberated. After the initial supply of epinephrine is exhausted, it would appear that more norepinephrine than epinephrine is secreted.

Epinephrine (Adrenalin)

Source and general characteristics. Epinephrine can be prepared synthetically, but most of that used in medicine is obtained from the adrenal glands of domestic animals. This preparation contains about 18 per cent levarterenol. Chemically, epinephrine is an amine and reacts with acids to form salts. Epinephrine hydrochloride solutions are unstable, react to light, and should be kept in the refrigerator. Both epinephrine and norepinephrine are inactivated in the tissues by enzymes, one of which is aminoxidase.

Action and result. Epinephrine is capable of producing both local and systemic effects.

Local. Epinephrine has no effect on the skin, but when applied to mucous membranes or wounds, or when injected into tissues (in the usual dosage), vasoconstriction is rapid and may last as long as two hours.

Systemic. Epinephrine acts upon the effector cells (muscle and gland cells) connected with the adrenergic nerve fibers. For the most part, its action is the same as that resulting from stimulation of the sympathetic nerve to the part acted upon. If stimulation of the part causes contraction of the muscle, epinephrine causes contraction. If stimulation causes relaxation, epinephrine causes relaxation. An exception exists in the response of the sweat glands and the pilomotor muscles, neither of which is affected in the human being, although there is increased sweating in many of the animals and also pilomotor activity. Mydriasis is not secured after therapeutic doses of epinephrine except under special conditions. *Epinephrine exerts its main action upon the heart, the blood vessels, and some of the smooth muscle of the body.*

ON HEART. Epinephrine accelerates the heart rate by stimulating the myocardium and the conduction tissue.[*] This results in stronger contraction and a more complete emptying of the chambers and usually a prompt rise in blood pressure. The increased cardiac output is thought to be the main reason for the rise in blood pressure. After a short time the increase of blood pressure reflexly slows the heart by stimulation of the vagus center. Small doses accelerate and strengthen the heart. Large doses may cause so great an acceleration that efficiency is temporarily lessened, and if the heart muscle is weak, as may be true in disease or when certain drug effects are present, it may strain it sufficiently to cause acute dilatation, disturbances in rhythm, or ventricular fibrillation. Oxygen consumption by the myocardium is markedly increased.

ON BLOOD VESSELS. Epinephrine acts chiefly on the smooth muscle of the arterioles and, to a lesser extent, on the capillaries and veins. It stimulates the smooth muscle in the vascular beds in much the same way as the sympathetic nervous system does. Small doses produce vasodilatation in the skin and skeletal muscles but not in the viscera or splanchnic regions. Thus in a moderate emergency, secretion of epinephrine favors blood flow through the skeletal muscles and elimination of heat. When larger doses of epinephrine are given, there is marked peripheral vasoconstriction of the blood vessels of the skin and skeletal muscles as well as of the splanchnic regions. This is associated with a marked rise in blood pressure. The cerebral vessels, those of the eye, and, to some extent, those of the lungs also constrict. Reports about the effect on the coronary circulation are contradictory.

The most striking response to the administration of epinephrine when

[*]Goodman, L., and Gilman, A.: The Pharmacological Basis of Therapeutics, New York, 1955, The Macmillan Co., p. 483.

given intravenously is a dramatic rise in blood pressure. Subcutaneous injection results in a slower rise in pressure. *Epinephrine is one of the most powerful vasoconstrictors known.* However, many factors, such as dosage, channel of administration, presence of disease, and action of drugs, act to modify the responses obtained. When the blood pressure subsides, it lowers to a brief period of hypotension before it becomes normal. This explains the period of nasal congestion which occurs after the use of epinephrine in nasal drops and sprays.

ON SMOOTH MUSCLE. Epinephrine relaxes the smooth muscles in the respiratory tract, especially if they are hypertonic. The action, which is immediate and very effective, relieves bronchial constriction, as seen when used for relief of acute asthma.

The smooth muscle of the stomach and intestine is relaxed by large doses of epinephrine, and the sphincters are usually contracted, although the sphincter action depends on the state of tonus. Intestinal tone is decreased and peristalsis is diminished. The emptying time of these organs would thus be increased. However, therapeutic doses rarely produce these effects.

Epinephrine stimulates the musculature of the splenic capsule, thereby increasing contractions of that organ. This action results in increasing the number of red cells and the viscosity of the blood.

ON GLANDS. The glandular action of epinephrine is relatively unimportant. Its action on the salivary gland resembles the effect of stimulation of the sympathetic nerve, i.e., the secretion obtained is of the sympathetic type—thick and rich in organic matter. Little or no effect is seen on the glands along the rest of the digestive tube, with the exception of the liver. Epinephrine causes glycogenolysis and a rise in the blood sugar. This effect is sometimes utilized in the treatment of insulin shock if there is reason to believe the glycogen stores are normal.

ON UTERUS. The action of epinephrine on the human uterus does not seem to have any therapeutic significance.

Absorption and excretion. Although epinephrine is readily absorbed from mucous membranes, it is destroyed by digestive enzymes and therefore useless if given by mouth. Rapid effects may be noted when the drug is given hypodermically or intramuscularly and almost immediate effects occur when it is given intravenously. The drug is rapidly excreted.

Uses. An important use of epinephrine is to prevent capillary bleeding. It may also be used to diminish hyperemia of the conjunctiva, to reduce congestion in nasal membranes, and to check or reduce hemorrhage of mucous membrane in surgery of the eye, ear, nose, mouth, or throat. One reason for giving it with procaine at the time of a tooth extraction is to prevent excessive bleeding and permit a clot to form. Epinephrine is effective only in checking bleeding of the smaller arterioles or capillaries; it has no value in controlling hemorrhage from larger vessels.

Epinephrine is probably *the* most valuable drug for the relief of acute bronchial asthma. The subcutaneous administration of 0.2 to 0.3 ml. (3 to 4½ ℳ) of a 1:1,000 solution provides rapid relief. Dosage may be repeated hourly if necessary. It is likewise of great value to relieve the acute symptoms of allergic conditions seen in acute anaphylactic shock, serum reactions, angioneurotic edema, hay fever, urticaria, etc. Dose is 0.3 to 0.5 ml. of a 1:1,000 solution.

Epinephrine enhances the action of local anesthetics when given with them by constricting the blood vessels in the field of operation and thereby checking bleeding, preventing widespread absorption of the anesthetic, and intensifying the anesthetic in the region where it is needed.

In heart block 0.3 to 0.5 ml. of a 1:1,000 solution may be given subcutaneously if fainting attacks occur.

Epinephrine is a powerful drug and requires great caution when used as a heart stimulant. In certain conditions of heart failure 0.25 to 0.5 ml. of a 1:1,000 solution is given subcutaneously or occasionally very small amounts are added to intravenous fluids. If too much epinephrine is given when the heart is in a weakened condition, ventricular fibrillation and death may result. Cases have been reported in which patients whose heart had stopped beating for several minutes have been brought back to life by injecting directly into the heart or into veins close to the heart and by massaging the organ in such a way that the epinephrine circulates through it. Intracardiac injection should be used only as a last resort.

Preparation, dosage, and administration.

Epinephrine Solution, U.S.P. This 1:1,000 aqueous solution is applied topically as required.

Epinephrine Injection, U.S.P., B.P. This 1:1,000 solution is available in ampule form. Dosage is 0.2 to 1 mg. (1/300 to 1/60 gr.) given subcutaneously or intramuscularly. This preparation is sterile and contains 1 mg. of drug in each milliliter of solution.

Epinephrine Inhalation, U.S.P. Epinephrine solution 1:100. This should be administered with a special nebulizer to provide a fine mist for inhalation. Epinephrine is not well absorbed from mucous membranes. The effectiveness of this preparation for the asthmatic patient is explained on the basis of achieving a relatively high concentration of the drug in the throat and respiratory passages rather than from a systemic action. Special precautions should be observed to avoid confusing the 1:100 solution with the 1:1,000 solution.

Sterile Epinephrine Suspension, U.S.P. (Epinephrine in Oil Injection.) Dosage is 0.4 to 3 mg. ($\frac{1}{150}$ to $\frac{1}{20}$ gr.) intramuscularly. It is available in 1 ml. ampules (1:500).

Epinephrine Bitartrate, U.S.P. This form should be applied topically as a 1 per cent ophthalmic ointment, as required.

Epinephrine Bitartrate Ophthalmic Ointment, U.S.P. This ointment consists of epinephrine bitartrate in a petrolatum base in a concentration of 1:100.

Adrenaline Injection, B.P. This is a 1:1,000 solution for injection. The dosage is 0.2 to 0.5 ml. (3 to 8 ♏) subcutaneously.

Adrenaline Solution, B.P. This is a 1:1,000 solution of adrenaline tartrate for topical application.

Solutions of epinephrine do not keep well; deterioration is evidenced by formation of sediment and brownish discoloration.

As mentioned above, epinephrine is given either locally or parenterally. When given orally it is destroyed by enzymes in the digestive tract. The subcutaneous route is the one most often employed. The intravenous route is rarely used, but if employed the drug must be given very slowly and in a very low concentration. Epinephrine in oil is usually given intramuscularly. Epinephrine may be applied topically or given by inhalation in the form of nasal sprays.

Because epinephrine is such a potent drug, the nurse must be particularly careful to give the right dose. If the preparation at hand is an ampule containing 1 ml. of the drug, it does not follow that 1 ml. is the usual dose. Usually, or very often, the dose is only a few minims. To be sure, the order for the drug will have been written by the doctor, but sometimes his handwriting is not the best and the nurse is expected to recognize an obvious error.

Side effects and toxic effects. Mild symptoms of poisoning are most often seen in nervous patients, those with hypertension or exophthalmic goiter. Symptoms usually consist of increased nervousness, muscular tremor, pallor, anxiety, headache, palpitation, respiratory difficulty, and precordial pain.

More dangerous effects may result from large doses or from the administration of the drug intravenously. These include cardiac dilatation, pulmonary edema, and cerebral accident. Death may also result from ventricular fibrillation.

The milder symptoms usually disappear with rest, reassurance, and discontinuance of the medication. The more serious symptoms must be treated symptomatically. They are best avoided by cautious use of the drug. Epinephrine should be avoided in patients with heart disease, hyperthyroidism, and nervous instability. Gormsen[*] reported a death following the subcutaneous injection of 60 mg. of epinephrine given by

*Abst. J. A. M. A. 112: 2644, 1939.

mistake. A 10 per cent solution for use by inhalation was used. Death resulted in a few minutes. The symptoms were immediate pain in the neck, anxiety, pallor, vomiting, dyspnea, increased pulse rate, marked rise in blood pressure, and collapse. Necropsy showed hyperemia of all organs, but neither macroscopic nor microscopic changes were specific.

The minimum fatal dose of epinephrine subcutaneously seems to be about 10 mg.

Isoproterenerol (Isuprel)

$$HO-\underset{}{\bigcirc}\overset{OH}{|}$$

OH   CH₃

— CH — CH₂ — NH — CH

CH₃

Isoproterenerol hydrochloride is a white, odorless, slightly bitter, crystalline solid.

Action and result. It is closely related to epinephrine and levarterenol, although it exhibits much less effect on smooth muscle of blood vessels and does not cause much change in blood pressure. It accelerates the heart and severe tachycardia can develop. Its most outstanding therapeutic effect is on the bronchial musculature, which is relaxed in asthmatic conditions. When given orally the drug tends to liquefy tenacious mucus and thus aids expectoration.

Uses. Isoproterenerol hydrochloride is used to increase the ventricular rate in patients with heart block and to prevent cardiac arrest. It is used to prevent and to treat bronchospasm and laryngospasm during anesthesia. It is used for mild to moderately severe asthma to relieve bronchial spasm, shrink swollen mucous membranes, and reduce the secretion of mucus. It is also used for the patient who is no longer benefited by the use of epinephrine or the patient in status asthmaticus.

Preparation, dosage, and administration.

Isoproterenerol Hydrochloride, U.S.P. (Isuprel Hydrochloride, Aludrine Hydrochloride). This preparation is usually administered sublingually and by oral inhalation. It is available in 10 and 15 mg. tablets for sublingual administration and in solution, 1:100 and 1:200, for oral nebulized inhalation. It is occasionally given parenterally (intramuscularly) in 1:5,000 concentration.

Isoproterenerol Sulfate (Norisodrine Sulfate, Isonorin Sulfate); *Isoprenaline Sulfate,* B.P. This is available in the form of a powder for inhalation, 10 and 25 per cent; as a solution for inhalation, 1:100; and in tablets, 10 mg., for sublingual administration.

For bronchial asthma, 10 mg. (5 to 20 mg.) are given sublingually three or four times daily; 0.5 ml. of a 1:200 solution may be nebulized and given for each dose by inhalation, and 0.02 to 0.15 mg. of a 1:5,000 concentration may be injected intramuscularly.

Side effects and toxic effects. Untoward effects include precordial pain, heart palpitation, anginal pain (pain down one or both arms), headache, nausea, tremor, nervousness, and excitement, and there may be a fall in arterial blood pressure. It is contraindicated for patients who have insufficient coronary blood flow.

Levarterenol Bitartrate (Levophed Bitartrate)

$$HO \left\langle \bigcirc \right\rangle - \overset{H}{\underset{OH}{C}} - \overset{H}{\underset{H}{C}} - \overset{H}{\underset{H}{N}} \cdot COOH - (CHOH)_2 - COOH \cdot H_2O$$

Source. Levarterenol bitartrate is a grayish white, crystalline powder, freely soluble in water. It darkens on exposure to light and air. It has been synthesized, but, like epinephrine, levarterenol is obtained chiefly from the medullary portion of the adrenal glands of animals.

Action and result. Levarterenol bitartrate differs from epinephrine chiefly in its over-all vasoconstrictor effect, in its ability to slow the heart when the patient is in a horizontal position, and in its failure to increase the cardiac output.* It causes a rise in blood pressure as a result of its peripheral effects on blood vessels rather than by its action on the heart. It has only a slight effect on blood sugar and no effect on bronchial musculature.

Uses. Levarterenol bitartrate is used to maintain blood pressure in acute hypotensive conditions caused by vasomotor depression, trauma, and shock. It does not take the place of intravascular fluids if the fall in blood pressure is due to diminished blood volume. Its therapeutic value appears to be limited.

Preparation, dosage, and administration.

Levarterenol Bitartrate Injection, U.S.P. (Levophed Bitartrate). It is available in 4 ml. ampules containing 0.2 per cent solutions of the drug. This amount (4 ml.) is usually added to 1,000 ml. of 5 per cent glucose in distilled water or to 5 per cent glucose in physiologic saline solution and administered slowly by intravenous infusion with a control drip bulb, 2 to 3 ml. per minute at first, decreased to 0.5 to 1 ml. per minute, depending on the response of the patient. The drug is also available in 2 ml. ampules of 0.02 per cent solution.

During administration of the agent the blood pressure of the patient must be taken frequently (every 2 to 5 minutes), and someone must

*N.N.D., 1960, p. 219.

be with the patient continuously. Great care must be taken that the drug does not leak into the subcutaneous tissue since it is irritating and will cause the tissues to slough. Sudden changes in the patient's blood pressure can occur.

Side effects and toxic effects. Symptoms of hypersensitivity (rash, hives, and itching) have occasionally been observed. Overdosage can produce marked hypertension, severe headache, photophobia, pain in the chest, pallor, and vomiting. Although it is thought to be a safer drug than epinephrine because it has less effect on the heart, some physicians have discontinued using it, believing that agents such as Neo-Synephrine are safer drugs. The constant attention which must be given to the patient adds to the problems of nursing service.

Ephedrine

$$\langle = \rangle - \underset{\underset{OH}{|}}{\overset{\overset{H}{|}}{C}} - \underset{\underset{CH_3}{|}}{\overset{\overset{H}{|}}{C}} - \underset{\underset{CH_3}{|}}{\overset{\overset{H}{|}}{N}}$$

Source. Ephedrine is the name given to an active principle isolated from an Asiatic drug, ma huang (*Ephedra vulgaris* var. *helvetica*), which has been used in the practice of medicine in China for more than five thousand years. In chemical composition it is an amine, closely allied to epinephrine, and it is also an alkaloid.

Action and result. Ephedrine is a sympathomimetic or adrenergic drug which resembles epinephrine but, in addition, it stimulates the central nervous system. It differs from epinephrine in a number of ways. It can be given both parenterally and orally since it is absorbed from the gastrointestinal tract, as well as from parenteral sites, of injection. Ephedrine has a more prolonged action on the heart and blood vessels, although its action is slower and weaker. Vasodilation does not ordinarily follow vasoconstriction as may occur after epinephrine. The central action of the drug is exerted mainly on the cortex and medulla. It stimulates the respiratory center in the medulla. It acts as a mydriatic in the eye, by acting on the radial muscles of the iris. It does not affect the muscle of accommodation.

Ephedrine relaxes hypertonic muscle in the bronchioles and in the gastrointestinal tract. Emptying time of the stomach and intestine is delayed. Sphincter muscles in the urinary as well as in the gastrointestinal tracts are stimulated. The effect on metabolism is similar to that of epinephrine. It exhibits a tendency to increase the tone of skeletal muscle.

Uses. Ephedrine is used to combat low blood pressure in certain hypotensive states, e.g., during spinal anesthesia.

314

In the treatment of bronchial asthma, ephedrine is useful in preventing acute attacks. Epinephrine is preferable when attacks are acute because of its more rapid effect.

As a constituent of nasal drops, jellies, and sprays, ephedrine relieves acute congestion of hay fever, sinusitis, head colds, and vasomotor rhinitis. Shrinkage of mucous membranes begins immediately and lasts for several hours.

Ephedrine is also effective for the treatment of narcotic poisoning. It stimulates the respiratory center as well as the cerebral cortex. It has been used in treatment of narcolepsy, a state in which the patient persistently falls off to sleep.

Ephedrine is used in the treatment of muscle weakness associated with myasthenia gravis. It is most effective, however, when combined with prostigmine.*

Ephedrine may be used in solution as a mydriatic when a cycloplegic action is not necessarily desired.

Preparation, dosage, and administration.

Ephedrine Sulfate Tablets, U.S.P.; *Ephedrine Sulfate Tablets,* N.F. These are available in 25 and 50 mg. for oral administration. Usual dose is 25 mg. (⅜ gr.).

Ephedrine Sulfate Injection, U.S.P. This is available in 1 ml. ampules containing 25 or 50 mg. (⅜ to ¾ gr.) of drug in solution for injection. Usual dose is 25 mg. (⅜ gr.).

Ephedrine Hydrochloride, N.F., B.P. This is available in capsule and tablet form. Usual dose is 25 mg. (⅜ gr.).

Ephedrine Sulfate Solution, N.F. A 3 per cent solution of the drug in 0.36 per cent sodium chloride solution, which is further diluted with an equal amount of isotonic saline before use.

Ephedrine Sulfate Syrup, N.F. The syrup contains 16 mg. of drug in 4 ml.

Ephedrine Sulfate and Phenobarbital Capsules, N.F. Each capsule contains 25 mg. of ephedrine sulfate and 30 mg. of phenobarbital.

(The main difference between the hydrochloride and the sulfate salts of ephedrine is that the latter are more freely soluble in water.)

Racephedrine Hydrochloride, N.F. This is a synthetic preparation that contains both the dextrorotatory and the levorotatory portions of ephedrine, and its uses and effects are similar to ephedrine sulfate or ephedrine hydrochloride. It is available in the form of a solution and as capsules (25 mg.).

Salts of ephedrine are effective when given orally, subcutaneously, intramuscularly, or intravenously. The oral channel of administration is

---

*Goodman, L., and Gilman, A.: The Pharmacological Basis of Therapeutics, New York, 1955, The Macmillan Co., p. 515.

used in preference to any other when systemic effects are desired. Local application is made in the form of drops or sprays to mucous membranes, or the drug may be applied in the form of an aqueous or oily solution or as a jelly or ointment. A 3 to 4 per cent solution is used for eyedrops, and the oral range of dosage is 20 to 50 mg. ($\frac{1}{3}$ to $\frac{3}{4}$ gr.) every 3 or 4 hours.

Side effects and toxic effects. Toxic doses are likely to cause insomnia, nervousness, dizziness, tremor, headache, heart palpitation, and sweating. Occasionally a patient will exhibit symptoms of hypersensitivity. The same precautions are recommended for the use of ephedrine as for epinephrine. Barbiturates or some type of sedative is sometimes prescribed for the patient who is receiving the drug over a period of time. This is to counteract the central stimulating effect of ephedrine. Some degree of tolerance to ephedrine develops, but it has not been known to cause addiction.

Amphetamines

$$\langle\!\!\!\bigcirc\!\!\!\rangle - CH_2 - \underset{\underset{CH_3}{|}}{CH} - NH_2$$

Amphetamine

The amphetamines were discussed under central nervous system stimulants; hence only their adrenergic effects will be emphasized in this chapter. Although amphetamine is a more potent stimulant of the cerebral cortex it resembles ephedrine in a number of ways.

Amphetamine constricts peripheral blood vessels, elevates the blood pressure, stimulates the heart, relaxes bronchial and gastrointestinal muscles, delays the emptying of the stomach, and dilates the pupil of the eye (after topical application). It does not produce vasodilation following vasoconstriction and in this way differs from epinephrine.

It is used because of its sympathomimetic action in the symptomatic treatment of orthostatic hypotension, for the treatment of nasal congestion associated with colds, sinusitis, vasomotor rhinitis, and hay fever. Its use is not recommended for pylorospasm or spastic colitis. It should be given with caution to patients with cardiovascular disease or to those manifesting restlessness, anxiety, or hyperexcitability.

Preparation and dosage for the various preparations of amphetamine have been listed in Chapter 9.

Phenylephrine Hydrochloride (Neo-Synephrine Hydrochloride)

Source. Phenylephrine hydrochloride is a synthetic sympathomimetic drug chemically related to epinephrine and levarterenol as well as ephedrine.

316

$$\text{(benzene ring with OH)} - \overset{\overset{\text{H}}{|}}{\underset{\underset{\text{OH}}{|}}{\text{C}}} - \overset{\overset{\text{H}}{|}}{\underset{\underset{\text{H}}{|}}{\text{C}}} - \overset{\overset{\text{H}}{|}}{\underset{\underset{\text{CH}_3}{|}}{\text{N}}}{}^{+} - \text{HCl}^-$$

Action and result. Phenylephrine hydrochloride is relatively nontoxic and exhibits fewer side effects than epinephrine, and its therapeutic effects are longer lasting. It has no effect on the central nervous system. When given parenterally it produces vasoconstriction and a rise in arterial blood pressure and the heart is reflexly slowed. It is one of the more useful adrenergic drugs. When applied topically to mucous membranes, it reduces swelling and congestion by constricting the small blood vessels.

Uses. It is useful in the treatment of sinusitis, vasomotor rhinitis, and hay fever. It is sometimes combined with local anesthetics to retard their systemic absorption and to prolong their action. Like ephedrine, this drug can be used to combat hypotension due to vasomotor depression, although it is not indicated when the fall in blood pressure is due primarily to diminished blood volume.

Phenylephrine hydrochloride is used as a mydriatic for certain conditions where dilatation of the pupil is desired without cycloplegia (paralysis of the ciliary muscle).

It is occasionally used for patients who have allergic symptoms and used alone or with other drugs for the relief of bronchial asthma.

Preparation, dosage, and administration.

Phenylephrine Hydrochloride, U.S.P., B.P. (Neo-Synephrine Hydrochloride). This drug is marketed in 10 and 25 mg. capsules for oral administration, as a 0.2 and a 1 per cent solution for injection, and in a number of forms for topical application—solutions, an ophthalmic solution, a jelly, and as an emulsion. *Phenylephrine Hydrochloride,* U.S.P. (2 and 10 mg. per milliliter) and *Phenylephrine Hydrochloride Solution,* U.S.P. (0.25, 0.5, and 1 per cent) are official preparations.

For topical application to the nasal mucous membrane, 0.25 per cent solution is ordinarily used. For parenteral injection, 0.1 to 1 ml. of a 1 per cent solution is used. The intravenous dose should be about $\frac{1}{10}$ the subcutaneous or intramuscular dose. As a mydriatic, 1 or 2 drops of the 1 per cent solution or emulsion or the 2.5 per cent ophthalmic solution are used. The oral dose needs to be about 50 times the subcutaneous dose—30 to 75 mg. (in divided doses) daily for allergic conditions.

Mephentermine Sulfate (Wyamine Sulfate)

$$\text{(benzene ring)} - \text{CH}_2 - \overset{\overset{\text{CH}_3}{|}}{\underset{\underset{\text{CH}_3}{|}}{\text{C}}} - \text{NH} - \text{CH}_3 \cdot \tfrac{1}{2}\ \text{H}_2\text{SO}_4 \cdot \text{H}_2\text{O}$$

Mephentermine sulfate is a white, crystalline powder which is freely soluble in water.

Action. Its effects are similar to those of the amphetamines and ephedrine. It produces vasconstriction, which is reasonably prolonged. It brings about less cerebral stimulation than amphetamine or methamphetamine, although it is sometimes used to dispel feelings of lethargy and fatigue and to elevate the mood. It has little effect on smooth muscle. Local application in the eye produces dilatation of the pupil.

Uses. Mephentermine sulfate is used topically to relieve nasal congestion in allergic or nonallergic rhinitis and sinusitis. It is also used for its vasoconstrictor effects to prevent and treat hypotensive states not associated with hemorrhage.

Preparation, dosage, and administration.

Mephentermine Sulfate, U.S.P. (Wyamine Sulfate). It is administered topically for nasal congestion and orally, intramuscularly, and intravenously for systemic effects. It is available in 1 and 2 ml. ampules containing 15 mg. per milliliter for injection; as an elixir, 5 mg. per milliliter; in tablets, 12.5 and 25 mg., for oral administration; and as a solution, 0.5 per cent, for topical administration to nasal membranes (2 or 3 drops every 4 hours as needed). Dosage for systemic effect varies from 20 to 80 mg., although the usual dose given by slow intravenous injection ranges from 15 to 30 mg.

Other adrenergic drugs

There are a number of other adrenergic drugs listed in the last edition of *New and Nonofficial Drugs.* Students are likely to recognize them more easily by their trade names, which are indicated in parentheses: *cyclopentamine hydrochloride* (Clopane Hydrochloride), *isometheptene hydrochloride* (Octin Hydrochloride), *metaraminol bitartrate* (Aramine Bitartrate), *methoxamine hydrochloride* (Vasoxyl Hydrochloride), *methoxyphenamine hydrochloride* (Orthoxine Hydrochloride), *methylhexaneamine* (Forthane), *naphazoline hydrochloride* (Privine Hydrochloride), *nylidrin hydrochloride* (Arlidin Hydrochloride), and others.

Minor differences exist in their actions, uses, advantages, and disadvantages. With certain exceptions, sympathomimetic drugs produce dilatation of the pupils, sometimes relaxation of the ciliary muscles of the eye, decreased tone of the muscle in the bronchial tubes, stomach, intestine, bladder, and ureters, contraction of smooth muscle sphincters, constriction of blood vessels other than coronary, inhibition of secretion of a number of glands, and increased heart rate.

The choice of one drug over another depends largely on the purpose for which it is given. The side effects of insomnia, tension, restlessness, tremor, weakness, and palpitation of the heart may at times interfere with clinical use. These drugs are to be avoided or used with considerable caution if patients have hyperthyroidism or hypertensive heart disease.

Many more drugs are likely to appear on the market and in the drug rooms of the hospital wards. It is important to read labels carefully and make the names mean as much as possible. Note the similarity in many of their names, especially the ending. Read the literature which accompanies a new drug. If it states that the drug is a sympathomimetic amine or an adrenergic agent you can predict some things about it since these drugs as a group have points of similarity.

Adrenergic blocking agents
Sympatholytic drugs

Sympatholytic drugs exert an effect antagonistic to drugs such as epinephrine. They lower the blood pressure because of extensive vasodilation, increased muscular tone, and activity of the gastrointestinal organs but inhibit the action of the heart only after very large doses. These drugs may be obtained from natural sources, e.g., ergot and its derivatives, or they may be synthesized. The latter group of agents include the following: *azapetine phosphate* (Ilidar Phosphate), *dibenzyl-β-chlorethylamine* (Dibenamine), *phenoxybenzamine* (Dibenzyline), *phentolamine hydrochloride* (Regitine Hydrochloride), *piperoxan*, and *tolazoline hydrochloride* (Priscoline Hydrochloride).

These drugs are used in the treatment of peripheral vascular disease such as Raynaud's disease, frostbite, trench foot, and other conditions with an associated condition of vasospasm. Phentolamine and piperoxan are valuable in diagnosing pheochromocytoma (tumors of the medullary portion of the adrenal gland which secrete large amounts of epinephrine and norepinephrine). They are also useful in controlling the hypertension before and after the surgical removal of such tumors.

The adrenergic blocking agents are not the drugs of choice in the treatment of essential hypertension, because their action is too transient, and side effects are troublesome.

Cholinergic drugs (parasympathomimetic agents)

Cholinergic drugs fall into two main groups: one group is chemically related to acetylcholine and produces effects similar to those of acetylcholine; members of the other group are cholinesterase inhibitors, which prevent the rapid inactivation of acetylcholine.

The effects of cholinergic drugs as seen in man are similar to those produced by the electric stimulation of cholinergic nerves. Since the chemical mediator released at the terminals of both preganglionic and postganglionic nerve fibers of parasympathetic nerves is acetylcholine, it is apparent why these drugs which behave so much like acetylcholine are often referred to as cholinergic.

Since acetylcholine is also released at the terminals of certain fibers of the sympathetic nervous system as well as at the terminals of efferent fibers to skeletal muscles, sweat glands, and the adrenal gland, it became customary to use terms to differentiate the effects of this complex drug. The effect of acetylcholine on peripheral effector cells (cardiac, smooth muscle cells, and cells of exocrine glands) is similar to the effects produced by an alkaloid, muscarine. Hence such effects of acetylcholine are said to be its muscarinic effects. The action of acetylcholine on autonomic ganglia and skeletal muscle cells resembles the action of nicotine; hence they are called the nicotinic effects of acetylcholine.

Muscarinic effects include slowing of the heart, increased gastrointestinal peristalsis and secretion, increased contractions of the urinary bladder, sweating, miosis, and, to some extent, peripheral vasodilatation. Tone of the bronchial musculature may also be increased.

Nicotinic effects include increased power of contraction of skeletal muscle and sometimes an elevation in blood pressure.

Since acetylcholine is so rapidly destroyed or inactivated in human tissues, its effects are too transitory to be of therapeutic value. Effort has been made to find chemical compounds that are more stable and less easily inactivated but will at the same time produce desired effects. Various esters of choline have been synthesized and some differ from acetylcholine in that they may exhibit more muscarinic effects than nicotinic effects, or vice versa. They may also differ in that some of the newer preparations can be administered orally and are more stable.

$$CH_3-\overset{\overset{\displaystyle CH_3}{|}}{\underset{\underset{\displaystyle CH_3}{|}}{N^+}}-CH_2-CH_2-O-\overset{\underset{\displaystyle O}{\|}}{C}-CH_3$$

Acetylcholine

$$CH_3-\overset{\overset{\displaystyle CH_3}{|}}{\underset{\underset{\displaystyle CH_3}{|}}{N^+}}-CH_2-\overset{\underset{\displaystyle CH_3}{|}}{CH}-O-\overset{\underset{\displaystyle O}{\|}}{C}-CH_3$$

Methacholine

$$CH_3-\overset{\overset{\displaystyle CH_3}{|}}{\underset{\underset{\displaystyle CH_3}{|}}{N^+}}-CH_2-CH_2-O-\overset{\underset{\displaystyle O}{\|}}{C}-NH_2$$

Carbachol
(carbamylcholine)

$$CH_3-\overset{\overset{\displaystyle CH_3}{|}}{\underset{\underset{\displaystyle CH_3}{|}}{N^+}}-CH_2-\overset{\underset{\displaystyle CH_3}{|}}{CH}-O-\overset{\underset{\displaystyle O}{\|}}{C}-NH_2$$

Bethanechol
(carbamyl-β-methylcholine)

Choline derivatives

Methacholine Chloride (Mecholyl Chloride)

Methacholine was one of the first cholinergic drugs to be synthesized.

Action and result. It resembles acetylcholine but the duration of its action is longer since it is less easily inactivated by cholinesterase. Although effects are related to dosage and route of administration, methacholine can be expected to slow the heart, to produce a lowering of blood pressure, and to increase the tone of muscle in the bronchioles, the gastrointestinal organs, and in the urinary bladder. Secretion of gastric juice, sweat, tears, and bronchial mucus is also increased.

Uses. Methacholine chloride is used to terminate attacks of paroxysmal tachycardia in selected cases which do not respond to the usual forms of therapy. It is considered inferior to quinidine for this purpose, however. It has been used to relieve vasospasm and improve circulation in Raynaud's disease and also for chronic ulcers, scleroderma, and arthritis, but its value is very limited. It has also been tried for relief of urinary retention, but better derivatives have been found, e.g., bethanechol chloride.

Preparation, dosage, and administration.

Methacholine Chloride, N.F. (Mecholyl Chloride). This drug is available as a sterile powder for subcutaneous injection and as a powder for oral administration. The therapeutically effective oral dose is 200 to 500 mg. two or three times a day. The drug, to some extent, is destroyed by gastric juice. The subcutaneous dose is usually limited to 10 mg. and then gradually increased to 25 mg., depending on the patient's tolerance. It is occasionally given by ion transfer (iontophoresis),* in which case a 0.2 to 0.5 per cent aqueous solution is used.

Side effects and toxic effects. Symptoms of overdosage usually begin with nausea and vomiting but may also include asthmatic attacks (in susceptible persons), substernal pain, dyspnea, and fainting. Atrial fibrillation, heart block and cardiac arrest can develop. Atropine is considered the best antagonist to use in treatment.

Methacholine Bromide (Mecholyl Bromide)

Methacholine Bromide, N.F. This preparation is similar to methacholine chloride, but its properties are such that it lends itself to tablet formation for oral administration. It is given in doses of 200 to 600 mg. two or three times a day.† If patients are receiving 2 Gm. of the drug daily without satisfactory effect, it is recommended that the oral treatment be abandoned in favor of methacholine chloride subcutaneously or local application by iontophoresis.

Carbachol

Carbachol is a synthetic derivative of choline.

Action and result. It resembles methacholine but is even more stable because it is entirely nonsusceptible to hydrolysis by cholinesterase. It is a potent cholinergic agent which exerts its main action on the urinary bladder and the gastrointestinal organs. As a result of its action the pa-

---

*A method whereby an electric current is used to force ions of the drug through the skin.
†N.N.D., 1960, p. 252.

tient experiences a sense of warmth, flushing of the face, increased flow of saliva, increased peristaltic activity, and increased contractions of the urinary bladder and sometimes of the uterus. It seems to have less effect on the heart than does methacholine. Severe abdominal cramps may develop. It shows some nicotinic effects similar to acetylcholine.

Uses. Carbachol has been used to relieve postoperative urinary retention. It promotes contractions of the musculature of the bladder and brings about relaxation of the sphincter of the bladder. It is also used to relieve postoperative distention of the bowel, since it increases intestinal peristalsis.

Carbachol is occasionally used to improve circulation in certain peripheral vascular diseases, but its value for such conditions is said to be limited. It is sometimes used as a miotic in the treatment of glaucoma.

Preparation, dosage, and administration.

Carbachol, U.S.P. The only dosage form of carbachol that is official and available in the United States is the powder for ophthalmic use. Ampules and tablets have been withdrawn from the market. The ophthalmic preparation is applied topically to the conjunctiva as 0.75 to 1.5 per cent solution or ointment two to six times daily. The ophthalmic powder is marketed under the name of Carcholin.

Carbachol, B.P.; *Carbachol Injection,* B.P. The subcutaneous dose is 0.25 to 0.5 mg.

Side effects and toxic effects. Carbachol produces many of the same toxic effects as mentioned for methacholine, although the gastrointestinal symptoms are especially prominent, e.g., abdominal cramps, diarrhea, nausea, belching, as well as malaise, headache, drop in blood pressure, and asthmatic attacks.

Atropine antagonizes the effects of carbachol but may do so rather slowly. Carbachol is contraindicated in the very ill patient and for those who are subject to asthmatic attacks.

Bethanechol Chloride (Urecholine Chloride)

The drug exhibits properties similar to methacholine chloride but differs from acetylcholine in that it does not exhibit any ganglion-stimulating effect. It is not destroyed by cholinesterase; hence its action is of comparatively long duration. It is less potent than some of the other choline derivatives but also less toxic. Cardiovascular effects are minimal. Its chief effects are seen on the musculature of the gastrointestinal organs and the urinary bladder.

Uses. This compound alleviates conditions which are relieved by stimulation of the parasympathetic nervous system. It is used to treat gastric retention following vagotomy or gastric surgery, for postoperative abdominal distention, and for urinary retention. It is sometimes used to prevent paralytic ileus and urinary retention in patients receiving certain drugs for hypertension (ganglion blocking agents).

Preparation, dosage, and administration.

Bethanechol Chloride, U.S.P. (Urecholine Chloride). It is available in 1 ml. ampules containing 5 mg. of the drug and also in 5 and 10 mg. tablets. Bethanechol chloride is administered orally, sublingually, or subcutaneously. It must not be given intramuscularly or intravenously.

Oral and sublingual doses of 10 to 30 mg. three or four times daily will usually control symptoms. The effect of the drug can usually be observed in about 30 minutes. The usual subcutaneous dose is 2.5 to 5 mg.

Side effects and toxic effects. Side effects are sometimes seen after subcutaneous administration and include headache, flushing, abdominal cramps, sweating, asthmatic attacks, and sometimes a drop in blood pressure. Parenteral administration of atropine promptly abolishes side effects. The major advantage of bethanechol over other choline derivatives is its greater margin of safety and low incidence of severe toxic effects.

Pilocarpine

Source. Pilocarpine is an alkaloid obtained from the leaves of South American plants called *Pilocarpus jaborandi* and *Pilocarpus microphyllus*. It was one of the first compounds known to exert cholinergic effects.

Action and result. Pilocarpine stimulates effector cells (smooth muscle and gland cells) innervated by postganglionic cholinergic nerves. The action is highly selective on the reactive substance of these cells, especially the cells of the sweat and salivary glands. The sweat glands are under control of sympathetic nerves anatomically, but their response to drugs would indicate that these nerves are cholinergic. It brings about constriction of the pupil, reduction of intraocular tension, and increased secretion tears. Other actions of pilocarpine in the body are rarely therapeutically useful and are likely to constitute side effects.[*]

Uses. The chief use of pilocarpine is for its miotic effect in early stages of a disease of the eye called glaucoma. The production of miosis promotes better drainage of the aqueous humor through the canal of Schlemm and thus reduces the intraocular pressure. Pilocarpine was once used to promote sweating in patients with renal insufficiency, but this practice is now obsolete since safer and better methods of dealing with this condition have become available. It is occasionally used to overcome paralysis of the muscle of accommodation (ciliary muscle) after the use of a drug such as atropine.

[*]Goodman, L., and Gilman, A.: The Pharmacological Basis of Therapeutics, New York, 1955, The Macmillan Co., p. 471.

Preparation, dosage, and administration.

Pilocarpine Nitrate, U.S.P., B.P. This is the salt most frequently used. It is applied locally in 0.5 to 3 per cent solutions to the conjunctiva every 2 to 3 hours.

Pilocarpine Hydrochloride, U.S.P. This form is also available and the dosage is the same as that for pilocarpine nitrate. Preparations of pilocarpine hydrochloride are available in plastic containers suitable for dropping the solution into the eye (Drop-tainers). The solution contains the drug in 0.5 per cent methylcellulose to which a preservative has been added.

Side effects and toxic effects. Poisoning from pilocarpine does not occur frequently, but overdosage can cause weakness, an excessive flow of saliva and tears, blurred vision, nausea and vomiting, diarrhea, slow weak pulse, and rapid difficult breathing. Death is usually due to respiratory failure or pulmonary edema. Atropine is given parenterally in the way of treatment along with measures to support circulation and respiration.

Anticholinesterase drugs

Some drugs act as cholinergic agents not by directly affecting the cells innervated by postganglionic cholinergic nerves but by inactivating or inhibiting the enzyme which normally degrades acetylcholine. In this way the activity of acetylcholine is prolonged and its concentration at the myoneural junction is increased.

Physostigmine (Eserine)

Source. Physostigmine is an alkaloid obtained from the seed of the *Physostigma venenosum.* This seed is also known as the Calabar or "ordeal" bean. It has been so called because natives of the Calabar coast of Africa often used it in what was known as "trial by ordeal." The person suspected of crime was compelled to swallow some of the powdered bean. If he survived, he was declared innocent; if he died, he was pronounced guilty, and there was no escape from the verdict.

Action and result. Physostigmine produces its effects indirectly by inactivating (temporarily) the enzyme which ordinarily is responsible for the hydrolysis of acetylcholine in body fluids and tissues.

The effects of physostigmine are not always predictable and may be complex because the drug acts at the autonomic ganglia and on skeletal muscle, as well as on the peripheral effector cells associated with postganglionic fibers of the parasympathetic nerves. However, when a therapeutic dose of physostigmine is given to man, the most significant effects are on the eye and the bowel.

In eye. After local application of the drug to the conjunctiva, the pupil constricts and the muscle of accommodation (ciliary muscle) goes into spasm. This action occurs within a few minutes. Vision may be distorted for a short time because of the effect on the ciliary muscle. Intraocular pressure is usually reduced because of the more favorable resorption of aqueous humor.

In gastrointestinal tract. Tone and motility are increased, which may result in bowel evacuation.

On skeletal muscle. There is no noticeable effect after therapeutic doses. Large doses may produce muscular twitching. Observation of this action of the drug led to studies of its use for myasthenia gravis. Its use for myasthenia gravis has been replaced by neostigmine.

Uses. Physostigmine is used principally as a miotic to relieve intraocular tension in glaucoma. It is also used to relieve mydriasis (dilated pupils) after the use of drugs that produce this effect and to break adhesions between the iris and the crystalline lens. It is occasionally used to increase the motility of the bowel and thus aid in the relief of gaseous distention.

Preparation, dosage, and administration.

Physostigmine Salicylate, U.S.P., B.P. (Eserine Salicylate). It is administered topically to the conjunctiva in solutions which vary from 0.02 to 1.0 per cent concentration. Oral doses of 1 to 3 mg. may be given as often as three times a day. The subcutaneous dose is 0.5 to 1 mg.

Side effects and toxic effects. Symptoms of poisoning develop quickly and soon reach their peak effect. Symptoms include nausea and vomiting, diarrhea, abdominal cramps, muscular twitching, pin-point pupils, excessive sweating, salivation and flow of tears, dyspnea, urinary urgency, rapid weak pulse, and low blood pressure. The patient feels faint and apprehensive. Death is usually due to respiratory failure or pulmonary edema.

Atropine is the physiologic antidote and should be given intravenously or subcutaneously. Endotracheal intubation and the administration of oxygen may be indicated. Artificial respiration may also prove lifesaving. An attempt should be made to keep the patient warm and dry.

Neostigmine (Prostigmin)

Source. Neostigmine is a synthetic drug similar pharmacologically to physostigmine. It is available only in the form of its salts which are freely soluble in water and stable in aqueous solutions.

Action and result. The action of neostigmine is similar to that of physostigmine, but it has the advantage of being more stable. It is also an anticholinesterase but has little effect on circulation, the eye, or the activity of glands. It exhibits a selective action primarily on the bowel, the urinary bladder, and the skeletal muscle. Its effect on skeletal muscle

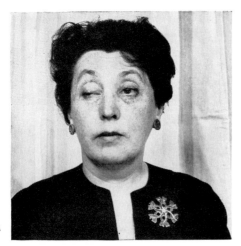 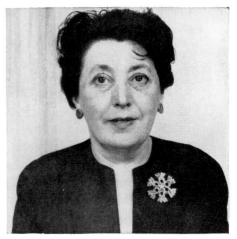

A

B

Fig. 31 A, A patient with myasthenia gravis, before treatment. Note ptosis of eyelids. B, The same patient after treatment. (Reprinted, by permission, from the film Myasthenia Gravis, produced by Sturgis-Grant, Inc., for the Myasthenia Gravis Foundation, Inc., and Hoffmann-La Roche, Inc.; from Osserman, Kermit E.: Myasthenia Gravis, New York, 1958, Grune & Stratton, Inc.)

is believed to be due to both its anticholinesterase activity and a direct stimulating action on the muscle.

Uses. Neostigmine is used to relieve abdominal distention caused by accumulation of gas and insufficient peristaltic activity following surgical operations. It is preferred to physostigmine for this purpose because it has fewer side effects.

It is also used for the prevention and treatment of atonic conditions of the urinary bladder. It will enable the patient to empty the bladder completely.

Myasthenia gravis is a rare chronic disease manifested by extreme fatigability of the skeletal muscles. Although any skeletal muscle may be involved, those concerned with movement of the eyeballs, eyelids, and face, and those used in chewing, swallowing, and speech are most likely to show involvement. Ptosis of the eyelids is an almost constant symptom. Diplopia is also likely to be present. The cause of this disease is not known. Nothing has been found in the muscle or nerve tissue to account for the muscular weakness, but a curare-like block seems to occur at the myoneural junction and interferes with stimulation of muscle cells. The disease is usually subject to remissions and exacerbations (periods of improvement followed by periods of decline). Judicious use of neostigmine or other anticholinesterase drugs may produce dramatic results, but overdosage tends to aggravate the muscular fatigue and cause side effects such as nausea and vomiting, abdominal cramps, diarrhea, and muscle twitching. It is important that the patient have sufficient therapy

326

to maintain function of the chewing and swallowing muscles to avoid malnutrition.

Neostigmine has several other uses; e.g., it is used as a test for pregnancy. It is given intramuscularly for three days, and if the patient is not pregnant bleeding will occur usually within 72 hours.

Neostigmine (ophthalmic solution) is sometimes used as a miotic for patients with glaucoma.

Preparation, dosage, and administration.

Neostigmine Bromide, U.S.P., B.P. (Prostigmin Bromide). This drug is available in 15 mg. tablets and also in the form of a slow-release tablet for oral administration. Dosage is 15 mg. three times a day, depending on the needs of the patient. This preparation is also available as a 5 per cent ophthalmic solution. The slow-release dosage form decreases the need for administration of the drug at night.

Neostigmine Methyl Sulfate Injection, U.S.P., B.P. This is available in 1 ml. ampules containing 0.25 mg. (1:4,000), 0.5 mg. (1:2,000), and 1 mg. (1:1,000) solution. The total daily dosage must be determined in accordance with the severity of the symptoms and the response of the patient. A dose of 0.5 mg. of neostigmine intramuscularly is said to be equivalent to 15 mg. given orally. In the treatment of myasthenia gravis 1 to 2 mg. intramuscularly every 3 hours is generally satisfactory when the patient is unable to swallow. Sometimes neostigmine bromide is given orally and neostigmine methylsulfate is given intramuscularly to re-enforce the oral dosage when symptoms are severe. Sometimes patients will require only one 15 mg. tablet two or three times a day and other patients may require 20 or more tablets a day. Increased physical activity and/or emotional strain usually causes the patient to require more medication.

Side effects and toxic effects. The toxic effects are essentially the same as those produced by physostigmine, and the treatment is also similar. Excessive doses of any of the anticholinesterase compounds may cause severe weakness accompanied by parasympathetic side effects and various degrees of muscular tightness and twitching. Atropine is given when overdosage from these drugs is apparent, but care must be exercised to avoid overdosage with the atropine.

Other drugs used for myasthenia gravis

Pyridostigmin (Mestinon) and *ambemonium* (Mytelase) are two anticholinesterase compounds which are being used for myasthenia gravis. They differ from neostigmine mainly in their longer action and decreased severity of side effects. The longer duration of their action often makes it possible for the patient to sleep undisturbed without the administration of the drug during the night.

Both drugs are available in tablet form for oral administration. Mestinon Bromide is available in a slow-release dosage form.

Edrophonium chloride (Tensilon) is a cholinergic drug which is discussed further in Chapter 11, Skeletal Muscle Relaxants and Their Antagonists. It is mentioned here because its action resembles that of neostigmine and because it is used in the emergency treatment of patients with myasthenia gravis and as a diagnostic agent. When given to a patient suspected of having myasthenia gravis, he will show prompt improvement in muscular strength should the disease be present. The duration of the action of the drug is too brief to be of value for maintenance therapy.

As a diagnostic agent, 10 mg. of the drug are administered intravenously. In myasthenic crisis, the drug is given by continuous intravenous drip. Edrophonium chloride is listed in the U.S.P. and is available in 10 ml. vials containing 10 mg. per milliliter.

Benzpyrinium Bromide (Stigmonene Bromide)

Benzpyrinium bromide is similar to neostigmine in both its action and uses. It is one of the inhibitors of cholinesterase.

Uses. This drug is used to relieve postoperative abdominal distention and urinary retention and also for the treatment of simple delayed menstruation.

Preparation, dosage, and administration.

*Benzpyrinium Bromide** (Stigmonene Bromide). It is available in 1 ml. ampules containing 0.5 or 2 mg. in each milliliter. It is administered intramuscularly in doses of 2 mg. for postoperative abdominal distention, followed in about 30 minutes with a low enema. The dosage may be repeated every 2 to 3 hours until effective results are obtained. The same dosage is recommended for the relief of urinary retention but should be accompanied by heat (hot-water bottle) over the lower part of the abdomen. For simple delayed menstruation 2 mg. daily for 1 to 3 successive days is recommended.

Isoflurophate (Floropryl)

Isoflurophate is one of the cholinergic organic phosphates which is chemically related to certain poisonous insecticides, hexaethyl tetraphosphate (HETP) and tetraethyl pyrophosphate (TEPP).

Isoflurophate is a liquid which forms hydrogen fluoride and loses its anticholinesterase activity when in the presence of moisture.

Action and result. Isoflurophate is a potent antagonist of cholinesterase and produces permanent inhibition of this enzyme. Its effects are more prolonged than those of physostigmine and similar drugs whose

*Described in annual publication of A. M. A. Council on Drugs, N.N.D., 1960.

inhibition of cholinesterase is reversible. The miotic action of isofluro-phate is more potent than that of pilocarpine or physostigmine. Because of its toxic potential it cannot be administered for systemic effects. Systemic effects sometimes result from absorption of the drug through the skin.

Uses. It is used chiefly as a miotic in the treatment of certain types of glaucoma and for certain kinds of strabismus. It has also been used for myasthenia gravis.

Preparation, dosage, and administration.

Isoflurophate (Floropryl). U.S.P. preparations of this drug are available as a 0.025 per cent ophthalmic ointment and a 0.1 per cent ophthalmic solution. They are applied to the conjunctival sac of the eye. Care should be exercised to avoid washing the eyedropper with water or allowing it to touch the conjunctiva. Caution should also be observed so that this preparation is not mistaken for an oral preparation.

In glaucoma, 1 to 3 drops of the 0.1 per cent solution every 8 to 72 hours is the usual dose. Administration at bedtime helps to minimize the inconvenience of blurred vision.

Side effects and toxic effects. Systemic administration may precipitate severe and potentially fatal effects similar to those of other potent cholinergic drugs. Toxic symptoms include nausea and vomiting, intestinal cramps and diarrhea, profuse flow of tears, bronchial constriction, shock, convulsions, and collapse.

Side effects include aching of the eyes, twitching of the eyelids, headache, photophobia, and blurred vision.

Poisonous effects are treated with intravenous administration of atropine sulfate to combat general cholinergic effects. Anticonvulsant drugs are indicated for the control of convulsive seizures.

Cholinergic blocking agents (anticholinergic drugs, parasympatholytic agents)

The drugs discussed under this heading produce effects similar to those produced when parasympathetic nerves are severed. The drugs block the effect of acetylcholine at myoneural junctions of tissues and organs supplied by postganglionic cholinergic nerves. The cells affected are chiefly the smooth muscle, cardiac muscle, and exocrine gland cells. Since these cells are unable to respond normally to acetylcholine, the heart rate can be expected to become more rapid, the smooth muscle to become relaxed, secretions of duct glands to be inhibited, and the pupil of the eye to be dilated.

Atropine and scopolamine are two important cholinergic blocking agents. They block especially the muscarinic effects of acetylcholine.

When atropine or similar drugs are given for one effect, all other actions tend to become side effects, and many times they are undesirable. The synthetic substitutes for atropine tend to have fewer side effects, although each drug exhibits individual characteristics.

Cholinergic blocking agents—belladonna group

A number of plants belonging to the potato family (Solanaceae) contain similar alkaloids. Included are the *Atropa belladonna* (deadly nightshade), *Hyoscyamus niger* (henbane),* *Datura stramonium* (Jimson weed or thorn apple),† and several species of Scopola. The principal alkaloids of these plants are atropine, scopolamine (hyoscine), and hyoscyamine.

Atropa belladonna was the name conferred on one of these plants by Linnaeus in 1753. The first part of the name was selected because of the poisonous qualities of the plant and is called Atropa after Atropos, the eldest of the Greek Fates who supposedly cut the thread of life.‡ The second part of the name, belladonna, means "beautiful lady" and was chosen because of the custom practiced by certain Roman ladies of placing belladonna preparations in their eyes to make them appear larger and more lustrous.

Atropine and hyoscine resemble each other closely, both in effects and in chemical structure, as can be seen in the accompanying formulas.

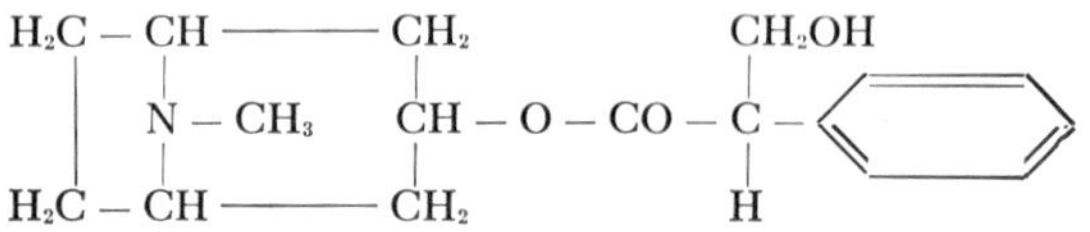

Atropine

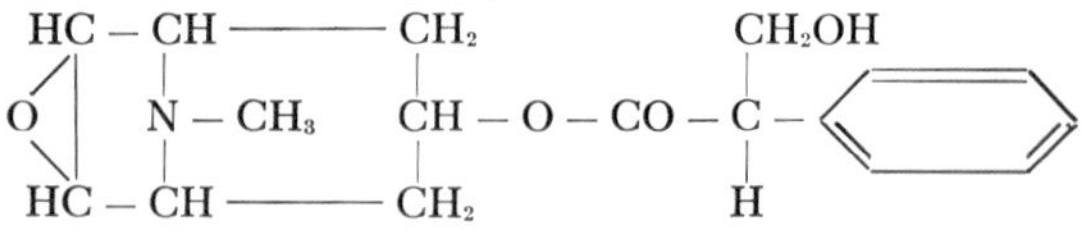

Hyoscine

*Henbane is thought to be a corruption of henne-bell, which suggests a musical instrument. In medieval Latin, henbane was referred to as *Symphoniaca herba;* Symphoniaca being a rod with many bells on it. (Wootton.) Henbane is the bane of domestic fowl.

†Jimson weed is a corruption of Jamestown weed, so called because it was early observed as a weed in Jamestown, Virginia. It is given its other name, thorn apple, because of its spiny capsule.

‡Name of *Atropa belladonna* from Greek and Roman mythology.

THREE FATES	CONTROLLED THE DESTINIES, HUMAN AND DIVINE
Clotho	Held the spindle or distaff
Lachesis	Drew out the thread
Atropos	Cut the thread of life

Atropine

Source. Atropine is the chief alkaloid of the plant *Atropa belladonna,* which is grown for commercial purposes in Germany, England, Austria, and America. It is also synthesized.

Action and result. There may be a local, central, or peripheral action.

Local. There is a slight amount of absorption when atropine or belladonna is applied to the skin, especially if it is in an oily or alcoholic preparation or in the form of a plaster. Belladonna ointment or suppositories were sometimes used on mucous surfaces. The local effect for the relief of pain is slight, however, and these preparations are seldom used.

When an aqueous solution of atropine is dropped into the conjuctival sac of the eye, it rather quickly produces dilatation of the pupil, diminished secretion of tears, and impaired ability to focus objects close to the eye. If the eye is normal there is little change in intraocular tension, but it may increase in patients who have glaucoma. These effects are mentioned again under peripheral action.

Central action. This refers to the action of atropine on the central nervous system.

ON CEREBRUM. Small or moderate doses of atropine have little or no effect. Large or toxic doses cause the patient to become restless, wakeful, and talkative, a condition that may develop into delirium and finally stupor and coma. The exalted, excited stage has sometimes been called a "belladonna jag." A rise in temperature is sometimes seen, especially in infants and young children, but this is now thought to be caused by the suppression of sweating rather than by an action on the heat-regulating center.

Atropine is thought to have a depressant effect on motor mechanisms which affect muscle tone and movement. For this reason, atropine and especially scopolamine have been used to diminish tremor in Parkinson's disease. The precise mechanism of this action is unknown.

ON MEDULLA. Therapeutic doses of atropine stimulate the respiratory center and make breathing faster and sometimes deeper. When respiration is seriously depressed atropine is not always reliable as a stimulant; in fact it may deepen the depression. Large doses stimulate respiration but they can also cause respiratory failure. Death is usually due to failure of respiration.

Small doses stimulate the vagus center in the medulla, causing primary slowing of the heart. The vasoconstrictor center is stimulated briefly and then depressed. Because depression follows rather soon after stimulation, atropine has been called a borderline stimulant of the central nervous system.

Peripheral action. The main therapeutic uses of atropine are due to its peripheral action rather than to its central action. The more important effect is on the smooth muscle, cardiac muscle, and gland cells, which are supplied by postganglionic cholinergic nerves. These cells are so affected by atropine that they become insensitive to acetylcholine. The drug apparently does not interfere with the formation of acetylcholine nor does it combine with acetylcholine. To some extent, atropine brings about effects similar to those produced by stimulation of postganglionic fibers in the sympathetic nervous system. The following results of peripheral action are seen.

IN EYE. The pupil is dilated (mydriasis) and the muscle of accommodation is paralyzed (cycloplegia). The sphincter muscle of the iris and the ciliary muscle are both innervated by cholinergic nerve fibers and hence are affected by atropine. Since the sphincter muscle is unable to contract normally, the radial muscle of the iris causes the pupil to dilate. These effects in the eye are brought about by both local and systemic administration of atropine, although the usual single therapeutic dose of atropine given orally or parenterally has little effect on the eye. After the pupil is dilated photophobia occurs, and when the drug has reached its full effect the usual reflexes to light and accommodation disappear.

IN RESPIRATORY TRACT. Secretions of the nose, pharynx, and bronchial tubes are decreased and the mucous membrane is made more dry. This is particularly true if the action of atropine has been preceded by a period of excessive secretion. The muscles of the bronchial tubes relax, which tends to increase the ease of breathing. Atropine and scopolamine are less effective than epinephrine as bronchodilators and are seldom used for asthma.

IN HEART AND BLOOD VESSELS. When the usual clinical doses are given, the cardiac rate is temporarily and slightly slowed because of the central action of the drug on the cardiac center in the medulla. Moderate to large doses accelerate the heart by interfering with the response of the heart muscle to vagal nerve impulses. The latter is a peripheral action. In therapeutic doses atropine has little or no effect on blood pressure, although large doses and sometimes ordinary doses cause vasodilatation of vessels in the skin of the face and neck. Reddening of the face and neck is seen, especially after large or toxic doses.

IN GLANDS. Since the sweat glands of the skin are supplied by cholinergic nerves, atropine decreases or abolishes their activity. This causes the skin to become hot and dry.

In the mouth, salivary and mucus secretions are decreased and the mouth feels dry. The patient experiences marked thirst and sometimes has difficulty in swallowing. Postoperative patients sometimes have the desire to rinse their mouth a great deal because they received atropine preoperatively and have developed this reaction.

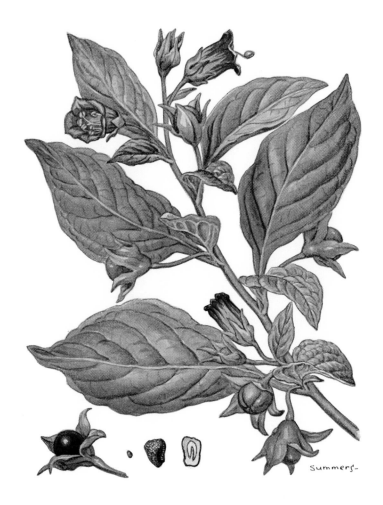

Plate 4

Atropa belladonna (deadly nightshade). (From Jackson, D. E.: Experimental Pharmacology and Materia Medica, St. Louis, The C. V. Mosby Co.)

Although some difference of opinion exists among authorities as to the effect of atropine on the activity of gastric glands, it appears that the amount and character of the gastric secretion are little affected by atropine, at least when it is given in ordinary therapeutic doses. Effects which are produced in laboratory animals have not always been confirmed in human tissues. The secretion of acid in the stomach is presumably less under vagal control than under hormonal or chemical control. The effect of atropine on the secretion of the pancreas and intestinal glands is not therapeutically significant.

IN SMOOTH MUSCLE. Atropine and other belladonna alkaloids decrease motility and tone, as well as peristalsis in the stomach and the small and large intestine.

Atropine does not affect the secretion of bile, but it exerts a mildly antispasmodic effect in the gallbladder and bile ducts.

It exerts a relaxing effect on the ureter, especially when it has been in a state of spasm. Therapeutic doses decrease the tone of the fundus of the urinary bladder. When the detrusor muscle is hypertonic it is relaxed by atropine.

The power of atropine to decrease the activity of uterine muscle is thought to be negligible. It is at best only mildly antispasmodic. However, atropine is said to have a relaxing effect on the circular muscle of a hypertonic uterus, which probably explains its use for dysmenorrhea.

Uses. Atropine is especially useful as a preliminary medication prior to surgical anesthesia. It decreases secretions of the mouth and respiratory passages. It is effective in the prevention of laryngospasm.

Atropine may be used as a mydriatic and cycloplegic in examinations of the eye and in the treatment of certain conditions of the eye. It is used especially for the refractions of the eyes of children who need a potent drug to paralyze the muscle of accommodation. Homatropine, a shorter acting cycloplegic and mydriatic, is usually satisfactory for adults.

Atropine is sometimes given with morphine to relieve biliary and renal colic. Atropine tends to relieve the muscular spasm induced by morphine.

Preparations of belladonna or its alkaloids are administered for their antispasmodic effects in conditions characterized by hypermotility of the stomach and bowel, e.g., pylorospasm, spastic colon, biliary and renal colic, and hypertonicity of the urinary bladder and ureters. These drugs are also found in certain cough remedies (antiasthmatic mixtures), in which case they are given to relieve mild conditions of bronchial spasm and excessive secretions.

Belladonna derivatives are sometimes useful for the relief of painful menstruation.

Symptoms in selected cases of Parkinson's disease are also relieved, that is, the tremor, muscular rigidity, and cramps. However, scopolamine is thought to be superior to atropine for this use.

Preparation, dosage, and administration.

Atropine Sulfate, U.S.P., B.P. Tablets are available, containing 0.3, 0.4, 0.5, 0.6, and 1.2 mg. of drug. This corresponds to 1/200, 1/150, 1/120, 1/100, and 1/50 gr., respectively. The drug is also available in multiple-dose vials (1/150 gr. per milliliter) for injection and in the form of atropine sulfate ophthalmic ointment. Atropine sulfate is usually administered subcutaneously, orally, or topically (in the eye). The usual subcutaneous or oral dose is 0.5 mg. (1/120 gr.), although 0.4 mg. (1/150 gr.) is frequently ordered. The ophthalmic solution and the ointment are usually used in a 0.5 or 1 per cent concentration.

Belladonna Extract, N.F., B.P. The extract is prepared from belladonna leaf and contains alkaloids of the belladonna leaf. It is given orally, usually in doses of 15 mg. (¼ gr.).

Belladonna Tincture, U.S.P., B.P. The usual dose is 0.6 ml. (10 minims), although the range of dosage may be from 0.3 to 2.4 ml. It is given orally.

A number of additional preparations of belladonna are listed in N.F.

Absorption, distribution, and excretion. Atropine (and also scopolamine) is readily absorbed after oral and parenteral administration. It is also absorbed from mucous membranes, as is noted when ophthalmic solutions escape through the lacrimal ducts to the mucous membrane of the nose. To a lesser extent, atropine is also absorbed from the skin. The drug is widely distributed in the fluids of the body and easily passes the placental barrier to the blood of the fetus. It is excreted chiefly by way of the kidney. Some is excreted through the bile. The remainder is apparently metabolized in the liver. Traces are found in other secretions, such as the milk.

Side effects and toxic effects. Atropine is a potent alkaloid but it has a wide margin of safety. Poisoning occurs but is rarely fatal. The fatal dose is said to be about 100 mg. for adults and 10 mg. for children. Survival has occurred after much larger doses.

Symptoms develop rapidly after overdosage and consist of dry mouth, great thirst, and difficulty in swallowing and talking. Vision becomes blurred, pupils are dilated, and photophobia (sensitivity to light) is present. A rash may develop which is seen chiefly over the face, neck, and upper trunk. Rash is seen particularly in children, although it may be seen also in adults. The body temperature is elevated, and in young children and infants it may reach 107° F. and more. The skin of the face and neck is flushed; the pulse becomes rapid and may be weak. Urinary urgency and difficulty in emptying the bladder may be noted. The patient becomes restless, excited, talkative, and confused. This may progress to delirium and mania and may be mistaken for an acute psychosis. The patient may also experience giddiness, staggering stupor, coma, and respiratory and circulatory failure.

Young children who are given atropine or scopolamine as a preanesthetic medication often have a pronounced cutaneous flush after administration of the drug. Parents may be much disturbed about this and think that the child is ill with an acute disease. This is a side effect and is not seen as often in adults as in children.

Goodman and Gilman state that a patient who shows an acute onset of bizarre mental and neurologic symptoms should be suspected of having symptoms of drug poisoning and atropine poisoning in particular.

Contraindications. Atropine and related alkaloids are usually contraindicated for patients with glaucoma because of the tendency of drugs which are mydriatics to increase intraocular tension in the eyes.

Treatment. If the drug has been taken by mouth the stomach should be lavaged promptly with tannic acid solution. Administration of the Universal Antidote or activated charcoal will help to inhibit further absorption of the drug. Pilocarpine is sometimes ordered to be given subcutaneously in doses of 10 mg. until the mouth is moist. Artificial respiration, oxygen, or oxygen and carbon dioxide may be indicated. Short-acting barbiturates, chloral hydrate, or paraldehyde may be given to relieve excitement. Cautious use of central nervous system stimulants is recommended should the patient become stuporous. Ice bags and alcohol sponge baths aid in reducing the fever.

Scopolamine (Hyoscine)

Action. Scopolamine resembles atropine in its peripheral effects but it differs in its central action, since doses of the drug given parenterally depress the central nervous system, producing drowsiness, euphoria, relief of fear, relaxation, and sleep. Little sedative action is observed after oral administration of scopolamine. It produces amnesia. It is not an analgesic, however, and in the presence of pain it may cause delirium unless accompanied by an analgesic. Scopolamine frequently stimulates rather than depresses the respiratory center and is believed to counteract the respiratory depressant effects of morphine when given with that drug. On the other hand, in some persons scopolamine is observed to cause respiratory depression and to increase the respiratory depression caused by morphine.*

Uses. Scopolamine is used as a preanesthetic medication, usually

*Cullumbine, H.: Cholinergic Blocking Agents. In Drill, V. A. (editor): Pharmacology in Medicine, New York, 1958, McGraw-Hill Book Co., Inc., p. 411.

along with morphine or one of the barbiturates, to check secretions and to prevent laryngospasm, as well as for its sedative effect.

In obstetrics it is used to produce obstetric amnesia (twilight sleep) and analgesia when combined with a barbiturate, meperidine, or morphine.

It is one of the drugs used for motion sickness. When given orally it does not cause sedation, which may be an advantage.

It is employed as a sedative for certain maniacal and delirious patients.

It is used for postencephalitic parkinsonism and paralysis agitans.

It is also used as a mydriatic and cycloplegic. Its effects appear more promptly and disappear more rapidly than atropine. Scopolamine is less likely to cause irritation in the eyes than atropine.

Preparation, dosage, and administration.

Scopolamine Hydrobromide, U.S.P.; *Hyoscine Hydrobromide*, B.P. This drug is available in 0.6 mg. (1/100 gr.) tablets which can be given orally or parenterally. Ophthalmic solutions are applied topically to the eye in 0.2 per cent concentration.

Hyoscine Eye Ointment, B.P. The ointment contains 0.25 per cent hyoscine hydrobromide.

Scopolamine Hydrobromide Injection, U.S.P.; *Hyoscine Injection*, B.P. The injection is available in ampules containing 0.3, 0.4, and 0.6 mg. in 1 ml. and 0.4 mg. in 0.5 ml. Dosage is 0.3 to 0.6 mg. subcutaneously.

Hyoscyamus and Stramonium

A number of preparations of Hyoscyamus as well as of Stramonium are listed in the *National Formulary*. They are seldom used in modern therapy.

Synthetic substitutes for atropine—mydriatics and cycloplegics

Homatropine Hydrobromide

Action. Homatropine hydrobromide is a synthetic alkaloid which resembles atropine, but larger doses are required to produce effects equivalent to atropine. When it is instilled in the conjunctival sac, the pupil is dilated as rapidly as with atropine but the duration of effect is shorter. Cycloplegia is usually satisfactory if repeated applications to the eye are made. Accommodation or the ability of the eye to focus objects clearly is usually normal within 20 to 24 hours. Homatropine is not as effective as a cycloplegic in the eyes of children as atropine. Homatropine is used in preference to atropine when mydriasis of short duration is desired and when cycloplegia need not be complete for ocular examination. Solutions of cocaine are sometimes used in addition to homatropine to increase mydriasis.

Preparation, dosage, and administration.

Homatropine Hydrobromide, U.S.P., B.P. It is used in 1 to 2 per cent aqueous solution and is instilled in the conjunctival sac a drop at a time until the pupils are satisfactorily dilated.

Eucatropine Hydrochloride (Euphthalmine Hydrochloride)

Action. Eucatropine hydrochloride is a prompt-acting mydriatic which has little or no effect on the muscle of accommodation. It is effective within 30 minutes, and the iris returns to normal within a few hours.

Uses. It is said to be safe and convenient for use in examinations of the eye. Its systemic effects resemble atropine, but it is much less potent. As is true of other mydriatics, its use should be avoided in patients with glaucoma or in those who have a predisposition to its development.

Preparation, dosage, and administration.

Eucatropine Hydrochloride, U.S.P. (Euphthalmine Hydrochloride). This is a white, crystalline powder. Two or 3 drops of a 2 per cent aqueous solution are instilled in the conjunctival sac of the eye.

Cyclopentolate Hydrochloride (Cyclogyl Hydrochloride)

Action. Cyclopentolate hydrochloride is a synthetic agent which produces rapid intense mydriasis and cycloplegia of moderate duration when instilled in the eye. It is said to be nonirritating and nonsensitizing and that it does not produce undesirable systemic effects.

Preparation, dosage, and administration.

Cyclopentolate Hydrochloride, U.S.P. (Cyclogyl Hydrochloride). Administration is only in the form of ophthalmic solutions for instillation in the conjunctival sac of the eye. It is effective for persons of all ages who have highly pigmented irises. Solutions of 0.5 to 1 per cent are used for refractive studies and for the treatment of keratitis, adhesions, and other conditions of the eye.

Synthetic substitutes for atropine—antispasmodics

The usefulness of atropine is limited by the fact that it is a complex drug and produces effects in a number of organs or tissues simultaneously. When it is administered for its antispasmodic effects it will also produce prolonged effects in the eye, causing dilated pupils, blurred vision, etc., as well as dry mouth and possibly a rapid heart rate. When the antispasmodic effect is the one desired, other effects become side effects and sometimes they are distinctly undesirable.

A large number of drugs have been synthesized in an effort to capture the antispasmodic effect of atropine without its other effects. Drugs of this type are frequently used to relieve hypertonicity and hypersecretion in the stomach. Belladonna and atropine in the amounts usually prescribed are believed to have relatively little influence on gastric secretion in man. In recent years more potent drugs have been synthesized, but their usefulness is sometimes limited because of their side effects. A number of these preparations reduce gastrointestinal motility as well as secretion and are used as a part of the treatment for patients with gastric and duodenal ulcers.

Although such drugs are only a part of the total treatment of the patient with an ulcer, effective treatment with drugs is dependent on certain qualifications of the drug.

The ideal drug for the management of peptic ulcer should block the mechanism of gastric secretion without producing blockage in the autonomic ganglia and without causing curariform effects (muscular weakness). It should be relatively nontoxic and palatable and should reduce both the volume and the acidity of the gastric secretion over long periods of time. It should be effective when given orally. It should not produce troublesome or adverse side effects. The ideal drug has not been found which probably explains why so many different preparations are available. Seemingly no single preparation excels all others.

Continued synthesis of new anticholinergic drugs takes place, and if the claims for longer action and greater effectiveness are substantiated after long trial, more useful therapeutic agents may become available.

Like most of the cholinergic blocking agents they are contraindicated for patients with glaucoma, pyloric obstruction, and prostatic hypertrophy.

Homatropine Methylbromide (Novatrin, Mesopin)

Action. Homatropine methylbromide is one of the older cholinergic blocking agents used in the United States. Its effects are similar to those of atropine, but it is without the latter drug's effect on the central nervous system. Its anticholinergic potency is said to be considerably less than that of atropine, but it is also less toxic. Its effect on gastric secretion, hypermotility, and the duration of its action is said to be much the same as that for atropine.

Uses. Homatropine methylbromide is used for the treatment of gastrointestinal spasm and as an adjunct in the treatment of patients with peptic ulcer.

Preparation, dosage, and administration.

Homatropine Methylbromide, U.S.P. (Novatrin, Mesopin). The drug is available in 2.5, 5, or 10 mg. tablets and as an elixir (2.5 mg. per 4 ml.). The usual oral dose is 5 to 10 mg. three or four times daily.

Side effects. Side effects include dryness of the mouth and blurring of vision.

338

Methscopolamine Bromide (Pamine Bromide, Lescapine Bromide)

Action. Methscopolamine bromide is an anticholinergic drug which produces antispasmodic and antisecretory effects. It is said to suppress both volume and acidity of the gastric secretion. It slows the emptying of the stomach and reduces peristalsis in the bowel. It decreases secretion of saliva and sweat. Tolerance to the medication does not seem to develop.

Uses. Methscopolamine bromide is used as an antispasmodic in the treatment of patients with hypermotility of the gastrointestinal tract, for peptic ulcer, and for forms of gastritis associated with hypermotility and hyperacidity. It is also occasionally used to relieve excessive salivation and sweating.

Preparation, dosage, and administration.

*Methscopolamine Bromide** (Pamine Bromide, Lescapine Bromide). This is available in 2.5 mg. tablets and in solution for injection (1 mg. per milliliter). The usual dosage for adults is 2.5 to 5 mg. administered before meals and at bedtime. The usual parenteral dose is 0.25 to 1 mg. intramuscularly or intravenously every 6 to 8 hours as needed to control symptoms.

Side effects and toxic effects. The side effects most frequently encountered include dry mouth, constipation, and blurred vision. Other effects encountered less frequently may include dizziness, palpitation, flushed dry skin, difficult urination, headache, and nausea.

Overdosage may bring about a ganglionic blocking action and a curare-like effect on skeletal muscle.

Methscopolamine Nitrate (Skopolate Nitrate)

Methscopolamine nitrate* has the same action, uses, and side effects as given above for methscopolamine bromide. The usual oral dose for adults is 2 to 4 mg. before meals and at bedtime. Tablets containing 2 mg. of the drug are available for oral administration, as well as enteric-coated tablets for delayed action. It is also marketed in vials (0.5 mg. per milliliter) for intramuscular or subcutaneous injection.

Methantheline Bromide (Banthine Bromide)

Action. Methantheline bromide has an anticholinergic action similar to that of atropine and a ganglionic blocking action in the autonomic nervous system, as well as a curare-like effect on skeletal muscle.

Early studies seemed to show that this drug produced favorable inhibitions of hypertonic muscle in the gastrointestinal tract and genitourinary organs as well as diminished gastric secretion, but later results appeared to be disappointing. Apparently it does not inhibit gastric

*Described in annual publication of A. M. A. Council on Drugs, N.N.D., 1960.

secretion consistently and effectively when the drug is given orally.* However, it does delay the emptying of the stomach and acts as an antispasmodic in the treatment of patients with pylorospasm, hypermotility of the intestine, spastic colon, and spasm of the ureter and urinary bladder. Some degree of pupillary dilatation accompanies the antispasmodic effect.

Preparation, dosage, and administration.

Methantheline Bromide, N.F. (Banthine Bromide). This is available in 50 mg. tablets for oral administration and in ampules, each containing 50 mg. The content of the ampule is dissolved in physiologic saline solution for the purpose of injection (intramuscularly or intravenously). Parenteral administration is not recommended if the patient can take the drug orally. The tablets should not be chewed because they have an unpleasant taste.

The usual initial dose for adults is 50 mg., although the usual effective dose is 100 mg. four times a day. Some patients require more, some less, than this amount. The recommended dosage is the smallest amount that will effectively relieve the symptoms.

Side effects and toxic effects. Patients may experience side effects in the form of dryness of the mouth, dilated pupils, and inability to read fine print. Some may develop constipation and require a laxative. Varying degrees of urinary retention have been observed in patients with hypertrophy of the prostate gland. A small percentage of patients complain of general malaise and weakness and do not tolerate the drug well. The curare-like effect (muscular weakness) may be counteracted by artificial respiration and prompt administration of oxygen.

Propantheline Bromide (Pro-Banthine Bromide)

Action. Propantheline bromide is an analogue of methantheline bromide and is said to be more effective than the latter drug to reduce the volume and acidity of gastric secretions. It is also said to produce less severe effects. It has come to replace the older drug to a great extent.

Preparation, dosage, and administration.

Propantheline Bromide, U.S.P., B.P. (Pro-Banthine Bromide). Tablets (15 mg.) are available for oral administration, as well as ampules containing 30 mg. of the drug. The content of the ampule is dissolved in not less than 10 ml. of water for injection prior to intravenous administration. Parenteral administration is reserved for patients who cannot take the drug orally.

Propantheline bromide is also available in tablets that contain 15 mg. of propantheline bromide and 15 mg. of phenobarbital.

*Kirsner, J. B., Ford, H., and Kassriel, R. S.: Anticholinergic Drugs in Peptic Ulcer, M. Clin. North America, p. 506, March, 1957.

The dosage of Pro-Banthine must be carefully adjusted to the needs of individual patients. The initial dose that is recommended is 1 tablet (15 mg.) with meals and 2 tablets at bedtime, with subsequent adjustment depending on the patient's reaction and tolerance to the medication. The bitter taste of methantheline bromide (Banthine Bromide) has been controlled by sugar-coating the Pro-Banthine tablet.

Side effects. Propantheline is thought to show less severe side effects than methantheline bromide but not less frequent side effects.

Diphemanil Methylsulfate (Prantal Methylsulfate)

Action. Diphemanil methylsulfate is a synthetic drug that exhibits characteristic anticholinergic effects on gastrointestinal motility and secretion, heart action, and activity of sweat glands. It also exhibits some ganglionic blocking activity.

Uses. Diphemanil methylsulfate has been used as a part of the total treatment for patients with peptic ulcer. Results appear to be variable, especially after oral administration. The drug has also been employed for the relief of excessive sweating which aggravates certain dermatologic conditions.

Preparation, dosage, and administration.

*Diphemanil Methylsulfate** (Prantal Methylsulfate). This drug is marketed in 100 mg. tablets for oral administration, as a 2 per cent topical cream, and as a solution for injection (2.5 mg. per milliliter).

The usual oral dose for adults is 100 mg. every 4 to 6 hours (between meals). Enteric-coated tablets are available which are said to prolong the action as much as 8 hours. A dose of 15 to 25 mg. may be injected subcutaneously or intramuscularly, although dosage must always be adjusted according to the needs of the patient. Oral administration is recommended for use as soon as expedient.

Side effects and toxic effects. Side effects are usually mild but are similar to those produced by atropine; they include dry mouth, dilated pupils and blurred vision, tachycardia, constipation or diarrhea, and urinary retention.

Oxyphenonium Bromide (Antrenyl Bromide)

Action. Oxyphenonium bromide is a cholinergic blocking agent that inhibits gastric and salivary secretions and gastrointestinal motility. It relaxes the detrusor muscle of the urinary bladder. Its postganglionic blocking activity is similar to that of atropine.

Uses. Oxyphenonium bromide has been used as an adjunctive agent in the treatment of patients with duodenal ulcer or for spastic and hypertensive conditions of the gastrointestinal tract. It is used mainly for

*Described in annual publication of A. M. A. Council on Drugs, N.N.D., 1960.

its antispasmodic effect. Occasionally it is used as a substitute for atropine or scopolamine as a preanesthetic drug.

Preparation, dosage, and administration.

*Oxyphenonium Bromide** (Antrenyl Bromide). It is available in 5 mg. tablets and as a syrup (1.25 mg. per milliliter) for oral administration and in solution (2 mg. per milliliter) for subcutaneous and intramuscular injection. The usual oral dose is 10 mg. four times a day. When immediate action is desired, 1 to 2 mg. are injected every 6 hours. Dosage must be adjusted according to the response of the patient and the severity of the side effects.

Side effects. Side effects are similar to those associated with other anticholinergic agents and include dry mouth, blurred vision, constipation, and difficulty in emptying the urinary bladder. Large doses produce ganglionic blocking effects and a curariform effect on skeletal muscle. These effects are similar to those produced by large doses of Banthine (weakness, dizziness, tachycardia, etc.).

Although oxyphenonium bromide is a useful antispasmodic, it does not seem to exhibit any advantages over other drugs of this category. With continued therapy some degree of tolerance is said to develop to the antispasmodic effects of this compound.

---

*Tricyclamol chloride** (Tricoloid Chloride), *trihexethyl chloride** (Pathilon Chloride), and *hexocyclium methylsulfate** (Tral) are said to be similar to oxyphenonium bromide in pharmacologic effects, side actions, and chemical structure.

Trihexyphenidyl Hydrochloride (Artane Hydrochloride)

Action. Trihexyphenidyl hydrochloride is a synthetic preparation which exerts an antispasmodic effect on smooth muscle similar to that of atropine. It also relieves spasm of skeletal muscle partly by an action on the cerebral cortex of the brain and partly by an anticholinergic action. Its more potent action is that of a muscle relaxant. It has much less effect on the eye, heart, and salivary glands than has atropine.

Uses. It is used to reduce the muscular rigidity, mental depression, and inertia found in patients with Parkinson's disease. It is especially effective in reducing rigidity due to muscle spasm, although it is useful in all forms of parkinsonism.

Preparation, dosage, and administration.

Trihexyphenidyl Hydrochloride, U.S.P. (Artane Hydrochloride). This drug is available in 2 and 5 mg. tablets and as an elixir (0.4 mg. per milliliter) for oral administration. Dosage is carefully determined for

*Described in annual publication of A. M. A. Council on Drugs, N.N.D., 1960.

each individual patient. The usual initial dose is 1 mg. for the first day. If the patient is not receiving other medication the dosage may be increased to 2 mg. on the second day with further increases of dosage until the patient is receiving 6 to 10 mg. Some patients may require more. The total dosage is divided into three parts and given close to mealtime (before or after meals).

Side effects and toxic effects. If dosage is kept within therapeutic limits this drug seldom produces severe side effects. Some patients have mild side effects such as dryness of the mouth, dizziness, blurred vision, mild nausea, and nervousness. These tend to disappear with continued use. Some degree of tolerance seems to develop. It does not tend to precipitate glaucoma.

There are a number of other anticholinergic drugs listed in N.N.D. that are used to relieve symptoms of Parkinson's disease. These include *cycrimine hydrochloride* (Pagitane Hydrochloride), *ethopropazine hydrochloride* (Parsidol Hydrochloride), *benztropine methanesulfonate* (Cogentin Methanesulfonate), and *procyclidine hydrochloride* (Kemadrin). These drugs share a certain similarity of structure and exhibit peripheral effects similar to atropine. They are administered orally.

Ganglionic blocking agents

Ganglionic blocking agents prevent the passage of nerve impulses from the preganglionic nerve fibers to the postganglionic nerve fibers. Autonomic ganglia both in the sympathetic and parasympathetic divisions are all activated by acetylcholine, and complete blocking at the ganglion level would produce paralysis of the entire autonomic nervous system.

These drugs frequently produce stimulation, which is followed by depression, and large or toxic doses are required to produce complete absence of activity in the ganglia. These drugs tend to be complex and confusing because they act on both the sympathetic and parasympathetic ganglia and are likely to affect other structures of the body as well, causing widespread effects.

Nicotine

Nicotine is a liquid alkaloid, freely soluble in water. It turns brown on exposure to air. It is the chief alkaloid found in tobacco.

It has no particular use but is of great pharmacologic interest and toxicologic importance. Its use in experiments performed on animals has helped to increase our understanding of the autonomic nervous system.

Absorption. Nicotine is readily absorbed from the gastrointestinal tract, respiratory mucous membrane, and the skin.

Action and result. Nicotine produces a temporary stimulation of all sympathetic and parasympathetic ganglia. This is followed by depression which tends to last longer than the period of stimulation. It affects skeletal muscle in a way similar to the way it affects the ganglia, i.e., a depressant phase follows stimulation. During the depressant phase nicotine exerts a curare-like action on skeletal muscle.

In addition, nicotine stimulates the central nervous system, especially the medullary centers (respiratory, emetic, and vasomotor). Stimulation is followed by depression. Death is due to respiratory failure, although it may be caused more by the curariform action of nicotine on skeletal muscle than from the central action on the respiratory center. Large doses of nicotine may cause tremor and convulsions due to the central stimulating action.

The actions and effects of nicotine on the blood-vascular system are complex. The rate of the heart is frequently slowed at first, but later it may beat faster than usual. Various disturbances in rhythm have been observed. The small blood vessels in peripheral parts of the body constrict and the blood pressure will fall. The latter condition is observed in nicotine poisoning.

Repeated administration of nicotine causes tolerance to develop.

Toxic effects. Acute or chronic poisoning can result.

Acute poisoning. Nicotine is a rapid-acting, extremely toxic drug. Cases have been reported of gardeners who were poisoned while handling the drug as an insecticide. Death occurred in a few minutes. Black Leaf 40 is a commercial preparation that contains nicotine and is used as a spray to kill various types of insects.

Symptoms of poisoning include increased flow of saliva, nausea, vomiting, abdominal cramps, diarrhea, cold sweat, confusion, fainting, drop in blood pressure, rapid pulse, prostration, and collapse. Convulsions sometimes occur. Death is due to respiratory failure.

Treatment is directed toward keeping the patient breathing. Artificial respiration with oxygen is said to be more effective than central respiratory stimulants. If life can be prolonged to give the tissues an opportunity to detoxify the drug, the patient may recover.

If the poison has been swallowed, gastric lavage with solution of potassium permanganate (1:10,000) is recommended. Other forms of treatment indicated depend upon the symptoms presented.

Chronic poisoning. The effect of tobacco in the individual who smokes is a subject about which there is considerable difference of opinion. The effects of excessive smoking seem to afford more agreement than the effects of mild or moderate use of tobacco. Excessive smoking is known to cause irritation of the respiratory tract, and there is a real possibility that tobacco smoke exerts carcinogenic effects in the lungs of man. Chronic dyspepsia may develop in heavy smokers and patients with gastric ulcer are usually advised to avoid overindulgence.

In patients with peripheral vascular disease such as thromboangiitis obliterans (Buerger's disease), nicotine is generally believed to be a contributing factor in the disease and may precipitate spasms of the peripheral blood vessels and thus reduce the blood flow through the affected vessels. Vasospasm in the retinal blood vessels of the eye, associated with smoking of tobacco, is thought to be the cause of a serious disturbance of vision.

Roth found that nicotine in cigarettes must be reduced more than 60 per cent before vascular effects of smoking fail to appear or are only slight.

Some physicians recommend that patients with hypertension and peripheral vascular disease sharply limit their smoking habits or discontinue smoking entirely. Others feel that the treatment of patients must be on the basis of individual study of each patient.

Tetraethylammonium Chloride (Etamon Chloride)

Action and result. Tetraethylammonium chloride is a synthetic compound that resembles nicotine in that it is a generalized ganglionic blocking agent. It partially blocks the transmission of motor impulses through the ganglia of both the sympathetic and parasympathetic divisions of the autonomic nervous system. This may result in increased blood flow through certain blood vessels, reduced arterial blood pressure, decreased motility in the gastrointestinal tract, loss of accommodation in the eye, and disturbed function of the urinary bladder.

Uses. Tetraethylammonium chloride is of limited clinical usefulness as a therapeutic and diagnostic agent in the treatment of peripheral vascular disease. Although it lowers the blood pressure of both the normal and the hypertensive patient, its action is short-lived and frequently its action is accompanied by undesirable side effects. These include dyspnea, weakness, lightheadedness, slowing of speech, dryness of the mouth, and difficulty with muscular movement. Patients who experience these symptoms should be kept horizontal until the symptoms are relieved.

Preparation, dosage, and administration.

*Tetraethylammonium Chloride** (Etamon Chloride). The drug is administered intravenously and intramuscularly. The intravenous dose is 200 to 500 mg. and should not exceed 7 mg. per kilogram of body weight. The intramuscular dose is 1 to 1.2 Gm. and should not exceed 20 mg. per kilogram of body weight.

*Described in annual publication of A. M. A. Council on Drugs, N.N.D., 1960.

Other ganglionic blocking agents

A number of other ganglionic blocking agents, including hexamethonium chloride, hexamethonium bromide, pentolinium tartrate, and mecamylamine hydrochloride, are discussed in Chapter 16 under drugs used for hypertension.

Questions
for review and study

1 What is the usual dosage and the usual route of administration for each of the following?

Drug	Dosage	Administration
a. epinephrine hydrochloride	————	————
b. amphetamine sulfate	————	————
c. bethanechol chloride	————	————
d. atropine sulfate	————	————
e. propantheline bromide	————	————

2 What effect might you expect from the action of an adrenergic drug on the following?
a. heart:
b. blood pressure:
c. bronchial muscle:
d. nasal mucosae of a patient with hay fever:
e. peristaltic activity of the stomach and intestine:

3 What drug is considered to be especially effective for the following? Indicate reason for your answer.
a. acute asthma:
b. hypotension and shock:
c. myasthenia gravis:
d. excessive appetite:
e. postoperative gaseous distention of abdomen:
f. urinary retention:
g. a drug to produce mydriasis and cycloplegia in the eyes of a child:
h. for refraction of the eyes of an adult:
i. for relief of rigidity in a patient with Parkinson's disease:

4 **Single choice**
Encircle the letter in front of the drug of your choice for each of the following:

a. Hyoscine is an active principle of which of the following?
(1) opium
(2) belladonna
(3) physostigmine
(4) atropine

b. Scopolamine differs from atropine chiefly in its action on which of the following?
(1) medullary centers
(2) smooth muscle
(3) cerebrum
(4) eye

c. Which of the following is an example of an anticholinergic drug?
(1) carbachol
(2) dextro amphetamine sulfate
(3) bethanechol chloride
(4) propantheline bromide

d. Dry mouth, dilated pupils, blurred vision, talkativeness, and restlessness are side effects associated with which of the following?
(1) neostigmine
(2) epinephrine
(3) levarterenol
(4) atropine

e. If a physician expected to give emergency treatment to a patient with myasthenia gravis, which of the following preparations would you attempt to have ready?
(1) neostigmine bromide
(2) neostigmine methylsulfate
(3) epinephrine hydrochloride
(4) physostigmine sulfate

f. Atropine is frequently given as a preanesthetic drug not only to inhibit oral and bronchial secretions but also to prevent:
(1) cardiac arrest
(2) respiratory failure
(3) laryngospasm
(4) hypotension

g. Anticholinergic drugs are frequently

346

given to patients with peptic ulcer for which of the following reasons?
   (1) to control the gastric acidity
   (2) for their direct analgesic effect
   (3) to soothe and coat the ulcer
   (4) to diminish hypermotility and hypersecretion of the stomach
h. Patients with hypertension and cardiovascular disease are often encouraged to stop smoking for which of the following reasons?
   (1) nicotine stimulates the central nervous system
   (2) nicotine has a tendency to cause vasospasm
   (3) tobacco smoke contains substances thought to be carcinogenic
   (4) tobacco smoke is irritating to the respiratory mucous membrane
i. If the stock supply of atropine sulfate is in solution and the vial is labeled 0.4 mg. per milliliter, how many minims (approximately) would be required to give gr. 1/200?
   (1) 11
   (2) 15
   (3) 20
   (4) 7½

References

A. M. A. Council on Drugs: New and Nonofficial Drugs, Philadelphia, 1960, J. B. Lippincott Co.

Beckman, H.: Drugs, Their Nature, Action and Use, Philadelphia, 1958, W. B. Saunders Co.

Clagett, O. T.: Myasthenia Gravis, Am. J. Nursing 51: 654, 1951.

Goodman, Louis, and Gilman, Alfred: The Pharmacological Basis of Therapeutics, New York, 1955, The Macmillan Co.

Grimson, K. S., Hendrix, J. P., and Reardon, M. J.: Report to the Council on Pharmacy and Chemistry: Newer Adrenolytic, Sympathetic and Ganglion Blocking Drugs, J. A. M. A. 139: 154, 1949.

Grimson, K. S., Lyons, C. H., and Reeves, R. J.: Clinical Trial of Banthine in 100 Patients With Peptic Ulcer, J. A. M. A. 143: 873, 1950.

Haggerty, R. J.: Levartenenol for Shock, Am. J. Nursing 58: 1243, 1958.

Harvey, A. M.: Myasthenia Gravis. In Cecil, R. L., and Loeb, R. F.: A Textbook of Medicine, Philadelphia, 1959, W. B. Saunders Co., pp. 1474-1480.

Longino, F. H., Grimson, K. S., Chittum, J. R., and Metcalf, B. H.: An Orally Effective Quaternary Amine, Banthine, Capable of Reducing Gastric Motility and Secretion, Gastroenterology 14: 301, 1950.

McGee, K. R.: Myasthenia Gravis, Am. J. Nursing 60: 336, 1960.

Osserman, K., and Shapiro, E.: Nursing Care in Myasthenia Gravis, Nursing World 130: 12, 1956.

Roth, Grace: The Effects of Smoking Tobacco on the Cardiovascular System of Normal Persons and Patients With Hypertension, Collected Papers of the Mayo Clinic 45: 435, 1953.

Roth, Grace, McDonald, John B., and Sheard, Charles: The Effect of Smoking Cigarettes, J. A. M. A. 125: 761, 1944.

Salter, W. T.: A Textbook of Pharmacology, Philadelphia, 1952, W. B. Saunders Co.

Schwab, R. S., Osserman, K. E., and Tether, J. E.: Treatment of Myasthenia Gravis, J. A. M. A. 165: 671, 1957.

Schwartz, I. R., Lehman, E., Ostrove, R., and Seibel, J. M.: A Clinical Evaluation of a New Anticholinergic Drug, Pro-Banthine, Gastroenterology 25: 416, 1953.

Sollmann, Torald: A Manual of Pharmacology, Philadelphia, 1957, W. B. Saunders Co.

Swan, H. J. C.: Noradrenaline, Adrenaline and the Human Circulation, Brit. M. J. 1: 1003, 1952.

Chapter 11

Skeletal muscle relaxants
and their
antagonists

Skeletal muscle relaxants are drugs used to prevent and relieve muscular spasm associated with conditions such as anterior poliomyelitis, back strain, fibrositis, and various states of spasticity. They are also used to produce relaxation during surgical anesthesia, orthopedic manipulation, and ocular and rectal surgery and for protection against traumatic injury which may occur during electric shock therapy. Their most important use is probably as an adjunct to general anesthesia, because they permit the achievement of good muscle relaxation without necessitating the deeper levels of general anesthesia.

A number of these drugs act at the myoneural junction. The preparation d-tubocurarine and its derivatives interfere with the depolarization of the muscle portion of the end plate by acetylcholine. Other preparations, such as succinylcholine, produce muscular relaxation by depolarizing the end plate and keeping it in that state until the agent is eliminated. In other words, the latter agents act essentially like acetylcholine except that they have a longer duration of effect and are not destroyed as is the natural mediator, acetylcholine. This prevents repolarization of the end plate and the subsequent passage of nerve impulses. Because of the differing mechanism of action by the latter type of compound, it is no longer spoken of as a "curare-like" drug. Other agents act to produce muscular relaxation by inhibiting certain reflexes in the central nervous system, e.g., mephenesin, zoxaxolamine, and methocarbamol. Because the first group of skeletal muscle relaxants act at the myoneural junction, i.e., in the muscle itself, they are sometimes called the group of "peripheral" relaxants, in contrast to the second group which are called "central" because of their site of action in the central nervous system.

Some of the more potent skeletal muscle relaxants may cause undesirable side effects, such as respiratory paralysis, circulatory collapse, and untoward effects in the central nervous system. The patient requires constant, close attention while receiving a drug of this type and sometimes for a time after administration has been discontinued.

Since these are potent drugs, not without danger, their use is recommended only by those thoroughly familiar with their effects and under conditions where adequate equipment, antidotes and measures for prompt treatment of overdosage are readily available.

Curariform blocking agents

Curare

Curare is a generic name for a number of arrow poisons used by the South American Indians. Crude curare is a gummy, tarlike material, dark brown or black. For a time it was classified according to the container in which it was stored and was known as pot curare, tube curare (stored in bamboo tubes), and calabash curare (stored in gourds). However, manufacture of curare is said to be fast becoming a lost art, and the active alkaloids are now extracted from the various species of climbing vines whose bark and leaves contain these substances. A number of alkaloids are extracted from the plant species Strychnos, e.g., *Strychnos toxifera*, and certain species of chondodendron, e.g., *Chondodendron tomentosum*, which is a source of *d*-tubocurarine. The latter alkaloid was isolated by King in 1935 and is available as a pure crystalline compound of known chemical structure.

Action and result. In therapeutic doses curare blocks transmission at the myoneural junctions of skeletal muscle. Curare interrupts the functional connection between the peripheral nerve endings and the striated muscle in much the same way as atropine affects the response of certain smooth muscle to parasympathetic nerves. The muscle can be made to respond to direct electric stimulation or certain chemical agents but not to nerve stimulation. When large doses are given, one muscle after another becomes weak and flaccid, until complete paralysis occurs.

After therapeutic doses of curare the patient notices the first effects in the short muscles, similar to those found in the eyes, eyelids, fingers, and toes. The muscles least affected appear to be those that contain the largest amount of utilizable oxygen.* Within 2 to 3 minutes after an intravenous injection of an ordinary clinical dose the patient experiences haziness of vision, difficulty in talking and swallowing, ptosis of the eyelids, and weakness of the muscles of the jaw, neck, and legs; then follow ptosis, relaxation, and finally paralysis of the muscles of the neck, spine, legs, arms, and abdomen. With larger doses the last muscles to be affected are the intercostals and the diaphragm. In recovery after the

*Sollman, T.: A Manual of Pharmacology, Philadelphia, 1957, W. B. Saunders Co., p. 445.

ordinary clinical dose, the paralysis disappears in reverse order and may require 15 to 20 minutes.

A secondary action of curare is that of blockage of transmission in the autonomic ganglia. This means that the nerve impulses cannot get through or that the chemical mediator is ineffective in the ganglia. In some persons the predominant effect is on the parasympathetic nerves, and in others it is on the sympathetic nerves. This action is similar to that of nicotine, although it occurs to a lesser degree and without the initial stimulant action of nicotine or its ability to stimulate respiration. The action of curare does not extend to structures beyond the autonomic ganglia, and thus the smooth muscle and gland cells are not directly affected.

Absorption and excretion. Because of its poor absorption, curare may be swallowed (ordinary doses) without ill effect, provided there are no wounds or abrasions along the digestive tract. It is rapidly excreted by the kidney and also rapidly destroyed by the liver. For this reason the patient who has paralysis of the muscles of respiration can be kept alive with artificial respiration, particularly if an airway is used.

Uses. Curare is used to enhance muscular relaxation during anesthesia, particularly when certain of the lighter anesthetic agents are used; or to permit adequate relaxation without subjecting patients to deep planes of anesthesia which border on medullary paralysis. The margin of safety between the dose which produces good relaxation of voluntary muscle and the one producing paralysis of respiratory muscles, however, is small.

It is used to prevent trauma and excessive muscular contraction in electroshock therapy and to provide muscular relaxation during endoscopy and the reduction of fractures and dislocations.

With curare it is possible to relieve spasticity of muscles in tetanus, in convulsive states, and in certain neuromuscular conditions.

It is sometimes used as a diagnostic agent in myasthenia gravis.

Preparation, dosage, and administration.

Tubocurarine Chloride, U.S.P., B.P. (*d*-tubocurarine). This drug is available in vials of solution for intravenous injection (3 mg. per milliliter). It is also available in 5 ml. vials in which it is contained in a slow-release menstruum and sold under the name of *Tubadil Injection.*

*Dimethyl Tubocurarine Chloride** (Mecostin Chloride). This form is administered by slow intravenous injection. It is available as a solution (10 mg. in 10 ml.).

Dimethyl Tubocurarine Iodide Injection, N.F. (Metubine Iodide). This form is administered intravenously in physiologic saline solution. The dimethyl derivatives of *d*-tubocurarine are comparable to the

*Described in annual publication of A. M. A. Council on Drugs, N.N.D., 1960.

parent compound, *d*-tubocurarine, in general characteristics.

Dosage must be determined individually for each patient. It varies with the preparation used, as well as with the anesthetic to be administered. With ether anesthesia the total dose must be reduced because ether itself has a curare-like effect on skeletal muscle. A test dose prior to a curarizing dose is recommended. After 3 to 5 minutes an additional dose may be given, and small supplemental doses are injected as needed.

Side effects and toxic effects. If large doses are injected rapidly, histamine is apparently released from muscle tissue, resulting in hypotension, circulatory collapse, and occasionally bronchospasm. Depression of the muscles of respiration causes hypoxia and possibly death. Treatment includes early establishment of an open airway (endotracheal tube) and the use of positive-pressure artificial respiration with oxygen.

Neostigmine methylsulfate (Prostigmine Methylsulfate) and edrophonium chloride (Tensilon Chloride) are used as antidotes under certain conditions but only as supplements to artificial respiration with oxygen. These antidotes inactivate cholinesterase and permit acetylcholine to be built up, and unless large overdoses of curare have been given this increased level of acetylcholine tends to overcome the paralysis. However, overdosage with the antidote can also produce untoward effects. Effective doses of neostigmine are likely to produce increased flow of saliva, slowing of the heart, hypotension and increased motility of the intestine. Atropine is sometimes given to counteract the latter effects. The anticurare drugs are said to be most safely used when employed in small and (if necessary) repeated doses.

Contraindications. Patients with myasthenia gravis are very sensitive to curare and show a pronounced response to small doses of the drug. It is therefore contraindicated for such patients except as a diagnostic agent. It is also contraindicated for patients with respiratory depression, pulmonary disorder, and liver and renal disease.

Gallamine Triethiodide (Flaxedil Triethiodide)

Gallamine triethiodide is a synthetic compound whose action, uses, and contraindications are similar to those of the curare drugs. Advantages claimed for this preparation include the following: (1) it has no effect on autonomic ganglia, (2) it does not cause bronchospasm because of the release of histamine, and (3) it affords a high degree of flexibility because of rapid onset and short duration of action.

Preparation, dosage, and administration.

*Gallamine Triethiodide** (Flaxedil Triethiodide). This is administered intravenously in an aqueous solution. It may be mixed with a 2.5 per cent thiopental sodium solution. The average dose of 50 to 60 mg. is

*Described in annual publication of A. M. A. Council on Drugs, N.N.D., 1960.

effective for approximately ½ to 1 hour. Dosage must be individually adjusted for each patient.

Side effects and toxic effects. This drug may produce an allergic reaction in patients sensitive to iodine and a marked tachycardia due to its acetylcholine blocking action in the myocardium. It must be used with the same precautions as other potent skeletal muscle relaxants. It is said not to be the relaxant of choice for patients with cardiovascular disease.

Quinine

Quinine sulfate is prescribed for the relief of "night cramps" of the extremities. For this effect it is given in doses of 200 to 500 mg. after the evening meal and before retiring. The work of Harvey (1939) showed that quinine has a slight curare-like action on skeletal muscle. This effect is obtained rapidly after intravenous injection of the drug. It is also used for relief of muscle spasm in patients who have a condition known as *myotonia congenita*. Quinine increases muscular weakness in patients with myasthenia gravis.

Antagonists of curariform drugs

Edrophonium Chloride (Tensilon Chloride)

Edrophonium chloride is an antagonist of skeletal muscle relaxants such as tubocurarine and similar preparations which act by preventing the depolarization of the end plate at the myoneural junction. Edrophonium chloride probably displaces the curariform drugs from their sites of attachment to the muscle cell and thus allows the normal transmission of nerve impulses to be restored.

Uses. Edrophonium chloride can be used to terminate the effects of curariform agents when muscular relaxation is no longer desired or to reverse respiratory muscle paralysis produced by overdosage. Its use as a diagnostic agent for myasthenia gravis is mentioned on p. 328. It is not used as an antidote for succinylcholine chloride or decamethonium.

Preparation, dosage, and administration.

Edrophonium Chloride Injection, U.S.P. (Tensilon Chloride). It is administered intravenously. The dosage employed for antagonism of appropriate curariform drugs varies from 5 to 10 mg. or more. It should not be given if apnea is present. To counteract overdosage of appropriate muscle relaxants, therefore, it should be used along with artificial respiration and oxygen therapy and only when some definite sign of voluntary respiration can be observed.

Side effects and toxic effects. Side effects of edrophonium chloride include increased flow of saliva (salivation), bronchiolar spasm (especially in asthmatic patients), slow pulse, and disturbance of cardiac rhythm (especially in elderly patients). When edrophonium chloride is used in large doses it intensifies the peripheral effects of the curariform drugs instead of antagonizing them. Furthermore, it does not combat circulatory collapse which is associated with respiratory depression.

Neostigmine and other cholinesterase inhibitors are also useful in combating the effects of the compounds of curare. Like edrophonium chloride, they promote the accumulation of acetylcholine by competing with acetylcholine for the enzyme cholinesterase.

A word of extreme caution should be given regarding the use of oxygen in patients with severe respiratory disease who have become resistant to the usual respiratory stimulating effect of carbon dioxide and who are stimulated to breathe primarily by anoxemia. If one indiscriminately administers nasal oxygen to this person, his last stimulus to breathe is removed and death may ensue.

Agents that act as relaxants by prolongation of depolarization

Decamethonium Bromide (Syncurine)

Action. Decamethonium bromide is a very potent relaxant of skeletal muscle, with a rapid onset of action but rather short duration of effect. It blocks motor impulses at the myoneural junction by acting as a depolarizing agent, i.e., it acts as such a potent depolarizing agent that nerve impulses cannot be sent through the end plate.

It should be noted that agents which appear to have opposite physiologic actions may have the same final effect, i.e., muscular relaxation and paralysis. The curare group of drugs makes it more difficult for normally secreted acetycholine to depolarize the myoneural plate, whereas the decamethonium group maintains a prolonged depolarization. Normal muscle contraction requires depolarization, but somehow in a way that is not precisely understood, excessive and continued depolarization will also prevent contraction.

Decamethonium is more potent than tubocurarine but the duration of its effect is said to be intermediate between that of tubocurarine and succinylcholine. It does not produce a ganglionic blocking action and it does not cause bronchospasm from a liberation of histamine. It has no cumulative effect even after repeated dosage.

Uses. Decamethonium bromide is a useful agent to produce marked relaxation which lasts for a short time and can be used in connection with procedures such as endoscopy, endotracheal intubation, and closure of the peritoneum during surgical procedure.

Preparation, dosage, and administration.

*Decamethonium Bromide** (Syncurine). The usual dose varies from

*Described in annual publication of A. M. A. Council on Drugs, N.N.D., 1960.

0.5 to 3 mg., depending on the response of the patient and the degree of relaxation desired. It is administered by a single intravenous injection which may be repeated as necessary.

Side effects. Despite its relative short duration of action, this drug may cause respiratory depression. Neostigmine and edrophonium chloride are of no value as antagonists; hence facilities for controlled artificial respiration with oxygen are essential.

Succinylcholine Chloride (Anectine Chloride)

Action and result. Succinylcholine chloride is an ultrashort-acting myoneural blocking agent. Although the end result of its action is similar to that of curare, the mechanism of its action is thought to be different. Its action is apparently the same as that of decamethonium, i.e., it intensifies the depolarizing effect of acetylcholine to such an extent that repolarization of the end plate, which is necessary for muscle contraction, does not occur.

Its action is of shorter duration than is that of tubocurarine chloride. This is explained by the fact that it is easily hydrolyzed by cholinesterase to form choline and succinic acid. Alkaline solutions of the drug undergo rapid hydrolysis; therefore succinylcholine chloride should not be mixed with alkaline solutions of anesthetics such as thiopental sodium. The intensity of its effect can be modified readily by varying the rate of its administration.

Clinical doses do not seem to produce significant effects on the circulatory system and autonomic ganglia and cause no significant liberation of histamine.

Uses. Some authorities are of the opinion that succinylcholine approaches the ideal muscle relaxant. It is the relaxant of choice whenever it is important to terminate a skeletal muscle relaxant effect rapidly.

It is used to produce muscular relaxation during anesthesia and in conjunction with electroshock therapy. Because of the short duration of its action, it is particularly well suited to procedures of short duration such as endotracheal intubation and endoscopy.

Preparation, dosage, and administration.

Succinylcholine Chloride, U.S.P. (Anectine Chloride). This is available as *Succinylcholine Chloride Injection,* U.S.P., and is administered intravenously, either in separately repeated injections or as a continuous drip infusion. The optimum dose is between 10 and 30 mg. for an adult when used for short procedures. Relaxation occurs in about 1 minute and lasts for about 2 minutes, after which there is rapid recovery. Sustained relaxation for prolonged procedure is obtained by continuous drip infusion in which approximately 2.5 mg. are given per minute. Succinylcholine chloride is said to require closer attention during its administration than other muscle relaxants, but it also affords greater ease of control.

Side effects and toxic effects. Succinylcholine chloride exhibits a low level of toxicity and is characterized by a lack of undesirable side effects on vital organs of the body. On the other hand, large doses produce respiratory depression; hence, facilities to combat respiratory paralysis must be at hand. There is no effective antagonist. Neostigmine and edrophonium chloride prolong the effect of succinylcholine chloride and are therefore contraindicated as antidotes in case of overdosage. However, because it loses its potency rapidly when administration is discontinued, it is a relatively safe drug. The patient must be observed closely to prevent undue respiratory depression. The drug is not well tolerated by patients with severe disease of the liver, severe anemia, or malnutrition.

Skeletal muscle relaxants that act centrally

A number of skeletal muscle relaxants act centrally and are known as polysynaptic depressants. Following are some of these drugs.

Mephenesin

Action. Mephenesin exhibits a selective depressant action on the basal ganglia, brain stem, and synaptic connections in the spinal cord. Large doses produce a temporary paralysis of skeletal muscle, although it does not directly influence muscle as is true of curare. It also has a local anesthetic action, although it is too irritating to be used for this effect.

Mephenesin has a sedative action which produces a temporary improvement in certain psychotic conditions.

Uses. The transient action of mephenesin seriously limits its usefulness. It has been of value as an experimental tool and has also prompted an active search for drugs more effective for motor disturbances. It has been used to relieve spasticity of muscle associated with back injuries, bursitis, cerebral palsy, tetanus, Parkinson's disease, and various neurologic disorders, but its beneficial effects are brief.

Preparation, dosage, and administration.

Mephenesin, N.F. This drug is marketed under a number of trade names* and in a number of dosage forms for oral administration and in a solution for intravenous injection. It is given orally in doses of 1 to 3 Gm. three to five times daily. As a diagnostic aid it is given intravenously (2 per cent solution).

Side effects and toxic effects. Untoward effects are said to be infrequent, but the following have been noted after intravenous administra-

*Some are Tolserol, Tolansin, Myoten, Spasmolyn, and Daserol.

tion of mephenesin: weakness, nystagmus, diplopia, nausea and vomiting, anorexia, and muscular incoordination. Side effects are usually absent after oral administration, although lassitude has resulted occasionally and leukopenia, rarely.

Meprobamate (Equanil, Miltown)

Action. Meprobamate was discussed under the subject of ataractics (Chapter 9) and is mentioned here because it is chemically related to mephenesin and shares the central interneuronal blocking action of the latter drug. However, the duration of its action is much longer than that of mephenesin.

Uses. Meprobamate is thought to have an inhibiting effect on certain cases of abnormal motor activity and for conditions in which muscular spasm is characteristically present, e.g., fibrositis, back injuries, and rheumatic disorders. Its use for emotionally disturbed patients exceeds by far its use as a skeletal muscle relaxant.

Preparation, dosage, and administration.

Meprobamate, U.S.P. (Equanil, Miltown). It is administered orally. It is available in sustained-release capsules, 200 mg.; oral suspension, 40 mg. per milliliter; and in tablets, 200 and 400 mg. The usual dose is 400 mg. three or four times daily.

Side effects. For side effects see Chapter 9.

Carisoprodol (Soma)

Carisoprodol is a derivative of meprobamate and has been found to possess both analgesic and muscle-relaxant properties. It is undergoing clinical investigation at the present time. Its ability to relieve muscular spasm and pain associated with fibrositis, bursitis, sprains, strains, etc. is being studied.

It is available in 250 mg. capsules and 350 mg. tablets for oral administration. The usual adult dose is 350 mg. three times daily and at bedtime. Drowsiness seems to be one of its side effects, which is said to be easily controlled by adjustment of dosage.

Zoxazolamine (Flexin)

Action. Zoxazolamine is a skeletal muscle relaxant which blocks the transmission of nerve impulses through synaptic pathways, especially in the subcortical areas of the cerebrum, brain stem, and spinal cord. It apparently does not affect skeletal muscle directly, and it has no effect on the myoneural junction. The duration of its effect is longer than mephenesin (several hours), and its ability to relieve spasm is greater. It is more effective orally than mephenesin. Its action as a uricosuric agent is mentioned elsewhere (see Index).

Uses. Zoxazolamine is used to relieve muscular spasm associated with sprains, low back pain, fibrositis, bursitis, myositis, etc. Relief of spasm may be produced with concomitant production of muscular weakness not only of the spastic muscles but of the normal muscles as well.

Patients suffering from muscular spasm associated with musculo-skeletal disorders are said to receive more benefit than those with neuro-logic disease, with the possible exception of cerebral palsy and spastic paraplegia.

Zoxazolamine seems to be of little benefit to patients with Parkinson's disease or convulsive disorders.

Preparation, dosage, and administration.

Zoxazolamine* (Flexin). This drug is available in 250 mg. tablets (plain or enteric coated) for oral administration. The usual adult dose is 250 to 500 mg. three or four times daily. It should be administered after meals or with food, to minimize gastric irritation.

Side effects. Zoxazolamine has a relatively wide margin of safety. Side effects are likely to be frequent and may be unpleasant, but they are reversible as soon as administration of the drug is discontinued; they are not serious. They include anorexia, nausea and vomiting, malaise, weakness, drowsiness, and skin rash, which is usually transient.

Chlorzoxazone (Paraflex)

Chlorzoxazone is a derivative of zoxazolamine and has actions and uses similar to the parent drug. It produces higher blood levels after oral administration than does zoxazolamine but does not have the uricosuric activity exhibited by zoxazolamine. Its clinical toxicity is thought to be less, however.

Preparation, dosage, and administration.

Chlorzoxazone* (Paraflex). Administered orally, the dosage ranges from 250 to 750 mg. three or four times a day. It is available in 250 mg. tablets.

Methocarbamol (Robaxin)

Uses. Methocarbamol is a new synthetic skeletal muscle relaxant which is being used for the relief of muscular spasm associated with traumatic conditions, fractures, dislocations, herniated discs, arthritis, fibrositis, etc. It is said to inhibit polysynaptic spinal reflexes but does not directly affect skeletal muscle.

Preparation, dosage, and administration.

Methocarbamol† (Robaxin). The drug is available in 500 mg. tablets for oral administration. The average dose is 6 Gm. daily given in divided

---

*Described in annual publication of A. M. A. Council on Drugs, N.N.D., 1960.

†Council on Drugs, J. A. M. A. **172:** 69, 1960.

doses. It is also available as a preparation for intravenous and intramuscular administration.

Side effects. No serious side effects have been reported. Lightheadedness, headache, nausea, mild drowsiness, and fatigability have been reported, but reduction of dosage effectively relieves the symptoms.

References

A. M. A. Council on Drugs: New and Non-official Drugs, Philadelphia, 1960, J. B. Lippincott Co.

Beckman, H.: Drugs, Their Nature, Action and Use, Philadelphia, 1958, W. B. Saunders Co.

Brotman, M., and Cullen, S. C.: The Muscle Relaxants. In Hale, D. H. (editor): Anesthesiology, Philadelphia, 1955, F. A. Davis Co.

Drill, V. A.: Pharmacology in Medicine, New York, 1958, McGraw-Hill Book Co., Inc.

Forsyth, H. Francis: Methocarbamol (Robaxin) in Orthopedic Conditions, J. A. M. A. **167**: 163, 1959.

Miller, J. (editor): The Pharmacology and Clinical Usefulness of Carisoprodol, Detroit, 1959, Wayne State University Press.

Park, H. W.: Clinical Results With Methocarbamol, A New Interneuronal Blocking Agent, J. A. M. A. **167**: 168, 1958.

Sollmann, Y.: A Manual of Pharmacology, Philadelphia, 1957, W. B. Saunders Co.

Chapter 12

Histamine, antihistamines,
and drugs used
for motion sickness

Histamine

Histamine, like epinephrine, norepinephrine, and 5-hydroxytryptamine, is a compound of pharmacologic and physiologic interest, since in contrast to most drugs it occurs naturally in the body. Like the other natural body constituents named above, it is an amine possessing the basic group NH_2. Histamine is derived from the amino acid histidine, by the removal of the carboxyl group as carbon dioxide, a reaction that takes place in the body cells as well as in the intestinal contents.

$$H - C = C - CH_2 - CH - COOH \qquad\qquad H - C = C - CH_2 - CH_2$$
$$H - N \qquad N \qquad NH_2 \qquad\longrightarrow\qquad H - N \qquad N \qquad NH_2 \quad + CO_2$$
$$\backslash C \diagup\!\!/ \qquad\qquad\qquad\qquad\qquad \backslash C \diagup\!\!/$$
$$H \qquad\qquad\qquad\qquad\qquad\qquad H$$

Histidine   Histamine

Although histamine was discovered in animal tissues many years ago (it was first found in the rye fungus, ergot), there is still question as to its normal function in the body. Its interest to medicine is multiple; the compound itself can be used to produce certain pharmacologic effects, employed chiefly for diagnostic tests. Much more important than this use, however, is the fact that certain compounds that prevent the pharmacologic action of histamine (histamine antagonists, antihistaminics) have very useful effects, including the prevention or relief of allergic symptoms and the relief of motion sickness.

Action and result. When given orally, histamine is destroyed in the intestinal tract. After parenteral administration it produces a direct stimulation of certain smooth muscles and is a powerful vasodilator in the capillary beds. In man, a noticeable dilation of the arterioles is also seen. Circulatory effects differ, however, in different species of animals.

The marked dilation of the arterioles and capillaries by histamine produces a definite flushing of the skin, rise in skin temperature, and fall in blood pressure. Vasodilation in the meningeal vessels is accompanied by an increase in intracranial pressure, which may cause headache. The fall in blood pressure after small doses of histamine is followed by rather quick recovery, due to the release of epinephrine and the activity of the cardiovascular reflexes.

Uterine and intestinal muscle is stimulated as well as the smooth muscle of the bronchial tubes. Bronchial spasm may be induced in man after large doses of the drug, especially if the patient suffers from chronic conditions of the respiratory tract, such as asthma and bronchitis.

Histamine stimulates the gastric, salivary, pancreatic, and lacrimal glands. The chief effect in man, however, is seen in the gastric glands. The resulting secretion in the normal stomach is high in acid because of the selective action on the acid-forming cells.

A marked fall in blood pressure may follow a large dose of histamine, and the same vascular changes that take place in surgical shock may occur. The permeability of the capillary beds increases and sufficient blood proteins are lost to the tissues so that blood volume cannot be maintained and circulation is slowed.

Some investigators maintain that histamine is liberated in the body in large amounts as a result of extensive tissue damage or of antigen-antibody reactions. Attempts to demonstrate that histamine tolerance can be achieved by desensitization of the patient have been inconclusive.

Histamine and hypersensitivity. Because the symptoms of acute histamine poisoning and those of anaphylactic shock are quite similar, it was suggested long ago that acute allergic reactions (resulting from the exposure of a sensitive individual to an antigen) resulted in the release of histamine. Since then it has been found that when allergic shock is produced either in the whole animal or in an isolated organ (such as a guinea pig uterus), histamine is released. The thesis is now well accepted that abnormal release of histamine from a stored inactive form in the body accompanies acute allergic reactions, both mild and severe, and accounts for at least some of the changes observed in the patient. A further convincing finding has been that antihistaminics can modify and significantly lessen the picture of an acute allergic reaction.

Uses. Histamine is rarely used therapeutically but has occasionally been used for diagnostic purposes.

One diagnostic use is concerned with gastric acid production. Histamine is a potent stimulus to the secretion of gastric hydrochloric acid and there is some evidence suggesting that it may be the natural trigger that starts the secretion of hydrochloric acid. Accordingly, it can be used to reveal the absence of gastric acid (achlorhydria), a diagnostic aid for certain of the anemias. If a patient does not respond with a significant secretion of gastric acid to the challenge of a small dose of histamine, it is likely that he cannot make gastric acid. This is believed to be due to a degenerative change in the gastric mucosa.

Another use is in the diagnosis of pheochromocytoma. Tumors of the medullary portion of the adrenal gland which secrete epinephrine and norepinephrine are rare, but their discovery is important since they represent one type of hypertension which can be permanently cured by surgery. Small doses of histamine stimulate the secretion of the adrenal medulla; in the normal individual the pressor amines secreted by the adrenal gland are not sufficient to produce a marked rise in blood pressure, but in the patient with pheochromocytoma, histamine may lead to a very prominent secretion of medullary amines with a resultant striking rise in blood pressure. The histamine test is one of several "pharmacologic" provocative tests for pheochromocytoma.

Histamine may also be used to test the capacity of capillaries to dilate in certain peripheral vascular diseases.

Preparation, dosage, and administration.

Histamine Phosphate, U.S.P., B.P. (also known as histamine diphosphate and histamine acid phosphate). It is available in ampules, 0.275, 1, and 2.75 mg. per milliliter, in vials, and in bottles. When used for a gastric function test, 0.275 mg. to several times this amount have been used. It is administered subcutaneously.

Side effects and toxic effects. Symptoms of overdosage include rapid drop in blood pressure, intense headache, dyspnea, flushing of the skin, vomiting, diarrhea, shock, and collapse. The toxic symptoms are rarely dangerous, although they may be alarming. If the patient goes into shock, the blood volume may need to be restored. Elevation of the foot of the bed is often sufficient treatment. Epinephrine is a specific physiologic antagonist and will prevent or counteract symptoms if administered promptly.

Ordinarily, histamine is destroyed in the body partly by oxidation and partly by an enzyme, diamine oxidase. Diamine oxidase is now the name given to an enzyme formerly called histaminase, since it is recognized that the enzyme is not specific for histamine but will attack a number of compounds having two amine groups in the same molecule just as histamine with its "primary" NH_2 group and its "secondary"— NH—group in the imidozole ring. Diamine oxidase is present in greatest amounts in the intestinal mucosa and kidney. It acts slowly to inactivate histamine. It has been reported that serum sickness, bronchial asthma, and anaphylactic disorders have responded favorably to enzyme therapy, but further study and observation of its effects in living tissues have resulted in the conclusion that it neither prevents nor relieves anaphylactic reactions.

Histamine-antagonizing drugs

Histamine can be antagonized by other drugs in two ways: (1) by the use of drugs that produce pharmacologic effects opposed to those of histamine, of which the best example is epinephrine, and (2) by the use of drugs that have no prominent opposing pharmacologic actions themselves but in some way prevent histamine from showing its typical actions. The latter drugs are the group generally called antihistaminics.

Epinephrine

Epinephrine is a lifesaving drug in anaphylactic shock. The most serious effects of anaphylaxis (or severe acute allergic reactions) in man are the extensive arteriolar dilatation with hypotensive shock and collapse and the marked constriction of bronchial tubes which can lead to extreme respiratory difficulty and even suffocation. By promoting vasoconstriction and by dilating the bronchial tubes, epinephrine can antagonize the physiologic effects of anaphylaxis or of histamine poisoning.

Antihistaminics

Antihistaminics are believed to act not by opposing but by preventing the physiologic action of histamine, and although no really detailed picture of this effect in chemical terms can be given, it is postulated that the antihistaminics act by preventing the combination of histamine with some chemical substance in the cell, a combination that leads to the observed effects on smooth muscle and glands. The first antihistaminic was found in 1933 as a result of a conscious attempt to discover a compound with this activity. Although the initial compounds were quite toxic and therefore not very useful, hundreds of antihistaminics have been synthesized and tested. Many of these compounds have similar chemical features, represented by three typical compounds:

Diphenhydramine (Benadryl)

Tripelennamine (Pyribenzamine)

Chlorpheniramine (Chlor-Trimeton)

It can be seen that a common structural feature is the short straight chain terminating in a tertiary amine: $-C-C-N\begin{smallmatrix} R' \\ \diagup \\ \diagdown \\ R'' \end{smallmatrix}$ and it has been suggested that this portion of the antihistaminics is an analogue of the $-C-C-NH_2$ chain of histamine.

Pharmacologically it is known that the antihistaminics block histamine action somewhat selectively. These drugs tend to prevent the muscular (circulatory and bronchiolar) action of histamine but are not as effective against the secretory actions of histamine. For example, antihistaminics do not prevent the normal gastric acid secretory response to histamine.

During the past few years histamine antagonists of various types have been tried for histamine shock, anaphylactic reactions, and allergy. The antihistamine compounds have the greatest therapeutic effect on nasal allergies, particularly on seasonal hay fever. They relieve symptoms better at the beginning of the hay fever season than at the end, and they fail to relieve the asthma which frequently accompanies hay fever. These preparations have a palliative usefulness, however, rather than an ability to immunize the patient or even protect him over a period of time against allergic reactions. Their benefits are therefore comparatively short lived and provide only a relief of symptoms. They must be regarded only as adjuncts to more specific methods of treatment of allergic conditions. They do not begin to replace such remedies as epinephrine, ephedrine, and aminophylline. In acute asthmatic reactions the antihistamine drugs serve only as supplements to these older remedies. Furthermore, relief of various symptoms of allergy is obtained only while the drug is being taken. They do not appear to have a cumulative action and can therefore be taken over a period of time.

One peculiar and unanticipated action of many of the antihistaminics is their ability to relieve or abolish the symptoms of motion sickness both in animals and in man. Thus a number of anti-motion sickness agents are also potent antihistaminics. The commonly used compound, dimenhydrinate (Dramamine), for example, is simply diphenhydramine (Benadryl) with a different salt neutralizing the basic nitrogens of the antihistaminic itself.

The most common untoward effect of these preparations is drowsiness which may become so marked that deep sleep may result. Other symptoms of untoward nature include dizziness, dryness of the mouth and throat, nausea, disturbed coordination, lassitude, muscular weakness, and gastrointestinal disturbances. Sedation sometimes disappears after two or three days of treatment. However, in some patients symptoms of excitation may occur: insomnia, nervousness, and even convulsions.

Patients receiving these preparations, especially those under continuous treatment, should have the benefit of periodic medical examinations.

Preparation, dosage, and administration.

Antazoline Hydrochloride, B.P. This is one of the milder antihistaminics and is less irritating to tissues than other drugs of this group. Nausea and drowsiness are the side effects most commonly encountered. The usual range of oral dosage is 50 to 100 mg. three or four times daily (for adults). A 0.5 per cent solution made with isotonic saline solution can be instilled in the nose or given with a nebulizer every 3 or 4 hours. *Antazoline Phosphate,* N.F. (Antistine Phosphate) is used for ophthalmic solutions (0.5 per cent).

Chlorcyclizine Hydrochloride, U.S.P., B.P. (Di-Paralene Hydrochloride, Perazil). Advantages claimed for chlorcyclizine hydrochloride are a prolonged action and low incidence of side effects. A dose of 50 mg. or more is given orally up to four times a day. *Chlorcyclizine Hydrochloride Tablets,* U.S.P., are available in 25 and 50 mg. each.

Chloropheniramine Maleate, U.S.P. (Chlor-Trimeton Maleate). This preparation produces a low incidence of side effects but compares favorably with other antihistaminics in therapeutic usefulness and does so after comparatively low dosage. The effect of the drug is prolonged by the use of a special tablet form which contains twice the average single dose, half of which is contained in an enteric-coated core that delays absorption. The drug is available in dosage forms suited for parenteral as well as oral administration. Its action tends to be slow. The usual adult oral dose is 2 to 8 mg. The repeat-action tablet is available in 8 and 12 mg. The usual parenteral dose is 5 to 10 mg.

Diphenhydramine Hydrochloride, U.S.P., B.P. (Benadryl Hydrochloride). This compound is similar to other members of the group. In addition to its antihistaminic activity it has a moderate antispasmodic action. This is sometimes significant in cases of bronchial asthma. When given in full therapeutic doses, it causes a high incidence of sedation. The average oral dose for adults is 25 to 50 mg. given three or four times daily. It is available in a number of dosage forms suited for topical, oral, and parenteral administration. The usual intravenous dose is 10 to 50 mg.

Doxylamine Succinate, U.S.P. (Decapryn Succinate). This preparation is an effective antihistaminic but produces a high incidence of sedation when used in full therapeutic dosage. It is administered orally in tablet form or as a syrup. The usual adult dose is 12.5 to 25 mg.

Promethazine Hydrochloride, U.S.P., B.P. (Phenergan Hydrochloride). This drug exhibits a number of pharmacologic effects and therefore has a number of clinical uses. It is a potent antihistaminic; it can be used for the relief of motion sickness, and it relieves apprehension.

It potentiates the action of drugs which depress the central nervous system, making possible a reduction of their dosage. It has a relatively prolonged action. Its sedative action is utilized clinically for surgical and obstetric patients. Promethazine hydrochloride is administered orally, parenterally, and rectally. The usual oral dose is 25 mg., although the range of dosage may be 6 to 50 mg. Parenterally, the dosage is up to 1 mg. per kilogram of body weight. It is available in 12.5 and 25 mg. tablets, as a syrup, and as a sterile solution for injection (25 mg. per milliliter).

Pyrilamine Maleate, U.S.P. (Neo-Antergan Maleate); *Mepyramine Maleate,* B.P. This compound is available in 25 and 50 mg. tablets and as a syrup, 2.5 mg. per milliliter, for oral administration. The usual adult dose is 25 to 50 mg. three or four times daily. The incidence of sedation is low, but it may cause gastrointestinal irritation.

Tripelennamine Hydrochloride, U.S.P. (Pyribenzamine Hydrochloride). This drug is therapeutically effective, and the incidence of untoward reactions is low. Stimulation of the nervous system does occur, as well as gastrointestinal irritation, but the latter is not severe. Sedation is moderate. This agent is available in a number of dosage forms for topical, oral, and parenteral (subcutaneous, intramuscular, and intravenous) administration. The usual adult dose is 50 mg. up to three times a day when given orally, although doses of 100 to 150 mg. are tolerated by most patients.

Tripelennamine Citrate, U.S.P. (Pyribenzamine Citrate). This preparation is more palatable than the hydrochloride when administered in a liquid form. It provides the same therapeutic action as does the hydrochloride. The dosage is greater for the citrate than for the hydrochloride preparation of the drug because of the difference in the molecular weights of the compounds.* The usual adult dose is 50 mg. four times a day.

There are a number of additional antihistaminic agents listed in N.F. and N.N.D. These include *brompheniramine maleate* (Dimetane), *carbinoxamine maleate* (Clistin), *chlorothen citrate* (Tagathen), *methapyrilene hydrochloride* (Thenylene Hydrochloride), *pheniramine maleate* (Trimeton Maleate), *pyrathiazine hydrochloride* (Pyrrolazote), *pyrrobutamine phosphate* (Pyronil), and *thonzylamine hydrochloride* (Anahist).

Drugs used for motion sickness

Motion sickness is a reaction to certain kinds of movement, sometimes any kind if it is sufficiently severe. Most persons are well adjusted

*N.N.D., 1960, p. 30.

to horizontal movements, but some are unable to tolerate continuous up and down (vertical) movements. Such persons are prone to become ill when traveling in cars, trains, airplanes, or ships. Disturbance of the cells in the labyrinth of the ear is believed to be the cause of motion sickness. As a result of this disturbance, contact is made with parts of the brain including the vomiting center in the medulla. The person usually becomes pale, perspires, feels chilly (or warm), and salivates freely. If he continues to be subjected to the motion, symptoms usually progress to nausea and vomiting.

A number of drugs have been used for motion sickness, including sedatives such as barbiturates, autonomic drugs such as scopolamine, as well as a number of others. Promethazine, mentioned previously, has been widely tested and found effective. The following agents have also been found useful for prevention of motion sickness and vestibular dysfunction (disturbance of functions of the inner ear). The exact mechanism of their action is not clear, but most of them appear to depress the central nervous system and decrease sensitivity of the labyrinth of the ear. Like other antihistaminics they should be used with caution by persons who are responsible for the operation of power machines, e.g., automobiles.

Preparation, dosage, and administration.

Cyclizine Hydrochloride, U.S.P. (Marezine Hydrochloride). This is an antihistaminic drug which has been found effective, in a high percentage of cases, in the prevention of nausea and vomiting associated with motion sickness.

Although dry mouth, drowsiness, and blurred vision can be observed after large doses, these symptoms seldom appear after ordinary therapeutic doses.

Cyclizine hydrochloride is administered orally. The usual adult dose is 50 mg. one-half hour before departure and 50 mg. three times daily before meals. Reduction of dosage may be indicated after the initial dose. depending on the duration of the trip, type of travel, and reaction of the individual person. For the relief of dizziness and associated symptoms of vestibular disorder (in conditions other than motion sickness) the usual dose is 50 mg. three times a day.

Cyclizine hydrochloride is available in 50 mg. tablets. Cyclizine lactate* has the same effects as cyclizine hydrochloride but is suited for intramuscular injection. The dosage is the same as that for the hydrochloride.

Dimenhydrinate, U.S.P. (Dramamine). As mentioned previously, this drug is chemically related to diphenhydramine (Benadryl). It produces mild sedation. It is effective for a high percentage of persons who suf-

*Described in annual publication of A. M. A. Council on Drugs, N.N.D., 1960.

fer from motion sickness. It is also used to control nausea, vomiting, and dizziness associated with a number of conditions such as fenestration operations, radiation sickness, and Meniere's disease. It has also been employed for the relief of postoperative nausea and vomiting. Its status as an antemetic for this purpose is not well established because of the variety of factors that contribute to the illness.

Dimenhydrinate is available in a number of dosage forms for oral, rectal, or intramuscular administration. The usual oral dose is 50 mg. 30 minutes before departure, to prevent motion sickness. Dosage up to 100 mg. every 4 hours may be prescribed not only for motion sickness but also for the control of nausea and vomiting associated with other conditions. The usual intramuscular dose is 50 mg.

Meclizine Hydrochloride, U.S.P. (Bonamine Hydrochloride). This drug exerts a mild but prolonged antihistaminic action and is effective in the prevention of motion sickness. The duration of its effects may be as long as 24 hours. It appears to affect the central nervous system and the inner ear like other members of this group of drugs.

The incidence of its side effects seems to be low, although like most other antihistaminic drugs it can cause drowsiness, blurred vision, dryness of the mouth, and fatigue.

It is administered orally. The usual adult dose is 25 to 50 mg. once a day for the prevention of motion sickness (1 hour before departure). For the relief of nausea and vomiting due to other reasons, the dosage is similar or the same. The drug is available in tablets, 25 mg.; as an elixir, 2.5 mg. per milliliter; and as a chewing gum, 25 mg.

References

A. M. A. Council on Drugs: New and Nonofficial Drugs, Philadelphia, 1960, J. B. Lippincott Co.

A. M. A. Council on Pharmacy and Chemistry: Status Report on Antihistaminic Agents in the Prophylaxis and Treatment of the Common Cold, J. A. M. A. **142:** 566, 1950.

Beckman, H.: Drugs, Their Nature, Action and Use, Philadelphia, 1958, W. B. Saunders Co.

Goodman, L., and Gilman, A.: The Pharmacological Basis of Therapeutics, New York, 1955, The Macmillan Co.

Rainey, J. J.: Histamine in the Treatment of Meniere's Syndrome, J. A. M. A. **122:** 850, 1943.

Chapter 13

Drugs that affect
the
gastrointestinal organs

Drugs affecting the digestive tract exert their action mainly on the muscle and the gland tissue. The action may be directly on the smooth muscle and gland cells or indirectly on the autonomic nervous system. Both divisions of the autonomic system discharge nerve impulses into the tissues of the digestive tube more or less constantly, and under normal conditions they maintain a delicate balance of control of functions.

Drugs may bring about increased or decreased function of involved structures, e.g., increased or decreased tone, emptying time, or peristaltic action of the stomach or bowel. In addition, drugs may be used as diagnostic aids or given to relieve enzyme deficiency, counteract excess acidity or gas formation, or produce or prevent vomiting.

Drugs that affect the mouth

On the whole, drugs have little effect upon the mouth. Good oral hygiene which includes adequate measures of mechanically cleansing the mouth and teeth has more influence than most medicines.

Flavoring agents

Oral medications that have an unpleasant taste are usually encapsulated, but occasionally it is necessary to give a drug in a liquid or powder form. If the taste is disagreeable the patient may refuse to take it and in some instances it may cause nausea and vomiting. It is frequently difficult to coax children to take a second dose of an obnoxious-tasting preparation.

Cocoa syrup is one of the more effective vehicles in which to disguise the taste of a medicine. It is especially liked by children. Other syrups also popular are raspberry syrup and cherry syrup. Licorice syrup is particularly effective to disguise the taste of a saline substance because of its colloidal properties and because the taste lingers in the mouth.

Unpleasant-tasting drugs which are disguised in a suitable flavoring agent are further improved (psychologically at least) by the addition of a coloring agent. A chocolate-colored medicine is often thought to have the taste of chocolate even when the flavoring agent actually added is something entirely different.

Much credit should be given to the pharmacist who skillfully disguises an unpleasant-tasting drug. The nurse, too, can sometimes decrease the taste of a liquid preparation by pouring it over chipped ice to make it very cold. Sometimes simply diluting the medicine with water or a fruit juice will diminish the annoying aftertaste of the substance.

Simple bitters

Bitters are substances with a bitter taste, given to improve the appetite. Stimulation of the taste buds and reflex stimulation of the gastric glands has been thought to be an effective way of improving a poor appetite. This is likely to be more effective in the person who has no need for them than in the sick person. Bitters are much less frequently prescribed today than formerly. Their administration has to a great extent been supplanted by the administration of certain vitamin concentrates. When prescribed by the physician, bitters should be given shortly before meals and in solution, but they should not be diluted to the extent that the bitter taste is markedly diminished.

Preparation, dosage, and administration.

Compound Gentian Tincture, N.F. One hundred milliliters contain 10 Gm. of gentian, with bitter orange peel and cardamon seed. The dose is 4 ml.

Iron, Quinine, and Strychnine Elixir, N.F. Both the quinine and the strychnine are very bitter substances. The dose is 4 ml.

Mouthwashes and gargles

The efficacy of a mouthwash or gargle depends largely on the length of time it is allowed to remain in contact with the tissues of the mouth and throat. Ordinarily, these preparations cannot be used in sufficient concentration or over a period of time that will ensure germicidal effects.

Preparation, dosage, and administration. A 1 per cent solution of sodium bicarbonate (½ teaspoonful in a glass of water) is useful to remove mucus from the mouth and throat. A 0.9 per cent sodium chloride solution is probably as good a gargle as most mixtures used.

Sodium perborate is a white, odorless, salty-tasting powder which contains not less than 9 per cent available oxygen. It is used in 2 per cent solution as a mouthwash and local disinfectant. Its action results from the liberation of oxygen. It may be obtained in flavored preparations which disguise the salty taste. It is a popular ingredient of tooth powder and is said to be particularly effective against Vincent's infection and pyorrhea infection of the gums. *Potassium permanganate* (0.1 per cent), *potassium chlorate* (1 per cent), or *hydrogen peroxide* (1:4) may also be used. They are oxidizing agents.

Other substances used in the treatment of stomatitis include boric acid, formalin, gentian violet, and zinc chloride.

Many hospital pharmacies prepare the mouthwash which is used in that particular institution. Nurses should inquire regarding the content of the preparation which she gives to patients and should know whether or not the mouthwash should be diluted prior to administration.

Dentifrices, tooth powders, or abrasives

The ordinary dentifrice contains one or more mild abrasives, a foaming agent, and flavoring materials made into a powder or paste to be used as an aid to the work of the toothbrush in the mechanical cleansing of such parts of the teeth as are accessible. The N.F.° Dentifrice contains hard soap and precipitated calcium carbonate, along with several flavoring agents.

The most used dentifrices, abrasives, and cleaners are the following preparations, alone or mixed in various proportions:

N.F. Dentifrice	Soap
Precipitated calcium carbonate	Sodium borate
Pumice (flour)	Milk of magnesia

The essential requirement of a tooth powder or cleaner is that it must not injure the teeth or surrounding tissues. Probably the most that a dentifrice can do is to clean the teeth mechanically.

Therapeutic dentifrices. The Council on Dental Therapeutics of the American Dental Association does not recognize any dentifrice on the market at the present time as being therapeutic. The effectiveness of the so-called ammoniated dentifrices in the control of tooth decay has not yet been established. Dentifrices containing soluble chlorophyll derivatives have appeared on the market in considerable numbers, but evidence that they prevent dental caries seems to be lacking. Claims made that they deodorize the mouth for several hours are probably untrue, partly because chlorophyll derivatives are quickly diluted with saliva. A more recent approach to developing a therapeutic dentifrice consists in the use of antienzymes to block production of acid in the oral cavity by inhibiting the carbohydrate-splitting enzymes. Again, there is at pres-

°N.F. X.

ent no acceptable evidence that daily use of such a dentifrice will prevent tooth decay.

On the other hand, intensive research over a period of twenty-five years seems to show that drinking water containing a proper amount of fluoride reduces dental decay by about 65 per cent.* The American Dental Association as well as the American Medical Association has recommended the fluoridation of public water supplies. The cost is only a few cents per person per year. Sodium fluoride is effective when added to water supplies in a concentration of one part of fluoride to a million parts of water. Research has shown that this amount is perfectly safe and causes no bodily harm. A 2 per cent solution may be applied directly to the teeth of children.

In those parts of the country where fluoridation of water supplies is not technically feasible or has been legally blocked, various vehicles have been proposed for the systemic administration of fluoride. The most important of these seem to be milk, table salt, and fluoride tablets; the feasibility of all of these is undergoing investigation.

Drugs that affect the stomach

Drugs affecting the stomach include (1) antacids, (2) digestants, (3) carminatives, (4) emetics, (5) antemetics, and (6) drugs used for diagnostic purposes.

Peptic ulcer is an erosion of the mucosal lining of the stomach or duodenum. Ordinarily the stomach is resistant to the digestant action of its acid and pepsin due to several factors such as (1) the protective effect of the mucus which coats the gastric lining, (2) regurgitation of the alkaline secretions from the duodenum, and (3) the effect of enterogastrone on gastric secretion and motility. When the mucosa is eroded the underlying tissues are subjected to a penetrating process or action of the acid and pepsin which produces pain and tenderness and may eventually result in perforation and/or hemorrhage.

The precise cause of acute peptic ulcer is not understood. Some authorities believe that the patient possesses a constitutional factor which predisposes him to the formation of ulcers. That a strong emotional component is present is usually conceded. In fact it is observed that freedom from fear, worry, and emotional and physical tension probably play a more important role in the treatment of patients with peptic ulcer than do drugs per se. On the other hand, drugs do have a place in medical treatment, to bring about relief of pain as well as to reduce hypersecretion and hypermotility.

One of the aims of medical therapy is to control the gastric acid over

*Flemming, Arthur S.: Fluoridation, Pub. Health Rep. 74: 511, 1959.

relatively prolonged periods of time and thus give the ulcer an opportunity to heal. Reduction of acidity and relief of hypermotility of the stomach helps to relieve pain and promote healing. This often means that the patient must receive nighttime administration of antacids along with small amounts of milk to maintain control of gastric acidity. Drugs that are used in the treatment of the patient with peptic ulcer include antacids, antispasmodics (like the belladonna drugs), and other anticholinergic preparations, sedatives, and tranquilizers. In addition, attention is given to the diet and dietary restrictions (alcohol, coffee, and sometimes tobacco).

Antacids

Gastric antacids are chemical substances which lower the acidity of the gastric secretion. They are used to buffer the gastric acid to a pH of 3 or 4 (the pH of the gastric juice is usually 1 or 2). At this pH the proteolytic action of pepsin is greatly reduced and the gastric juice loses its corrosive effect. As the pH approaches 7 or 8 pepsin becomes completely inactive. The stomach empties rapidly, and this is followed by a rebound of gastric secretion. Hence it is thought to be preferable to lower gastric acidity rather than to raise the pH to a state of neutral or above. However, antacids are effective only for the period of time they are in the stomach, and when the stomach empties, the effect of any excess antacid is lost. Furthermore the stomach continues to secrete more acid.

Antacids tend to be widely used by the general public for a variety of supposed gastric ailments. This is probably due in part to the type of advertisement with which the public is bombarded. Goodman and Gilman state the situation thus:

"As a result of wide advertising the belief has been fostered in the minds of both the public and the physician that man is constantly fighting a battle against acidity and should he digress from the alkaline side in an unguarded moment, the results would be catastrophic."[*]

The fact of the matter is that excess alkalinity can cause an uncompensated alkalosis characterized by a number of symptoms which often are not recognized.

Following are properties of an ideal antacid:

1. It should be efficient so that a small amount of the antacid will control a relatively large amount of gastric acid.

2. It should not interfere with the electrolyte balance when given in therapeutic amounts. It should not produce systemic alkalosis.

[*]From Goodman, L., and Gilman, A.: The Pharmacological Basis of Therapeutics, New York, 1955, The Macmillan Co., p. 1029.

3. It should exert a prolonged effect and not stimulate a secondary increase of gastric secretion. In many instances it is important that the acid of the gastric juice should be controlled during the entire twenty-four-hour period of the day.

4. It should not be unpleasant to take and should cause neither constipation nor diarrhea.

5. It should be inexpensive since the patient may need to take it over relatively long periods of time.

6. It should not release carbon dioxide after reacting with hydrochloride acid of the gastric content since this would increase gastric distention and discomfort and also, in certain instances, increase the danger of perforation.

Action of antacids

In the stomach antacids exhibit any one or more of the following properties or actions.

1. Chemical neutralization, e.g., the reaction of an acid with a basic:

$$2 \ HCl + Mg(OH)_2 = Mg(Cl)_2 + 2 \ H_2O$$

Some antacids that raise the pH to a point below neutral are spoken of as buffer antacids in contrast to those antacids that elevate the pH to a point above 7.

2. Physical adsorption is a process whereby hydrochloric acid and possibly other substances are physically bound by certain colloidal substances.

3. Antacid preparations frequently exhibit other effects such as an astringent effect, which means that it shrinks the membrane (gastric mucous membrane) with which it comes in contact.

4. Some antacids contain or form a gelatinous material which coats and protects the surface of the ulcer (demulcent effect).

Classification

Antacids may be classified as systemic and nonsystemic. A systemic antacid is one that is soluble in gastric and intestinal secretions and is readily absorbed. It therefore is capable of altering the electrolyte balance and of producing systemic alkalosis. It will also bring about increased work of the kidney since that organ must bear the burden of electrolyte readjustment. The nonsystemic antacids form relatively insoluble compounds which are not readily absorbed and hence are unlikely to produce alkalosis.

Systemic antacids

Systemic antacids, as previously mentioned, are readily soluble and easily absorbed. When they are given in large amounts they are likely to produce systemic alkalosis. They are found in many widely advertised proprietary preparations but are prescribed by the physician much less than they were at one time. They are avoided particularly for the patient who has pyloric obstruction or renal disease. However, patients sometimes seem to experience more relief of distress from the systemic antacids and physicians sometimes prescribe them in conjunction with one or more of the nonsystemic preparations.

Sodium Bicarbonate and Sodium Citrate

$$NaHCO_3 + HCl \rightarrow NaCl + H_2CO_3(H_2O \text{ and } CO_2)$$

Sodium bicarbonate is a typical systemic antacid. It is readily soluble and easily absorbed, and the duration of its action is short.

Although it has a number of therapeutic uses, it has been greatly overused by lay persons. It is easily accessible and far too many people feel justified in using it for any number of ailments. Many persons have a fear of an "acid stomach" and fail to recognize that gastric digestion is dependent upon a certain amount of acid being present in the gastric secretion.

It should be remembered that when the amount ingested exceeds that which is needed to neutralize the acid in the stomach at the time of administration, the excess rather readily passes into the intestine from which it is absorbed and contributes to a disturbance in the electrolyte balance in the blood. Likewise, a too frequent use of sodium bicarbonate, even in small quantities, may seriously interfere with electrolyte balance because of more or less constant neutralization of the gastric acids. This results in an increased burden on the kidney as it attempts to maintain the blood in stable acid-base reaction. Furthermore, gastric digestion of protein is likely to be inhibited because pepsin works best in an acid medium. (The latter is less serious since protein is also digested in the intestine.)

The reaction of sodium bicarbonate and hydrochloric acid results in the liberation of carbon dioxide. The resulting gastric distention may be quite undesirable, especially if an ulcer is present.

Preparation, dosage, and administration.

Sodium Bicarbonate, U.S.P., B.P. (Baking Soda). This is a white crystalline powder. The official dose is 2 Gm. (30 gr.) three times a day or more often (hourly) when symptoms are acute.

Sodium Citrate. This is also an absorbable systemic antacid similar to sodium bicarbonate. It differs from the latter substance in action in that it does not release carbon dioxide. It is seldom prescribed as an antacid in the treatment of peptic ulcer but it is commonly found in proprietary preparations recommended to relieve gastric distress. Sodium citrate is subject to oxidation, which results in the formation of sodium bicarbonate and is therefore capable of causing alkalosis when given in large amounts.

Nonsystemic antacids

Aluminum Hydroxide Gel

Aluminum hydroxide gel is one of the more popular of the nonsystemic antacids. In water it is insoluble but forms a white colloidal suspension which has practically no taste. It does not interfere with electrolyte balance nor does it produce alkalosis or a compensatory rise in free gastric acid. It is not absorbed from the gastrointestinal tract and therefore is not toxic when given orally. Its chief action is believed to be chemical neutralization of the hydrochloric acid of the stomach.

$$Al(OH)_3 + 3\ HCl \rightarrow AlCl_3 + 3\ H_2O$$

It has been found to buffer the gastric secretion to a maximum pH of about 4. It does not therefore completely suppress peptic digestion. It is thought to possess some absorptive properties, but evidence is not conclusive that acids, bacteria, gases, and toxins are absorbed. It has mild astringent and demulcent properties which are believed to be of some significance because of their local effect on an ulcer. The formation of aluminum chloride is responsible for both the astringent and constipating effects of aluminum hydroxide gel. The use of a mixture of aluminum hydroxide and either magnesium trisilicate or magnesium hydroxide helps to prevent the development of constipation.

The aluminum ion combines readily with phosphate to form an insoluble compound which is not absorbed in the intestine. Thus the intestinal excretion of phosphate is increased. This is of consequence only when the intake of phosphate is limited and the dosage of aluminum hydroxide is large. The diet of the patient with peptic ulcer is usually high in phosphorus.

Uses. Aluminum hydroxide gel is used alone or in combination with other antacids in the treatment of patients with peptic ulcer. It is also used to relieve gastric irritation associated with other conditions. It does not seem to affect the total output of gastric acid, and its activity is limited to the time it is actually in the stomach.

Preparation, dosage, and administration.

Aluminum Hydroxide Gel, U.S.P., B.P. (Amphojel, Creamalin, Al-U-Creme, Alkagel). This compound is available in the form of a liquid suspension and as tablets (300 and 600 mg.). The tablets should be chewed slowly. The patient may prefer the tablet form but the liquid preparation affords a better antacid effect. Aluminum hydroxide gel is given orally in doses of 4 to 8 ml. every 2 to 4 hours, although as much as 15 to 30 ml. may be given hourly. Some physicians like to have their patients take the aluminum hydroxide gel diluted in a small amount of water or milk or else drink a small amount of liquid after swallowing the antacid. Unless some fluid is taken with a small amount of the antacid, it may only coat the esophagus and little or none of it reach the stomach. It may also be administered by continuous drip through a stomach tube, in which case it is diluted and given 1 part to 2 or 3 parts of water at the rate of 15 to 20 drops per minute (1,500 ml. in 24 hours).

Aluminum Phosphate

The properties of this preparation are similar to those of aluminum hydroxide gel, but it does not interfere with absorption of phosphate. Larger doses of this preparation are necessary because its acid-combining power is less than one half that of aluminum hydroxide gel of the same concentration.

Uses. Aluminum Phosphate Gel is a preparation of choice for patients with ulcer who are unable to be maintained on a high phosphate diet or who suffer an accompanying diarrhea.

Preparation, dosage, and administration.

Aluminum Phosphate Gel, N.F. (Phosphaljel). This preparation is available as a 4 per cent suspension for oral administration. During the active phase of the ulcer, 15 to 30 ml. may be given alone or with milk every 2 hours. Later the dose may be reduced and given after each meal, at bedtime, and between meals if necessary.

There are a number of other aluminum compounds used as antacids, such as *dihydroxyaluminum aminoacetate* (Alglyn is one of many names under which it is sold) and *basic aluminum carbonate* (Basaljel). They are not believed to have any marked advantage over aluminum hydroxide.

Magnesium Trisilicate

Magnesium trisilicate is a compound of silicon dioxide and magnesium oxide with water.

$$MgO \cdot 3\ SiO_2 \cdot n\ H_2O$$

It occurs as a white, odorless, tasteless powder insoluble in water but partially soluble in acids. It is said to compare favorably with other nonsystemic antacids. It acts effectively as an adsorbent as well as providing chemical neutralization. In the stomach it has a gelatinous consistency which explains its ability to coat and protect the crater of the ulcer. In therapeutic amounts it apparently does not affect the motility of the gastrointestinal tract.

$$2 \text{ MgO} \cdot 3 \text{ SiO}_2 \cdot \text{n H}_2\text{O} + 4 \text{ HCl} \rightarrow 2 \text{ MgCl}_2 + 3 \text{ SiO}_2 + (\text{n} + 2)\text{H}_2\text{O}$$

In the intestine the magnesium chloride reacts with the bicarbonate in the intestinal secretions to form magnesium carbonate (which is excreted) and sodium chloride (which is subject to absorption). This follows a pattern similar to that of the neutralization of the bicarbonate by the hydrochloric acid of the stomach under normal circumstances and helps to explain why electrolyte balance is not disturbed. The magnesium chloride formed after neutralization of the hydrochloric acid is also responsible for a cathartic action in the bowel. Large doses may produce diarrhea, although therapeutic doses do not seem to disturb normal motility of the gastrointestinal tract.

Uses. Magnesium trisilicate is an effective antacid for the relief of gastric hyperacidity and for pain associated with peptic ulcer. A judicious combination of magnesium trisilicate and aluminum hydroxide has resulted in an antacid preparation which is efficient, safe when given in large amounts over prolonged periods, and relatively free from constipating effects.

Preparation, dosage, and administration.

Magnesium Trisilicate, U.S.P., B.P. This is available in 500 mg. tablets and in powder form. The usual dose is 1 Gm., four times a day, but as much as 2 to 4 Gm. may be given hourly during the treatment of the acute phase of an ulcer. The tablets should be chewed before they are swallowed.

A combination of magnesium trisilicate and aluminum hydroxide gel is available under the trade name *Gelusil* (tablet and liquid form). The dosage of this preparation varies with the severity of the symptoms to be controlled; 4 to 8 ml. is an average dose, although more may be prescribed.

Mucin, aluminum hydroxide, and magnesium trisilicate (Mucotin) is an antacid mixture which provides an additional protective coating to the ulcer and the gastric mucosa because of the mucin content. The preparation is available in tablets which should be well chewed before they are swallowed. The dose recommended is 2 tablets every 2 hours.

The following antacids are well-known preparations which act by chemical neutralization of gastric acid.

Calcium Carbonate

Calcium carbonate (chalk) is a fine white powder which is practically insoluble in water but is somewhat soluble in water containing carbon dioxide. It is decomposed by acids, forming a salt of calcium and carbonic acid which in turn yields water and carbon dioxide.

$$CaCO_3 + 2\ HCl \rightarrow CaCl_2 + H_2CO_3\ (CO_2 + H_2O)$$

The calcium chloride will react with the sodium bicarbonate in the intestinal secretions to form calcium carbonate and sodium chloride. The sodium chloride is absorbable but the calcium carbonate is excreted.

Uses. Calcium carbonate is used chiefly as an antacid and as a protective for patients with hyperacidity, gastritis, and peptic ulcer.

Preparation, dosage, and administration.

Precipitated Calcium Carbonate, U.S.P., B.P. This preparation is administered orally in doses of 2 to 4 Gm. hourly when acute symptoms are to be controlled. Thereafter the dosage may be lowered. The official (U.S.P.) single dose is 1 Gm.

Side effects. Calcium carbonate has a tendency to cause constipation, a disadvantage which may be avoided by alternating the administration of calcium carbonate with the use of magnesium oxide. The release of carbon dioxide may be dangerous if an ulcer is close to perforation. Large doses and prolonged administration may cause an accumulation of chalky formations in the bowel. Difference of opinion has been expressed as to whether calcium carbonate causes a gastric rebound of acid secretion.

Magnesium Oxide

Magnesium oxide is a widely used nonsystemic antacid. It is a bulky white powder which is relatively insoluble in water. It reacts with hydrochloric acid to form magnesium chloride and water.

$$MgO + 2\ HCl - MgCl_2 + H_2O$$

In the intestine, magnesium chloride acts as a saline cathartic and eventually reacts with sodium bicarbonate to form magnesium carbonate which is excreted and sodium chloride which may be absorbed. The neutralizing capacity of magnesium oxide is outstanding among the various antacids. It does not act rapidly but its effect is prolonged. Its chief disadvantage is that it may cause diarrhea in certain patients. It has therefore become a frequent practice to utilize the laxative effect of magnesium oxide to counteract the constipating effect of certain other antacids.

Magnesium oxide is not likely to cause alkalosis since little is absorbed, but it may cause the urine to become alkaline.

Preparation, dosage, and administration.

Magnesium Oxide, U.S.P., B.P. (Light Magnesia); *Magnesium Oxide* U.S.P., B.P. (Heavy Magnesia). These are two compounds which are identical in chemical composition but differ in physical properties, the former being lighter and five times more bulky than the latter. The light magnesia is more difficult to administer but affords a greater surface for reaction with the gastric content because of its greater capacity for dispersion. Recommended antacid dose (U.S.P.) is 250 mg. (300 to 600 mg., B.P.).

Following are other magnesium compounds.

Magnesium Carbonate, U.S.P., B.P. This preparation has antacid properties almost identical with those of magnesium oxide except that it liberates carbon dioxide upon neutralization of hydrochloric acid. It is a bulky white powder. The official dose (U.S.P.) as an antacid is 0.6 Gm. (600 mg.) (300 to 600 mg., B.P.).

Magnesia Magma, U.S.P. (Milk of Magnesia); *Mixture of Magnesium Hydroxide*, B.P. These exhibit the characteristic antacid effect of the basic salts of magnesium. The usual antacid dose is 5 ml. *Maalox* is a trade name for a mixture of aluminum hydroxide gel and magnesium hydroxide. It is comparable to *Gelusil* (aluminum hydroxide and magnesium trisilicate). The usual dosage of Maalox is 8 ml. It should be given with a little water, or a small quantity of water or milk should be swallowed after the dose.

Sippy Powders

Sippy Powders contain a mixture of antacids. They were introduced by Dr. Sippy and, in the original form, powder No. 1 contained 0.6 Gm. of magnesium oxide and 0.6 Gm. of sodium bicarbonate. Powder No. 2 contained 0.6 Gm. of bismuth subcarbonate and 2 to 3 Gm. of sodium bicarbonate. The powders were given alternately and in conjunction with a milk and cream diet. These powders are frequently modified by individual physicians both as to content and quantity of ingredients. However, they are then no longer known as Sippy Powders.

Polyamine-Methylene Resin (Exorbin, Resinat)

Polyamine-methylene resin is a synthetic substance that acts like an antacid by temporarily binding the hydrochloric acid and pepsin of the gastric juice. The acid and pepsin are later released in the intestine, thus causing no alteration in electrolyte balance. The resin itself is insoluble, unabsorbed, and is eliminated by the bowel.

Uses. The use of this agent is recommended only as an adjunct for the symptomatic relief of peptic ulcer.

Preparation, dosage, and administration.

*Polyamine-Methylene Resin** (Exorbin, Resinat). This is marketed in 250 and 500 mg. tablets and 250 mg. capsules for oral administration. The dosage recommended is 0.5 to 1 Gm. every 2 hours. Excessive doses may produce nausea and vomiting.

*Described in annual publication of A. M. A. Council on Drugs, N.N.D., 1960.

Digestants

Digestants are drugs that promote the process of digestion in the gastrointestinal tract and constitute a type of replacement therapy in deficiency states.

Hydrochloric acid

Hypochlorhydria is a term that denotes decreased secretion of hydrochloric acid in the stomach. *Achlorhydria* means an absence of hydrochloric acid, and when both acid and enzymes are absent in the gastric secretion the condition is known as *achylia gastrica*. A deficiency of acid is said to occur in aproximately 10 to 15 per cent of the population. It is more commonly found in elderly persons. Achlorhydria is associated with gastric carcinoma, pernicious anemia, some types of gastritis, and a number of other conditions. It is occasionally found in apparently normal individuals.

The hydrochloric acid of the stomach has several important functions. It is essential for the conversion of pepsinogen to active pepsin, which is important for the digestion of protein; it has a germicidal effect of numerous bacteria; it affects absorption in the upper part of the bowel; and it neutralizes bicarbonate of the intestinal secretions and thus helps to maintain electrolyte balance.

Uses. Hydrochloric acid is administered to relieve symptoms that result from gastric achlorhydria.

Preparation, dosage, and administration.

Hydrochloric Acid Diluted, N.F.; *Dilute Hydrochloride Acid,* B.P. This preparation contains 10 per cent hydrochloric acid, which should be further diluted in at least ½ glass of water and should be administered through a tube to avoid injury to the enamel of the teeth. The usual dose is 4 ml., although some physicians recommend doses up to 10 ml. The acid may be sipped with the meal or taken just after the meal. Even though the acid is diluted well, the taste is very sour. Food should be eaten after the last swallow of the acid or the mouth rinsed with an alkaline mouthwash.

Glutamic Acid Hydrochloride, N.F. (Acidulin). This is a combination of glutamic acid and hydrochloric acid. The hydrochloric acid is released when the preparation comes in contact with water. It is available in capsules containing 0.3 Gm., which is equivalent to 0.6 ml. of dilute hydrochloric acid. The preparation is usually administered before meals.

Betaine Hydrochloride (Normacid). This is a mixture of betaine hydrochloride, pepsin, and methylcellulose. The mixture releases hydrochloric acid in the stomach. It is available in tablets, each containing the equivalent of 15 minims of dilute hydrochloric acid. The usual dose is 1 or 2 tablets with or just after the meal.

Gastric and pancreatic enzymes

Pepsin

Pepsin is an enzyme secreted by the stomach, which initiates the hydrolysis of protein. It has been employed in the treatment of gastric achylia, but it is now believed that the symptoms associated with this condition are better relieved by the administration of dilute hydrochloric acid. Proteolytic enzymes in the intestinal and pancreatic secretions are capable of digesting proteins completely so that gastric pepsin is not an indispensable enzyme. Pepsin is seldom used today, but when given, the dose is 0.5 to 1 Gm. and is taken after meals. Pepsin, N.F., contains the proteolytic enzyme obtained from fresh hog's stomach.

Pancreatin

Pancreatin, N.F., B.P., is a powdered substance obtained from the pancreas of the hog or ox. It contains principally pancreatic amylase, trypsin, and pancreatic lipase. It has been employed in the treatment of conditions such as pancreatitis in which there may be a deficiency of the pancreatic secretion. However, some doubt has been expressed as to its therapeutic usefulness. Pancreatin should be dispersed in enteric-coated capsules to avoid destruction in the stomach. The recommended dose is 500 mg.

Bile and bile salts

Bile is composed chiefly of water, bile salts, bile pigments, cholesterol, lecithin, and inorganic salts. Bile is essential for the normal digestion of fats as well as for the absorption of digested fats and fat-soluble substances such as the fat-soluble vitamins. The principal bile salts are sodium glycocholate and sodium taurocholate. They represent combinations of bile acids with amino acids. Both bile salts and bile acids are normally absorbed from the intestine, pass through the portal blood to the liver, are re-excreted by the liver, then pass through the bile ducts, and again enter the intestine. Bile exerts a mild cathartic effect in the bowel, and the bile acids stimulate the production of bile by the liver. The latter is known as a choleretic action. Patients with derangement of the liver, gallbladder, and bile ducts are prone to have nutritional and digestive disturbances.

Uses. Bile and bile salts are used for patients with various hepatic disorders to aid digestion and absorption and to increase biliary drainage.

Preparation, dosage, and administration.

Ox Bile Extract, N.F. This is a dry powder made from the fresh bile of the ox. It is available in enteric-coated tablets and in capsule form. The average dose is 300 mg. It is administered after meals.

Dehydrocholic Acid, U.S.P. (Decholin). This compound increases the volume of bile and is used to facilitate biliary drainage. It is not recommended for patients with biliary obstruction. The usual dose is 250 to 500 mg. two or three times daily.

*Florantyrone** (Zanchol). This is a synthetic substance chemically unrelated to the natural bile salts but one that produces an increased volume of bile similar to the effect of dehydrocholic acid and related compounds. The bile produced is low in sediment and is of low viscosity. The usual dose for adults is 750 mg. to 1 Gm. daily. It is available in 250 mg. tablets.

Carminatives

Carminatives are mild irritant drugs which are given to increase gastrointestinal motility and thus aid in the expulsion of gas from the stomach and intestine. The active ingredients are, with few exceptions, aromatic substances such as volatile oils. They are sometimes used to lessen irritation of cathartics, abdominal distention, and colic. In the mouth they tend to increase the flow of saliva; in the stomach they promote a feeling of warmth and relaxation; and in the bowel they relieve gaseous distention. In cases of gastrointestinal paresis which sometimes develops after surgical operation, carminatives are of little value compared to the more powerful stimulants of smooth muscle, e.g., neostigmine. Carminatives are more likely to be used in the home than in the hospital. Elderly patients may prefer them, partly because they may be accustomed to using them for the relief of mild symptoms. Whisky or brandy in hot water and a few drops of peppermint in hot water are remedies commonly used in the home. The following are official preparations:

Peppermint Water, U.S.P.; *Concentrated Peppermint Water*, B.P., 0.3 to 1 ml.

Peppermint Spirit, U.S.P., B.P. (Essence of Peppermint), 1 ml.

Rhubarb and Soda Mixture, N.F., 4 ml.

Emetics

Emetics are agents given to produce vomiting. Their use has been supplanted to a great extent by gastric lavage. They occasionally are used as a first-aid measure when prompt evacuation of the stomach is essential.

*Described in annual publication of A. M. A. Council on Drugs, N.N.D., 1960.

Vomiting is a complex reflex mechanism, and drugs given to induce vomiting may act at one or more locations in the reflex arc. Vomiting can sometimes be brought about simply by tickling the back of the throat with a finger. A number of household substances can also be used to produce emesis. They include the following: mustard water (1 level teaspoonful of mustard to a glass of tepid water), mild soapsuds solution, warm salt water, or plain starch in warm water. Copious amounts of warm or tepid water will usually induce vomiting. Other emetics include copper sulfate, zinc sulfate, and ipecac fluidextract.

Emetics are also presented in Chapter 28, Toxicology.

Preparation, dosage, and administration.

Apomorphine Hydrochloride, U.S.P., B.P. This drug acts by direct stimulation of the vomiting center. The dose is 5 mg. (2 to 8 mg.), and it is administered subcutaneously or intramuscularly. Vomiting is usually produced in a few minutes. Large doses produce central depression so that the drug should be avoided for patients who are already depressed. Since the drug is prepared from morphine, conformity with regulations of the Harrison Narcotic Law is essential.

Antemetics

Antemetics are drugs given to produce symptomatic relief of nausea and vomiting. Control of vomiting is important and often difficult. Numerous preparations have been used, but effective treatment usually depends upon the removal of the cause. A number of factors influence vomiting. Some individuals vomit very easily and the reaction may be brought on by emotional stress and strain. Vomiting is sometimes associated with malingering. Other factors include motion sickness, endocrine disturbances, the action of certain drugs, gastrointestinal pathology, e.g., carcinoma of the stomach, reaction to roentgen treatments, heart disease, severe pain, etc.

When there is reason to believe that the nausea and vomiting is associated with a mild disturbance of some kind, a cup of plain hot tea will often relieve a nauseated patient. Carbonated drinks are popular remedies. Gastric lavage at other times may be indicated to empty the stomach of irritating material. A glass of warm solution of sodium bicarbonate may provoke emesis and empty the stomach with much the same result as gastric lavage. Salts of bismuth, magnesium oxide, and calcium carbonate may be employed as antacids and protectives to relieve irritation and vomiting. Vomiting due to other conditions may be relieved by central nervous system depressants, e.g., bromides, scopolamine, and the barbiturates. More recently, some of the antihistaminics and ataractics have been used to relieve vomiting and nausea. *Chlor-*

promazine is regarded as an unusually potent antemetic. *Dimenhydrinate* (Dramamine), *meclizine* (Bonamine), and several others are employed effectively for motion sickness. These are discussed elsewhere (see Index).

Diagnostic aids

Agents used to determine gastric acidity

Histamine

Histamine is such a potent stimulant of the gastric glands that when injected subcutaneously or intramuscularly in doses of approximately 0.3 to 0.5 mg., its failure to stimulate secretion of hydrochloric acid is considered proof of achlorhydria (inability of the stomach to produce acid). The injection may produce side effects such as a wheal at the site of injection (more marked if the injection is given subcutaneously), headache, vertigo, flushing, and sometimes a drop in blood pressure.

Preparation, dosage, and administration.

Histamine Phosphate, U.S.P., B.P. This drug is also known as histamine diphosphate or histamine acid phosphate. Dosage may vary from 0.275 mg. to several times this amount.

Betazole Hydrochloride, U.S.P. (Histalog). This preparation is an analogue of histamine which is coming to be used as a substitute for histamine phosphate. The drug stimulates the secretion of hydrochloric acid but causes a lower incidence of side effects. When side effects occur, however, they are similar to those produced by histamine. A 50 mg. dose is considered standard for individuals of normal weight. It is administered subcutaneously.

Azuresin (Diagnex Blue)

Azuresin is a preparation used to detect gastric anacidity (achlorhydria) without intubation. It has come to replace the older quinine carbacrylic resin for tubeless gastric analysis. The blue dye in the resin can be displaced by the hydrogen ions of the hydrochloric acid (if acid is present). A part of the displaced dye is excreted in the urine within 2 hours after the administration of the resin. The dye content of the urine is usually estimated and taken as a measure of the amount of acid secreted by the stomach.

Preparation, dosage, and administration.

Azuresin, U.S.P. (Azure A Carbacrylic Resin, Diagnex Blue). Two grams constitute a single test dose, which is administered orally in the form of granules. A gastric stimulant such as caffeine or histamine phosphate is given about 1 hour prior to the administration of the resin. The urine must be collected carefully according to directions.

Agents used for roentgenographic studies

Barium Sulfate

Barium sulfate is a fine, white, colorless, tasteless, and bulky powder free from grittiness. It is insoluble in water, in organic solvents, and in aqueous solutions of acids and alkalies. Its property of insolubility explains the safety which accompanies its use, for all soluble salts of barium are exceedingly poisonous. It is more impermeable to x-rays than are the tissues and for that reason it is used in roentgenography of the organs of the gastrointestinal tract. The patient is usually examined first by means of the fluoroscope, and flat plates are taken later to determine the rate of passage of the barium through the digestive tract and to locate sites of abnormality. A number of conditions may be discovered by a series of roentgenographs following the administration of barium sulfate. Among them are peptic ulcer, carcinoma, diverticula, and adhesions.

Preparation, dosage, and administration.

Barium Sulfate, U.S.P., B.P. This compound is given in doses of 300 Gm. for examination of the stomach. The dose is suspended in water and given orally. If the large bowel is to be examined, the barium sulfate must be given as an enema in quantity sufficient to fill the lumen of the organ. The patient is usually given a cleansing enema following the test.

Organic iodine compounds for cholecystography

A number of organic iodine compounds are used as diagnostic aids in examination of the liver, gallbladder, and bile ducts. These compounds are excreted by the liver into the bile and concentrated in the gallbladder. Since they cast a shadow on x-ray film they can be used to visualize the outline of the gallbladder, to determine the presence of stones, and to determine whether the organ fills and empties normally. It is recommended that iodinated compounds be used cautiously, if at all, for patients with severe renal disease. They are contraindicated for patients sensitive to iodine, and their use will also interfere, for some ensuing time, with diagnostic tests for thyroid function based on measurement of iodine in the blood.

Preparation, dosage, and administration.

Iodophthalein Sodium, N.F. (Iodeikon). This compound belongs to the phenolphthalein dyes and contains 60 to 63 per cent iodine. It is a blue-violet powder which is freely soluble in water. Following intravenous or oral administration the substance appears in the normal gallbladder in sufficient quantity to cast a shadow when the roentgen examination is made. The drug may be toxic in large doses, and therefore patients who receive the drug must be carefully selected. The preferable route of administration is the oral one, since fewer reactions accompany this route of administration. It can be given in

Drugs that affect gastrointestinal organs 385

capsule form or dissolved in water and grape juice and given during and just after the evening meal. The usual dose for each 10 kilograms of body weight is 0.5 Gm. when the drug is given orally and 0.3 Gm. when it is given intravenously.

Iodoalphionic Acid, N.F. (Priodax). This drug produces fewer side effects than iodophthalein sodium. It is eventually excreted chiefly by the kidneys. Untoward effects include dysuria, nausea and vomiting, diarrhea, dryness of the mouth, and general weakness. The drug is available in 0.5 Gm. tablets for oral administration. The usual adult dose is 3 Gm. This should be taken with several glasses of water during or after a light, fat-free meal in the late afternoon. Nothing further should be eaten until the examination is made the next morning.

Iopanoic Acid, U.S.P., B.P. (Telepaque). This is another radiopaque medium used in cholecystography. It is claimed that undesirable side effects seldom occur. When they do occur they include nausea, diarrhea, and dysuria. The usual dose is 3 Gm. given orally 10 hours before the roentgenogram is to be made. The patient should have a fat-free meal the evening before administration of the medication and allowed nothing by mouth until all roentgenograms are complete. The drug is available in 500 mg. tablets.

Iophenoxic Acid, U.S.P. (Teridax). This agent is an organic iodine compound for oral administration. The dose for an individual of average weight (150 pounds) is 3 Gm. It seems to produce a low incidence of unpleasant side effects. It is available in 750 mg. tablets.

Agent used for liver function test

Sulfobromophthalein Sodium

Sulfobromophthalein sodium is a water-soluble, white crystalline powder. It is used in connection with a test for liver function. It is normally rapidly removed from the blood stream and excreted in the bile. The time required for removal depends upon the size of the dose and the functional capacity of the liver.

Test doses of 2 or 5 mg. per kilogram of body weight should be completely removed from the blood within 20 and 45 minutes, respectively. In liver disease much longer time is required for removal.

Preparation, dosage, and administration.

Sulfobromophthalein Sodium, U.S.P. This is administered intravenously in 5 per cent solution. The usual dose is 5 mg. per kilogram of body weight, and the amount of dye in the blood is estimated at the end of 1 hour. Normally less than 6 per cent should be retained at the end of 1 hour.

Drugs that act in or upon the intestine

Drugs acting on the intestine which are included in this chapter include cathartics and antidiarrheics.

Cathartics

Misconceptions about the function of the bowel and the use of cathartics have long been harbored by mankind. Almy and Steinberg aptly put it thus:

"Drugs have been used since time immemorial for the purpose of promoting defecation. Such agents are widely self-administered by lay persons. Whatever the psychological basis, there is a durable attitude, spanning many centuries and many cultures, that associates excrement with evil and its elimination with the expiation of guilt. The practical result is that most people in our society still regard even transitory constipation as something to be directly and promptly treated with a cathartic. In the past the medical profession has abetted these tendencies by the empiric and nonspecific use of purgation in the treatment of systemic disease (even the common cold) and has been slow to disown the theory of intestinal autointoxication. As a consequence, more patients now consult the physician because of the untoward effects of chronic use of cathartics than for any condition that can be relieved by them."*

Constipation is a condition associated with a functional impairment of the bowel which prevents it from producing stools of normal consistency and frequency. Chronic constipation is sometimes due to organic disease such as tumors (benign or malignant), which produce obstruction in the bowel, megacolon, hypothyroidism, anal and rectal disorders, and diseases of the liver and gallbladder. Patients who suffer from disorders of the gastrointestinal tract frequently complain of constipation. On the other hand, many persons complain of constipation when no organic disease or lesion can be found. A number of factors may operate to cause constipation in such persons.

1. Faulty diet and faulty eating habits. A diet which provides inadequate bulk and residue will contribute to the development of constipation. A "meal" composed of a soft drink and a cigarette will do little to stimulate intestinal peristalsis. A gastrointestinal tract should function normally if fluids and residue are supplied sufficient to keep the stool formed but soft.

2. Failure to respond to the normal defecation impulses and insufficient time to permit the bowel to produce an evacuation. Hurry and worry are not conducive to a normal response on the part of the bowel.

3. Sedentary habits and insufficient exercise. Bedridden patients may be constipated because of inactivity, unnatural position for defecation, and numerous other reasons.

*From Almy, T. P., and Steinberg, H.: The Choice of Drugs for Gastrointestinal Disturbances. In Modell, W. (editor): Drugs of Choice, 1960-1961, St. Louis, 1960, The C. V. Mosby Co., p. 361.

4. The effect of drugs. The use of morphine, codeine, or some of the ganglionic blocking agents often explains why constipation is encountered in hospitalized patients.

5. Other conditions. There are a number of other conditions sometimes associated with constipation, such as febrile states, psychosomatic disorders, anemias, sick headaches, etc. Constipation can be a symptom of disorders of both the body and the mind.

6. Atonic and hypertonic conditions of the musculature of the colon. These may result from habitual use of cathartics.

The only treatment that will relieve constipation is to remove the cause. Since the cause is often related to faulty habits, many persons find relief when more attention is paid to simple hygienic rules, i.e., adequate exercise, food, fluids, freedom from excessive tension and worry, and prompt attention to the call for defecation. If these measures do not afford the desired relief, it is important that a physician be consulted, since a physical examination may uncover a serious disease which demands prompt attention and treatment. Symptoms associated with constipation and often attributed to self-intoxication are debility, lassitude, vertigo, mental depression, headache, loss of appetite, coated tongue, etc. There is evidence, however, that these symptoms are the result of distention of the lower bowel and not to the absorption of toxic products.

Responsibilities of the nurse in relation to use

As is true for all medications, the nurse must exercise caution in giving advice about cathartics. Persons who seek help because they are becoming increasingly dependent upon cathartics need the advice of a physician and should be persuaded to go to one. Not only should the cause of the constipation be found and removed but the patient should in most instances also be helped to overcome his dependence on the medication.

No cathartic should be needed by a healthy individual, and the sick person should take the drug prescribed by the physician. This is likely to be one which allows the patient to return gradually to a normal defecation pattern.

The nurse should direct her efforts toward the teaching of basic facts of good hygiene; she should help the patient to understand what is meant by an adequate diet, what constitutes plenty of fluids, and how to develop regular bowel habits. She may be able to help some patients by persuading them to eat all the food that is served to them, by providing plenty of drinking water and encouraging them to drink it, and by providing as much exercise as the patients are allowed. She may also be of assistance in helping patients reduce the emotional strain under which they may be living.

Conditions for which use may be indicated

Cathartics are used justifiably for the following:

1. In the preparation of abdominal viscera prior to roentgen examination.

2. To produce some degree of dehydration in cases of edema (cerebral, cardiac, etc.).

3. In cases of food and drug poisoning to promote the elimination of the offending substance from the gastrointestinal tract. Saline cathartics are considered useful for this purpose.

4. To keep the stool soft when it is essential to avoid the irritation that accompanies the passage of a hardened stool; e.g., patients who have a colostomy, a rectal disorder, or irritated polyps in the bowel, or cases in which straining should be avoided, as after the repair of a hernia or after a cerebral accident. The type of cathartic selected is likely to be one of the emollients such as liquid petrolatum.

5. To expel parasites and toxic anthelmintics. Cathartics are routinely prescribed after certain anthelmintics for the purpose of expelling the parasites as well as the anthelmintic that may be toxic.

6. To secure a stool specimen to be examined for parasites. A saline cathartic is often preferred.

Cathartics are not necessarily indicated for constipation, although the occasional and temporary use of one may be necessary. If used, the cathartic should be chosen judiciously and in accordance with the patient's needs. What may be suitable for one person may not be at all satisfactory for another. The important thing is that the right preparation be chosen and that some recognition be made of its limitations.

Elderly persons who have some degree of constipation cannot be treated the same as younger adults. They cannot be expected to change the habit patterns of a lifetime or to subject themselves to tiresome diets that disturb the calm and peace required by the elderly person in his later years. After an examination the doctor can select a laxative for more or less regular use, and if it produces satisfactory results (no griping, gaseous distention, etc.), there is probably little need to worry about the cathartic habit. It may be decidedly unwise to urge an elderly person to increase the roughage of his diet. He or she may not have the teeth or the type of bowel to make such an adjustment happily. The best plan is to choose a preparation which experience has proved to be nonirritating but effective.

Conditions for which use may be contraindicated

There are a number of conditions for which cathartics should be given with caution, if at all.

1. Inflammatory disorders of the alimentary tract, such as appendicitis, typhoid fever, and chronic ulcerative colitis.

2. Cases of undiagnosed abdominal pain. Should the pain be due to an inflamed appendix, a cathartic may bring about a rupture of the appendix by increasing intestinal peristalsis.

3. Following certain surgical operations. Cathartics may be contraindicated after some operations, at least for a time, e.g., after repair work on the perineum or rectum.

4. For pregnant and severely anemic or debilitated patients.

5. Chronic constipation and spastic constipation.

6. For patients with bowel obstruction, hemorrhage, or intussusception.

A number of ill effects may follow the use or overuse of irritant cathartics in particular; one of these is a disturbance of electrolyte balance. The small intestine contains an abundance of sodium, potassium, chloride, and bicarbonate ions which will be lost when the bowel is emptied vigorously. This can result in alkalosis or acidosis, dehydration, and potassium deficiency. Young and healthy individuals may recover from the purgation without noticeable ill effect but the same may not be true in the elderly or the debilitated patient or the patient with renal impairment.

Classification

Cathartics are drugs given to induce defecation, and they may be classified according to their source, site of action, degree of action, and method of action. The latter two classifications will be described.

A. According to degree of cathartic action
   1. Laxatives—cathartics that cause few movements of the bowel; stool formed and normal in appearance and unaccompanied by griping
   2. Purgatives—cathartics that produce frequent movements with soft or liquid stools which may or may not be accompanied by griping

This classification is not a hard and fast one because dosage is frequently the determining factor. A small dose of some cathartics may have a laxative effect, whereas a larger dose may cause a purgative effect.

Drastic purgatives such as croton oil, jalap, colocynth, etc., exert such a severe irritation in the gastrointestinal tract that their use is no longer considered justifiable.

B. According to method of action
   1. Cathartics that stimulate peristalsis by increasing fluid, gaseous, or solid bulk of the intestinal content
   2. Emollient cathartics that act somewhat like bulk-forming cathartics—coat food and liquid particles, delay absorption, and delay drying of the fecal content of the bowel
   3. Cathartics that act as wetting agents by lowering surface tension and by preventing desiccation (drying) of stool

390

4. Chemical irritation—another method by which cathartics bring about increased intestinal peristalsis; results in more rapid propulsion of contents along alimentary canal

Bulk-forming cathartics

Hydrophilic colloids stimulate peristalsis by increasing bulk, thus modifying the consistency of the stool. They apparently do not interfere with absorption of food, but they can cause fecal impaction and obstruction. It is important to give them with adequate fluid. Mention should also be made of suppositories, e.g., glycerine suppositories and suppositories that bring about release of carbon dioxide in the rectum (Pharmalax).

Agar

Agar is a dried mucilaginous substance obtained from several varieties of seaweed. It may be obtained in the powdered, granular, or flaked form. The granular preparation is the one most desirable, as a rule. Agar is rich in indigestible cellulose. When moistened, it swells, forming a mass of material which passes through the intestine without being affected by the digestive juices and by its blandness and bulk makes the stool large and soft so that it is easily moved along the colon and into the rectum.

The effect of agar is not noticed immediately. It may require a week or two to establish satisfactory evacuation, but as soon as results seem satisfactory, the dose should gradually be reduced to the smallest amount needed for a satisfactory bowel movement. Doses should then be omitted occasionally until its use is no longer necessary. This gradual reduction and cessation of dosage should constitute a principle underlying the use of all laxative cathartics to avoid undesirable reactions and habit formation.

Preparation, dosage, and administration.

Agar, U.S.P. This compound is best taken twice daily in doses of 4 to 16 Gm. accompanied by plenty of fluid. Some find agar more palatable when it has been allowed to soak in hot water and is then added to such food as cereal, soup, or mashed potatoes or is merely taken in the soft semisolid form. When the dry agar is used, it likewise may be added to soup, cereal, potatoes, pudding, etc. It also may be emulsified with liquid petrolatum (Petrogalar). Cascara, phenolphthalein, or milk of magnesia is sometimes added to the emulsified form.

The mineral oil and agar emulsions are widely advertised but are of little value because the agar content is so small (2 to 6 per cent). The laxative effect of these emulsions is usually due to the addition of some other cathartic.

Plantago Seed (Psyllium Seed)

Plantago seed is the dried ripe seed of the *Plantago psyllium, Plantago indica,* or *Plantago ovata.* The seeds are small, brown or blonde seeds which contain a mucilaginous material that swells in the presence of moisture to form a jellylike indigestible mass. The main disadvantage lies in the fact that although the seeds swell, their ends remain sharp and may be the cause of irritation in the alimentary tract. At present, only the preparation of the extracted gums are available, and these have the advantage of causing less mechanical irritation.

Preparation, dosage, and administration.

*Psyllium Hydrophilic Mucilloid** (Metamucil). This is a white to cream-colored powder containing about 50 per cent powdered muci-laginous portion (outer epidermis) of bland psyllium seeds and about 50 per cent dextrose. This mixture is used in the treatment of constipation because it promotes the formation of a soft, water-retaining gelatinous residue in the lower bowel. In addition, it has a demulcent effect on inflamed mucosa. The dose is 4 to 7 Gm. one to three times daily. It should be stirred into a glass of water or other fluid and followed by an additional glass of fluid.

*Plantago Ovata Coating** (Konsyl). This form is a cream- to brown-colored granular powder obtained from the *Plantago ovata* (blond psyllium). The dose is 5 to 10 Gm. three times daily before meals in a glass of water or milk. It should be swallowed before it thickens.

Methylcellulose (Cellothyl)

Methylcellulose is a synthetic hydrophilic colloid. It is a grayish white, fibrous powder which, in the presence of water, swells and produces a viscous, colloidal solution in the upper part of the alimentary tract. In the colon this solution loses water and forms a gel which increases the bulk and softness of the stool.

Preparation, dosage, and administration.

Methylcellulose, U.S.P. (Cellothyl, Hydrolose, Methocel, Syncelose). This preparation is available in 500 mg. tablets or as a syrup (200 mg. per milliliter). It is administered orally two to four times daily in doses of 1 to 1.5 Gm. It should be accompanied by 1 or 2 glasses of water. The dosage is gradually reduced as normal defecation reflexes establish a normal pattern for the behavior of the bowel.

Sodium Carboxymethylcellulose (Carmethose)

Sodium carboxymethylcellulose is a synthetic, hydrophilic, colloid gum. It is similar to methylcellulose in that it forms a soft bulk in the intestine after oral ingestion. It is insoluble in gastric juices which is not

*Described in annual publication of A. M. A. Council on Drugs, N.N.D., 1960.

true of methylcellulose. It is a satisfactory agent to use, along with constructive, re-educative measures in the treatment of chronic constipation.

Preparation, dosage, and administration.

Sodium Carboxymethylcellulose, U.S.P. (Carmethose, CMC Cellulose Gum, Thylose Sodium). This is available in 225 and 500 mg. tablets and in 5 per cent solution for oral administration. The usual oral dose is 1.5 Gm. three times daily with 1 or 2 glasses of water.

Saline cathartics

The saline cathartics are soluble salts which are only slightly absorbed from the alimentary canal. The speed of their action depends upon the nature of the solution administered and whether the stomach is empty at the time of administration. An isotonic solution will inhibit absorption of water from the bowel and will therefore increase the total fluid bulk. Peristalsis will be increased and several liquid or semiliquid stools will result. A hypertonic solution will cause diffusion of fluid from the blood in the wall of the bowel into the lumen of the organ until the solution has been made isotonic. This type of fluid is especially effective in relieving edema, although the action may prove exhausting to the patient. Catharsis results in 1 to 4 hours.

The intestinal membrane is not entirely impermeable to the passage of saline cathartics. Some find their way into the general circulation only to be excreted by the kidney, in which case they act as saline diuretics. Hypertonic saline solutions in the bowel may result in so much loss of fluid that little or no diuretic effect will be possible. Some ions may have a toxic effect if they accumulate in the blood in sufficient quantity. This may occur with magnesium ions if a solution is retained in the intestine for a long time or if the patient suffers from renal impairment. It may also occur when large doses of the salt are given intravenously.

Uses. The saline cathartics are the agents of choice for the relief of edema (cerebral, cardiac, etc.) and for securing a stool specimen for examination, as well as for use with certain anthelmintics and in certain cases of food and drug poisoning.

When the object is merely to empty the intestine, magnesium citrate, magnesium sulfate, sodium phosphate, or milk of magnesia is effective. Milk of magnesia (magnesium hydroxide) is the mildest of the salines and is best suited for children. Heavy magnesium oxide is better for adults, as a rule. Magnesium sulfate is probably the best to relieve edema, although it has a disagreeable taste. Sodium sulfate is the most disagreeable and not much used except in veterinary practice. The effervescent preparations are the most agreeable to take.

Preparation, dosage, and administration.

Sodium Sulfate, N.F., B.P. (Glauber's Salt). This compound occurs as

Drugs that affect gastrointestinal organs 393

glassy crystals or as a white powder which is readily soluble in water. It has a strong disagreeable saline taste. It is one of the cheapest of the saline cathartics. The usual dose is 15 Gm.

Magnesium Sulfate (Epsom Salt), U.S.P.; *Magnesium Sulfate* (Epsom Salts), B.P. This agent occurs as glassy needlelike crystals or as a white powder and is readily soluble in water. It has a bitter saline taste. The usual dose for cathartic effect is 15 Gm. (½ ounce), although the range of dosage may be from 10 to 30 Gm.

Magnesia Magma, U.S.P. (Milk of Magnesia); *Magnesium Hydroxide Mixture*, B.P. This preparation is also used as an antacid. In the stomach the magnesium hydroxide reacts with the hydrochloric acid to form magnesium chloride, which is responsible for the cathartic effect. The usual dose for adults is 15 ml. (½ fluidounce), although the range of dosage is 5 to 30 ml. *Magnesium Hydroxide Tablets*, N.F., contain 0.3 Gm. of the drug.

Magnesium Oxide, U.S.P.; *Heavy Magnesium Oxide*, B.P. This preparation depends on the conversion of the oxide into soluble salts of magnesium which are themselves responsible for the cathartic effect.

$$MgO \; + \; 2 \; HCl \; - \; MgCl_2 \; + \; H_2O$$

The usual laxative dose is 1 to 4 Gm.

Heavy Magnesium Carbonate, B.P.; *Light Magnesium Carbonate*, B.P. This cathartic is a bulky white powder practically insoluble in water. It is used as an antacid as well as a cathartic. Cathartic effect is dependent upon the formation of a soluble salt of magnesium. The usual dose is 2 to 4 Gm.

Magnesium Citrate Solution, N.F. This preparation is not very soluble; hence the need for a relatively large dose. It is not unpleasant to take because it is carbonated and flavored. The usual dose is ½ to 1 bottle (6 to 12 ounces).

Sodium Phosphate, N.F., B.P. This is a white crystalline substance readily soluble in water. It tastes less disagreeable than either sodium sulfate or magnesium sulfate. The usual dose is 4 Gm.

Effervescent Sodium Phosphate, N.F. This preparation is made effervescent by the addition of sodium bicarbonate and citric and tartaric acids. The usual dose is 10 Gm.

A concentrated aqueous solution of sodium biphosphate and sodium phosphate is available under the name of Phospho-Soda. The usual dose as a cathartic is 4 to 15 ml. It is also marketed in a disposable enema unit.

Potassium Sodium Tartrate, N.F. (Rochelle Salt). Dose is 10 Gm. (⅓ ounce) orally. This preparation occurs as crystals or white powder, is very soluble, and has a not unpleasant taste.

Compound Effervescent Powders, N.F. (Seidlitz Powders). Dose consists of the contents of a blue and a white paper dissolved separately in about ⅓ glass of water and the solutions mixed at the bedside or just prior to swallowing. The blue paper contains sodium and potassium tartrate and sodium bicarbonate. The white paper contains tartaric acid. The effervescence is caused by the liberation of carbon dioxide when the sodium bicarbonate and tartaric acid interact. The effervescence does much to increase the palatability of the mixture.

Sodium sulfate is the basis of many proprietary saline cathartics such as Sal Hepatica. Mineral waters are usually artificially prepared solutions made in a factory and contain magnesium sulfate or sodium sulfate or both. Their use in the treatment of constipation is thought inadvisable.

The above-mentioned salts when given for their cathartic effect are usually given orally. Certain of them may be given rectally as an enema. The salts tend to have a rapid action, especially if administered in the morning before breakfast. Patients sometimes complain of gaseous distention after taking saline cathartics. All preparations should be accompanied by a liberal intake of water since the salts do not readily leave the stomach unless well diluted. On the other hand, if the saline is given to reduce edema, the patient's total daily intake of fluids will probably be restricted.

When a salt such as magnesium sulfate is administered to a patient, it should not only be dissolved in an adequate amount of water but it should also be disguised in fruit juice. Grape juice is excellent unless the patient is nauseated, in which case it is better to give it in plain water (chilled) or on chipped ice since the grape juice, if vomited, will stain bedclothing, etc.

Emollient cathartics

Liquid Petrolatum

Liquid petrolatum or mineral oil is a mixture of liquid hydrocarbons obtained from petroleum. The oil is not digested and absorption is minimal. It softens the fecal mass and prevents excessive absorption of water. It is especially useful when it is desirable to keep feces soft and when straining at stool must be reduced, as after rectal operations, repair of hernias, or cerebrospinal accidents. Because it acts as a laxative it may be useful for patients who have a chronic type of constipation that is due to prolonged inactivity. Such might be the case in patients with certain orthopedic conditions.

Some physicians object to the use of mineral oil on the basis that it dissolves certain of the fat-soluble vitamins and bile salts and inhibits their absorption. Others maintain that only the precursor to vitamin A (carotene) is so affected and that natural vitamin A is quantitatively absorbed from the intestine in the presence of mineral oil.° Another objection to its use is that in large doses it tends to seep from the rectum and soil clothing or destroy rubber sheets on hospital beds. Furthermore, leakage from the rectum may interfere with healing of postoperative wounds in the region of the anus and perineum. Although absorption of mineral oil is very limited, it is said to give rise to a chronic inflammatory reaction in tissues where it is found after absorption.†

Preparation, dosage, and administration.

Liquid Petrolatum, U.S.P.; *Liquid Paraffin,* B.P. It is administered in doses that range from 15 to 30 ml. (adults) and is best given between meals or at bedtime. It should not be given immediately after meals, as it may delay the passage of food from the stomach. Most patients may have a slice of orange just after swallowing the oil, to relieve the oily taste in the mouth. When mineral oil is purchased it is important to get an oil of official standard.

Other emollients

Olive oil and cottonseed oil are digestible oils, but if given in sufficient quantity they may act as emollient cathartics, since part of the oil will escape hydrolysis. Corn oil is sometimes given to relieve constipation in children.

Olive Oil, U.S.P., B.P. When administered in doses of 30 ml., olive oil acts as a laxative. It may be given orally or rectally.

Corn Oil, U.S.P. This emollient is given to children in doses of 2 to 4 ml.

Fecal moistening agent

Dioctyl Sodium Sulfosuccinate

Dioctyl sodium sulfosuccinate is not classified as a cathartic but as a wetting agent or fecal moistening agent. When taken internally it acts in a manner similar to that of detergents and permits water and fatty substances to penetrate and to be well mixed with the fecal material. Thus, this agent promotes the formation of soft, formed stools and is a useful aid in the treatment of constipation.

This preparation is said to have a wide margin of safety and negligible toxicity. There is some question about advisability of giving it with mineral oil since there is a possibility that it may promote absorption of the oil.

Uses. It is indicated for patients with rectal impaction, chronic con-

°Davison, F. R.: Handbook of Materia Medica, Toxicology and Pharmacology, St. Louis, 1949, The C. V. Mosby Co., p. 177.

†Goodman, L. S., and Gilman, A.: The Pharmacological Basis of Therapeutics, New York, 1955, The Macmillan Co., p. 1060.

stipation, and painful conditions of the rectum and anus and for those who should avoid straining at the time of defecation.

Preparation, dosage, and administration.

Dioctyl Sodium Sulfosuccinate, N.F. (Colace, Doxinate). This preparation is available in 50, 60, 100, and 240 mg. capsules; in solution, 10 mg. per milliliter; and as a syrup, 4 mg. per milliliter. The average adult dose is 10 to 60 mg. daily; 10 to 20 mg. for infants and children.

Cathartics that act by chemical irritation

Castor Oil (Oleum Ricini)

Castor oil is obtained from the seeds of the castor bean, *Ricinus communis,* a plant that grows in India but is also cultivated in a number of places where the climate is warm. Castor oil is a bland colorless emollient which passes through the stomach unchanged, but, like other fatty substances, it retards the emptying of the stomach and for this reason is usually given when the stomach is empty. In the intestine the oil is hydrolyzed, like other esters, to glycerol and a fatty acid, which in this instance is ricinoleic acid. This fatty acid is responsible for the irritation of the bowel, especially the small intestine. It rarely reaches the large intestine before causing irritation. The site of action may be observed with a fluoroscope. Its irritating effect causes a rapid propulsion of content from the small intestine, including any of the oil that may have escaped hydrolysis. This helps to make its effect somewhat self-limiting. A therapeutic dose will produce several copious semiliquid stools in from 2 to 6 hours. Some persons have little or no griping or colic-like distress, whereas others may experience considerable abdominal cramping and exhaustion. Patients who have an irritable bowel or lesions in the bowel may be made very ill.

The fluid nature of the stool is due to the rapid passage of the fecal content rather than to a diffusion of fluid into the bowel. Castor oil tends to empty the bowel completely; hence no evacuation is likely to occur for a day or so, a point which patients sometimes do not understand. Castor oil is excreted into the milk of nursing mothers.

Uses. Castor oil is used much less often today than formerly. It continues to be used in the preparation of certain patients who are to have a roentgen examination of abdominal viscera. Because of its irritant action, however, it is usually contraindicated for patients who have ulcerative lesions of the bowel.

It may be used for the treatment of food or drug poisoning or for the relief of diarrhea, unless the patient is already dehydrated. When given for diarrhea it is given to empty the bowel and put it at rest.

Castor oil has been used to help initiate labor in obstetric patients, but present-day authorities do not agree that this use is justifiable.

Preparation, dosage, and administration.

Castor Oil, U.S.P., B.P. (Oleum Ricini). The usual adult dose is 15 ml. and it is given orally. As much as 60 ml. may be ordered.

In sensitive individuals the natural oil may be unpleasant and nauseating. This may be overcome by the use of fruit juices or pharmaceutic mixtures to emulsify and disguise the oil. Some care should be exercised, especially in children, to prevent untoward conditioning of the child against such things as orange juice. Each hospital is likely to have its own particular way of administering castor oil and the nurse should learn the recipe of the institution in which she is employed.

The anthracene cathartics (emodin cathartics)

The principal members of the anthracene group of cathartics are cascara, senna, rhubarb, and aloe. They are obtained from the bark, seed pods, leaves, and roots of a number of plants. They contain glycosidal compounds which are inactive as such, but in the alkaline portion of the small intestine these compounds yield the anthraquinones, emodin and chrysophanic acid, which are absorbed and later excreted into the lumen of the large intestine where they produce irritation. Chemical substances other than anthraquinones are also found in these cathartics and help to explain individual differences and characteristics. After absorption, a number of the active ingredients of these drugs find their way into body fluids, e.g., milk and urine. Some are responsible for the color of the urine (a yellowish brown if the reaction is acid or a reddish violet if the urine is alkaline).

The anthracenes exert their main action on the large bowel; hence they have a tendency to produce griping. They require from 6 to 12 hours or more to produce evacuation.

Cascara Sagrada

Cascara sagrada is obtained from the bark of the *Rhamnus purshiana,* a shrub or small tree. It was once called "sacred bark" by the Indians who lived in the region of the Pacific coast. It is one of the most extensively used cathartics. Its action is mainly on the large bowel, and although its effects are comparatively mild it does act by irritation. It is less likely to cause griping than some of the other cathartics belonging to this group of compounds. When given occasionally and in therapeutic doses it tends to improve the tone of the muscle of the intestine.

Preparation, dosage, and administration.

Aromatic Cascara Sagrada Fluidextract, U.S.P.; *Cascara Elixir*, B.P. This compound is made more palatable than the plain fluidextract by extraction with boiling water and by the addition of magnesium oxide

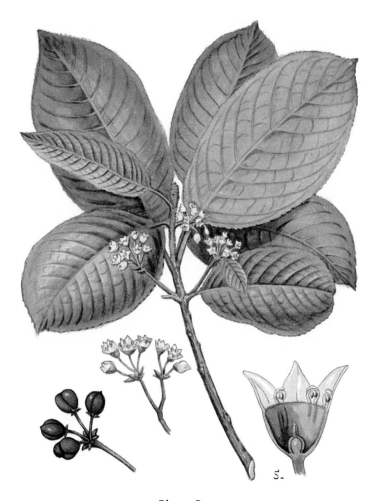

Plate 5

Rhamnus purshiana. (From Jackson, D. E.: Experimental Pharmacology and Materia Medica,
St. Louis, The C. V. Mosby Co.)

as well as a number of flavoring agents. The magnesium oxide is used to form insoluble anthraquinone derivatives which are then removed. This makes this preparation less harsh than the fluidextract. The dose is 2 to 12 ml., and it is given orally. The dose of Cascara Elixir, B.P., is 2 to 4 ml.

Cascara Sagrada Fluidextract, N.F.; *Cascara Liquid Extract*, B.P. This preparation has a very bitter taste. The adult dose is 2 to 4 ml.

Cascara Sagrada Extract Tablets, N.F.; *Cascara Tablets*, B.P. These forms are available in 120, 200, and 300 mg. tablets. The average dose is 300 mg. (5 gr.) for adults. *Cascara Tablets*, B.P., 120 to 250 mg.

Aloe

Aloe is the dried juice of leaves of a plant that grows in Africa and the West Indies. It contains a glycoside known as aloin, which is subject to hydrolysis in the intestine like the other emodin cathartics. Aloe is the most irritating of the emodin cathartics. Its action is accompanied by considerable griping, and in large doses it is capable of causing pelvic congestion. It has a very bitter taste. Both the crude drug and aloin are used as cathartics. Aloin is often incorporated into preparations that contain other cathartics, e.g., A.S.B. and C. pills—A for aloin, S for strychnine, B for belladonna, and C for cascara. Several other proprietary preparations contain aloin along with a little bile and other substances—Carter's Little Pills, Hinkle's Pills, and Alophen Pills.

Preparation, dosage, and administration.

Aloe (Aloes), U.S.P., B.P. The preparation listed in U.S.P. is used as a constituent of Compound Benzoin Tincture. The dosage as listed in B.P. is 120 to 300 mg.

Aloin, Belladonna, Cascara, and Podophyllum Pills, N.F. (Hinkle's Pills). This preparation contains cascara sagrada extract, aloin, podophyllum resin, belladonna extract, ginger oleoresin, glycyrrhiza, and liquid glucose. The usual dose is 1 pill. Preparations of aloe are given orally.

Rhubarb

Rhubarb is obtained from the dried roots of several species of Rheum plants which grow in China. The American variety of rhubarb does not exert a cathartic action. This drug contains tannin and hence an astringent effect accompanies and sometimes masks the cathartic action. Its action is not accompanied by severe griping and discomfort. A bowel evacuation usually occurs 4 to 8 hours after the administration of a cathartic dose.

Preparation, dosage, and administration.

Aromatic Rhubarb Tincture, N.F.; *Compound Rhubarb Tincture*, B.P. This form is given orally in doses of 2 to 4 ml.

Rhubarb and Soda Mixture, N.F. This preparation includes the following: rhubarb fluidextract, ipecac fluidextract, sodium bicarbonate, peppermint spirit, glycerin, and distilled water. The usual dose is 4 ml. It serves both as a cathartic and as an antacid. It is sometimes effective in relieving a gastrointestinal upset after overindulgence in food.

Senna

Senna is obtained from the dried leaves of the Cassia senna plant, a cathartic well known to the Arabians. The dried leaves have been used to make a homemade infusion of the drug which is decidedly potent. It produces a thorough bowel evacuation in from 4 to 6 hours and is likely to be accompanied by griping. It resembles cascara but is more powerful. It is found in the proprietary remedies, Castoria and Syrup of Figs.

Senna tea is an infusion of senna leaves made from a teaspoonful of leaves to a cup of hot water. Senna is sometimes cooked with equal parts of prunes or figs and the mixture is given as a purgative.

Preparation, dosage, and administration.

Compound Senna Powder, N.F. (Compound Licorice Powder). This compound contains senna, glycirrhiza (licorice), washed sulfur, oil of fennel, and sugar. The usual dose is 4 Gm. It is mixed with a little water and given orally. It should be followed by a generous drink of water (as is recommended for most cathartics).

Senna Syrup, N.F. Usual dose is 8 ml. orally.

Senna Fluidextract. Also official in the N.F. Usual dose is 2 ml. orally.

Phenolphthalein

This phenol derivative is a synthetic substance, the cathartic action of which is similar to that of the anthracene group. It is a white powder insoluble in water but soluble in the juice of the intestine where it exerts its relatively mild irritant action. Evacuation is produced in from 8 to 12 hours, unaccompanied by griping. It acts upon both the small and large bowel, particularly the latter. When given orally, part of the drug is absorbed and resecreted into the bile. When given parenterally, large amounts are secreted into the bile and thus a prolonged cathartic action may be obtained.

Repeated doses may cause nausea, and in some susceptible individuals a skin rash may appear. In other cases a prolonged and excessive purgative effect may indicate individual idiosyncrasy. Obviously susceptible individuals should avoid the use of phenolphthalein. However, because the drug is odorless and tasteless and relatively pleasant to take, it is found in a number of proprietary preparations and is sold in a candylike form and in a chewing gum. Children should not be allowed free access to these preparations, as they are likely to regard them as ordinary candy or gum and may get an overdose of the drug. Deaths have been reported from such accidents, although the dose causing toxicity is large.

Preparation, dosage, and administration.

Phenolphthalein Tablets, N.F. B.P. The tablets are available in 60 and 120 mg. amounts. The usual dose is 60 mg. (orally).

Phenolphthalein is found in some proprietary preparations with other cathartics such as agar, liquid petrolatum, as well as with other irritant cathartics.

Antidiarrheics

Diarrhea is a symptom of a disorder of the bowel associated with too rapid a passage of intestinal content, frequent fluid stools, and griping. The remedies selected or ordered to relieve diarrhea are selected on the basis of what is causing the diarrhea. The causes may be many and varied and include (1) the eating of contaminated or partially decomposed food, (2) bacterial or protozoan infection, (3) certain nervous disorders, (4) disturbances of gastric physiology, such as absence of hydrochloric acid or the effects of resectional surgery of the stomach, (5) inflammatory processes of the intestine or adjacent viscera, and (6) the effects of certain drugs in the intestine, e.g., some of the broad-spectrum antibiotics.

The antidiarrheic drugs are less likely to be used without medical supervision than are the cathartics. Diarrhea may at times have serious consequences in terms of dehydration, loss of electrolytes, vitamins, and food materials, and exhaustion. In view of the numerous possible causes, it is evident that effective treatment depends on discovering the cause and removing it if possible. In a few instances the administration of a cathartic which brings about the emptying of the entire bowel may be the best way of relieving the diarrhea because it brings about the elimination of the material that is irritating the bowel. Since diarrhea is looked upon as a defense mechanism on the part of the bowel against irritants or toxins which may be present, the diarrhea preferably should not be checked until the cause has been determined.

The drugs used in the treatment of diarrhea include (1) demulcents, (2) adsorbents, (3) astringents, (4) carminatives, (5) antiseptics, and (6) sedatives and antispasmodics.

Demulcents

The demulcents are preparations that have a soothing effect on the irritated membrane of the gastrointestinal tract. The demulcents in common use are salts of bismuth, calcium carbonate, and magnesium oxide. The bismuth preparations supposedly coat the irritated membrane and act mechanically as a protective.

Preparation, dosage, and administration.

Bismuth Subcarbonate, U.S.P.; *Bismuth Subnitrate*, N.F.; *Bismuth Subgallate*, N.F. These compounds are available in powder form or in tablets for oral administration. The usual dose is 1 to 4 Gm. four times a day. Large doses of bismuth subnitrate may be responsible for a nitrite reaction and it is administered less often than the subcarbonate.

Precipitated Calcium Carbonate, U.S.P. The usual dose is 1 to 2 Gm. two or four times a day.

Bismuth Magma, N.F. (Milk of Bismuth).

Adsorbents

Preparations that adsorb gas or toxic substances from the stomach and bowel have been used extensively, but their value in the control of diarrhea has come to be questioned. If they are effective adsorbents they adsorb not only undesirable substances but desirable ones such as enzymes and food nutrients as well. Hydrophilic substances such as psyllium hydrophilic mucilloid (Metamucil) are sometimes combined with adsorbents for use as antidiarrheics. They contribute adhesiveness to the stool but do not necessarily stop the diarrhea. Adsorbents have an advantage of being inexpensive and nontoxic.

Preparation, dosage, and administration.

Activated Charcoal, N.F. In a dry state this is one of the most effective adsorbent substances. The usual dose is 1 Gm.

Kaolin, N.F.; *Light Kaolin*, B.P. This is a naturally occurring aluminum silicate, long used by the Chinese for the relief of diarrhea. It is given suspended in water in doses of 15 to 60 Gm. every 3 or 4 hours until relief is obtained.

Kaolin Mixture with Pectin, N.F. (Kaopectate). This mixture contains kaolin and pectin and acts as both an adsorbent and demulcent. Pectin is a coarse, yellowish powder which, when mixed with water, has a mucilaginous consistency. Ground raw apples constitute a good source of it and have been used in the treatment of diarrhea, especially of children. Kaopectate is effective but must be given in relatively large doses, 15 to 30 ml. several times a day.

Astringents

Astringents are substances that shrink swollen and inflamed tissues such as the intestinal mucosa of the patient suffering from diarrhea. Astringents precipitate proteins and form an insoluble substance (a protein salt) over the mucous membrane and thus protect it from irritating substances. Astringents also inhibit secretions. Tannic acid has long been used as an astringent in the treatment of diarrhea, but there is some doubt as to its effectiveness beyond the stomach because it may combine with food substances and be destroyed by hydrolysis.

Preparation, dosage, and administration.

Tannic Acid, N.F., B.P. When given orally the preparation is best given in a capsule since it may otherwise cause gastric irritation, nausea, and vomiting. The usual dose is 1 Gm.

The bismuth salts, mentioned under demulcents, also exert an astringent effect.

Carminatives

A number have been mentioned earlier in this chapter.

Antiseptics

Sulfonamides

Several of the sulfonamide compounds which are poorly absorbed from the intestine have been used in the treatment of certain cases of bacillary dysentery. These have included sulfaguanadine and succinylsulfathiazole. However, sulfadiazine (which is absorbed from the bowel) has come to be the preparation of choice. It is also the preparation of choice for the treatment of cholera. The usual full doses of the drug are employed. The initial dose is usually 2 to 4 Gm. followed by 1 Gm. every 4 to 6 hours. Adequate fluid intake should be provided for the patient.

Salicylazosulfapyridine (Azulfidine) is employed in the treatment of secondary infections of patients who suffer from chronic ulcerative colitis. One gram is administered every 4 hours around the clock, or when the patient becomes ambulatory 1 Gm. may be given after meals and at bedtime for a period of one or two weeks.

Antibiotics

Several of the antibiotics are bactericidal when administered orally, e.g., streptomycin, chloramphenicol, and the tetracyclines. Combinations of penicillin and streptomycin may also be given intramuscularly for certain infections of the bowel.

Other drugs

A number of other drugs have been used for their antiseptic effect in the intestine and they include drugs such as methylene blue, gentian violet, and phenylsalicylate (Salol). Certain arsenicals, emetine, the iodohydroxyquinoline compounds, as well as certain antibiotics, are used in the treatment of amebic dysentery. See Chapter 22.

Sedatives and antispasmodics

The sedatives most often used to relieve diarrhea are preparations of opium such as camphorated opium tincture (paregoric) and opium tincture (laudanum). The dosage of opium tincture is usually 0.3 to 1 ml. (5 to 15 minims), and the dosage of the camphorated opium tincture is 4 to 8 ml. (1 to 2 fluidrams) three or four times daily. Codeine and morphine are sometimes used but should not be employed for chronic conditions because of the hazard of producing addiction.

Belladonna and its alkaloids, either natural or synthetic, are employed for their antispasmodic action on the intestine. Belladonna tincture, 10 drops, and phenobarbital are frequently prescribed for the relief of tenesmus (painful persistent desire to empty the rectum).

Patients who have suffered from persistent diarrhea invariably have need for the replacement not only of fluids but also of vitamins, electrolytes, and food lost by excessive peristalsis.

Questions
for study and review

1 What organs make up the alimentary tract?
2 Explain how flavoring agents may promote the desirable action of a drug.
3 Why is it impossible to use as a tooth powder or dentifrice a substance that is capable of marked power of disinfection? What is the most we may expect of a dentifrice?
4 When using a salt solution for a gargle, why is it preferable to use a normal salt solution rather than a strong salt solution?
5 Mention some of the ways drugs may affect the stomach.
6 Name several simple emetics.
7 Name several preparations that are useful to check vomiting.
8 What are several popular misconceptions about constipation?
9 Name several conditions in which cathartics are contraindicated.
10 When a person walks into a drugstore and asks for a cathartic, why is a good druggist likely to inquire whether the person has any nausea or abdominal pain?
11 What are three ways by which cathartics may act upon the intestine?
12 Indicate the method of action for each of the following:
 a. magnesium sulfate
 b. mineral oil
 c. castor oil
 d. milk of magnesia
 e. cascara
 f. dioctyl sodium sulfosuccinate
 g. psyllium seed
13 How does a laxative differ from a purgative?
14 What group of cathartics are particularly indicated for patients with edema?
15 In case of food poisoning, why would castor oil be a more suitable cathartic than cascara?
16 What suggestions would you give to a person who asked you what could be done to overcome habitual constipation?
17 What special care must be taken of rubber sheets when bed patients are given mineral oil? What advantage does a mixture of agar and mineral oil have over mineral oil alone?
18 Evaluate the claims made for cathartics on present-day television and radio programs.

Single choice
Encircle the answer of your choice.

19 For which of the following reasons is saccharin sometimes used in medicines?
 a. as an antacid
 b. to increase caloric content
 c. as a flavoring agent
 d. as a digestant
20 Which of the following is a good example of a systemic antacid?

a. calcium carbonate
b. sodium bicarbonate
c. lime water
d. rhubarb and soda

21 Which of the following is a good example of a nonsystemic antacid?
a. aluminum hydroxide
b. calcium chloride
c. sodium bicarbonate
d. sodium carbonate

22 Which of the following represents the most outstanding precaution to observe when giving hydrochloric acid to a patient?
a. dilute well with water
b. give with meals
c. give after meals
d. follow administration with a drink of water

23 A potent stimulant of gastric secretions is:
a. hydrochloric acid
b. alcohol 7 per cent
c. histamine phosphate
d. glutamic acid

24 All of the following preparations act both as an antacid and as a cathartic except:
a. rhubarb and soda mixture
b. magnesium hydroxide
c. magnesium oxide
d. bismuth subcarbonate

25 Kaopectate can be expected to relieve diarrhea by producing which of the following effects?
a. cathartic and demulcent
b. adsorbent and demulcent
c. adsorbent and astringent
d. carminative and sedative

26 In which of the following classifications would essence of peppermint belong?
a. digestant
b. antemetic
c. carminative
d. antidiarrheic

27 Which of the following substances is responsible for the cathartic effect when milk of magnesia is administered?
a. magnesium citrate
b. magnesium chloride
c. magnesium carbonate
d. magnesium hydroxide

28 Methylcellulose is a cathartic that acts in which of the following ways?
a. irritation of the intestine
b. formation of bulk
c. stimulation of bile flow
d. detergent action

29 The active ingredients in compound licorice powder are:
a. phenolphthalein and sulfur
b. sulfur and senna
c. aloin and senna
d. cascara and aloe

30 Of the following cathartics which would you say is the one of choice for children?
a. castor oil
b. senna syrup
c. milk of magnesia
d. sodium sulfate

31 The usual therapeutic dosage of Aromatic fluidextract of Cascara Sagrada is:
a. ounces ½ to 1
b. fluidrams 1 to 2
c. 10 to 15 ℳ
d. gr. 5 to 15

32 A sulfonamide of choice for bacillary dysentery is:
a. sulfadiazine
b. sulfathiazole
c. Azulfidine
d. Sulfasuxidine

33 If an acquaintance of yours remarks as follows: "I see nothing wrong with (a certain popular, widely advertised irritant cathartic). I find these pills very effective." Which of the following statements would you consider the most suitable reply?
a. "They are all right if you want to be taken in by high-pressure advertising."
b. "I don't doubt that they act as a cathartic but they are known to contain a strong irritant and the best cathartics are mild in action."
c. "You really ought to see your doctor if you have constipation. You may have something seriously wrong with you."
d. "Well I can't take the responsibility for advising you, but I guess they can't hurt you if you don't use them too often."

34 If a young mother approached you for advice regarding her 7-year-old son, saying: "Johnny seems to be perfectly well but he has not had a bowel movement for two days. What kind of a cathartic do you think I should give him?" which of the following replies would you consider the safest and the most helpful?
a. "You had better see your doctor; cathartics can be dangerous if used at the wrong time."

b. "A dose of castor oil should take care of him nicely."

c. "The use of a glycerine suppository will probably take care of his immediate needs, and then see that he gets plenty of fruits and vegetables in his diet."

d. "A teaspoonful of milk of magnesia is a mild cathartic and well suited to the needs of children."

35 If you were to accompany a patient into a part of the world where the weather will be warm, and the patient suggests taking along some simple medicinal substances among which is bismuth subcarbonate, which of the following statements would, in your opinion, be most appropriate?

a. "I don't think it would be advisable for us to plan to dose ourselves for things we may encounter in the course of our travels."

b. "I think it would be better for you to get your doctor to prescribe some paregoric."

c. "Bismuth subcarbonate is harmless and easy to carry. I think it would be a good idea to take some if it meets with your doctor's approval."

d. "Sulfonamides are likely to be more effective, and they are also easy to carry."

36 If a young woman tells you that she is accustomed to taking a tablespoon of a certain saline cathartic every other day and expresses an interest in your opinion of the practice, which of the following replies would you consider the most helpful and appropriate?

a. "This cathartic contains a salt fit only for animals."

b. "This cathartic contains sodium sulfate which is one of the most disagreeable of the salines."

c. "This preparation acts like most of the salines, but I am concerned that you find you must take it at all."

d. "Widely advertised cathartics such as this one are frequently overrated products."

37 If a patient tells you that she insists that all of her children eat plenty of bran for breakfast so that they will never have trouble with constipation, which of the following replies would you consider most pertinent and helpful?

a. "Bran is an easy way to add bulk to the diet."

b. "Bran is likely to cause an intestinal obstruction and you should be careful about urging anyone to take it.'"

c. "Have you consulted your doctor about the use of bran?"

d. "Bran can be irritating to the bowel and really is not needed by normal individuals."

Multiple choice
Encircle all the suitable answers.

38 Effects that antacids may produce include:
a. depression of gastric glands
b. chemical neutralization of acid
c. stimulation of sphincter muscles of the stomach
d. soothing effect on gastric mucosa
e. formation of bulk
f. adsorption of acid
g. relaxation of gastric muscle
h. astringent effect

39 Characteristics of a good antacid:
a. inexpensive
b. does not alter the pH of the blood easily
c. effective in controlling gastric acid
d. does not cause acid rebound
e. does not form gas in the stomach
f. helps to control diarrhea or constipation
g. long acting

40 Check the cathartics that act in the intestine by irritation:
a. mineral oil and milk of magnesia
b. methylcellulose
c. cascara
d. compound licorice powder
e. phenolphthalein
f. oleum ricini
g. Epsom salt
h. milk of magnesia

41 Ways by which the bulky content of the intestine may be increased:
a. formation of isotonic solutions in the bowel
b. ingestion of indigestible material
c. accumulation of gaseous material
d. osmotic conditions which cause fluid to be drawn into the intestine
e. irritation of the intestinal mucosa

42 Conditions for which cathartics are usually contraindicated:
a. undiagnosed abdominal pain
b. food poisoning

c. edema
d. intestinal obstruction
e. chronic constipation
f. prolonged diarrhea
g. bowel surgery (immediate postoperative period)
h. pregnancy

References

Alvarez, W. C.: Gastro-Enterology, New York, 1949, Paul B. Hoeber, Inc.

A. M. A. Council on Drugs: New and Nonofficial Drugs, Philadelphia, 1960, J. B. Lippincott Co.

Bard, Philip: Medical Physiology, St. Louis, 1956, The C. V. Mosby Co.

Beckman, H.: Drugs, Their Nature, Action and Use, Philadelphia, 1958, W. B. Saunders Co.

Best, Charles H., and Taylor, Norman B.: The Physiological Basis of Medical Practice, Baltimore, 1955, Williams & Wilkins Co.

Carlson, A. J., and Johnson, V.: The Machinery of the Body, Chicago, 1953, University of Chicago Press.

Collins, E. N.: Use of Aluminum Hydroxide and Other Nonabsorbable Antacids in the Treatment of Peptic Ulcer, J. A. M. A. 127: 899, 1945.

Drill, V. A. (editor): Pharmacology in Medicine, New York, 1958, McGraw-Hill Book Co., Inc.

Editorial: Which Tooth Paste to Use, Consumer's Research Bulletin, March, 1954, pp. 22-26.

Editorial: Is There a Therapeutic Dentifrice? J. A. M. A. 155: 366, 1954.

Frohman, I. P.: Constipation, Am. J. Nursing 55: 65, 1955.

Gambill, E. E.: Drugs in Peptic Ulcer, Minnesota Med. 37: 787, 1954.

Goodman, Louis, and Gilman, Alfred: The Pharmacological Basis of Therapeutics, New York, 1955, The Macmillan Co.

Help Your Doctor to Help You When You Have Constipation, New York, 1942, Harper & Bros.

Knutson, J. W.: Fluoridation, Where Are We Today? Am. J. Nursing 60: 196, 1960.

Modell, W.: Drugs of Choice, 1960-1961, St. Louis, 1960, The C. V. Mosby Co.

Morgan, J. W.: The Harmful Effects of Mineral Oil Purgatives, J. A. M. A. 117: 1335, 1941.

Salter, W. T.: A Textbook of Pharmacology, Philadelphia, 1952, W. B. Saunders Co.

Sollman, Torald: A Manual of Pharmacology, Philadelphia, 1957, W. B. Saunders Co.

Chapter 14

Drugs that affect
the
circulatory system

The circulatory system, like the nervous system and the respiratory system, can be considered as a single physiologic unit, the ultimate function of the circulation being to maintain the proper composition of the medium that bathes all cells (extracellular fluid) by providing for the continuous supply of oxygen and nutrients and the continuous removal of potentially toxic products of metabolism such as carbon dioxide, ammonia, and organic acids. Failure of the circulation, even for a short period, can produce irreversible changes in certain cells (notably those of the brain), leading to death of the individual; failure of the circulation in cardiac failure or in shock, therefore, represents a therapeutic emergency.

The circulation in its simplest mechanical terms can be considered to include a muscular pump (the heart) and a system of vessels which divide and subdivide to the dimensions of the capillaries, tiny tubules through whose thin walls the critical diffusion of gases and other chemicals in solution actually takes place.

In its system of controls, however, the circulatory system is amazingly complex; the flow of blood can be altered by changes in the rate of the heart, in the force of ejection of the blood, or by changes in the diameter of the blood vessels. Individual drugs may be used to affect any or all of these functions in different directions, and the exact site at which a given drug may act can be quite diverse even in accomplishing the same overall effect. Thus some drugs may influence the heart rate by a direct action on the heart muscle, others by an effect on the brain centers controlling heart rate, and still others by action on some of the reflex centers of the medulla (vagal centers). Drugs may lower blood pressure by acting through quite different mechanisms; by blocking autonomic ganglia (hexamethonium) which send adrenergic impulses to the heart, or by producing direct relaxation of blood vessels, thereby increasing the capacity of the vascular bed. The intelligent nursing student should try to understand what is known of the mechanism by which a drug produces a certain effect on the circulation (or on any other system) so that the reasons for using one or another agent may be clearer to her and so that she can understand the basis for certain side actions or toxic actions as these develop.

Anatomy and physiology of the heart (points of review)

The heart is a complex muscular pump of remarkable efficiency. Fortunately the heart muscle is tough and strong. It pumps nine to ten tons of blood daily through 60,000 to 100,000 miles of blood vessels.*

It has four chambers with a complete septum between the two sides. The efficiency of it depends on accurate timing and sequence of contraction of the ventricles in relation to the atria. Being highly specialized, with thick muscular walls, in the mammal, it requires a circulation of its own for nutrition and oxygen supply. This is furnished by the coronary circulation.

Special tissues

Special tissues include (1) the sinoatrial node, (2) the functional tissue between the atria and ventricles, including the atrioventricular node, (3) the atrioventricular bundle or bundle of His, and (4) the right and left septal divisions of the bundle and their branches.

The efficiency of the heart as a pump is a matter of great importance in both health and disease. Muscular work that lasts more than a few seconds demands renewed circulation. The brain deprived of circulation for a few minutes is damaged permanently. The heart itself fails almost instantly if the coronary supply is shut off. Both the timing of the atria and the coronary circulation are frequently damaged by disease.

Heart muscles resemble other muscles in the possession of three qualities: tone or maintained mild contraction, irritability or readiness to respond to stimulation, and contractility. The contractility of heart muscles differs from that of other muscles in that it is rhythmic and depends upon certain intrinsic properties of the muscle itself and not alone upon impulses received through nerves. Moreover, the atria and ventricles of the heart can contract independently of one another; the atria are capable of beating three times as fast as the ventricles whose intrinsic rate is 30 to 40 beats per minute. The contraction wave begins in the atria and is transmitted by the atrioventricular bundle to the ventricles, which pump the blood into the arteries and determine the pulse. Normally the beat of its atria is followed in about a fifth of a second by the beat of the

*Soehren, Irene: New Treatment for Coronary Disease, Today's Health, p. 22, Feb., 1957.

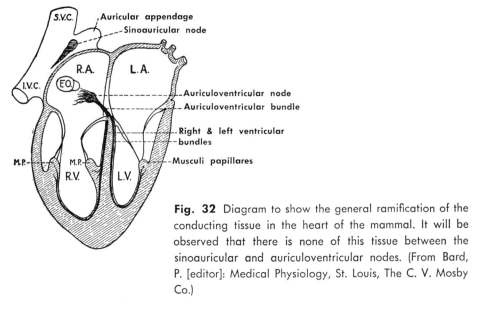

Fig. 32 Diagram to show the general ramification of the conducting tissue in the heart of the mammal. It will be observed that there is none of this tissue between the sinoauricular and auriculoventricular nodes. (From Bard, P. [editor]: Medical Physiology, St. Louis, The C. V. Mosby Co.)

ventricles, the whole contraction forming the systole which occurs about 72 times a minute. Each systole or contraction is followed immediately by a period of relaxation called the diastole.

Heart muscle differs from skeletal muscle in that its refractory period is relatively long. This means that heart muscle will not respond to a second stimulus as long as its fibers are in a contracted state.

The long refractory periods of cardiac muscle help to preserve the cardiac rhythm. Although the muscle is only relatively refractory during diastole, response to further stimulation is discouraged until complete relaxation of the muscle fibers has occurred.

Blood supply

The blood which flows through the chambers of the heart nourishes only the cells of the endocardium. The pericardial arteries supply the pericardium. The right and left coronary arteries are the important sources of blood for the heart muscle itself. The flow of blood through the coronary arteries is greatest during diastole and least during systole, although the coronary outflow is greatest during ventricular systole. Consequently, prolonged rapid heart action is prone to result in a poorly nourished and hence a weakened heart muscle. The coronary vessels are supplied with nerve fibers from both divisions of the autonomic nervous system.

Nerve supply

The contractions of the heart muscle are regulated by the accelerator nerves of the sympathetic nervous system and by the inhibitory nerves, the vagi of the parasympathetic division. Stimulation of the accelerator nerves causes the heart to beat stronger and faster. The impulses originate in the cardio-accelerator center of the medulla, pass over the nerves, and activate the sinoatrial node or the pacemaker of the heart. The periods of rest and diastole are therefore shortened. Stimulation of the inhibitory nerves causes the heart to beat more slowly and weakly. The period of relaxation or diastole is longer. Activation of the vagus nerve may result from stimulation of the vagus center in the medulla or anywhere along the course of the nerve or in the endings and myoneural junctions. The vagus is the only nerve the stimulation of which directly slows the heart. High blood pressure from any cause tends to slow the heart by reflex stimulation of the vagus center in the medulla.

Blood pressure

In order that the circulation of blood through the body be continuous, it is essential that the blood exert a certain force against the walls of the vessels in which it is contained. This force is measured by changes in blood pressure. Blood pressure is modified by the following:

1. The rate and force of the heartbeat. A forceful heartbeat tends to raise blood pressure, whereas a weak beat tends to lower blood pressure.

2. The resistance which the blood vessels offer to the passage of blood. Vasoconstriction tends to increase blood pressure while vasodilation lowers blood pressure.

3. Other factors, such as the total volume of blood and its viscosity, also affect blood pressure.

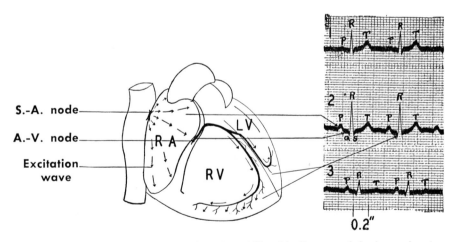

Fig. 33 Electrocardiogram. Leads I, II, and III, with diagram of the heart showing schematically the origin of the waves. (From Bard, P. [editor]: Medical Physiology, St. Louis, The C. V. Mosby Co.)

Circulatory disease

Diseases of the heart and blood vessels as a cause of death have assumed greater and greater proportions, until now they are the leading cause of death in this country. About one out of every two deaths has been reported to be due to cardiovascular disease in one or more of its various ramifications.* This is primarily a reflection of the fact that the death rate from other causes, particularly infections, has dropped.

Congestive heart failure

The symptoms of cardiac insufficiency of which a patient is likely to complain are due to the inability of the heart muscle to function efficiently as a pump. Failure of the circulation due to failure of the heart as a pump is one of the most common kinds of heart disease and can occur as a late event following various kinds of underlying disease of the heart and/or blood vessels. Structural deformities of the heart valves caused by rheumatic fever or by degenerating aging changes (arteriosclerosis) can impair the efficiency of the heart; insufficient coronary circulation can lead to scarring and weakening of the heart muscle; or hypertension can lead to enlargement of the heart to the point where it can no longer pump efficiently. If blood is not forced out of the heart, it will be dammed back in the great veins and into the organs drained by these veins. If the left ventricle fails, the lungs become congested, and symptoms of dyspnea and cough appear. Failure of the right ventricle causes congestion in the systemic veins, giving rise to generalized edema. Inefficiency in both ventricles will cause inadequate oxygenation of blood and the appearance of cyanosis. Either the right or the left ventricle may fail, and usually there are manifestations of failure in both. This type of circulatory failure is called "congestive" because of the distended veins and the tendency to edema (either in the lungs or the extremities or both) which is quite characteristic.

Coronary disease

When the coronary arteries become thrombosed, narrowed, or sclerosed, certain portions of the heart muscle will receive an insufficient supply of blood. This will give rise to pain in the heart or cardiac region. Pain due to the narrowing of the coronary arteries is called *angina pectoris*. When the coronary circulation is suddenly reduced, a portion of the heart muscle supplied by the occluded vessel may become necrotic (die) and be replaced by scar tissue. This event, called a "coronary occlusion" or "myocardial infarct," is usually accompanied by extreme pain and distress, often collapse and shock, and, not infrequently, sudden death.

*White, Paul D.: Heart Disease, New York, 1951, The Macmillan Co., p. 268.

Auricular fibrillation

Auricular fibrillation is a type of arrhythmia in which a region of atrial structure transmits nerve impulses with such extreme rapidity that only portions of the atrial wall are able to respond. As a result, the atrial walls quiver or "fibrillate." Likewise all of the impulses are not transmitted to the walls of the ventricles, causing them to beat rapidly but irregularly and at a slower rate than the atria. This condition is serious because the rapid rate of contraction may cause the heart to fail.

Atrial flutter

Atrial flutter is a form of arrhythmia similar to atrial fibrillation except that the rate of contraction of the atria is not as extreme. They respond to each impulse, however, so that the rate of contraction is very fast. All of the impulses are not conducted to the ventricles, but they may respond to every second or third beat with more or less regularity.

Heart block

Impairment of the conduction mechanism between the atria and the ventricles may result in some impulses getting through and some failing to get through. This is known as *partial heart block*. When no impulses get through, *complete heart block* is said to be present. The ventricles then beat according to a rhythm of their own, independently from the atria, and more slowly.

One of the causes of heart block is death of a critical region of heart muscle (containing the conduction tissue) due to coronary insufficiency.

Effect of drugs upon the heart

Drugs may change the rate, the force, and the rhythm of the heart.

Heart stimulants

Many of the heart stimulants have been discussed in greater detail elsewhere and will be only mentioned here. They increase the rate of action of the heart.

Atropine

Atropine makes the heartbeat stronger and faster because of its action which causes the nerve impulses along the vagi to be ineffective. Since the inhibitory action of the vagus is removed, the heart beats faster and stronger.

Caffeine

Caffeine stimulants the myocardium directly and produces a rapid, strong pulse for a short time. It is used in treatment of collapse, or heart failure to improve breathing and pulse. Other members of the caffeine group are sometimes valuable to relax coronary blood vessels in attacks of coronary disease.

Epinephrine

Epinephrine may be given intravenously or intramuscularly as a powerful emergency circulatory stimulant. When given intravenously it must be well diluted, given slowly, and in small quantities. Its effects appear to be due chiefly to its power as a vasoconstrictor, although some authorities maintain that it stimulates the myocardium directly and also the conduction tissue.*

Drugs that improve quality of the heart's action (cardiotonics)
Cardiac glycosides

The digitalis family of drugs is among the oldest and most important groups of compounds available to the physician. Their use in medicine, dating from the thirteenth century, was made rational toward the end of the eighteenth century. At present they are indispensable drugs in the treatment of heart disease, particularly in the treatment of heart failure.

Chemically, all digitalis-like compounds are closely related in that they are made up of a sugar portion and a steroid portion, linked together in glycosidic linkage. This group of compounds is therefore sometimes referred to as the "cardiac glycosides." The steroid portion of the cardiac glycosides is similar in general structure to the chemical nucleus making up the sex hormones (testosterone, estradiol, etc.) and the adrenal cortical hormones (corticosterones). A third chemical feature required for the typical action of the cardiac (or digitalis) glycosides is a five-membered *lactone* ring attached to carbon 17 of the steroid nucleus. These structures are illustrated in the accompanying structural formula of digitoxin, one of the therapeutically important pure glycosides present in the foxglove, *Digitalis purpurea*.

When the sugar or sugars are removed from a glycoside, the remainder of the compound is called an *aglycone* or *genin*. Thus when digitoxin which contains three molecules of a peculiar monosaccharide called digitoxose is treated so as to cleave off the sugar portions, the remainder of the molecule (steroid plus lactone) is called digitoxigenin.

Many of the digitalis glycosides have their typical cardiac action even

*Goodman, L., and Gilman, A.: Pharmacological Basis of Therapeutics, New York, 1955, The Macmillan Co., p. 481.

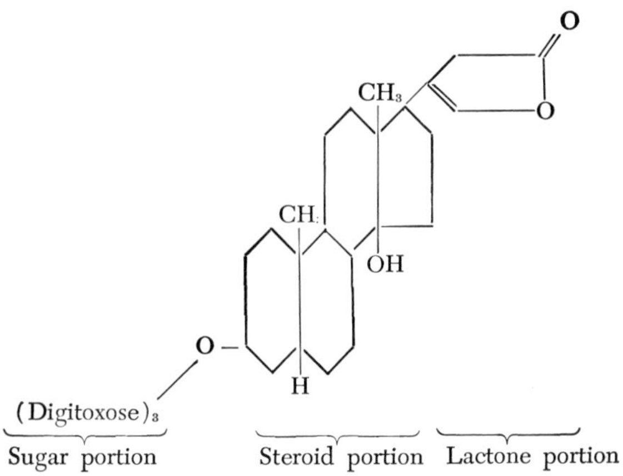

Sugar portion   Steroid portion   Lactone portion

(Digitoxose)₃

Digitoxin

when the sugar residues are removed, although often to a less potent and less prolonged degree than if the sugar(s) are present. The lactone portion, however, is absolutely required for typical cardiac action. The presence of the sugar or sugars in the molecule of the glycosides is thought to affect such things as permeability of cell membranes, solubility, and cellular distribution.

The digitalis series

Many substances, of which digitalis is the most important, are characterized by their action on the heart. These substances belong to many different botanical families. For ages they have been used empirically in therapeutics. The action of each is fundamentally the same, so that the description for digitalis, with minor differences, will apply to all.

The most important plants that contain digitaloid substances are as follows:

Digitalis purpurea	Purple foxglove
Digitalis lanata	White foxglove
Strophanthus hispidus—S. kombé	(An African arrow poison)
Scilla maritima	Squills or sea onion

Source. Digitalis is the dried leaves of *Digitalis purpurea*, or purple foxglove. This plant is cultivated for the drug market in England, America, and Germany, and grows wild in Europe, the United States, and Australia. Early investigators gave the plant the name of "Digitalis purpurea" because the flower is purple and resembles a finger. William Withering of England, physician and botanist, recognized and recorded the pharmacologic actions of digitalis (1785) and brought about the discovery of its value in treatment of cardiac failure. Digitalis leaves contain a number of glycosides, the most important being digitoxin, gitoxin, and gitalin.

Drugs that affect circulatory system   415

Action and result. There may be a local or a systemic action.

Local. Local irritation is marked. If a small quantity of digitalis is placed in the eye, intense pain, redness and congestion of the conjunctiva, and all the symptoms of inflammation follow. When a solution is held in the mouth, it is frequently followed by burning pain. When it is swallowed, the local irritation of the stomach may cause vomiting. If drawn into the nostrils, it elicits sneezing, coughing, hoarseness, and, in many instances, marked swelling of the mucous membranes. When injected hypodermically, it produces pain and sometimes abscess formation, which forbids this method of administration. Intramuscular injections are sometimes used, although they are not painless and not advisable, since in many cases abscess follows.

Systemic. Systemic effects are brought about by action on several mechanisms, and experimental analyses of these are made by studying the isolated heart, a heart in situ, and isolated parts of the cardiac muscle. The cellular or biochemical mechanisms by which digitalis glycosides have their prominent effects on the heart's rate and muscular action are not well understood. It is believed by some students of the subject that digitalis affects the electric properties of the membrane of heart-muscle cells, perhaps by altering the tendency of cells to hold potassium ions. However, it should be noted that a clear explanation of the action of digitalis at the molecular level is not yet available.

The beneficial effects from this drug are to be seen particularly in the patient with congestive heart failure, in whom the following may be observed:

1. Digitalis *stimulates the heart muscle, causing an increased force of systolic contraction, improved tone, and increased irritability of the heart muscle.* This is apparently the most important action of the drug. The increased force of contraction in the failing heart causes the ventricles to empty more completely and allows the heart to receive an increased amount of venous blood, thus relieving increased venous pressure associated with the failing heart. Increased power of contraction also promotes coronary circulation which favors recuperation of the myocardium.

2. Digitalis *brings about stimulation of the vagus mechanism whereby an increased number of inhibitory impulses is sent to the heart and to the bundle of His.* Although this action tends to result in a slower heartbeat, the present concept of the action of digitalis minimizes the slowing effect as a beneficial factor as compared to the value of increased power of muscle contraction. Improvement of symptoms of congestive heart failure in man has been noted without apparent slowing of the cardiac rate. Slowed heart action and partial heart block are often seen, however, particularly after the administration of large doses.

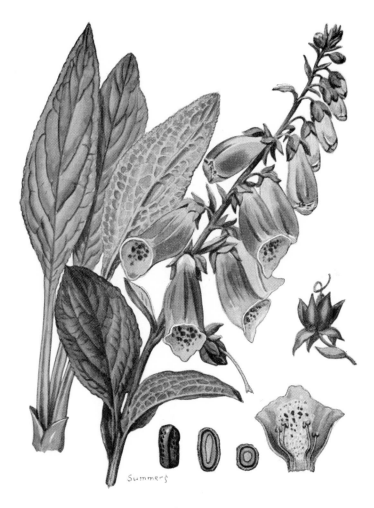

Plate 6

Digitalis purpurea (foxglove). (From Jackson, D. E.: Experimental Pharmacology and Materia Medica, St. Louis, The C. V. Mosby Co.)

The effect of digitalis in a patient with congestive heart failure and in a normal person can, of course, be quite different. This is the difference between a therapeutic and a physiologic action. In the patient for whom the drug is prescribed the heart beats stronger and more forcefully, increasing the cardiac output and improving the circulation to all organs, including the heart itself. Disappearance of edema from the lungs makes breathing easier, from the abdomen ascites gradually disappears, and from all tissues of the body there is relief of the waterlogged condition which may be present. Improved circulation means that more oxygen is brought to the tissues and cyanosis can be expected to disappear. The dilated inefficient heart is frequently reduced in size.

Digitalis is not a diuretic in the sense that it acts primarily on the renal tissue, but marked diuresis may be observed in the edematous patient as a result of the improved heart action and better general circulation. The edema, which forms because of venous congestion, is eliminated by way of the kidney.

In the patient with heart failure the blood pressure may be raised or lowered or not affected at all. Therapeutic amounts of digitalis produce no significant changes in blood pressure of normal persons.

Absorption, excretion, and administration. When digitalis is given by mouth, the active glycosides are absorbed from the intestine. Local irritation of gastric mucosa is decreased by giving the drug with meals or just after meals. The rate at which cardiac effects can be noted depends upon the preparation that is given.

Preparations of digitalis are frequently given by mouth, although several of the purified or crystalline preparations are suitable for intravenous injection. Parenteral injection, however, is usually reserved for cases of emergency. Even purified digitalis preparations tend to be irritating to subcutaneous or muscular tissues. Rectal administration has been used for patients who do not tolerate well the drug by mouth.

The full effects of the digitalis glycosides develop rather slowly. This is true also of the preparations given intravenously, although some effects may be noted within a few minutes. The drug is taken up by all the tissues of the body and eliminated gradually. Repeated doses produce an accumulation of the drug and the eventual development of toxic symptoms. After the drug is stopped, cardiac effects persist for several days and even weeks. It is therefore necessary to know whether a patient has previously received digitalis in some form, the amount, and when, before giving additional drug.

Uses. Although digitalis is a cardiac drug of highest rank, it does not cure heart disease. It may, however, make it much easier for the patient to live within the physiologic limits of his heart action. It is particularly valuable to (1) relieve the symptoms of congestive heart failure and help prevent the recurrence of heart failure and (2) treat atrial fibrillation and atrial flutter when associated with heart failure.

Contraindications. Digitalis is contraindicated in severe myocarditis, heart block, and usually when ventricular tachycardia is present. Valvular disease, pneumonia, diphtheria, and thyrotoxicosis are not in themselves considered indications for digitalis therapy.

Standardization of digitalis preparations. Preparations of digitalis are assayed biologically. The United States Digitalis Reference Standard contains 1 unit of activity in 0.1 Gm. This is equal to the International Digitalis Standard.

The purified glycosides can be identified by chemical and physical means but must be assayed biologically because the amounts present in therapeutic dosage are too small to be accurately identified by physical or chemical means. Digitoxin is assayed (biologically) against the U.S.P. Digitoxin Reference Standard.

Digitalization and choice of preparations. In the treatment of heart failure, the aim is to give digitalis until optimum cardiac effects are achieved. When the patient has reached that state in which he has profited all that he can from the drug, he is said to be digitalized. The amount of drug required for digitalization may vary with each patient. It is associated with the appearance of mild toxic symptoms such as nausea and vomiting.

Usually digitalization is accomplished by giving the patient, over a period of hours or days, a total amount necessary to produce the desired cardiac effect—the "digitalizing" dose—and then keeping him on a smaller daily dose—the "maintenance" dose—designed to replace the daily loss of the drug from his body by destruction or excretion. For example, a common type of schedule for an average adult, using whole leaf digitalis, would include a digitalizing dose of 1.0 to 1.5 Gm., given in divided doses over 1 to 3 days, and then a maintenance dose of 0.1 Gm. daily. Naturally both the digitalizing and the maintenance doses must be adjusted to the particular patient in terms of toxic reactions and clinical signs of adequate digitalization. If digitoxin were administered, 1 to 1.5 mg. (orally) would constitute an average digitalizing dose of the drug and 0.1 to 0.2 mg., the maintenance dose.

Many patients who receive digitalis must continue to take the drug the rest of their lives. The maintenance dose represents the amount of the drug that ensures continued therapeutic effects without toxic symptoms. Again, the amount required varies with the needs of each patient but is always less than the dosage required for the initial digitalization.

Difference of opinion exists as to what is the best digitalis preparation for the treatment of heart disease. Some prefer the standardized preparations of the whole drug, such as the powdered leaf, and others prefer the purified glycosides.

Differences occur chiefly in absorption from the gastrointestinal tract, local emetic action, and speed of excretion.* The glycosides of digitalis are poorly absorbed when the whole drug is administered, which accounts for the fact that only one fifth as much of the intravenous preparation is required as the oral preparation. The digitalis glycosides are irritating to mucous membranes and subcutaneous tissues. Large oral doses of whole drug may produce nausea and vomiting shortly after administration. Smaller doses are less likely to produce emesis from local irritation. The nausea and vomiting occasioned by small doses are due to a central effect on the vomiting center and represent a toxic symptom. All preparations capable of exerting cardiac effects are capable of emetic action, and this untoward effect cannot be avoided by changing to other members of the digitalis group or by changing the method of administration. All preparations of digitalis or digitalis-like drugs have a cumulative action, although some are more cumulative than others. Digitoxin and digitalis leaf have an especially pronounced cumulative action.

In spite of differences of opinion, the use of the whole drug in the form of tincture of digitalis or powdered digitalis is being replaced by the use of refined preparations or by the use of the crystalline glycosides. These are frequently preferred because they are more stable and can be injected and the dosage can be determined more accurately. They are absorbed much more readily when given by mouth and cause less gastrointestinal irritation. Several glycosides are available in a high degree of purity, such as digitoxin, digoxin, and lanatoside C. These make rapid digitalization by an oral method of administration possible with a minimum of local irritant action due to nonabsorbable glycosides.

It should be emphasized that some of the purified digitalis glycosides are extremely potent compounds, and if looked upon as poisons, they are among the most powerful poisons known, some of the glycosides having a lethal dose for man of about 0.1 mg. per kilogram of body weight. The nurse should therefore handle these compounds with great care and respect.

Purple foxglove—preparation, dosage, and administration.

Powdered Digitalis, U.S.P.; *Prepared Digitalis*, B.P. This preparation is available in tablets and capsules. Usual initial dose is 1.5 Gm. divided over 24 to 48 hours. Usual maintenance dose is 0.1 Gm. (1½ gr.) daily.

Digitalis Tincture, N.F. This is the only acceptable form of liquid preparation for oral use; 1 ml. is equal to 1.0 U.S.P. Digitalis Unit. Dose is 1 ml. (15 minims). Calibrated medicine droppers or medicine glasses should be used to ensure accuracy.

*N.N.D., 1960, p. 296.

Gitalin (Amorphous), U.S.P.* (Gitaligin). This is a mixture of glycosides obtained from *Digitalis purpurea*. Its action and uses are the same as those of digitalis, and the same precautions should be taken with its administration. The rate of elimination or destruction is slower than that of digoxin but faster than that of digitoxin. Gitalin is administered orally or intravenously. Full effects are usually obtained from 2 to 3 tablets a day for 3 or 4 days or until 4 to 6.5 mg. are given, although individual requirements vary. The maintenance dose is usually 0.25 to 1 mg. daily. It is marketed in tablets (0.5 mg.), as a solution for injection (2.5 mg. in 5 ml.), and as a solution (drops) for oral administration.

Digitoxin, U.S.P. Digitoxin is the chief active glycoside of *Digitalis purpurea*. It is available in crystalline form and is readily absorbed from the intestinal tract. One milligram of digitoxin has the same effect as 1 Gm. of U.S.P. digitalis when given by mouth. It is available in tablet form as well as in ampules for intravenous therapy. It is extremely poisonous. Average daily oral dose is 0.1 mg. (1/600 gr.). Digitoxin is sold under a number of trade names; e.g., Crystodigin, Unidigin, Purodigin, and Digitaline Nativelle. *Digitoxin Tablets*, U.S.P., are available in amounts of 0.1 and 0.2 mg. Usual oral initial dose is 1.5 mg. over 24 to 48 hours. A dose of 0.5 to 1.2 mg. may be given intravenously for initial digitalization and followed by fractional doses (I.V.) at appropriate intervals or by oral therapy.

White foxglove—preparation, dosage, and administration.

Digilanid.† This is a mixture of the crystallized cardioactive glycosides, lanatoside A, lanatoside B, and lanatoside C, obtained from the leaves of the white foxglove, *Digitalis lanata*. The three components are present in this preparation in the same proportion as found in the crude drug. When these glycosides are hydrolyzed, they yield, respectively, digitoxin, gitoxin, and digoxin. The actions and uses of digilanid are similar to those of digitalis, U.S.P. It can be administered orally, intramuscularly, intravenously, and rectally. Dosage is 0.67 to 1.33 mg. (2 to 4 tablets) and is usually given daily in tablet form until desired effects are obtained, and then 1 to 2 tablets daily as maintenance dosage. Precautions to be observed are the same as those for any digitalis preparation. It is marketed in solution for injection (0.4 mg. in 2 ml.) and in tablets (0.33 mg.).

Lanatoside C, N.F. This glycoside of *Digitalis lanata* is thought to be more active, therapeutically, than the other two glycosides of the white foxglove. Lanatoside C is a white powder which is practically insoluble in water. It is marketed in tablets for oral administration. Lanatoside C tablets usually contain 0.5 mg. of the drug, and 0.5 mg.

*U.S.P. XVI Interim Admission.

†Described in annual publication of A. M. A. Council on Drugs, N.N.D., 1959.

(1/120 gr.) is the usual dose. It is sold under the trade name of *Cedilanid*.

Deslanoside (Desacetyl-Lanatoside C), U.S.P. (Cedilanid-D). This preparation is derived from lanatoside C and has the advantage of being more soluble and more stable than the parent substance. For practical purposes it constitutes the injectable form of lanatoside C. *Deslanoside Injection*, U.S.P., is marketed in 2 and 4 ml. ampules containing 0.4 mg. and 0.8 mg. of the drug, respectively. The initial dose varies from 1.2 to 1.6 mg., and the maintenance dose is 0.2 to 0.6 mg.

Digoxin, U.S.P., B.P. This is a hydrolytic product formed from lanatoside C. It has an advantage over digitalis for the patient who must be rapidly digitalized. Some patients seem to tolerate digoxin better than digitalis. The drug may be given intravenously, in which case saturation of the tissues may be accomplished much more rapidly than with digitalis. Digoxin may also be given orally. It should be administered with caution because it is extremely poisonous. It may bring about digitalization within a few hours when it is administered by mouth and within a few minutes when given intravenously. The usual initial dose when digoxin is administered orally is 1.5 mg. (0.5 to 2 mg.), and when it is given intravenously the usual initial dose is 1 mg. (0.5 to 1.5 mg.). The usual oral maintenance dose is 0.5 mg. daily (0.25 to 0.75 mg.), and the usual intravenous dose for maintenance therapy is 0.5 mg. daily (0.25 to 0.75 mg.). Dosage, of course, must be determined in terms of the needs and response of the patient. Official (U.S.P.) preparations of digoxin are available in tablets (0.25 and 0.5 mg.) and as an injectable solution (0.5 mg. in 2 ml.). The proprietary name *Lanoxin* has an advantage in that it helps to differentiate digoxin and digitoxin which are sometimes mistaken one for the other by the student.

Cardiac glycosides from other sources—preparation, dosage, and administration. Both strophanthin and ouabain are potent glycosides obtained from various species of the plant Strophanthus. Squill, also known as sea onion, contains active glycosides but there are no official preparations.

Strophanthin. This drug is highly similar to ouabain, and because its potency tends to be variable it is seldom used. It is no longer an official preparation.

Ouabain or G-Strophanthin. This preparation is obtained from *Strophanthus gratus*. For many years it was the standard against which all digitalis preparations were measured. It is not absorbed well from the gastrointestinal tract and hence must be given parenterally (usually intravenously). Its action is relatively rapid. Effects appear within about 30 minutes after intravenous injection, and the peak of effect is secured in about 90 minutes. Most of its effects have disappeared within 24 hours.* It is one of the preparations of choice for rapid digitalization. It is relatively soluble and not likely to cause venous thrombosis when given intravenously.

Ouabain Injection, U.S.P., B.P. This form is available in 1 and 2 ml. ampules containing 0.25 mg. per milliliter of solution. The usual dose is 0.5 mg. (120 to 250 mg., B.P.) which should not be repeated in less than 24 hours unless the dose is decreased.

Symptoms and treatment of overdosage. Anorexia, nausea, and vomiting are among the earliest symptoms of poisoning. The nausea and vomiting which follow customary doses of digitalis are due to a systemic action and represent a toxic symptom. The severity of the symptoms depends upon the general condition of the patient, dosage, and length of time the drug has been given. These symptoms alone, however, do not indicate overdigitalization. They are sometimes transient symptoms and are entirely absent in some patients.

Other symptoms include diarrhea and abdominal pain, and slow pulse, rate usually below 60, irregularity in rate and rhythm or a sudden change in the pulse. Partial heart block, extrasystoles, and coupled beats may be noted. Headache, malaise, drowsiness, hallucinations, and sometimes blurred vision or other visual disturbances may be present.

The treatment is to stop the drug and promote elimination if necessary. The patient should be kept absolutely quiet until decided improvement is seen. Atropine and morphine may be given to release the heart from strong stimulation of the vagi and to relieve abdominal pain. Sedatives are sometimes prescribed.

Since toxic effects are usually detected by careful observation of the pulse and the behavior of the heart, a patient who is receiving digitalis needs to be under vigilant medical observation.

Essentials of nursing care

Patients who have heart conditions that demand therapy with one of the cardiac glycosides usually require rest in bed and such anticipation of their needs as will cause them to expend a minimum of energy. An upright position in bed with adequate support will help to relieve dyspnea, and a table made high and wide enough to slip over the bed on which the patient can lean will afford change of position and greater comfort. Sometimes patients are much distressed if they are kept in bed, and in such instances it may be better to make them comfortable in a suitable chair. Other things expected of the nurse would include the following:

1. Careful measurement and record of intake and output of fluids.

*Modell, W. (editor): Drugs of Choice, 1960-1961, St. Louis, 1960, The C. V. Mosby Co., p. 403.

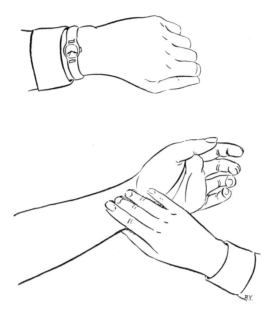

Fig. 34 Counting the pulse. This is done as a precautionary measure by the nurse when administering drugs that are likely to slow the action of the heart, e.g., members of the digitalis group.

2. Observation of the patient's color, degree of edema, and dyspnea.

3. Prompt and accurate administration of the drug with attention to symptoms and signs of early toxicity, especially as related to changes of the pulse. The pulse should be counted prior to giving each dose, and if it has slowed to a count below 60 beats per minute or if there is a sudden change in the beat, the drug should be withheld and the doctor notified.

4. Careful record of the patient's weight.

Understanding on the part of the nurse of the relationship between dosage and potency is fundamental to intelligent cooperation with the physician in the care of the patient who is receiving digitalis or related drugs. When medication is ordered in terms of a small fraction or a decimal fraction, the inference is not only that the drug is potent but also that a mistake in dosage can be especially dangerous even if the amount is small in terms of milligrams. Considerable difference exists among the following dosages of 1 mg., 0.1 mg., 0.15 mg., and 0.2 mg. Obviously 0.2 mg. is twice as much as 0.1 mg., and 1 mg. is ten times as much as 0.1 mg., whereas 0.15 mg. is halfway between 0.1 mg. and 0.2 mg. Differences of a fraction of a milligram can make a great deal of difference when dealing with a potent preparation. The nurse must exert particular care to see that the correct dosage is given.

Drugs that affect circulatory system 423

Heart depressants (anti-arrhythmic drugs)

Many patients with heart disease have, as their most disturbing symptom, changes in the rate of rhythm of the heartbeat, as in auricular fibrillation and auricular flutter. In addition to subjective disturbance and anxiety, these instances of altered heart action may lead to congestive failure, or increase the degree of failure already existing, because they make the circulation less efficient. It has already been noted that the digitalis glycosides frequently produce slowing of the heart rate, although their principal clinical action is to increase the force of contraction.

Another group of drugs (the "antifibrillatory" or "anti-arrhythmic" drugs) have a more selective effect on the heart rate, particularly when this is abnormally elevated. As with many drugs, this effect was discovered accidentally by a patient with auricular fibrillation who was taking quinine for malaria. We now know that quinidine, a compound closely related to quinine, is one of the most effective depressants used in treatment of disordered cardiac rhythm.

Quinidine Sulfate

Quinidine sulfate is the sulfate of the alkaloid quinidine, obtained like quinine from Cinchona bark.

Action. It acts directly on muscle of the auricles, decreasing its irritability and rate of conductivity. It slows the heart and lengthens the time of conduction between the atria and ventricles by increasing the refractory period in the sinoauricular node and auricular muscle. It thus changes a rapid irregular pulse to a slow regular one. The amplitude of contraction may be increased in the compensated heart, thus causing increased filling of the ventricles. Toxic doses, however, decrease the amplitude of contraction. Quinidine is a depressant, whereas digitalis is a stimulant or cardiotonic.

Uses. Quinidine sulfate is used to check both atrial and ventricular fibrillation and restore the normal rhythm of the heart. It is most successful in the treatment of cases of fibrillation of short duration or of a paroxysmal type. When the ventricular rate is rapid or there is evidence of cardiac insufficiency, the patient is frequently digitalized prior to the administration of quinidine. Some physicians expect the nurse to count the pulse before administering quinidine and to withhold the dose if there has been marked slowing or sudden change in the pulse rate.

Comparison of quinidine and digitalis effects. Digitalis increases cardiac irritability, whereas quinidine decreases it.

Quinidine rests the heart by depressing the abnormal auricular impulses, whereas digitalis prevents the impulses from reaching the ventricles as often. It is believed that certain types of cardiac rhythm are caused by an auricular excitation wave that travels in an abnormal circular path and more rapidly than the normal auricular wave. Quinidine, by its property of prolonging the refractory period of cardiac muscle can break the chain of excitation, and the heart may then revert to a normal rhythm.

Preparation, dosage, and administration.

Quinidine Sulfate, U.S.P., B.P. This drug is available in 200 mg. tablets (3 gr.). Quinidine sulfate is given orally in doses of 0.2 to 0.4 Gm. (3 to 6 gr.) and repeated every 4 hours if necessary for from 2 to 3 days. As a rule, its effects are established within that time and may last for several months. In some cases the drug is not effective and its use must be discontinued. A test dose is frequently given to determine whether or not the patient is sensitive to the drug.

Side effects and toxic effects. Untoward reactions to quinidine are believed to result from overdosage or hypersensitivity. Symptoms include the following: nausea and vomiting, dizziness, ringing in the ears, visual disturbances, headache, abdominal cramps, and diarrhea (many of these symptoms are similar to those seen after overdosage with quinine). Some symptoms which are seen reflect hypersensitivity on the part of the patient and include asthma, depression of breathing, drop in blood pressure, fainting, dermatitis, and vascular collapse. Cardiac arrhythmias and cardiac arrest have been known to occur.

Treatment is necessarily symptomatic. Artificial respiration and the use of circulatory and respiratory stimulants may be prescribed. Sometimes all that is required is that administration of the drug be stopped or the dosage reduced.

Successful treatment with quinidine depends upon the careful selection of patients who are to receive the medication and proper dosage of the drug.

Contraindications. It is contraindicated in patients who are hypersensitive or who have an acute infection or marked hyperthyroidism.

Procainamide Hydrochloride (Pronestyl Hydrochloride)

Action. Procainamide hydrochloride decreases the irritability of the muscles of the ventricles of the heart as does procaine hydrochloride, but the effect of procainamide hydrochloride is more prolonged and it is thought to be one half to two thirds as toxic. It has no significant effect on the central nervous system.

Uses. It is used in the treatment of auricular and ventricular arrythmias and for extrasystoles which may occur in the course of cardiac disease or in the course of general anesthesia. It can be administered orally, intravenously, or intramuscularly. When given intravenously it may precipitate hypotension of sufficient intensity to necessitate stopping the administration of the drug. Leukopenia and granulocytopenia have been reported in connection with its repeated use. Intravenously, its action is almost immediate; orally it acts within 30 to 60 minutes.

Preparation, dosage, and administration.

Procainamide Hydrochloride, U.S.P., B.P. (Pronestyl Hydrochloride). This preparation is available in 250 mg. capsules and in solution for injection (100 mg. per milliliter). It is usually administered orally or intravenously.

For ventricular tachycardia in conscious patients 1 Gm. is given orally followed by 0.5 to 1 Gm. every 4 to 6 hours. Intravenously, 0.2 to 1 Gm. (2 to 10 ml. of a solution containing 100 mg. in each milliliter) is administered at the rate of not more than 1 ml. per minute. During anesthesia, 0.1 to 0.5 Gm. is given at a rate not faster than 0.2 Gm. (2 ml.) per minute.*

Drugs that affect the blood vessels

In addition to action on the heart, other important drugs acting on the circulatory system have effects primarily on the blood vessels. Drugs producing vasoconstriction tend to increase the blood pressure, whereas those producing vasodilatation tend to lower the blood pressure. Increased blood flow to the extremities—often desirable in case of arteriosclerosis or of abnormal contraction of blood vessels (Raynaud's disease, for example)—can also be promoted by the use of drugs which increase the lumen of arterioles.

Drugs acting on the peripheral circulation can do so either directly or indirectly. Some of the drugs already considered under the heading of the autonomic nervous system act on blood flow not by a direct effect on the arterial muscle but by changing the number of impulses normally coursing from the autonomic ganglia to control the state of contraction or dilatation of blood vessels. Examples of this general group are the so-called ganglionic blocking agents which reduce or inhibit transmission of autonomic nerve impulses through all autonomic ganglia. Since abolishing autonomic tone completely tends to have greater relaxing than constricting effect on blood vessels, these drugs are vasodilators and lower the blood pressure. Other drugs affect vascular tone by action at still higher centers; e.g., reserpine produces vasodilatation and lowers blood pressure by acting at centers in the hypothalamus. Still other compounds, of which the nitrites are examples, do not appear to act on blood vessels through their nervous control but relax the muscle

*N.N.D., 1960, p. 303.

cells by direct action. As with many classes of other drugs, it should therefore be kept in mind that the same physiologic effect, e.g., vasodilatation with a resultant drop in blood pressure, may result from the action of a drug at one of several different sites—brain, autonomic ganglia, or the muscle cell itself.

Drugs are also used to sclerose and obliterate the lumen of blood vessels (veins) and in this way alter the course of the circulating blood in veins that have developed varicosities.

Vasoconstrictors

Vasoconstrictor drugs usually exert their effects by bringing about contraction of the muscle fibers in the walls of the blood vessels or by stimulation of the vasomotor center in the medulla. They may be used to stop superficial hemorrhage, relieve nasal congestion, raise and sustain the blood pressure, and sometimes increase the force of the heart action. The most important vasoconstrictors are epinephrine, norepinephrine (levarterenol), ephedrine, phenylephrine hydrochloride, and ergotamine tartrate. A number of other adrenergic drugs are used for their local vasoconstricting action.

Several sympathomimetic drugs which are used as vasoconstrictors are mentioned in Chapter 10, Autonomic Drugs.

Epinephrine (Adrenalin)

Action. Small doses of epinephrine will bring about vasodilatation in the skin and skeletal muscles, but larger doses produce a marked rise in blood pressure, due to vasoconstriction and stimulation of the myocardium. The peak of blood pressure is rarely sustained for more than a few minutes. Even after relatively large doses given intravenously, the blood pressure usually has returned to normal limits in 30 minutes. After subcutaneous injection, however, this may not be true because the local vasoconstriction slows the rate of absorption. A transient vasodilatation occurs in the coronary arterioles.

Uses. The chief therapeutic use of epinephrine is to constrict peripheral blood vessels following local application. In this way it is used to diminish hyperemia of the conjunctiva, reduce swelling of the nasal mucosa, and arrest hemorrhage from the mucosa of the upper respiratory tract and in operations on the eye, nose, or ear. It is used to check bleeding from capillaries or small arteries, but it does not stop hemorrhage from a large vessel. For the arrest of hemorrhage, it must be applied directly to the bleeding vessels or congested area. It should not be given for internal, concealed hemorrhage, in which case a rise in the blood pressure is not desirable.

A common use of epinephrine, or related adrenergic drugs, is in combination with a local anesthetic such as procaine (Novocain). Here the beneficial effect of producing local vasoconstriction is to check bleeding, prolong the action of the anesthetic, and also reduce the risk of systemic reactions to the local anesthetic. Both ends are accomplished by reducing absorption of the local anesthetic through drug-induced vasoconstriction in the region anesthetized. It is also used to treat hives, itching, and edema associated with severe allergic reactions.

Preparation, dosage, and administration.

Epinephrine, U.S.P., B.P. (Adrenalin). For subcutaneous or intramuscular injection 0.5 ml. (7 minims) or less of a 1:1,000 solution of epinephrine hydrochloride is used. The intravenous route of administration is not often used, but when it is, the drug must be adequately diluted and given slowly. For other preparations of epinephrine, see pp. 310 and 311.

Contraindications. It is contraindicated as a vasopressor drug in the treatment of shock. It may increase tissue anoxia by constricting arterioles, and it may produce excessive cardiac stimulation.

Levarterenol Bitartrate (Levophed Bitartrate)

Action. Levarterenol bitartrate is a potent pressor substance which differs from epinephrine in that its over-all action is that of vasoconstriction; it does not stimulate the heart to increased output and it tends to slow the pulse when patients are horizontal.* It is said to cause considerably more dilatation of the coronary arteries than does epinephrine.

Uses. It is being used to raise and sustain the blood pressure in acute states of hypotension such as may be seen in patients during or following surgical operation, as well as in traumatic states or after hemorrhage. It has also received some use in the treatment of profound shock occurring after myocardial infarction. In this instance it is far safer than epinephrine would be since the latter drug might produce dangerous ventricular fibrillation of the heart.

It should not be substituted for the administration of appropriate fluids when hypotension is due primarily to depleted blood volume.

Preparation, dosage, and administration.

Levarterenol Bitartrate, U.S.P. (Levophed Bitartrate). This is administered intravenously in 5 per cent dextrose in distilled water or 5 per cent dextrose in a saline solution. The dextrose protects against loss of potency because of oxidation. The drug is available in ampules containing 4 ml. of a 0.2 per cent solution. One ampule is usually added to 1,000 ml. of the fluid to be administered, and the rate of flow is carefully regulated to obtain and maintain the desired effect. The blood

*N.N.D., 1960, p. 219.

pressure should be determined frequently to avoid overdosage. The patient never should be left alone while receiving the drug.

Ephedrine

Ephedrine is the alkaloid of a plant of the genus Ephedra.

Action. Ephedrine affects structures supplied by the sympathetic nervous system much like Adrenalin. In small doses ephedrine stimulates the heart, increasing the rate and strength of the cardiac contractions and raising the blood pressure. In large and toxic doses the drug exerts a depressant action on the heart muscle. When given intramuscularly or intravenously it produces a rather prolonged rise of blood pressure due mainly to its constricting effect on the smooth muscles of the blood vessels. Applied locally, it contracts the capillaries to some extent and thus reduces the swelling of the turbinate bodies and lessens hyperemia.

Uses. Ephedrine is used to sustain the blood pressure in spinal anesthesia and in some types of hypotension, but it is of no benefit in shock, circulatory collapse, or hemorrhage.

Preparation, dosage, and administration. For local application to mucous membranes, ephedrine is used in the form of its official salts (*Ephedrine Sulfate*, U.S.P.; *Ephedrine Hydrochloride*, B.P.) in 0.5 to 2 per cent solutions. These solutions are applied as sprays. The usual dose for oral or parenteral use is 25 mg. For other preparations, see p. 315.

Phenylephrine Hydrochloride (Neo-Synephrine Hydrochloride)

Action. Phenylephrine hydrochloride is an adrenergic agent which is relatively nontoxic and produces a rise in blood pressure, which may be sustained for hours.

Uses. It is used to relieve local congestion of mucous membranes, retard systemic absorption of local anesthetics, and prevent or treat hypotension and shock, provided the hypotension is the result of vasomotor failure rather than loss of blood volume. Whereas phenylephrine is a less potent agent than levarterenol, there are occasions when it is a preferable drug, especially if prolonged intravenous administration is required. It is longer acting than levarterenol, fluctuations in blood pressure are less likely to occur (once blood pressure has been stabilized), and it does not produce slough of tissue in the event that some of the solution escapes from the needle into the subcutaneous tissue. It is sometimes used as a mydriatic and to relieve symptoms of an allergic reaction.

Preparation, dosage, and administration.

Phenylephrine Hydrochloride, U.S.P. (Neo-Synephrine Hydrochloride). This drug can be administered both orally and parenterally (subcutaneously, intramuscularly, and intravenously).

Drugs that affect circulatory system 429

Numerous preparations are available for topical application to mucous membranes of the nose and the eye. See p. 317.

Phenylephrine and Norepinephrine. A combination of norepinephrine and phenylephrine is sometimes used in the same infusion to combine the effects of the two vasopressor agents.

Ergotamine Tartrate

Action. Ergotamine tartrate shares with the other alkaloids of ergot the property of stimulating the smooth muscle of the uterus and the smooth muscle of blood vessels.

Uses. Ergotamine tartrate is of value in the treatment of migraine headache and has come to be considered almost a specific for this particular type of disorder. Its exact mode of action is not fully understood, but some authorities explain it on the basis of decreasing the amplitude of the pulsations of cranial arteries.

This drug also has been used to relieve intense itching and hives associated with jaundice, cirrhosis of the liver, or Hodgkin's disease. The dosage for migraine headache is 0.25 mg. given subcutaneously. Administration of the drug should be followed by bed rest for an hour or two. Best effects are secured if the drug is taken when the attack is just coming on. Since this drug has accumulative action it must be used with caution. It is capable of producing all the symptoms of ergotism: numbness and tingling of the fingers and toes, muscle pains and muscle weakness, as well as gangrene and blindness.

Preparation, dosage, and administration.

Ergotamine Tartrate, U.S.P., B.P. (Gynergen). Usual oral dose is 2 mg., and the usual intramuscular dose is 0.25 mg. Ergotamine tartrate is available in tablets for oral administration (1 mg.), ampules of solution for parenteral administration (0.25 mg. in 0.5 ml. and 0.5 mg. in 1 ml.), and as suppositories for rectal administration.

Ergotamine with Caffeine (Cafergot). Each tablet contains 1 mg. ergotamine tartrate and 100 mg. caffeine. Usual dose is 1 to 2 tablets for headache. Dosage may be repeated if necessary.

Dihydroergotamine (D.H.E. 45). This compound is prepared by hydrogenating ergotamine and is used in the treatment of migraine headache. It is available in 1 ml. ampules which contain 1 mg. of the drug. Administration is intramuscular, subcutaneous, or intravenous. It is said to produce fewer toxic effects than ergotamine tartrate.

Nasal decongestants

Perhaps the most commonly used attribute of the vasoconstricting drugs is their capacity to shrink the engorged nasal mucous membranes in mild upper respiratory infections. This use has already been noted

for some of the previously mentioned drugs which are also used to raise blood pressure. Many drugs, however, are used exclusively as nasal vasoconstrictors. Because of their wide popular use and lack of serious hazard (when used topically), a confusingly large number of preparations have been provided by the ethical pharmaceutical industry, as well as many patent preparations, for direct sale to the public. Some of the more widely used agents in this group are *phenylephrine hydrochloride* (Neo-Synephrine), *ephedrine sulfate, hydroxyamphetamine hydrobomide* (Paredrine), *methoxamine sulfate* (Wyamine Sulfate), *phenylpropanolamine hydrochloride* (Propadrine Hydrochloride), *prophylhexadrine* (Benzedrex), *phenylpropylmethylamine hydrochloride* (Vonedrine), and *naphazoline hydrochloride* (Privine). Students will recognize these drugs as adrenergic agents. They are used to shrink engorged mucous membranes of the nose and to relieve nasal stuffiness. However, there is a tendency on the part of patients to misuse them by using them in too large an amount and too frequently. Preservatives, antihistaminics, detergents, and antibiotics are sometimes added to the preparation of the decongestant. In some cases untoward reactions are believed to be due to the additive rather than to the decongestant.

Vasodilators and drugs used in treatment of hypertension

Drugs that bring about vasodilatation have a number of uses. They play a part in the treatment of peripheral vascular disease, coronary disease, and hypertension. A number of the older drugs act either on the smooth muscle of the blood vessels or on the vasomotor center in the medulla. Some of the newer hypotensive agents exhibit other actions or combinations of actions. These are indicated under the discussion on the individual drug. A good hypotensive agent preferably should exert an effect over a prolonged period (several hours at least) and in a large proportion of cases. It should not be toxic, should not have unpleasant or dangerous side effects, and should be practical for long-term usage. Tolerance should not develop, the drug should not interfere with sleep and preferably it should be suited to oral administration.

Although no one of the drugs being used at present is considered ideal, a number of them are effective in lowering blood pressure of hypertensive patients, especially when the drugs are used in combination.

A number of the older vasodilators will be presented first.

The nitrites

Certain members of the nitrite group of drugs have been used clinically for approximately one hundred years. A number of inorganic as well as organic compounds containing the nitrite (NO_2) or the nitrate

(NO$_3$) radical act as relaxants of smooth muscle. Bismuth subnitrate is an example of an inorganic compound which is changed to a nitrite in the intestine by the action of intestinal bacteria such as *Escherichia coli*, and sufficient absorption of nitrite ions can result in a lowering of blood pressure. Other inorganic nitrates, however, do not exhibit the typical nitrite effect. For a long time it was believed that the organic nitrates owed their pharmacologic effects to the formation of nitrites. It has been found, however, that both organic nitrates and nitrites can cause a prompt fall in blood pressure. This has caused some investigators to conclude that both nitrites and organic nitrates exert similar qualitative effects on the blood and circulatory system. Consequently, "nitrite" as used in the following discussion will include both nitrates and nitrites.

Action and result. The action of the nitrites on blood vessels is a direct one on the cells of smooth muscle, causing the muscle fibers to relax. The effect is seen particularly on the smaller vessels such as the arterioles, capillaries, and small veins. Thus the lumen of the vessel is increased, the blood pressure is reduced, and the capillary flow is increased. The heart is relieved of the extra work of overcoming excessive peripheral resistance. Relaxation and increased flow of blood through the coronary blood vessels is the basis for the greatest therapeutic use of the nitrites. Relaxation of blood vessels in the skin results in a deep flush and increased skin temperature. A similar effect in the meningeal vessels results in increased intracranial pressure which may be great enough to cause severe headache. Increased intraocular tension may result from dilated retinal vessels, hence the need for avoiding nitrites for patients with glaucoma. Blood vessels in the visceral organs are also relaxed.

The smooth muscle which is relaxed by the action of the nitrites is that of the bronchial tubes, the urinary system, the biliary tract, and the gastrointestinal tract. The spasmolytic effect, however, tends to be transient, and large doses are sometimes required to produce a desired effect. The muscle that is hypertonic or spastic gives the most marked response.

Tolerance. Tolerance to the nitrites is easily developed and necessitates the employment of the smallest dose of the drug that will give satisfactory results so that dosage may be increased as tolerance develops. Tolerance begins to appear within a few days and is well established within a few weeks. On the other hand, tolerance is rather easily broken by stopping administration, and the patient is again susceptible to the effects of the drug.

Uses. The nitrites are extensively used for patients with angina pectoris, both for an acute attack and for the prevention of a recurrence of an attack. The rapidly acting nitrites are the preparations of choice for an acute attack, in which the patient suffers severe pain from spasm of coronary vessels. Arteriosclerotic vessels may be unable to relax or change the size of their lumen, but benefit may be secured from better flow of blood through collateral vessels in the heart muscle. Nitroglycerin has come to be the preparation of choice, although 2 or 3 minutes may pass before the patient gets relief after sublingual administration. Amyl nitrite is effective within a few seconds after inhalation, but it is likely to cause a throbbing headache, flushing, and sometimes nausea and vomiting. It is also more expensive than nitroglycerin. Nitroglycerin or one of the longer-acting nitrites may be prescribed in the prophylactic treatment of patients who have anginal attacks.

Nitrites are sometimes used to relieve spasm of smooth muscle, e.g., for pylorospasm as well as biliary and renal colic. They are less effective than epinephrine or related drugs for acute attacks of bronchial asthma.

Nitrites have been employed in the symptomatic treatment of essential hypertension. Although the blood pressure may be lowered, the underlying cause of the condition is not changed and tolerance develops readily. Their use in treatment of hypertension has not been considered satisfactory.

Nitrites are used as an antidote in cyanide poisoning (see Index).

Preparation, dosage, and administration.

Amyl Nitrite, U.S.P. This preparation is available in glass ampules (pearls) which are placed in a loosely woven material that fits over the pearl so that the pearl can be crushed and the drug inhaled. Each pearl contains about 0.3 ml. (5 minims). It has a strong unpleasant odor, and the patient should not inhale more than two or three times to prevent overdosage. Amyl nitrite is very flammable.

Glyceryl Trinitrate Tablets (Nitroglycerin) U.S.P., B.P. These tablets are available in 0.3, 0.4, and 0.6 mg. The usual sublingual dose is 0.4 mg. (1/150 gr.) and may be repeated several times during the day. Hypodermic tablets of this preparation are used when it is desirable to give the drug subcutaneously.

Sodium Nitrite, U.S.P. The usual dose given intravenously as an antidote to cyanide poisoning is 10 ml. of a 3 per cent solution.

Sodium Nitrite Tablets, N.F. The usual oral dose is 30 to 60 mg.

*Mannitol Hexanitrate.** This drug is one of the longer-acting nitrites. It is given orally, and the usual dose is 30 mg. It is available in 16, 30, and 60 mg. tablets.

*Pentaerythritol Tetranitrate** (Peritrate Tetranitrate). This preparation is available in 10 and 20 mg. tablets. It is one of the longer-acting preparations. It is administered orally in doses of 10 to 20 mg. three or four times daily. It may prevent anginal attacks or decrease their severity.

The above preparations vary considerably in the duration of their

*Described in annual publication of A. M. A. Council on Drugs, N.N.D., 1960.

effects. The effects of amyl nitrite last only about 10 minutes, nitroglycerin about 30 minutes, and sodium nitrite 2 to 3 hours, whereas the longer-acting preparations (erythrityl tetranitrate, mannitol hexanitrate, and pentaerythritol tetranitrate) may exert effects over 6 hours or more.

Side effects and toxic effects. A sudden lowering of blood pressure may cause the patient to feel dizzy and faint. Headache may be a symptom which persists until some degree of tolerance is established. Large doses cause flushing of the face and neck, throbbing headache, fainting, drop in blood pressure, and a weak rapid pulse (nitrite reaction). Death from nitrite poisoning is rare but it has occurred. Large doses of nitrites cause hemoglobin to be converted to methemoglobin, which decreases the oxygen-carrying power of the blood. This results in hypoxia and contributes to circulatory collapse.

The patient should be placed with the head low and treated for shock. Oxygen is indicated if the patient is cyanosed. Blood tranfusion may relieve the state of shock.

Nitrites are used with caution, if at all, for patients with severe anemia, glaucoma, or increased intracranial pressure.

Papaverine

Action. Although papaverine is one of the alkaloids of opium, it is free of analgesic and sedative action, has a low level of toxicity, and neither tolerance nor habituation to its use has been reported. The main action of papaverine is seen in cardiac and smooth muscle, especially the smooth muscle of blood vessels.

Papaverine acts directly on cardiac muscle, depresses conduction, and increases the refractory period. It is capable of causing arrhythmias when given intravenously in large doses. Relaxation of muscle in blood vessels occurs especially if spasm has been present. Its effects are seen particularly in the coronary, peripheral, and pulmonary arteries.

Uses. Good results have been obtained by the use of papaverine for peripheral or pulmonary embolism. It acts by increasing the collateral circulation in vascular beds which have been reflexly constricted. When given intravenously in doses of 20 to 100 mg., disturbance of sensation or pain may be very well relieved. It has also been used to prevent threatened gangrene in patients suffering from ergotism. It is thought to increase the coronary blood flow in patients with anginal symptoms. However, it is not considered to be as reliable as nitroglycerin for angina pectoris.

Preparation, dosage, and administration.

Papaverine Hydrochloride, U.S.P., B.P. This drug is available in 1, 2, and 10 ml. ampules containing 30 mg. per milliliter and in 30, 60, 100, and 200 mg. tablets. It is given orally and parenterally (usually intravenously or intramuscularly). The usual range of dosage is 30 to 60 mg. intramuscularly, 60 to 200 mg. orally.

Dioxyline Phosphate (Paveril Phosphate)

Dioxyline phosphate is a synthetic analogue of papaverine which is said to resemble the action of papaverine but to exhibit fewer toxic effects in certain laboratory animals. Its status is at present uncertain. It is available in 200 mg. tablets.

The xanthine group

The xanthine derivatives, caffeine, theobromine, and theophylline, act on the nervous system, the kidneys, and the circulatory system. They are included here because of their circulatory effects. Caffeine and theobromine are less potent agents to relax blood vessels and are rarely used as such. Theophylline is not very soluble and is used almost exclusively in the form of its more soluble compound, aminophylline (theophylline ethylenediamine).

Aminophylline

Uses. Aminophylline is used for its effects as a vasodilator, although conflicting opinion is expressed as to its value. It is said to help prevent attacks of angina pectoris, but it is less suitable to bring relief of an acute attack. It has been employed by some physicians during the acute shock stage of coronary occlusion because of its tendency to stimulate the myocardium and elevate the blood pressure slightly.

Preparation, dosage, and administration.

Aminophylline, U.S.P., B.P. It is available in vials of solution for injection (250 or 500 mg. per vial); in suppositories, 125, 250, and 500 mg.; and as tablets, either plain or enteric-coated, 100 and 200 mg. Aminophylline is usually administered orally in doses of 200 mg., three or four times daily. Absorption after oral administration is said to be somewhat variable. A dose of 250 to 500 mg. may be administered intravenously or intramuscularly. Intravenous injection should be made slowly. The use of aminophylline as a diuretic and in the treatment of asthma is discussed elsewhere (see Index).

Alcohol (Ethyl)

Alcohol produces vasodilation, especially in the cutaneous vessels by a direct depression of the vasomotor center in the medulla. As a result the skin becomes warm and flushed. Alcohol is used for its vasodilating effect in the treatment of certain peripheral vascular diseases such as thromboangiitis obliterans, Raynaud's disease, etc. Some authorities consider moderate amounts of alcohol beneficial in the relief or prevention of attacks of angina pectoris because of its activity as a vasodilator. Evidence seems to indicate, however, that relief of anginal symptoms is due to a central depressant action in the brain rather than to a dilatation of its coronary arteries. Benefit may be secured by mild sedation, rest, and relaxation which an alcoholic beverage may produce. Whisky with soda is probably the alcoholic beverage of choice for cardiac patients.[*]

Nicotinic Acid (Niacin)

Although recognized as a specific form of treatment for pellagra, nicotinic acid also acts directly on the muscle of blood vessels to produce peripheral vasodilation, especially in regions of the head and neck. Intense flushing of the skin occurs about 15 to 60 minutes following an oral dose. It is accompanied by a sense of warmth, tingling, and itching of the skin. It is sometimes prescribed for patients who have recurring attacks of angina pectoris. It has also been used in treatment of Meniere's syndrome by those who believe that vasospasm is associated with this malady. Authorities do not agree about the usefulness of this agent as a vasodilator of clinical significance.

Recently a preparation has become available which has a more prolonged effect than nicotinic acid and is used in the treatment of peripheral vascular diseases. It is the tartaric acid salt of the alcohol corresponding to nicotinic acid and is sold under the trade name of *Roniacol.* It is available in 50 mg. tablets and as an elixir, 50 mg. per 5 ml. It is given orally in doses of 50 to 150 mg. three times a day after meals.

Thiocyanates

Both sodium and potassium thiocyanate were introduced into medicine for the symptomatic treatment of essential hypertension. They are more or less readily absorbed from the gastrointestinal tract and are excreted mainly by way of the kidneys. The rate of excretion is unpredictable, and hence it is necessary to determine the blood level of the drug in order to regulate dosage. The safe limit is said to be between 8 and 14 mg. per 100 ml. of blood.

The thiocyanates tend to be toxic and many patients exhibit symptoms of toxicity even when taking apparently safe doses. Mild symptoms include muscular weakness, fatigue, lethargy, cramping of the leg muscles, nervous irritability, and skin eruption. Severe reactions consist of vascular collapse, mental confusion, delirium, etc.

At present the thiocyanates are used only for the relief of hypertensive

[*]Goodman, L., and Gilman, A.: The Pharmacological Basis of Therapeutics, New York, 1955, The Macmillan Co., p. 110.

headache. Potassium thiocyanate is administered orally. The sodium salt can be given intravenously. Sixty milliliters of a 5 per cent solution are said to relieve headache in most cases in a matter of hours. The potency of these compounds as antihypertensive agents is low when compared to other agents presently available.

Drugs such as the nitrites have gradually been replaced by more potent agents for the treatment of hypertension. As mentioned previously, the ideal drug for this purpose should lower blood pressure effectively without producing undesirable side effects and it should be effective over relatively long periods of time. Tolerance to its effects should not develop, and adverse effects in vital body organs should not be produced. The ideal drug has not been found, although some of the newer preparations are more potent and less toxic than some of the older agents.

The use of sedatives, diets low in sodium chloride, and weight reduction continue to be advocated for hypertensive patients, although these measures alone are insufficient for many patients. Some patients do not respond well to treatment of hypertension with drugs, e.g., patients with severe renal insufficiency or severe psychiatric disturbance. On the other hand, many patients benefit from therapy and are spared damage to the heart, kidneys, and brain. The severity of hypertensive disease is often estimated in terms of the level of the diastolic blood pressure and the degree of change in the retinal vessels of the eye. Except for rare instances the cause of hypertension is unknown.

Among the drugs available for the present-day treatment of hypertension are the rauwolfia preparations, veratrum preparations, hydralazine, the ganglionic blocking agents, and chlorothiazide.

Rauwolfia alkaloids

Source. The shrub *Rauwolfia serpentina* has recently been rediscovered by Western medicine and is the source of a number of chemically distinct alkaloids, which are the compounds *reserpine, rescinnamine,* and *deserpidine.*

Action and result. The most dramatic effect of these compounds is their depressant action on the central nervous system, usually referred to as "tranquilizer" action; but they have an additional important pharmacologic action—they tend to lower blood pressure and have been widely used in the treatment of hypertension.

These compounds are recommended for the treatment of mild and moderate forms of hypertension. They exert their action centrally on the vasomotor center and thus decrease peripheral vasoconstriction. Their antihypertensive effects, however, are variable and not satisfactory in all patients.

Reserpine and its congeners (related compounds) are also thought to depress the hypothalamus and the central sympathetic centers, thus bringing about less predominance of activity of the sympathetic division of the autonomic system. Results of this action include gradual lowering of the blood pressure, relief of dizziness and headache, slowing of the pulse rate and increased motility of the bowel. Some patients experience drowsiness, increased appetite and a tendency to gain weight.

Preparation, dosage, and administration. Rauwolfia drugs may be administered alone or in combination with other antihypertensive agents.

*Rauwolfia** (Raudixin). This drug is the powdered whole root of *Rauwolfia serpentina*. It is administered orally. The daily oral dose for adults is 200 to 400 mg. It is usually divided into two doses. It is available in 50 and 100 mg. tablets.

*Alseroxylon** (Rauwiloid). This preparation is the fat-soluble alkaloidal fraction extracted from the root of the *Rauwolfia serpentina*. It is administered orally. The average adult dose is 2 to 4 mg. daily. Some physicians prescribe 1 to 6 mg. daily. It is available in 2 mg. tablets.

Reserpine, U.S.P., B.P. (Serpasil).† It is administered orally or by intramuscular or intravenous injection. The usual oral dose for adults for mild hypertension is 0.25 to 1 mg. daily in two or three divided doses. Intramuscular injection is said to afford no advantage over intravenous administration. It is a preparation of choice for most hypertensive emergencies, in which case doses of 2.5 to 5 mg. may be given.‡

*Rescinnamine** (Moderil) and *Deserpidine** (Harmonyl). Both are closely related to reserpine. They are administered orally in doses that range from 0.1 to 0.5 mg.

Side effects. Nasal stuffiness is the most common side effect and usually requires no special treatment. Other effects include drowsiness, bradycardia, nightmares, depression, increased secretion of gastric juice, myalgia, and parkinsonian rigidity. The most serious side effect is depression, which may be preceded by feelings of unreality and apprehension. Patients with a history of peptic ulcer or mental depression should not have these drugs. The parkinsonian rigidity occurs chiefly when large doses are administered. This symptom disappears when administration of the drug is discontinued.

---

*Described in annual publication of A. M. A. Council on Drugs, N.N.D., 1960.

†Reserpine is sold under many other trade names. See N.N.D.

‡Gifford, R. W.: Treatment of Hypertensive Emergencies Associated With Essential Hypertension, Collected Papers of the Mayo Clinic, Philadelphia, 1958, W. B. Saunders Co., p. 368.

Veratrum preparations

Source. *Veratrum viride* and *Veratrum album* (green and white helle-bore) are two species of plants which contain alkaloids that have the capacity to slow the heart and lower blood pressure. Protoveratrines A and B (Veralba) constitute a mixture of two alkaloids which have been isolated from *Veratrum album.* Alkavervir (Veriloid) is a preparation of the ester alkaloids of *Veratrum viride.*

Action and result. These drugs exert a depressant action on the vaso-motor center and bring about stimulation of the vagal nuclei which pro-duces slowing of the heart. They all have a central emetic effect as well as a hypotensive effect. The range between the toxic dose and the hypo-tensive dose is narrow and this limits their usefulness.

Uses. The veratrum drugs are said to be best used for hypotensive emergencies when parenteral administration is needed and rapid effects are desired. Patients with hypertensive encephalopathy may be given maintenance treatment by continuous slow infusion or by means of re-peated slow injections. Hypertensive encephalopathy refers to a symptom complex that resembles a convulsive seizure. It may or may not be pre-ceded by prodromal (warning) symptoms. The blood pressure rises dur-ing this period. The patient may be confused, complain of headache and drowsiness, and vomit. Convulsions can occur suddenly, and coma may ensue. The patient may recover or may be left with residual neurologic damage. However, *these preparations are now used chiefly when other drugs fail to be effective.*

Preparation, dosage, and administration. Little is stated in the follow-ing paragraphs about dosage since it must be determined by the physi-cian in relation to each patient.

Alkavervir* (Veriloid). This drug is administered orally and paren-terally (intramuscularly and intravenously). Dosage for parenteral ad-ministration is calculated on the basis of body weight. Blood pressure is taken periodically, and the rate and amount of injection are regulated accordingly.

Cryptenamine Acetates* (Unitensen Acetates). The acetate salts of alkaloids are derived from *Veratrum viride.* This preparation is given intravenously or intramuscularly.

Cryptenamine Tannate* (Unitensen Tannate). The usual oral dose is 2 to 5 mg. four times daily and is administered orally.

Protoveratrine A and B* (Veralba). This drug is administered orally, intravenously, and intramuscularly. The usual oral dose is 0.2 to 0.5 mg. after each meal and at bedtime.

Protoveratrine A and B Maleates* (Provell Maleate). These are ad-ministered orally. The usual dose is 0.2 to 0.5 mg. four times daily.

*Described in annual publication of A. M. A. Council on Drugs, N.N.D., 1960.

Drugs that affect circulatory system   439

Another preparation of *Veratrum viride* (purified alkaloids) is sold under the trade name of *Vergitryl*. It is administered orally. The usual dose is 1 to 4 units (tablets) three times daily.

Side effects and toxic effects. Side effects of the Veratrum preparations include epigastric distress, increased flow of saliva, nausea, vomiting, hiccoughing, and slow pulse. These effects may be abolished with atropine. Overdosage causes bradycardia, hypotension, respiratory depression, and collapse. Ephedrine is useful in overcoming the hypotension.

Contraindications. Veratrum products are contraindicated in patients with high intracranial pressure (which is not secondary to hypertension), in digitalis intoxication, and in patients with uremia (to be used cautiously because such patients have difficulty in adjusting to a lowered blood pressure).

Hydralazine Hydrochloride (Apresoline Hydrochloride)

Hydralazine hydrochloride is considered an antihypertensive agent of moderate potency. It appears to reduce blood pressure by an action on the midbrain and by inactivating a number of pressor substances found in the blood. It diminishes vascular tone and decreases both systolic and diastolic blood pressure. It helps to control essential and early malignant hypertension, especially when used in combination with other antihypertensive agents. Its effectiveness is diminished considerably by the presence of chronic glomerular nephritis or renal hypertension.

Uses. Some physicians prefer to use hydralazine hydrochloride in combination with other agents, such as ganglionic blocking agents, chlorothiazide or one of the Rauwolfia preparations. If it is added to one or more of these drugs several days after treatment has been started, the undesirable tachycardia, which is one of its side effects, is said to be avoided or decreased. Hydralazine hydrochloride when given parenterally is said to be frequently effective in the treatment of hypertensive emergencies associated with eclampsia and acute nephritis.

Preparation, dosage, and administration.

Hydralazine Hydrochloride° (Apresoline Hydrochloride). This drug is usually administered orally, although it may be given intravenously or intramuscularly when the patient is unable to take the drug orally. It is available in 10, 25, 50, and 100 mg. tablets and as a sterile solution for injection, 20 mg. per milliliter. As with other antihypertensive drugs, medication is started with small doses and the dosage increased gradually until desired effects are obtained or symptoms of toxicity appear. The initial oral dose for patients with moderate to severe hypertension is 10 mg. given after meals and at bedtime. Patients may receive larger

°Described in annual publication of A. M. A. Council on Drugs, N.N.D., 1960.

doses, depending on the severity of the hypertension and their response to the drug. Repeated blood pressure readings must be taken not only to determine the effect of the drug but also to avoid serious side effects.

Side effects and toxic effects. Side effects associated with hydralazine hydrochloride vary all the way from merely unpleasant effects to those that are serious and require cessation of administration. Headache, heart palpitation, anxiety, mild depression, dry mouth and unpleasant taste in the mouth, and nausea and vomiting are symptoms that are unpleasant but may not necessitate that the administration of the drug be stopped. More serious symptoms include symptoms of coronary insufficiency (pain in the region of the heart), edema of the feet and the legs, chills, fever, and severe depression. Other toxic symptoms which may result from prolonged administration of hydralazine hydrochloride in large doses resemble those of early rheumatoid arthritis or the more severe phase of the same syndrome—acute systemic lupus erythematosus.

Antihistaminic drugs, salicylates, or barbiturates are useful to control headache, palpitation, anxiety, and nausea and vomiting. The more severe symptoms require cessation of therapy with this drug. Fortunately the symptoms subside when the drug is withdrawn.

Ganglionic blocking agents

The ganglionic blocking agents referred to in the following discussion are agents that produce some degree of blockage in both the sympathetic and parasympathetic ganglia. The parent compound of this group of drugs is a quaternary nitrogen compound, tetraethylammonium chloride. It is not well suited for the treatment of hypertension because of the transient nature of its action and its side effects. A number of other ganglionic blocking drugs are available, e.g., hexamethonium chloride, pentolinium tartrate, chlorisondamine chloride, and mecamylamine hydrochloride. Some clinicians favor one drug over another because of greater absorption, longer action, and smoother hypotensive effects. Their action is similar in that they all block nerve impulses in both the sympathetic and parasympathetic ganglia. They therefore exhibit similar side effects. Their greatest hypotensive effect is secured when the patient is in upright position, because they suppress the vasoconstrictor reflexes which regulate blood pressure when posture is changed.* Therefore the patient should be in a semireclining position, with the head of the bed elevated, if maximal benefit is to be obtained in bedfast patients.

The ganglionic blocking agents are at present the most potent antihypertensive agents available. Severe and unpleasant side effects may be encountered when they are used. Blockage in the sympathetic ganglia is

*Spittel, J. A.: Selection of the Therapeutic Agent for the Patient, From Symposium on Medical Treatment of Hypertension, Proc. Staff Meet. Mayo Clin. **33:** 315, 1958.

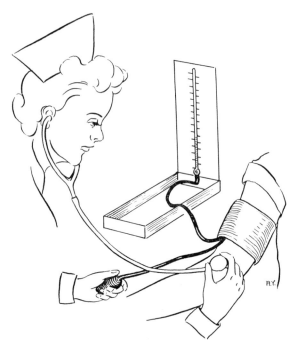

Fig. 35 Determining the blood pressure. This is done sometimes by the nurse prior to the administration of antihypertensive drugs such as hexamethonium chloride (Bistrium Chloride) or pentilinium tartrate (Ansolysen) in order that adjustments in dosage may be made according to the patient's response to the drug. Dosage may need to be increased, decreased, or omitted. It is important for the nurse to know the position of the patient at the time the blood pressure is taken, e.g., does the physician want the reading to be taken when the patient is standing, sitting, etc.

responsible for side effects such as nasal congestion and orthostatic hypotension. Blockage in the parasympathetic ganglia may give rise to symptoms such as constipation, blurred vision, dry mouth, paralytic ileus, urinary retention, and impotence. Constipation may be controlled or prevented by the use of cathartics such as Milk of Magnesia (30 to 45 ml. daily). It is important that the ganglionic blocking agents be administered on time to maintain consistent control of the hypertension. Dosage is modified according to the patient's blood pressure at the time the next dose is due. It is important for the nurse to know whether the blood pressure is to be taken when the patient is lying down, sitting, or standing up. The lowest pressure reading will be obtained after the patient has been standing for a few minutes. Some physicians say that the patient should stand for at least 3 minutes before the reading is taken.

Hexamethonium Chloride (Methium Chloride)

Action. Hexamethonium chloride inhibits transmission of nerve impulses at the ganglia of both the sympathetic and parasympathetic divisions of the autonomic nervous system. Interference with the passage of impulses through the sympathetic ganglia, where activity would normally bring about vasoconstriction, causes an increase in blood flow and a lowering of blood pressure. At the same time, interference with the passage of nerve impulses in the parasympathetic system is responsible for loss of visual accommodation or blurring of vision, decreased motility of stomach and intestine, and difficulty in emptying the bladder.

Uses. Hexamethonium chloride is useful in selected cases of hypertension. It is said to be more effective for controlling attacks of severe hypertension than for mild hypertension. Effects are achieved rather promptly and last 4 to 6 hours. It is absorbed slowly and less completely when given orally than when given parenterally.

Preparation, dosage, and administration.

*Hexamethonium Chloride** (Methium Chloride, also formerly sold under name of Bistrium Chloride). This is available in 125 and 250 mg. tablets and as a syrup, 62.5 mg. per milliliter, for oral administration and as a sterile solution, 250 mg. in 10 ml. and 1 Gm. in 10 ml., for parenteral administration (intravenous, intramuscular, or subcutaneous injection). The single oral dose may vary from 125 to 1,500 mg. The parenteral dose is usually 50 to 100 mg. injected in a single dose and repeated in 6 hours as necessary.

Hexamethonium Tartrate. Official preparation in the B.P.

Patients are sometimes taught to take their own medication and to determine their own blood pressure. They learn how to adjust dosage of the drug according to the blood pressure reading. In some institutions, patients are taught to stand erect for one minute before taking the drug and if they experience dizziness to reduce the dose by half.

Side effects. Undesirable side effects of hexamethonium chloride include severe hypotension, orthostatic hypotension, constipation, paralytic ileus, and difficulty in emptying the bladder. Retention catheters are often required for elderly men receiving this and similar drugs. The hypotension may be relieved by placing the patient in a recumbent position or by giving small doses of phenylephrine hydrochloride. Other side effects that may occur are dilated pupils, blurred vision, dryness of the mouth, faintness, and transient nausea. Laxatives may be given to relieve or prevent constipation. Sublingual administration of bethanechol chloride (Urecholine Chloride) also will receive constipation and urinary retention. Sometimes reserpine is alternated with a ganglionic blocking agent such as hexamethonium since reserpine is prone to increase in-

*Described in annual publication of A. M. A. Council on Drugs, N.N.D., 1960.

testinal motility. Tolerance develops, although not uniformly in all respects. Tolerance to the sympatholytic action develops more easily than does tolerance to the effects on the bowel and bladder.

Pentolinium Tartrate (Ansolysen Tartrate)

Action. Pentolinium tartrate is a ganglionic blocking agent the pharmacologic properties of which appear to be similar to those of hexamethonium chloride. It differs from the latter drug in degree and duration of activity. Pentolinium tartrate is said to be several times more active than hexamethonium chloride in blocking the transmission of impulses in both the sympathetic and parasympathetic divisions of the autonomic nervous system. However, activity is greater on the sympathetic than on the parasympathetic system. The effect of a single dose of pentolinium tartrate is more prolonged than one of hexamethonium chloride; this permits less frequent administration of pentolinium tartrate.

Uses. This drug is a potent substance and is indicated only for the treatment of hypertension that ranges from moderately severe to very severe and does not respond to milder treatment.

Preparation, dosage, and administration.

Pentolinium Tartrate,* B.P. (Ansolysen Tartrate). This preparation is administered orally, subcutaneously, and intramuscularly. It is available in 20, 40, 100, and 200 mg. tablets and as a sterile solution, 100 mg. in 10 ml. The total daily oral dosage may vary from 60 to 600 mg. The initial oral dose is usually 20 mg. The initial dose is made as small as possible and increased gradually while the patient is under careful medical supervision. The initial parenteral dose recommended is 2.5 to 3.5 mg.

Side effects and toxic effects. These effects are similar to the ones produced by other ganglionic blocking drugs, e.g., hexamethonium chloride.

Chlorisondamine Chloride (Ecolid Chloride)

Action. Chlorisondamine chloride is a ganglionic blocking agent the effects of which are similar to other agents in this category. It is more potent than hexamethonium chloride and pentolinium tartrate but less so than mecamylamine hydrochloride. Absorption after oral administration is said to be rapid but erratic and unpredictable. When given in adequate dosage it is said to lower effectively both the diastolic and systolic blood pressures.

Uses. Its use is recommended for severe types of hypertension rather than the mild forms of this disorder. The drug is potent and potentially toxic; hence it is important that the patient be under very close medical supervision.

*Described in annual publication of A. M. A. Council on Drugs, N.N.D., 1960.

Preparation, dosage, and administration.

Chlorisondamine Chloride* (Ecolid Chloride). This drug is administered orally, subcutaneously, and intramuscularly. It is marketed in 10, 25, and 50 mg. tablets and in a sterile solution for injection, 5 mg. per milliliter. Parenteral administration is usually reserved for the patient in acute hypertensive crises. All dosage is highly individualized. Initial doses are small and then are gradually increased until the desired therapeutic effects are achieved. When the drug is given subcutaneously or intramuscularly the beginning dose is not more than 2.5 mg., and this may be gradually increased, depending upon the response of the patient. An effective single parenteral dose is usually between 1 and 10 mg. Oral administration may be substituted for parenteral administration as soon as the blood pressure has been stabilized. The oral dose starts at 10 mg. and is taken in the evening. Next day, 10 mg. is given in the morning and 10 mg. in the evening. Dosage is increased until eventually it may be as much as 200 mg. daily, depending on the patient's response to the drug.

Side effects and toxic effects. The effects are the same or similar to those of other ganglionic blocking agents. They include blurring of vision, dryness of the mouth, postural hypotension, and urinary retention (especially in the presence of hypertrophy of the prostate gland). Constipation also may occur and must be treated or prevented.

Contraindications. The drug is contraindicated for patients with cerebrovascular accidents, myocardial infarction, or coronary or renal insufficiency.

Mecamylamine Hydrochloride (Inversine Hydrochloride)

Action. Mecamylamine hydrochloride is a potent ganglionic blocking agent similar to hexamethonium chloride except that it is well absorbed from the intestinal tract. It lowers the blood pressure of both normal persons and hypertensive patients. Its action is more prolonged than that of hexamethonium, and equivalent reduction of blood pressure is produced with a lower dose.

Tolerance develops after prolonged administration, although it is said to be somewhat less than that which develops after administration of hexamethonium chloride or pentolinium tartrate.

Uses. The indications for therapy with this drug are similar to those for the other members of the ganglionic blocking group of drugs.

Preparation, dosage, and administration.

Mecamylamine Hydrochloride, U.S.P. (Inversine Hydrochloride). This agent is marketed in 2.5 and 10 mg. tablets for oral administration. The dosage recommended is that which will reduce the blood pressure

*Described in annual publication of A. M. A. Council on Drugs, N.N.D., 1960.

and maintain it without the appearance of severe side effects. Treatment is usually started with a dosage of 2.5 mg. twice daily and is gradually increased. The average total daily maintenance dose is about 25 mg. (divided into three portions). Dosage must be determined in relation to readings of blood pressure.

Side effects and toxic effects. Side effects include blurred vision, dry mouth, constipation (which is sometimes preceded by diarrhea), loss of appetite, nausea and vomiting, urinary retention, fatigue, drowsiness, and orthostatic hypotension. The disturbance of bowel function may become severe and develop into paralytic ileus. The latter complication can be avoided usually with regular use of laxatives. Administration of the drug should be stopped if abdominal distention develops.

Contraindications. Its use is contraindicated for the same conditions for which other ganglionic blocking agents are contraindicated.

Trimethaphan Camphorsulfonate (Arfonad Camphorsulfonate)

Action. Trimethaphan camphorsulfonate is a rapid-acting ganglionic blocking agent which lowers blood pressure in both normotensive and hypertensive persons. The duration of its action is brief, which makes it unsuited to the treatment of hypertension.

Uses. This drug is used for the production of controlled hypotension during certain types of surgical procedures in which the production of some degree of hemostasis in capillary beds, arterioles, and venules helps to prevent excessive bleeding and increases visualization and exposure of the surgical field. It is used especially in neurosurgery and peripheral vascular surgery.

Preparation, dosage, and administration.

Trimethaphan Camphorsulfonate, U.S.P. (Arfonad Camphorsulfonate). This drug is administered by continuous intravenous infusion as a 0.1 per cent solution in 5 per cent dextrose in water or in isotonic salt solution.* It is available in 10 ml. ampules containing 500 mg.

Side effects and toxic effects. The use of this drug is recommended for administration only by experienced anesthetics. Respiratory depression is a complication, particularly when a muscle relaxant has been used. Tachycardia is a potential complication.

Contraindications. Contraindications are the same as those for other ganglionic blocking agents.

Chlorothiazide as a hypotensive agent

Action. Chlorothiazide, although introduced and primarily useful as a diuretic agent, has also been found to have significant blood pressure

*N.N.D., 1960, p. 328.

lowering action in hypertensive subjects, perhaps because of its effect in reducing the amount of sodium and chloride in the body. It also augments the effects of many of the other drugs used in treatment of hypertension.

Uses. Chlorothiazide is used either alone, as in cases of mild hypertension, or in combination with other antihypertensive drugs (such as the ganglionic blocking agents). In the latter case it is usually possible to lower the dose of the ganglionic blocking agent appreciably. This often means that the dose of the ganglionic blocking agent can be reduced sufficiently to produce no unpleasant side effects. Chlorothiazide is used in combination with hydralazine, Veratrum, the Rauwolfia drugs, as well as the ganglionic blocking agents. It also enhances their hypotensive effects.

Preparation, dosage, and administration.

Chlorothiazide, U.S.P. (Diuril). Tablets, 250 and 500 mg., are available for oral administration. When given alone, doses of 500 mg. may be prescribed to be given from one to three times daily. When combined with other antihypertensive drugs, the dosage is kept small, usually 250 mg. twice daily.

*Chlorothiazide Sodium** (Lyovac Diuril). This preparation is suited for parenteral administration since it is more soluble than the parent substance. Dosage is the same as that for chlorothiazide.

Side effects. Unlike many antihypertensive drugs, chlorothiazide produces few unpleasant side effects. Patients occasionally experience weakness, fatigue, nausea, abdominal pain, distention, and diarrhea. A fairly high percentage of patients have been known to show some disturbance of blood electrolytes. The blood urea may be elevated and the level of serum potassium lowered. Chlorothiazide should be administered cautiously to patients with renal insufficiency. Some physicians recommend that the patient on prolonged therapy with this drug be given supplemental amounts of potassium chloride. Skin rash has been observed occasionally.

Drugs that affect the blood

Blood consists of a straw-colored, slightly alkaline fluid, which is called plasma, and cells—red blood cells (erythocytes), white blood cells (leukocytes and lymphocytes), and blood platelets or thrombocytes. Red cells are found to the extent of between four and one half and five million cells per cubic millimeter, the number being slightly lower in women than in men. By volume, the red cells make up approximately half that of whole blood. The chief constituent of the red cell is an iron-

*Described in annual publication of A. M. A. Council on Drugs, N.N.D., 1960.

containing protein called hemoglobin. Hemoglobin has the important characteristic of being able to form an unstable combination with oxygen which enables it to transport that element to the tissues and to give it up readily. The amount of hemoglobin in the blood should be approximately 15 Gm. per 100 ml. of blood, again being somewhat less in women and slightly more in men. Hemoglobin also is able to form combinations with other substances such as carbon monoxide which may prevent the blood from carrying an adequate amount of oxygen to the tissues, or the iron in hemoglobin, normally in a reduced state (Fe^{++}), may be oxidized (Fe^{+++}) to form methemoglobin, which does not function in oxygen transport.

A deficiency in the red cells of the blood or in the total amount of hemoglobin constitutes *anemia.* An abnormal increase in red cells is known as *polycythemia.*

The number of white blood cells is usually between 5,000 and 7,000, although numbers up to 10,000 per cubic millimeter are not considered abnormal. Infectious diseases may cause a marked increase, which is called *leukocytosis.* Other diseases and certain drugs may deplete the normal number of white cells, in which case the deficiency is known as *leukopenia.*

The ability of the blood to clot is due to the presence of blood-clotting substances in the plasma derived from the platelets, which become active as soon as the blood is released from the blood vessel. The normal coagulation time is from 3 to 5 minutes, when venous blood is allowed to clot in a glass tube.

The normal reaction of blood is lightly alkaline, having a pH of 7.35 to 7.43, which is maintained with considerable constancy due to the presence of buffer substances and the ability of the kidneys and lungs to excrete substances that would otherwise change the pH. The chief buffer substances are the basic phosphates, the carbon dioxide-bicarbonate of the plasma, and the serum proteins.

Normal blood is about five times more viscous than water. The viscosity depends largely upon the presence of cells. The viscosity of the serum is about twice that of distilled water. The osmotic pressure of the blood is that of an 0.85 per cent solution of sodium chloride. A solution of this concentration is said to be isotonic with the blood. Shrinkage and distortion of cells will occur with the introduction of large amounts of hypertonic solutions into the blood, whereas hemolysis (rupture of red cells) is produced by hypotonic fluids.

The drugs we will consider in this section are those used in the treatment of certain specific anemias or those used to influence blood clotting. Other drugs such as the antifolic acid compounds, radioactive phosphorus, etc. are useful in the treatment of certain neoplastic disorders of the bone marrow, manifested largely by blood changes such as leukemia and polycythemia. Since these drugs are more closely related to the general group of agents used to treat neoplasms generally, they will be considered under that heading (see Chapter 25).

Antianemic or hemopoietic drugs

The formation of both red cells and hemoglobin is a complex process, and deficiency in any one of a number of constituents may result in a failure to produce the needed number of red cells or an adequate amount of hemoglobin. The hemoglobin molecule is composed of globin (a protein) and hematin, and iron-containing pigment portion. It is found in the muscle cells of mammals as well as in the red cells.

Some of the factors that promote the formation of red blood cells are as follows:

1. A diet which is adequate in the essentials for the making of red blood cells; namely, iron, vitamin C, and members of the vitamin B complex, the antianemic factor (vitamin B_{12}), and animal protein.

2. Normal activity of the gastrointestinal tract to assure adequate digestion and absorption of the needed essentials.

3. A liver which is able to store iron as well as the antianemic factor. It has been observed that chronic disease of the liver leads to anemia. Much of the iron needed for synthesis of hemoglobin is salvaged from erythrocytes. The antianemic factor is needed for the maturation and formation of normal red blood cells.

4. Normal activity of the blood-forming tissues of the body, particularly the red bone marrow of the adult.

Although an adequate diet is usually the preferable way to acquire the essential constituents for blood formation, various disease conditions require treatment that brings about more rapid results than can be obtained from diet alone. Anemia may arise from a number of causes. The aim of treatment is to strike at and remove the cause of the anemia if that is possible or to control the symptoms satisfactorily. Drugs may help to do this.

As indicated, many types of vitamin or hormonal deficiency may lead to anemia; specific examples are deficiency of ascorbic acid or of the thyroid or of the adrenocortical hormones. Replacement of any of these missing substances could then be considered a specific type of therapy for the corresponding anemia. In general usage, however, the antianemic "drugs" are those substances required in the formation of hemoglobin, the absence of which leads to anemia as the *principal clinical finding*. The major antianemic substances under this heading are iron, vitamin B_{12}, and folic acid.

Iron

Iron is a metallic element which is rather widely distributed in the body, being found not only in the hemoglobin of the blood but also in the chromatin of the cells and as a reserve supply in the blood-forming organs. Iron is essential to the normal transportation of oxygen in the body and to normal tissue respiration. Iron deficiency results in a form of anemia which is associated with symptoms of low vitality, pallor of the skin and mucous membrane, fatigue, poor appetite, etc.

Absorption of iron compounds. A number of different iron compounds are used in the treatment of secondary anemia. These include ferric and ferrous salts of iron, metallic iron, and inorganic and organic salts. The soluble salts of iron have a more unpleasant taste, are more likely to stain the teeth, and are more likely to cause gastrointestinal disturbance than the less soluble salts. The former, however, are absorbed more readily. The hydrochloric acid of the stomach acts to change many of the ferric salts to ferrous ones and also helps to prevent formation of insoluble salts. Absorption of iron seems to occur best in the duodenum and upper part of the jejunum regardless of the type of iron administered. The acidity of the upper part of the duodenum helps to prevent formation of insoluble iron compounds. The alkalinity of intestinal content does not promote good absorption of iron. The old idea that only organic iron can be utilized by the body has been disproved. In fact it is believed that much more rapid response is made by the body to the administration of inorganic rather than organic preparations.

Absorption of iron is influenced by a number of factors: (1) the presence of acid in the gastric content (the acid is thought to favor dissociation of iron compounds and the reduction of ferric to ferrous iron, although some doubt has been expressed about this); (2) the presence of reducing substances in the alimentary canal, such as ascorbic acid, which helps to keep iron in the ferrous state; and (3) the dietary intake of iron. Bile is no longer believed to have much effect on intestinal absorption of iron.

At best, the amount of iron that is actually absorbed is small. Most of it escapes absorption and is lost in the stool or is re-excreted through the mucosa of the large bowel and in the bile and urine.

Iron requirements in man. Ordinarily much of the iron that is salvaged from worn-out red cells is reused in the body; therefore only a small amount needs to be absorbed from the diet to maintain a positive iron balance (1 to 2 mg). During periods of rapid growth and development the body need for iron is correspondingly increased. Pregnancy, early adolescence (especially in girls), early childhood, and menopause constitute periods when the iron content should be increased either by increased dietary intake or medicinal iron or both. Women up through the age of menopause require two to four times as much iron as the adult male. This is due to pregnancy, loss of menstrual blood, excessive bleeding, etc. Although the body requirements are ordinarily met by making provision that the diet be adequate in red meats, green vegetables, eggs, whole wheat, and other foods rich in iron, during periods of increased need for iron the administration of medicinal forms may be necessary to maintain a positive iron balance.

The major and only significant way of losing iron from the body to such an extent that anemia develops is by blood loss: either the sudden blood loss of an acute large hemorrhage or the slow insidious loss which may occur from menorrhagia, hemorrhoids, or a silent ulcer or tumor of the gastrointestinal tract.

Action and result. The local action of iron salts constitutes a side action.

Local. When inorganic iron compounds are administered orally, iron acts as an irritant and astringent. It reacts with tissue proteins and forms an insoluble iron compound. Irritation and astringent effects along the gastrointestinal tract may cause nausea and vomiting, constipation or diarrhea, and abdominal distress. Organic forms do not cause the same irritation because of the fact that they dissociate with difficulty.

Systemic. The action for which iron is most often administered is its hemopoietic one. If the iron reserves of the body are depleted, they are restored when ample amounts are administered. It is believed that the action of iron in conditions of deficiency is largely to replace that which is needed for the hemoglobin molecule. The exact mechanism by which iron is utilized by the bone marrow is unknown. Iron is of value only in hypochromic anemias or those in which the color index is low. Iron therapy in this condition can be expected to result in increased vigor on the part of the patient, increased resistance to fatigue, improved condition of the skin and nails, improved appetite, and general feeling of well-being. In other words, it brings about a tonic effect. When administered to individuals with normal blood values it does not bring about an increase in the hemoglobin but only increases the reserve supply of iron in the body.

Uses. Hypochromic anemia is a form of iron-deficient anemia such as may be seen in patients after hemorrhage or in those with an inadequate supply of iron. This form of anemia is markedly benefited by the administration of medicinal iron, whereas it is useless in the treatment of pernicious anemia. Maximum response may be expected in the case of the former between the second and the fourth week. Favorable response may, however, be inhibited by vitamin deficiency, infection, achlorhydria, hepatic disorder, or disorders of absorption in the intestine. If the iron deficiency is a severe one, other forms of therapy may be needed to supplement the iron therapy. Blood transfusion will restore the blood more rapidly than anything else that can be done. Other measures include adequate diet, plenty of sunshine, and possibly the administration of hydrochloric acid, if there is evidence of deficient gastric acid.

Chlorosis, an iron-deficiency condition in its classical form, has largely disappeared, but a similar although mild grade of anemia in girls of adolescent years (14 to 20) is still a common finding. It responds well to iron therapy.

Solutions of ferric iron are sometimes used for their strong astringent properties. They are applied externally as styptics. Ferric solutions are also occasionally used as gargles for their astringent effects.

Preparation, dosage, and administration. Although many preparations of iron have been marketed, few have outstanding merit from the standpoint of effectiveness, tolerance, and ease of administration.

Ferrous Sulfate, U.S.P., B.P. ($FeSo_4 \cdot 7 H_2O$). This has come to be one of the most widely used preparations of iron. It is available in 200 and 300 mg. (3 and 5 gr.) enteric-coated tablets (Enseals). Dosage is 1 or 2 tablets after meals, and sometimes an additional dose is given at bedtime.

Ferrous Sulfate Syrup, N.F. The syrup contains 200 mg. of ferrous sulfate in each 5 ml. of the preparation. The usual adult dose is 8 ml. three times a day. *Ferrous Sulfate Elixir** is also available.

Exsiccated Ferrous Sulfate, U.S.P. (Feosol); *Dried Ferrous Sulfate*, B.P. This preparation contains not less than 80 per cent anhydrous ferrous sulfate. It is available in enteric-coated tablets, 200 mg., and as an elixir. Each 200 mg. tablet is equivalent to a 300 mg. tablet of ferrous sulfate. Usual dose is 200 mg. three times a day.

Ferrous Gluconate, U.S.P., B.P. (Fergon). Tablets are usually supplied in amounts of 300 mg. The usual dosage is 300 mg. three times a day. Ferrous gluconate is also available as an elixir.* It is said to have less tendency to cause gastric distress and is better tolerated by some patients than is ferrous sulfate.

Ferric Ammonium Citrate, N.F., B.P. This is one of the most soluble preparations of iron. It is commercially available in 500 mg. capsules, in an aqueous (50 per cent) solution, and as an elixir. The usual dose is 500 mg. three times daily after meals.

Ferroglycine Sulfate Complex (Ferronord). This compound represents a recent development in oral iron therapy. It is the complex formed between ferrous iron and the amino acid glycine. It has been reported that this form of iron provides just as thorough a blood response in the anemic patient as other forms of iron but causes considerably less dis-

*U.S.P. XVI Interim Admission.

comfort to the average patient. It is available in tablet form. The dose for an adult is 2 tablets two or three times daily.

*Ferrocholinate** (Chel-Iron, Ferrolip). This preparation, like the preceding preparation, is a chelated (bound) form of iron which is believed to be less toxic and better tolerated than some of the older preparations such as ferrous sulfate and ferrous gluconate. At the same time it is said to be clinically effective in the treatment of iron-deficiency anemia although clinical experience with the drug is limited to date. It is administered orally and can be given between meals. It is available in tablets (330 mg.), as a syrup (33.2 mg. per 1 ml.), and as a solution (208 mg. per 1 ml.). The proposed dose (adult) is 330 to 660 mg. three times daily.

There are a number of other iron compounds listed in the *National Formulary,* but all the beneficial effects of iron may be secured from adequate dosage of one or more of the mentioned oral preparations, at least for most patients who need iron.

Copper is thought to have a catalytic action in the utilization of iron in the formation of hemoglobin and is frequently given with iron. Most of the preparations of iron, however, contain traces of copper in sufficient amount. *Cupron* is a proprietary preparation which is composed of ferrous carbonate and cuprous carbonate.

Many of the inorganic preparations of iron, because they are irritant to the stomach, should be given after meals or with food. To avoid injury or staining of the teeth, solutions should be taken through a glass tube or straw. Because of the astringent property of these preparations, they may be combined with or be accompanied by a cathartic to ensure regular bowel exacuation. Iron stains silver; a silver spoon should never be used in giving iron. Such stains may be removed with strong ammonia water. Iron stains on linen and clothing may be removed with oxalic acid.

Preparations for injection. The preferable route of administration of iron is usually the oral one. However, the following conditions are indications for parenteral administration: (1) for patients with hypochromic anemia who do not tolerate iron preparations when given orally; (2) for those who do not absorb iron well from the gastrointestinal tract or have gastrointestinal complications such as ulceration or severe diarrhea; (3) for those who for one reason or another cannot be relied upon to take the iron orally, such as the aged or the mentally disturbed; and (4) for those in whom a maximal rate of hemoglobin regeneration is needed, such as patients with severe iron deficiency, e.g., patients prior to surgery for which there is immediate need or for patients in the last trimester of pregnancy.

*Described in annual publication of A. M. A. Council on Drugs, N.N.D., 1960.

Iron-Dextran Injection, U.S.P.* (Imferon). This is a colloidal suspension of ferric hydroxide in complex with partially hydrolized low molecular weight dextran. The preparation is stable, has a pH of 6, and contains 50 mg. of elemental iron per milliliter. It is available in 2 and 5 ml. ampules and in 10 ml. vials. Total dosage is calculated by determining the approximate extent of the hemoglobin deficit and adjusting the daily dose accordingly. The initial dose is usually 50 mg. on the first day, and amounts up to 250 mg. may be given every day or every other day thereafter until the amount needed has been given. This preparation is given by deep intramuscular injection into the gluteal muscle. The subcutaneous tissue should be pushed aside before insertion of the needle to prevent leakage along the tract of the needle. It is not administered intravenously. *For the present this preparation has been withdrawn from the market.*

Saccharated Iron Oxide (Proferrin). This preparation is marketed in ampules containing 5 ml. of solution of saccharated iron oxide for intravenous administration. The initial dose is usually small (50 mg.), and it must be given slowly. Systemic side effects may be observed.

Side effects and toxic effects. Long-continued administration of iron may cause headache, loss of appetite, gastric pain, nausea, vomiting, and constipation or diarrhea. Patients should be forewarned of the possibility of experiencing abdominal cramps and diarrhea when taking certain preparations of iron. If only the latter symptoms develop, the drug should be stopped for a day or two and then resumed. If many untoward symptoms develop, it may be necessary to take a longer rest period before resuming the dosage. Tolerance to iron is apparently not developed. Serious acute poisoning can result from ingestion of large doses of iron compounds. This is particularly true when it occurs in infants or young children. Preparations of iron should be kept out of the reach of children. The signs and symptoms of poisoning are those of gastrointestinal irritation, destruction of tissue, and shock.

Most cases of severe poisoning have occurred in young children who have swallowed many tablets of ferrous sulfate. Some deaths have been reported.

Toxic symptoms have occasionally been observed after parenteral administration of iron and include flushing, headache, nausea, vomiting, weakness, abdominal pain and aching of lower extremities, fever, and shock. Pain is sometimes experienced at the site of intramuscular injection. Injection of an iron preparation outside of a vein may cause a severe local reaction. When iron is administered orally there is a limit to which it will be absorbed, but when it is injected into the blood stream an overdose may be serious, partly because there is no

*U.S.P. XVI Interim Admission.

satisfactory way for the body to excrete the amount taken in, over and above what the body can use or can store as a normal reserve. It is deposited in organs such as the liver or pancreas and can be detrimental to these organs.

Cyanocobalamin (Vitamin B₁₂)

One of the major developments in nutrition in the past 30 years began with the recognition by Minot and Murphy in 1926 that a substance in liver could cure the hitherto fatal disease pernicious anemia. Their discovery led to the isolation of the pure compound, at first called "antianemic factor" in 1948, and in 1956, the elucidation of the structure of this molecule—vitamin B_{12}. Vitamin B_{12} is an extremely complex and large organic molecule, containing the metal ion cobalt. It has a structure similar to heme, the iron-bearing porphyrin in the hemoglobin molecule.

Today it is believed that persons with pernicious anemia (now a misnomer since the disease can now be arrested) lack the ability to absorb vitamin B_{12} from dietary sources, at least at the normal rate. They must therefore be supplied with enormous doses of the vitamin by mouth (so that a sufficient amount can be absorbed) or else be given rather small doses parenterally (since by this route all is made available to the tissues). The exact role of the vitamin in body chemistry is not well understood, but it is clearly required for some chemical step in the formation and normal development of the mature red cell.

Ham[*] states that the role of B_{12} is that of a coenzyme in the biosynthesis of nucleic acid, and that it is needed for the formation of DNA and RNA (desoxyribonucleic acid and ribonucleic acid).

The exact nature of the disease process in pernicious anemia which prevents the absorption of vitamin B_{12} is not well understood either. There is good evidence, however, that these patients fail to manufacture in their gastric mucous membrane a specific substance required for the normal absorption of vitamin B_{12}. The absorption factor has been called the "intrinsic" factor to distinguish it from vitamin B_{12} which (before its chemical nature was understood) used to be somewhat mysteriously identified as "extrinsic" factor.

There is no lack of vitamin B_{12} in a normal diet. Even without a dietary supply, evidence shows that there is sufficient formation of the vitamin by bacteria normally present in the intestine of man and other mammals. The patient with pernicious anemia therefore, in a sense, starves in the midst of plenty since he lacks the substance necessary for the absorption of vitamin B_{12}.

For this reason, it is also possible to supply the vitamin indirectly by

[*]Ham, A. W.: Histology, Philadelphia, 1957, J. B. Lippincott Co., p. 349.

giving the patient a preparation of dried gastric mucosa, containing the intrinsic factor, and thereby enabling him to absorb his own vitamin B_{12} from the diet. The surest way of remedying a deficiency, however, is to give the vitamin directly by needle, and this is the most common way of treating pernicious anemia.

When the body is deficient in vitamin B_{12} over a period of time, a series of characteristic symptoms and pathologic changes develop. The onset is gradual, and the early symptoms are usually fatigue, sore tongue, and achlorhydria. The patient develops a peculiar yellowish pallor, complains of increasing weakness, breathlessness, itching, dyspepsia, and diarrhea. Degenerative changes in the nervous system also occur, giving rise to incoordination of movement, loss of vibratory sense (due to changes in the dorsal columns of the spinal cord), peripheral neuritis, optic atropy, and, sometimes, psychosis. Death may result from the changes associated with pernicious anemia unless the changes are arrested. This is accomplished effectively with the administration of vitamin B_{12}.

Uses. Pernicious anemia is one of the macrocytic hyperchromic anemias for which the administration of vitamin B_{12} is effective either as the pure vitamin or in a preparation of liver. It constitutes a form of replacement therapy, and administration must be continued indefinitely. It corrects the abnormalities of the red blood cells, relieves the sore mouth and sore tongue, restores normal function of the peripheral nerves, and arrests the progression of changes in the central nervous system. In some cases the changes in the nervous system are reversed if the irreversible stage of degeneration has not been reached. Vitamin B_{12} is also used in certain nutritional macrocytic anemias and for tropical and nontropical sprue. Beneficial effects have been reported in a number of neurologic disorders, e.g., trifacial neuralgia. These effects have been secured only after very large doses.

Preparation, dosage, and administration. Cyanocobalamin is a red crystalline substance which contains cobalt, and it is obtained from cultures of *Streptomyces griseus* as a by-product in the manufacture of antibiotics. Because there is a group of closely related B_{12} factors, the activity of any preparation coming from natural sources may be due to several members of this group. Prior to the availability of pure vitamin B_{12}, liver was administered extensively since it contains B_{12}, but it is now considered scientifically obsolete since liver preparations have no advantage over the pure vitamin but have several distinct disadvantages— liver is more expensive, may be painful to give, and is allergenic in some persons.

Cyanocobalamin (Vitamin B_{12}) U.S.P., B.P. This is available in a variety of preparations for oral administration and in powder or solution for injection. The minimum effective dose is thought to be 1 microgram per day or multiples of this amount at appropriate intervals; e.g., 15 micrograms twice a month. The dosage may need to be larger or be given more frequently if the patient is very ill or has marked neurologic complications. Vitamin B_{12} is usually given intramuscularly. If it is administered orally, larger dosage is required, and the body response is slower than when it is given parenterally.

Vitamin B_{12} with Intrinsic Factor Concentrate, N.F. This is a mixture of vitamin B_{12} with preparations of gastric mucosa obtained from the stomachs of domestic animals used for food. The usual daily dose (oral) is 1 U.S.P. unit. It is available in capsule and tablet form. It is particularly desirable for patients for whom parenteral therapy is difficult or undesirable.

Side effects and toxic effects. No undesirable side effects or toxic effects have been reported following administration of vitamin B_{12} even after large parenteral doses.

Since nearly all patients with pernicious anemia have a lack of hydrochloric acid in the stomach, full doses of the official dilute hydrochloric acid may be prescribed for the patient, to be given with meals not only to aid digestion but also to act as a gastric antiseptic. The usual dose is ½ to 1 fluidram, which is well diluted with water (⅓ to ½ glass).

Other preparations

Although preparations of liver are no longer official in the *Pharmacopeia of the United States*, a number are listed in the *National Formulary*. They are believed to be of value because of their vitamin B_{12} content only and hence have, to a great extent, been replaced by preparations of cyanocobalamin.

Liver with Stomach, N.F. This is a powder which is made from dried defatted hog stomach mixed with an extract of liver. It contains vitamin B_{12} and intrinsic factor. The usual oral dose is 1 U.S.P. unit daily. An official preparation in the N.F. is Liver with Stomach Capsules.

Folic Acid

The chemical name for folic acid is pteroylglutamic acid. It is a member of the vitamin B complex and can be prepared synthetically. It is found only in small amounts in the free state in a number of foods. For a short time some years ago folic acid was used as a supplement to liver therapy in the treatment of pernicious anemia. It produces a response in the blood which is similar to that produced by liver extract. The hemoglobin and the red cells increase to normal, and the bone marrow returns to its normal state. The appetite improves, and the patient feels better in general. In most patients the blood response is apparently maintained indefinitely with folic acid. It does not, however, prevent the development or the progression of neurologic changes which are often a part of the disease, and it may in fact make them worse. Because of this, it cannot be recognized as adequate therapy for pernicious anemia and cannot replace vitamin B_{12}. Its use is therefore dangerous (when used alone for this condition), and the presence of folic acid in many multivitamin preparations adds to the hazard of this type of irrational therapy when used in the "treatment" of an undiagnosed anemia.

Uses. Although folic acid should not be employed in the treatment of pernicious anemia except possibly as a supplement to adequate therapy with vitamin B_{12}, it is used for the treatment of selected cases of macrocytic anemias and of nutritional and metabolic disorders associated with such anemia. It frequently is useful in the treatment of an anemia of pregnancy. It is sometimes used in the treatment of anemia associated with tropical sprue and celiac disease, although there is some question as to whether it constitutes complete therapy.

Preparation, dosage, and administration.

Folic Acid, U.S.P., B.P. (Folvite). This preparation is marketed in 5 mg. tablets and as an elixir, 1 mg. per milliliter, for oral administration and as a solution for injection, 15 mg. per milliliter. The usual oral dose is 5 to 15 mg. daily, in divided doses. The usual parenteral dose is 10 mg. once daily, intramuscularly. *Folic Acid Injection,* U.S.P., is the same as Sodium Folate.* It is the preparation preferred for parenteral therapy.

*Leucovorin Calcium.** This is referred to as the citrovorum factor or folinic acid. In man, folic acid is converted in the tissues to leucovorin before it exerts an effect on cellular elements of the blood. It is available in 1 ml. ampules containing 3 mg. of the drug and is used chiefly as an antidote for drugs that act as folic acid antagonists, e.g., aminopterin. It is administered intramuscularly in doses of 3 to 6 mg. daily.

Whole blood and its constituents

Blood transfusion plays an important although passive role in the treatment of anemic conditions. Transfusions do not apparently stimulate the bone marrow to greater activity but in times of crises they may save the patient's life when the patient cannot wait for iron or liver to become effective.

For blood transfusions to be used satisfactorily it is important that the blood be readily available and of the suitable type. It is also essential that a careful technic be developed and strictly adhered to, in order to help prevent reactions. The blood should be administered slowly, particularly if the patient's anemia is severe. Sometimes one transfusion of

*Described in annual publication of A. M. A. Council on Drugs, N.N.D., 1960.

whole blood will suffice, but under other conditions a series of small transfusions may accomplish better results.

Transfusions of whole blood are of value not only to replace red cells but also to restore blood volume and thereby restore blood pressure. The latter value is seen particularly in the treatment of shock. Whole blood, since it contains all of the necessary fluid-holding constituents, does not pass out of the vascular system as rapidly as most parenteral fluids.

Blood plasma

Blood plasma is the fluid part of the blood which may be procured by separating the blood cells from the whole citrated blood. Plasma may be given irrespective of the donor's group. Many authorities believe that blood plasma, since it contains the blood proteins, sugar, salts, etc., is an ideal transfusion medium to restore effective blood volume in the treatment of peripheral circulatory failure associated with severe burns, traumatic shock, or hemorrhage. Blood plasma can be used as it is for transfusion or it can be concentrated, dehydrated, and stored for long periods of time without deterioration. The addition of sterile distilled water is all that is needed to make it ready for immediate use. Plasma in the dried form is particularly stable and useful when transportation, storage, and contamination are problems that must be considered.

Normal Human Plasma, U.S.P., is obtained by pooling equal parts of citrated whole blood from eight or more adult human beings who qualify as donors by virtue of their having passed physical examinations and various clinical tests. The plasma is subjected to ultraviolet irradiation to destroy any possible bacterial or viral contaminants other than that of homologous serum jaundice.* Procedures are carried out under definite aseptic conditions and the cell-free plasma is obtained by centrifugation or by sedimentation. It is dispensed in liquid, dried, or frozen form. The usual amount given whole or restored is 500 ml. It is administered to combat surgical and traumatic shock, in the treatment of burned persons when much plasma has been lost, and in cases in which whole blood is not immediately available for the treatment of hemorrhage.

Blood proteins

Blood plasma can be further broken down to many useful parts. Albumin is just as effective as plasma in shock treatment and effective treatment requires less of the albumin than of the plasma.

Thrombin and fibrinogen also can be separated from plasma and then purified and concentrated into fine white powders. When put into solution they coagulate to form fibrin. The solution is sometimes applied

*N.N.D., 1960, p. 503.

locally to stimulate blood clotting and to provide a sort of glue in skin grafting.

Fibrinogen, U.S.P., is available as a powder for injection along with a suitable amount of diluent.

Normal Human Serum Albumin, U.S.P., is a brownish, viscous, clear liquid which is relatively odorless. It is obtained from the blood of healthy human donors. It is made free of the hazard of the virus of serum jaundice by heating at 60° C. for 10 hours.* It is available in a solution (25 Gm. in 100 ml.) or as a dried preparation. The normal unit is composed of 25 Gm. of human albumin to which sterile water or physiologic saline solution can be added before use. This is then equivalent to about 500 ml. of whole human plasma, in terms of protein osmotic pressure. It is used in the treatment of shock and in situations in which it is important to raise the serum protein of the blood. It is administered intravenously.

Plasma substitutes

Dextran (Expandex, Gentran, Plavolex)

Dextran is a glucose polymer made by the action of special bacteria *(Leuconostoc mesenteroides)* on sucrose. The resulting polysaccharide does not easily pass through capillary walls. As first made, the molecules are extremely large. When partially hydrolyzed, however, various preparations are made in which the molecules are of smaller size, more like those of serum albumin; these preparations have a molecular weight of about 75,000.

Uses. Dextran is used to expand plasma volume and maintain blood pressure in emergency conditions resulting from shock and hemorrhage. It is not considered a substitute for whole blood or its derivatives when the latter are needed for the treatment of anemia secondary to hemorrhage or when it is essential to restore blood proteins after traumatic injuries, burns, and so forth. The effect of an injection of 500 to 1,000 ml. of dextran (6 per cent) usually persists for a period of 24 hours. Thirty to 50 per cent is excreted in the urine and the remainder is metabolized in the body.

Preparation, dosage, and administration.

Dextran, U.S.P.† (Expandex, Gentran, Plavolex); *Dextran Injection*, U.S.P.,† B.P. This preparation is administered intravenously in isotonic solution of sodium chloride. The usual dose is 500 ml. of 6 per cent solution infused at the rate of 20 to 40 ml. per minute. Repeated injections can be given when necessary, if blood or its derivatives are not at hand or their use is not indicated. Solutions of dextran do not require refrig-

*N.N.D., 1960, p. 501.
†U.S.P. XVI Interim Admission.

eration and are easily stored. The 6 per cent solution of dextran is osmotically equivalent to serum albumin.

Side effects and toxic effects. Untoward effects are virtually unknown with the possible exception of an antigen-antibody type of reaction seen in certain persons. These are seldom encountered and tend to be mild with properly refined preparations. Renal and hepatic functions are not altered. Patients with cardiovascular disease who receive dextran infusions are watched for indications of congestive heart failure and pulmonary edema.

Special intravenous gelatine solution (Plazmoid)

This preparation is a 5 or 6 per cent sterile, pyrogen-free nonantigenic solution of gelatine in isotonic solution of sodium chloride.

Uses. It is used as an infusion colloid to support blood volume in various types of shock. It is excreted largely by the kidney and should not be used when renal impairment is present and should be used with caution in the presence of cardiac impairment. In the latter condition, an increase in fluid volume may become an excessive burden to the heart in its attempt to maintain circulation of the blood.

Preparation, dosage, and administration

*Special Intravenous Gelatine Solution** (Plazmoid). This solution should be warmed to about 122° F. and kept warm for prolonged intravenous administration. It will gel at temperatures lower than body temperature, although it is fluid at body temperature. A dose of 500 ml. is usually adequate for a single infusion and is given at the rate of 30 ml. per minute.

Polyvinylpyrrolidone (PVP)

Polyvinylpyrrolidone (PVP) is a nonofficial synthetic compound related to some of the plastics. Close to one half of the molecules are said to have a molecular weight of more than 50,000. It is available as a clear, amber-colored aqueous solution. It appears to have physical properties similar to those of blood plasma and its effect persists over at least a 12-hour period. About 50 per cent of it is said to be excreted in the urine. It can be stored without refrigeration. It is preferably administered by intravenous infusion. It is said to be nonantigenic.

Blood coagulation

Drugs affecting the clotting of blood are used both to hasten clotting (hemostatics) and to retard clotting (anticoagulants). In some instances normal components necessary for blood clotting must be supplied, much as are vitamins and hormones in the deficient individual.

*Described in annual publication of A. M. A. Council on Drugs, N.N.D., 1960.

The clotting reactions of plasma are a complex series of plasma protein transformations eventually leading to the formation of an insoluble fibrous meshwork of fibrin (the clot), which traps cells of the blood in its interstices and eventually contracts to form a firm seal. These reactions are not understood in entirety but can be presented as a series of three reactions complex.

1. *Formation of active plasma thromboplastin.* Ruptured blood platelets (thrombocytes) plus several plasma proteins interact to form thromboplastin.

2. *Formation of thrombin.* Thromboplastin plus a series of proteins in the plasma (prothrombin complex) interact to form thrombin. This step requires calcium ions.

3. *Formation of fibrin.* Thrombin, a proteolytic enzyme, cleaves off a portion of the protein fibrinogen. The altered fibrinogen forms an insoluble polymer called fibrin.

Drugs that retard coagulation may act at one of several steps in this linked chain of events. The simplest preparations are those used to produce hemostasis, partly by mechanical means and partly by assisting the terminal reactions of clotting.

Preparations that produce hemostasis

Absorbable Gelatin Sponge, B.P. (Gelfoam). This is an especially prepared form of gelatin which gives it a porous nature. It is used to control capillary bleeding and may be left in place in a surgical wound. It is completely absorbed in from 4 to 6 weeks. It should be well moistened with isotonic saline solution or thrombin solution before it is applied to a bleeding surface. Its presence does not induce excessive scar formation.

Fibrin Foam. This is a sterile dry preparation of human fibrin which, when applied to a bleeding surface, acts as a mechanical coagulant. In combination with thrombin it gives a chemical as well as a mechanical matrix for coagulation. It is used in surgery of organs where ordinary methods for the control of bleeding are ineffective or inadvisable, e.g., surgery of the brain, liver, or kidneys.

Tolonium Chloride* (Blutene Chloride). This preparation is also known as toluidine blue O, a dye that reduces the bleeding tendency in certain hemorrhagic conditions associated with excessive amounts of heparinoid substances in the blood. It is used in the treatment of idiopathic (cause unknown) functional bleeding from the uterus (prolonged or profuse menstruation or excessive or prolonged bleeding between periods). Tolonium chloride is administered orally in doses of 200 to 300 mg. daily. It is available in 100 mg. tablets. The urine of patients receiv-

*Described in annual publication of A. M. A. Council on Drugs, N.N.D., 1960.

ing the drug becomes blue-green. Some patients may experience nausea, tenesmus, and burning at the time of urination. Increased fluid intake or adjustment of dosage usually alleviates these symptoms.

Oxidized Cellulose, U.S.P., B.P. (Oxycel, Hemo-Pak). This is a specially treated form of surgical gauze or cotton which exerts a hemostatic effect but is absorbable when buried in the tissues. The hemostatic action is due to the formation of an artificial clot by cellulosic acid. Absorption of oxidized cellulose occurs between the second and the seventh day following implantation, although absorption of large amounts of blood-soaked material may take longer. Oxidized cellulose is of value in the control of bleeding in surgery of such organs as the liver, pancreas, spleen, kidney, thyroid, prostate, etc. Its hemostatic action is not increased by the addition of other hemostatic agents. It should not be used as a surface dressing except for the control of bleeding, because cellulosic acid inhibits the growth of epithelial tissue.

Thrombin, U.S.P. This is a preparation of thrombin, isolated from bovine or human plasma. It is intended as a hemostatic for topical application to control capillary bleeding. It may be applied as a dry powder or dissolved in sterile isotonic saline solution. It is not injected.

Vitamin K

Vitamin K was discovered by Dam of Copenhagen in 1935 as a result of a study of newly hatched chicks which had a fatal hemorrhagic disease. This condition he found could be prevented and cured by the administration of a substance found in hog liver and in alfalfa. It was later discovered that the delayed clotting time of the blood was due to a deficiency of prothrombin content. Vitamin K occurs naturally in two forms known as K_1 and K_2. Both have a naphthoquinone nucleus and exhibit similar physiologic properties.

Vitamin K-like compounds

In natural vitamin K (K_1 or K_2), R is a long alkyl chain of 20 or 30 carbons. In synthetic vitamin K (Menadione), R is only hydrogen, but this is as potent as the natural compound. These compounds are called *naphthoquinones* from the parent nucleus. The synthetic ana-

Drugs that affect circulatory system 463

logues greatly resemble the natural vitamin and have even greater physiologic activity. Certain of the analogues are water soluble, whereas the natural vitamin is fat soluble. The fat-soluble vitamin requires the presence of bile in the intestine to ensure adequate absorption after oral administration. This is not essential for the water-soluble preparations.

Vitamin K is widely found in foods; hence deficiency is rarely due to lack of it in the diet. It is also synthesized by intestinal bacteria.

Action and result. Vitamin K is essential to the synthesis of prothrombin by the liver. The exact mechanism of its action is not known, although it is thought to contribute to the activation of an enzyme necessary to the formation of prothrombin.

Prothrombin deficiency may occur because of inadequate absorption of vitamin K from the intestine (usually due to biliary disease in which bile fails to enter the intestine) or because of destruction of intestinal organisms, which may occur with antibiotic therapy. It is also encountered in the newborn in which case it is probably due to the fact that the intestinal organisms have not yet become established. It may result from therapy with certain anticoagulants.

Uses. Vitamin K is useful only in conditions in which the prolonged bleeding time is due to low concentration of prothrombin in the blood which is not in turn due to damaged liver cells. Vitamin K has been recommended for hemorrhagic conditions in the newborn for which prophylactic doses are administered during the last stages of pregnancy and first few weeks after birth.

It is also indicated in the preoperative preparation of patients with deficient prothrombin, particularly those with obstructive jaundice. In addition, it is given as an antidote for overdosage of systemic anticoagulants such as bishydroxycoumarin, as well as for hemorrhagic disorders and hypoprothrombinemia secondary to large doses, or overdosages, of drugs such as salicylates, quinine, sulfonamides, arsenicals, and barbiturates. Hemorrhagic conditions not due to deficiency of prothrombin are not successfully treated with vitamin K.

The natural concentrates have, to a great extent, been replaced by the synthetic preparations. It is important that the prothrombin activity of the blood be measured frequently when the patient is receiving a preparation of vitamin K. Parenteral preparations should be administered if for some reason the intestinal absorption is impaired.

Preparation, dosage, and administration

Menadione, U.S.P., *Menaphthone,* B.P. This drug is a synthetic substitute for natural vitamin K. The presence of bile is essential for adequate absorption after oral administration. *Menadione Tablets,* U.S.P., *Menadione Capsules,* N.F., and *Menadione Injection,*

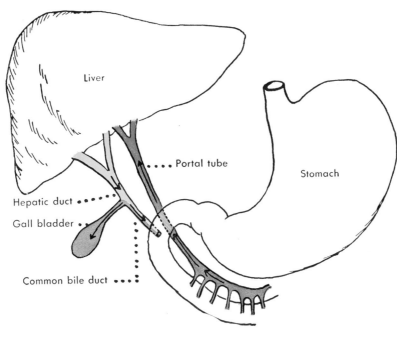

Plate 7

This diagram represents the pathway of the portal-biliary circulation of bile salts. After their passage into the duodenum, most of them are reabsorbed into the portal blood and are returned to the liver where they are again resecreted. This form of circulation is directly connected with the absorption of fats and fat-soluble vitamins.

N.F., are official preparations. The usual dose is 1 to 2 mg. daily.

Menadione Sodium Bisulfite, U.S.P. (Hykinone); *Menaphthone Sodium Bisulphite,* B.P. This form is similar to menadione but it is water soluble, and oral doses need not be accompanied by bile salts. It is available in tablet form for oral administration as well as in solution for injection (subcutaneous, intramuscular, and intravenous). *Menadione Sodium Bisulfite Injection,* U.S.P., and *Menapthone Sodium Bisulphite Injection,* B.P., are official preparations for injection. Average daily dose is 0.5 to 2 mg. daily. Dosage is determined in relation to the prothrombin level of the blood.

Various other commercial water-soluble vitamin K analogues are also available, e.g., *Synkamin,* which is marketed in 1 ml. ampules containing 1 mg. of the drug and in capsules containing 4 mg. of the drug.

Menadiol Sodium Diphosphate, U.S.P. (Synkayvite Sodium Diphosphate). This is a derivative of menadione and has the same action and uses as other analogues of vitamin K. It is water soluble and is adequately absorbed after oral administration without bile salts. It is administered orally, subcutaneously, intramuscularly, and intravenously. The dosage is approximately three times that of menadione. It is available in 5 mg. tablets for oral administration and in solution for injection. The usual dose is 5 mg. (4 to 75 mg.).

Phytonadione, U.S.P. (Vitamin K_1, Mephyton, Konakion). This preparation acts more promptly and over a longer period of time than the vitamin K analogues. It is a fat-soluble vitamin, and the presence of bile salts in the intestine is essential to adequate absorption. It will stop bleeding in 3 to 4 hours after intravenous administration and produce a normal prothrombin level in 12 to 14 hours. It is useful to reverse the effects of anticoagulant therapy which has produced a serious deficiency of prothrombin in the blood. Phytonadione is available in 5 mg. tablets and as an emulsion for injection. The emulsion is diluted with isotonic salt solution or sterile water before it is injected. Phytonadione is administered orally or parenterally, depending upon the severity of the condition being treated. The dosage varies greatly; 2 to 20 mg. may be given daily, although much larger doses have been given in emergency situations. However, small doses of vitamin K_1 orally administered will effectively correct the reduced prothrombin activity induced by certain anticoagulants (coumarin drugs). Effects are said to be less predictable when severe liver damage is present. The dosage of vitamin K_1 must be determined according to the level of prothrombin activity, the length of time during which the patient has received anticoagulant therapy, and the hazard of restoring the risk of thrombosis. Large doses of vitamin K_1 are said to make subsequent regulation of anticoagulant therapy with coumarin drugs more difficult.

Anticoagulants

It is of interest that diseases associated with abnormal clotting within vessels take a far greater toll of lives in our society than does hemorrhage. It is estimated that over a million persons suffer from thrombosis or embolism in the United States each year.* Diseases caused by intravascular clotting include some of the major causes of death from cardiovascular sources—coronary occlusion and cerebral accidents.

Drugs that might inhibit clotting are therefore correspondingly important; the last 20 years has seen the introduction of potent anticoagulants and their widespread prophylactic use in medicine.

Anticoagulants are used mainly for the following: (1) to prevent coagulation of blood which is to be used for transfusion or for laboratory and experimental work, (2) to prevent postoperative thrombosis and embolism, and (3) in the treatment of thromboembolic diseases to prevent extension of the clot and subsequent formation of emboli.

Sodium Citrate

Sodium citrate is used as an anticoagulant in blood which is to be used for a transfusion or in blood which is to be stored for a time. *Anticoagulant Sodium Citrate Solution,* U.S.P., is approximately a 4 per cent sterile solution of sodium citrate in water. It is used as an anticoagulant for blood plasma and for blood for fractionation. *Anticoagulant Acid Citrate Dextrose Solution,* U.S.P., is used as an anticoagulant for storage of whole blood.

Heparin

Heparin is a polysaccharide whose structure is only partly known. It is obtained commercially from the lungs of domestic animals slaughtered for food. It is effective in vitro and in vivo. In the presence of blood serum it is thought to increase the clotting time of the blood by preventing the formation of thrombin from prothrombin and also by exerting an antithrombin action which inhibits the conversion of fibrinogen into fibrin. It also prevents agglutination of platelets. The precise mechanism of these actions is not fully understood but it definitely prolongs the clotting time of the blood. It does not dissolve clots already formed but will help to prevent their extension and lessen the danger of the formation of emboli. Bleeding time is unaffected which decreases the danger of hemorrhage from superficial wounds or injuries in the patient who is receiving heparin. The effect of heparin is rapid but of short duration since it is rapidly inactivated in the blood.

Uses. Heparin appears to be of particular value in preventing post-

*Editorial: Anticoagulants, a Cooperative Effort, J. A. M. A. **169:** 1484, 1959.

466

operative thrombosis and embolism. It does not help the patient who develops a sudden and massive embolism but it helps to prevent the extension of a thrombus. Patients who have once had a phlebitis or nonfatal embolism are more likely to experience this mishap a second time than those who do not have this type of history, and hence they constitute a group of patients for whom the drug may be used with very satisfactory results.

The nurse should watch for bleeding in patients receiving heparin. This apparently does not occur often, but it may happen and usually means that administration of the drug must be discontinued. The postoperative patient may bleed from the wound or may develop hematuria. Male patients may be shaved or may be allowed to shave while receiving the drug because bleeding time is not affected, although the clotting time is prolonged.

Heparin is also used to provide a rapid anticoagulant action in cardiovascular surgery and to prevent clotting of blood during transfusions.

The main disadvantages associated with the use of heparin are its short action, its need for parenteral injection, and its high cost.

Preparation, dosage, and administration

Heparin Sodium Injection, U.S.P.; *Heparin Injection,* B.P. This drug is inactive orally and must be administered by injection (intramuscular or intravenous). It may be given by a single injection or continuous intravenous drip. The response to heparin occurs almost immediately and lasts for a relatively short time (3 to 4 hours) unless the dose is repeated. When administration is discontinued, the clotting time returns to normal rather quickly, and there is danger of massive clot formation should the drug be discontinued too soon. Dosage must be determined for each individual patient and maintained at a level that keeps the clotting time well above normal (15 to 20 minutes). The potency of heparin sodium is expressed in units. When it is given intravenously at spaced intervals, 50 mg. (5,000 units) may be given at a time. For continuous drip, 100 to 200 mg. (10,000 to 20,000 units) are added to 1,000 ml. of 5 per cent sterile glucose solution or to isotonic saline solution and the flow started at about 20 to 25 drops per minute. Dosage for the repository form is 20,000 to 40,000 units.

Intramuscular injection of heparin in a slowly absorbed medium repository form has been recommended, and this does reduce the frequency of the injections to one every 48 hours. There are accompanying disadvantages, however; namely, the injections may be painful and the absorption may not be even so that sometimes there is inadequate heparinization and at other times an excessive effect may be obtained; furthermore, the possibility of a local hematoma, tissue irritation, and concealed hemorrhage must be kept in mind.

Side effects and toxic effects. Toxic effects are due to overdosage and are manifested by bleeding from mucous membranes and open wounds. Reduction of dosage or frequency of injection or both are indicated. The effects of heparin on the clotting mechanism can be reversed by the administration of tolonium chloride (see p. 462) or protamine sulfate.

Therapy with heparin is expensive for the patient since the preparation is derived from animal tissues and it is difficult to purify it. It must be administered parenterally and the patient's clotting time must be determined daily.

Heparin antagonist—Protamine Sulfate

Protamine sulfate is a proteinlike substance derived from the sperm of the salmon and other fish.

Uses. It is used as a heparin antagonist, combating the bleeding tendency from an overdose of heparin.

Protamine by itself is an anticoagulant and will cause prolongation of clotting time; it is an antithromboplastin but is not as active as heparin. When protamine is given in the presence of heparin, they are attracted to each other instead of to the blood elements and each neutralizes the anticoagulant activity of the other.

When given intravenously to treat the bleeding tendency resulting from an overdose of heparin, protamine acts almost instantaneously, and its effects persist for about 2 hours. Its availability is therefore essential for safe management of a patient having anticoagulant therapy with heparin. It has been used to treat certain bleeding states which are believed to be characterized by increased amounts of heparin or heparin-like substances in the circulation; this use is experimental.

Preparation, dosage, and administration.

Protamine Sulfate Injection, U.S.P. This compound is administered intravenously and, occasionally, intramuscularly. In the treatment of overdosage of heparin, the extent of the overdosage can be determined from the amount of heparin given over the previous 3 or 4 hours; the amount of protamine needed is approximately equal to the amount of heparin overdosage. A 1 per cent solution is injected slowly in from 1 to 3 minutes intravenously. The dose should not exceed 50 mg. of protamine at one time. The commercial preparation of protamine sulfate consists of a solution containing 10 mg. in 1 ml.

Coumarin derivatives

When cattle are allowed to eat improperly cured sweet clover they may develop a hemorrhagic disorder which is believed to be due to a deficiency of prothrombin. In 1941 Link and his associates were able to show that the substance responsible for the prothrombin deficiency was a coumarin derivative. These workers later synthesized bishydroxy-coumarin (Dicumarol), and since that time several other coumarin derivatives have been synthesized. They are acenocoumarol, ethyl biscoumacetate, and warfarin sodium. These compounds differ mainly in their speed and duration of action.

Action and result. The coumarin compounds presumably act by suppressing the formation of prothrombin in the liver and also its stable conversion factor (proconvertin). Thus prothrombin time is prolonged because prothrombin activity is diminished. This action is achieved in vivo but not in vitro and only after a latent period of several hours. These compounds apparently have no effect on the circulating prothrombin but only on the production of it.

Although the coumarin drugs are referred to as anticoagulants they do not appreciably affect coagulation time or bleeding time when they are administered in therapeutic amounts.* Dosage is therefore not computed on the basis of these tests but on the determination of the plasma prothrombin time. Decreased prothrombin activity seems to act as a deterrent to intravascular clotting. Adequate and safe therapy therefore depends in part on accurate determinations of the patient's plasma prothrombin time.

Vitamin K and a coumarin compound like Dicumarol show similarity of structure, as indicated in the accompanying formulas. This has led to the supposition that the coumarin compounds act as antimetabolites to prevent the utilization of vitamin K by the liver.†

Bishydroxycoumarin (Dicumarol)   Menadione (vitamin K)

Uses. Coumarin compounds are used to decrease the incidence of postoperative venous thrombosis, pulmonary embolism, and thrombophlebitis and in the management of patients with coronary occlusion and myocardial infarction. They are also effective in treatment of arterial occlusion such as that associated with thromboangiitis obliterans and cerebrovascular disease (complete or partially occluded vessels).

Preparation, dosage, and administration

Bishydroxycoumarin, U.S.P. (Dicumarol). Official preparations of this drug are available in 25, 50, and 100 mg. tablets and also in capsules.

*Estes, J. E.: Long-Term Anticoagulant Therapy, Postgrad. Med. **22:** 326, 1957.
†Loomis, T. A.: Anticoagulant and Coagulant Drugs. In Drill, V. A. (editor): Pharmacology in Medicine, New York, 1958, McGraw-Hill Book Co., Inc., p. 753.

It is administered orally. The usual initial dose is 200 to 300 mg. daily. Subsequent dosage for a day or two depends on the prothrombin time of the patient and may vary from 50 to 200 mg. Some authorities attempt to keep prothrombin activity between 10 and 30 per cent of normal and others say 15 to 25 per cent of normal. In most patients, 25 to 50 mg. daily are required as maintenance doses. Dosage is determined not only by the prothrombin time but also by the direction in which it is changing. Bishydroxycoumarin requires 24 to 72 hours for its action to develop, and its action persists 24 to 72 hours after its administration is discontinued.

*Ethyl Biscoumacetate** B.P. (Tromexan Ethyl Acetate). This synthetic derivative of bishydroxycoumarin produces a similar anticoagulant action. It is available in 150 and 300 mg. tablets for oral administration. Its action and uses are similar to those of Dicumarol, but it is more rapidly absorbed, acts over a shorter period of time, is detoxified and excreted faster, and has less cumulative effect than Dicumarol. Average initial dose for a 24-hour period is 1.5 Gm. given at one time or in divided dosage. Subsequent doses of 600 to 900 mg. per day are usual, but maintenance dosage is regulated by determinations of prothrombin activity. This compound is more expensive than bishydroxycoumarin.

Cyclocumarol (Cumopyran). This preparation is similar to bishydroxycoumarin but it is more potent and its action is more prolonged. It is no longer available in the United States.

Warfarin Sodium, U.S.P.† (Coumadin Sodium, Prothromadin). This is available in 5, 10, and 25 mg. tablets for oral administration and as a powder from which a solution is made for injection (intravenous and intramuscular). Its action is more rapid than that of bishydroxycoumarin and it is more prolonged. The initial oral and intravenous dose is 25 to 50 mg.; then 5 to 10 mg. daily, depending on prothrombin activity.

*Acenocoumarol** (Sintrom). This is a synthetic coumarin type of anticoagulant. Its action is faster than that of bishydroxycoumarin but less rapid than that of ethyl biscoumacetate. It is available in 4 mg. tablets for oral administration. The initial dose is 16 to 28 mg. on the first day of therapy followed by 8 to 16 mg. on the second day. The average maintenance dose is 2 to 10 mg. daily, depending on the response of the patient as measured by frequent prothrombin time determinations.

Side effects and toxic effects. The coumarin compounds are relatively free of side reactions and can be used for prolonged therapy (several years) without untoward effects. Hemorrhage is the one effect which may be disastrous. It is almost always due to overdosage. Mild nosebleed, hematuria or small areas of bleeding into the skin are sometimes

---

*Described in annual publication of A. M. A. Council on Drugs, N.N.D., 1960.
†U.S.P. XVI Interim Admission.

470

seen. Patients should be instructed to notify their physician at once if bleeding occurs. Some physicians advise their patients to carry capsules of vitamin K_1 with them for use if prompt cessation of the effect of the coumarin drug is necessary. If it is necessary to return the plasma prothrombin activity to normal as quickly as possible, as in the case of hemorrhage, administration of the coumarin drug is stopped and a water-soluble preparation of vitamin K should be given, such as menadione sodium bisulfite or phytonadione (vitamin K_1). Transfusions of whole blood may be necessary if there has been a serious loss of blood volume.

Phenindione derivatives

Phenindione (Danilone, Hedulin, Eridione, Indon)

Phenindione* is a synthetic anticoagulant similar in action to bishydroxycoumarin but unrelated chemically. It acts more promptly than bishydroxycoumarin and in smaller doses. Therapeutic levels are obtained within 18 to 24 hours usually, and prothrombin time usually returns to normal 24 to 48 hours after administration of the drug has been discontinued.

This drug may produce an orange or reddish discoloration of the urine which patients may mistake for hematuria. Phenindione is administered orally in initial doses of 200 to 300 mg., one half being given in the morning and one half at bedtime. Continued dosage is adjusted as determinations of prothrombin activity indicate.

Periodic examinations of the blood have been recommended because this drug has been known to cause agranulocytosis.

Diphenadione (Dipaxin)

Diphenadione* is closely related to phenindione and is one of the most potent and prolonged-acting depressants of prothrombin activity. It is therefore effective in smaller doses than most oral anticoagulants. The initial dose is 20 to 30 mg. orally, followed by 10 to 15 mg. on the second day. Subsequent dosage is determined in accordance with the prothrombin time. The precautions to be observed for these drugs are much the same as those for the coumarin derivatives.

Effective anticoagulant therapy

Both heparin and coumarin derivatives are important anticoagulants. They can be used to complement each other. In some instances the administration of both heparin and one of the synthetic anticoagulants

*Described in annual publication of A. M. A. Council on Drugs, N.N.D., 1960.

such as bishydroxycoumarin is started simultaneously and the heparin is discontinued as soon as the prothrombin activity has been sufficiently reduced and the coumarin compound is producing a full therapeutic effect. Heparin is needed when rapid anticoagulant effect is required or when adequate facilities for determining the prothrombin time are not available, thus preventing the use of one of the synthetic anticoagulants.

In certain conditions when a rapid but not immediate anticoagulant effect is desired, bishydroxycoumarin and ethyl biscoumacetate are given together on the first day of therapy and only the former drug on successive days.

Contraindications for anticoagulant therapy

Heparin, Dicumarol, and related anticoagulants should not be used for the following: (1) patients with blood dyscrasias or those with a tendency to bleed; (2) patients with subacute bacterial endocarditis, because of their tendency to purpura; (3) patients undergoing spinal cord or brain surgery because the consequences of even minor bleeding may be attended with serious consequences; (4) patients with liver or kidney insufficiency because cumulative effects may develop (this does *not* apply to heparin); and (5) patients with ulcerative lesions or open wounds.

Anticoagulants are used with caution for patients with malnutrition, for those with hepatic and renal insufficiency, and for those with indwelling tubes or catheters.

Some physicians do not advocate long-term anticoagulant therapy for unreliable patients, e.g., patients who do not eat properly, go on alcoholic "binges," do not take their medicine as directed, and do not report for the test of their prothrombin activity (prothrombin time) as they have been directed to do.

Questions
for study and review

1 What symptoms would you look for in a patient with congestive heart failure? auricular fibrillation? heart block?
2 What do you think you need to understand about digitalis and its preparations in order to give intelligent nursing care to the patient getting the drug?
3 Which preparations of digitalis can be given parenterally? What advantage is there in giving them this way?
4 What special precautions would you ob-

serve and what observations would you be expected to make when caring for a patient getting digitalis for congestive heart failure?
5 For what conditions do heart depressants sometimes have therapeutic value?
6 Explain why, in treatment of patients with hypochromic anemia, different drugs are used than are used for treatment of patients with so-called pernicious anemia.
7 What is thought to be the role of vitamin B_{12} in the treatment of anemia? When is its use indicated rather than a preparation of iron? or folic acid?

8 Why would you encourage a patient to continue taking vitamin B₁₂ when he says that he feels perfectly well and sees no reason for spending his money this way, in spite of the fact that the doctor says he should continue taking it?

9 Name several characteristics of a good antihypertensive drug.

10 What side effects would you watch for in a patient receiving a drug such as hexamethonium chloride or hydralazine hydrochloride?

11 What laboratory test needs to be done frequently when a patient is receiving heparin? coumarin derivatives?

12 Why is long-term anticoagulant therapy with coumarin derivatives such as Dicumarol much less expensive than with heparin?

13 What should a patient, who is to be on long-term coagulant therapy with Dicumarol, have in the way of instruction before treatment is begun?

Single choice

Encircle one answer which in your opinion seems to be the best choice.

14 Which of the following laboratory tests is used in connection with the administration of bishydroxycoumarin (Dicumarol)?
a. sedimentation rate
b. prothrombin time
c. clotting time
d. bleeding time

15 Which of the following laboratory findings would indicate a favorable response of a patient to treatment with vitamin B₁₂?
a. increased hemoglobin
b. increased reticulocyte count
c. increased color index
d. increased white blood cell count

16 Which of the following preparations may produce a favorable hemopoietic response in a patient with pernicious anemia but will not arrest degenerative changes in the nervous system?
a. vitamin B₁₂
b. folic acid
c. liver extract
d. defatted hog stomach

17 If a patient's color index is 0.55, which of the following is likely to be ordered for him?
a. liver extract
b. ferrous sulfate
c. bishydroxycoumarin

d. vitamin K

18 If a patient's prothrombin activity is definitely below normal, which of the following drugs might you expect the doctor to order?
a. heparin sodium
b. vitamin K
c. liver or vitamin B₁₂
d. ferrous sulfate

19 Iron is best absorbed from the duodenum for which of the following reasons?
a. the duodenum has a better absorbing surface than the rest of the bowel
b. the duodenal secretions are alkaline in reaction
c. iron is best absorbed from an acid medium
d. the jejunum and ileum excrete the salts of heavy metals rather than absorb them

20 Which of the following drugs is most likely to be prescribed to relieve pain associated with spasm of coronary blood vessels?
a. ergotamine tartrate
b. nitroglycerin
c. histamine phosphate
d. atropine sulfate

21 Of the following antihypertensive agents, the one likely to be ordered for a patient with mild hypertension is:
a. hexamethonium chloride
b. hydralazine hydrochloride
c. reserpine
d. chlorothiazide

22 Which of the following symptoms is sometimes relieved by the action of ergotamine tartrate?
a. hypotension
b. headache and itching
c. pain of coronary disease
d. inadequate circulation due to a failing heart

23 If a patient has developed a thrombosis which of the following drugs would you expect the physician to order first?
a. menadione sodium bisulfite
b. bishydroxycoumarin (Dicumarol)
c. heparin
d. ethyl biscoumacetate (Tromexan)

Sample test situation

Mrs. Black, 70 years of age, is admitted to the hospital with a diagnosis of advanced arteriosclerosis and decompensated heart. She is edematous, cyanotic, dyspneic, restless, and nervous. The pulse is rapid, weak, and irregular. The blood pressure is 180/110. The following orders are left for her:

Phenobarbital gr. ½ t.i.d.

Digitoxin 0.4 mg. stat. and then 0.2 mg. q. 4 h.

Morphine Sulfate gr. ⅛ (H) q. 6 h. and p.r.n

Chlorothiazide 0.5 Gm. b.i.d.

Multiple choice

In relation to the above test situation, encircle the part or parts of the following which in your judgment constitute the best answers.

1 Which of the drugs ordered for Mrs. Black would you administer first?
   a. phenobarbital
   b. digitoxin
   c. morphine sulfate
   d. chlorothiazide

2 For which of the following effects is the morphine likely to have been ordered?
   a. to put the patient to sleep
   b. to make the pulse slower and stronger
   c. to bring about slow mobilization of the edema
   d. to relieve discomfort, stress, and strain

3 How would you expect to administer the digitoxin?
   a. rectally
   b. intramuscularly
   c. orally
   d. sublingually

4 You would expect the phenobarbital to act primarily as:
   a. an analgesic
   b. a cardiac depressant
   c. a sedative
   d. a hypnotic

5 The effect which could be expected from the chlorothiazide would be:
   a. relief of edema and hypertension
   b. potentiation of the morphine
   c. relief of apprehension
   d. increased urine output

6 The therapeutic action of digitoxin can be expected to result in:
   a. a slower rate of the heart
   b. a more forceful contraction of the heart muscle
   c. a better rhythm of the heart
   d. an increased urine output

7 A preparation obtained from the white foxglove which might have been ordered for this patient is:
   a. digitalis leaf
   b. strophanthin
   c. gitalin
   d. digoxin

8 Digitalization of the patient refers to:
   a. the development of early symptoms of digitalis poisoning
   b. a state in which the patient is free of symptoms of heart failure
   c. a state in which the failing heart is receiving maximum benefits from the digitalis preparation
   d. a condition in which the heart has been slowed to normal

9 Symptoms that may indicate cumulative effects of digitoxin:
   a. marked increase in urine output
   b. pulse rate below 60
   c. nausea and vomiting
   d. diarrhea

10 If symptoms of overdosage from digitoxin develop you would:
   a. stop the drug immediately
   b. give the drug and report the symptoms to the head nurse
   c. give the drug and chart the symptoms so that the doctor will see the record
   d. withhold the drug until the doctor knows of the symptoms and then proceed according to his further directions State reason for your choice.

11 Points in nursing care which if carried out will assist these drugs in obtaining desired results:
   a. provision for plenty of fluids
   b. provision for accuracy in records of intake and output
   c. provision for all factors possible which promote physical and mental rest
   d. accurate counting of the pulse before the administration of each dose of digitalis

References

A. M. A. Council on Drugs: New and Non-official Drugs, Philadelphia, 1960, J. B. Lippincott Co.

Best, C. H., and Taylor, N. B.: Physiological Basis of Medical Practice, Baltimore, 1955, Williams & Wilkins Co.

Drill, V. A. (editor): Pharmacology in Medicine, New York, 1958, McGraw-Hill Book Co., Inc.

Goodman, L., and Gilman, A.: The Pharmacological Basis of Therapeutics, New York, 1955, The Macmillan Co.

Anemia

Amerman, E. E., and others: Ferrous Sulfate Poisoning, J. Pediat. **53:** 476, 1958.

Franklin, M., and others: Chelate Iron Therapy, J. A. M. A. **166:** 1685, 1958.

Hagedorn, A. B.: Intramuscularly Administered Iron in the Treatment of Iron Deficiency Anemia, J. A. M. A. **164:** 1643, 1957.

Hagedorn, A. B.: The Parenteral Use of Iron in the Treatment of Anemia, Proc. Staff Meet. Mayo Clin. **25:** 706, 1957.

Hall, B. E., and Campbell, D. C.: Vitamin B$_{12}$ Therapy in Pernicious Anemia. I. Effect on Hemopoietic System: Preliminary Report, Proc. Staff Meet. Mayo Clin. **23:** 584, 1948.

Hall, B. E., and Campbell, D. C.: Vitamin B$_{12}$ Therapy in Pernicious Anemia. II. Effect on General, Clinical and Neurological Manifestations; Preliminary Report, Proc. Staff Meet. Mayo Clin. **23:** 591, 1948.

Cardiac drugs

Dry, T. J.: Treatment of Congestive Heart Failure, Collected Papers of the Mayo Clinic and the Mayo Foundation, Philadelphia, 1949, W. B. Saunders Co., pp. 241-249.

Frohman, I. P.: Digitalis and Its Derivatives, Am. J. Nursing **57:** 172, 1957.

Groom, D.: Drugs for Cardiac Patients, Am. J. Nursing **56:** 1125, 1957.

Kerkhof, A. C.: Effective Cardiac Drugs, Postgrad. Med. **25:** 255, 1959.

Antihypertensive drugs

Allen, E. V., and others: Medical Treatment of Hypertension, Proc. Staff Meet. Mayo Clin. **29:** 459, 1954.

Fairbairm, J., II, and others: Symposium on Medical Treatment of Hypertension, Proc. Staff Meet. Mayo Clin. **33:** 307, 1958.

Gifford, R. W.: Combined Drug Therapy in Hypertension: Methodology of Treatment With Sympathetic Depressants and Diuretics. Collected Papers of the Mayo Clinic and the Mayo Foundation, Philadelphia, 1958, W. B. Saunders Co., pp. 357-378.

Hoobler, S. W.: Seminars on Hypertensive Drugs, Treatment of Hypertension, Am. J. Med. **17:** 259, 1954.

Reinhardt, D. J., and Waldron, J. M.: Lupus Erythematosus-like Syndrome Complicating Hydralazine (Apresoline) Therapy, J. A. M. A. **155:** 1491, 1954.

Vakil, R. J.: A Clinical Trial of Rauwolfia Serpentina in Essential Hypertension, Brit. Heart J. **11:** 350, 1949.

Wilkins, R. W.: New Drugs for Hypertension With Special Reference to Chlorothiazide, New England J. Med. **257:** 1030, 1957.

Drugs used for shock

Haggerty, R. J.: Levarterenol for Shock, Am. J. Nursing **58:** 1243, 1958.

Simard, O. M.: Nursing Care During Levarterenol Therapy, Am. J. Nursing **58:** 1244, 1958.

Coagulants and anticoagulants

Allen, E. V., Barker, N. W., and Waugh, J. M.: The Preparation From Spoiled Sweet Clover, J. A. M. A. **120:** 1009, 1942.

Barker, N. W.: Anticoagulant Therapy, Collected Papers of the Mayo Clinic and the Mayo Foundation, Philadelphia, 1948, W. B. Saunders Co., pp. 372-376.

Barker, N. W.: The George E. Brown Memorial Lecture, Current Status of the Problem of Thrombosis, Circulation **17:** 487, 1958.

Cooley, D. G.: Men Behind Medical Miracles, Fate Walked in Clover, Today's Health **37:** 22, Jan., 1959.

Council on Pharmacy and Chemistry: The Use of Phytonadione, J. A. M. A. **163:** 38, 1957.

Estes, J. E.: Long Term Anticoagulant Therapy, Postgrad. Med. **22:** 323, 1957.

Priestley, J. T., and Barker, N. W.: Postoperative Thrombosis and Embolism: Their Treatment With Heparin. Collected Papers of the Mayo Clinic and the Mayo Foundation, Philadelphia, 1942, W. B. Saunders Co., pp. 130-142.

Schirger, A., Spittel, J. A., and Ragen, P. A.: Small Doses of Vitamin K for Correction of Reduced Prothrombin Activity, Proc. Staff Meet. Mayo Clin. **34:** 453, 1959.

Soehren, I.: Anticoagulants for Heart Disease, Today's Health **35:** 18, Feb., 1957.

Chapter 15

Drugs that affect
the
organs of the respiratory system

Respiration is necessary for and is a proof of life. The essential part consists in the utilization of oxygen and the elimination of carbon dioxide. It is important that all inspired air be warmed to body temperature and saturated with water vapor. In this manner, body heat and water are lost. The respiratory system in man includes the nasal cavity, larynx, trachea, bronchi, lungs, striped and unstriped muscles of the larynx, intercostal muscles and diaphragm, respiratory center in the medulla, and the blood.

Significant points of anatomy and physiology

The respiratory center

Respiration is under the control of a respiratory center in the medulla. This consists of an ill-defined group of cells in the reticular substance over an area bounded by the nucleus of the facial nerve anteriorly and by the calamus scriptorius below. It is bilateral but connected so that half a center may suffice for the continuation of bilateral respiratory movements. This center is sensitive to changes in carbon dioxide tension. The slightest rise in carbon dioxide increases respiration, and, thereby, the center tends to keep the carbon dioxide tension of the blood constant.

Carbon dioxide is the chief respiratory stimulant, although the respiratory center does respond to other stimuli, e.g., a fall in the pH of blood is also important in serving as a respiratory stimulant.

The lungs

The lungs may be regarded as elastic, membranous sacs the interior of which is in free communication with the outside air. The alveolar sacs are branches of the trachea > bronchi > bronchioles > alveolar sacs. The bronchiolar musculature is regulated by bronchoconstrictor fibers in the vagi and bronchodilator fibers in the sympathetic nervous system. The wall of each alveolus is composed of a single layer of respiratory epithelium. Across this layer and the endothelium of the capillaries, gaseous exchange occurs between the inhaled air and the blood. The total number of alveoli in the lungs of man has been estimated at about 725,000,000, and their total surface at about 200 square meters, or 100 to 130 times the surface area of the body. The surface area of the capillaries of the lungs is estimated to be about 90 square meters. The factor of safety, which may be taxed after pneumonectomy, is quite large.

Functions of respiration

The chief functions of respiration are (1) to supply oxygen to the body and to remove carbon dioxide and (2) to aid in evaporation of water in the respiratory passages, which assists in the regulation of the body temperature. The latter function is more important in animals like the dog, which have no sweat glands, than it is in man. In rise of temperature, as in man, however, increased respiration is a compensating factor.

Gaseous exchange in the lungs

The interchange of gases between the outside air and the blood depends on (1) the difference in tension of the gases, (2) the rate of blood flow through the lungs, (3) the area of the lungs, and (4) the resistance offered by the alveolar walls to the diffusion of gases. The tension of the gases depends on the composition of the air inspired and upon the rate and volume of inspiration. A man at rest may inspire 6 to 8 liters of air per minute, breathing 14 times per minute, whereas an athlete in maximal effort may inspire 30 times that volume and breathe 4 to 5 times as rapidly. This shows the great adaptive power of the respiratory mechanism.

Drugs that act on the respiratory center

Direct stimulation

The most important stimulants are carbon dioxide, caffeine, atropine, pentylenetetrazol and nikethamide.

Carbon dioxide

Carbon dioxide is a colorless, odorless gas which is heavier than air. It functions in the physiologic control of the respiratory center and can be used as a valuable respiratory stimulant. Whether it affects the respiratory center directly or by increasing the hydrogen ion concentration is not entirely agreed upon. The fact remains that inhalation of carbon dioxide increases both the rate and the depth of respiration.

Carbon dioxide is important in the field of therapeutics. When administered in from 2 to 5 per cent concentrations, it exerts a marked effect on the respiratory center. Inhalation of a 3 per cent concentration doubles the pulmonary ventilation and may be used to relieve Cheyne-Stokes breathing. In 5 to 7 per cent, mixed with oxygen, it may be used before, during, or after anesthesia. In the beginning it speeds up anesthesia by increasing pulmonary ventilation. By lessening the sense of asphyxiation, it reduces struggling. After the anesthesia, it hastens the elimination of many anesthetics.

Uses. Carbon dioxide is used as a respiratory stimulant in the treatment of certain types of asphyxia not including that which results from chronic pulmonary disease. Included are asphyxia neonatorum, carbon monoxide poisoning, cases of drowning, etc. As a respiratory stimulant it is administered along with a relatively high concentration of oxygen.

Carbon dioxide is used a great deal during and after anesthesia when it is useful to combat respiratory depression due to hyperventilation or excessive depression of the respiratory center.

Inhalation of carbon dioxide and oxygen mixtures is also thought to be effective in the treatment of postoperative hiccough. Relief of hiccough is apparently accomplished by stimulating the respiratory center and by making the contractions of the diaphragm more regular.

Postoperative pneumonia and its complications are believed to be prevented, at least in part, by increasing the depth of breathing and by preventing congestion in the lungs.

Administration. Carbon dioxide may be administered by means of a close-fitting mask, the gas coming from a storage tank. The patient should inhale the mixture until the depth of respirations is definitely increased, which is usually in about 3 minutes. For the postoperative patient the procedure should be repeated, for short periods every hour or two for the first 48 hours, and then several times a day for several days.

Another way of administering carbon dioxide is to allow the patient to hyperventilate with a paper bag held over the patient's face. He thus reinhales his expired air in which the carbon dioxide content is continually increased.

Signs of overdosage are dyspnea, breathholding, markedly increased chest and abdominal movements, nausea, and increased systolic blood pressure. The administration of the gas should be discontinued when these symptoms appear. The administration should, in fact, be stopped as soon as the desired effects on respiration have been secured.

The following respiratory stimulants have been discussed in greater detail elsewhere (see Index).

Atropine

Atropine has some action as a respiratory stimulant because it produces stimulation of the medullary centers. Ordinary therapeutic doses, however, seem to affect only the vagal center and the respiratory center, the latter to a mild degree. The rate and occasionally the depth of breathing are increased. When respiration is markedly depressed, atropine cannot be depended upon to produce stimulation of the respiratory center since large or continued doses of atropine may actually further depress the respiratory center.[*]

Atropine is commonly given with morphine in hypodermic injections to lessen the effect of the latter drug on respiration, as well as to check the secretion of mucus.

Caffeine

Caffeine when given in large doses or when given parenterally definitely stimulates the respiratory center. The effect is especially noticeable after the respiratory center has been depressed, as from morphine. Tolerance to caffeine, which is established in many individuals, is a disadvantage in the use of the drug as a respiratory stimulant.

Pentylenetetrazol (Metrazol)

Pentylenetetrazol stimulates the respiratory center in the medulla. It has been used particularly to overcome respiratory depression associated with barbiturate poisoning.

Nikethamide (Coramine)

Nikethamide apparently has its most marked effect upon the respiratory center when the center is in a state of depression. When used on experimental animals, the medullary centers give evidence of stimulation, resulting in increased rate and depth of respiration and peripheral vasoconstriction.

Acetazolamide, Aminophylline, Salicylates, Progesterone

Acetazolamide (Diamox), aminophylline, salicylates, and progester-

[*]Goodman, L., and Gilman, A.: The Pharmacological Basis of Therapeutics, New York, 1955, The Macmillan Co., p. 544.

one also act to stimulate the respiratory center and have been used alone or in combination with varying success to stimulate respiration in patients with severe respiratory disease and depression of the respiratory center.

Reflex stimulation

Usually respiration is increased by stimulation of the skin nerves and the endings of the olfactory and trigeminal nerves of the nose. Stimulation of the sciatic or almost any sensory nerve may stimulate respiration markedly. This explains why a dash of cold water may revive a fainting person or cause a newborn infant to inspire suddenly. It also explains the use of smelling salts or the dilatation of the anal sphincter as an emergency measure when a patient stops breathing.

Camphor, ammonia, and carminatives act as mild respiratory stimulants when taken by mouth. Ammonia, however, is the only drug given by mouth or inhalation for its action as a reflex respiratory stimulant. Ammonia is used as a heart and respiratory stimulant in the form of Aromatic Ammonia Spirit, U.S.P., 2 ml. in a half glass of water. It is the type of stimulant that could be safely kept in the home medicine chest. It would be suitable as a stimulant for treatment of fainting.

Respiratory depressants or sedatives

The most important respiratory depressants are the central depressants of the *opium group* and those of the *barbiturate group* of drugs. These drugs depress the respiratory center, thereby making the breathing slower and more shallow and lessening the irritability of the respiratory center. Respiratory depression, however, is seldom desirable or necessary, although it is sometimes unavoidable. It is sometimes a side action in otherwise very useful drugs. Occasionally a cough is so painful or harmful that an opiate is administered to inhibit the rate and depth of respiration. A greater value, however, lies in its action (codeine) to depress the cough reflex. Too high concentrations of carbon dioxide in inhalation mixtures may paradoxically act to depress respiration.

Drugs that affect the cough center and the mucous membrane lining of the respiratory tract

Preparations to relieve cough (antitussives)

A cough is a protective reflex which operates to clear the upper part of the respiratory tract of something irritating. A cough can be started by a variety of stimuli, such as cold air, a foreign substance, excessive mucus, inflammatory exudates, or the presence of a malignant growth. A cough is said to be "productive" when by it the irritating agent is expelled; then a cough is helpful. A nonproductive cough is irritating and exhausting. The coughing of asthmatic patients often is nonproductive and persistent. The cough associated with sinusitis is attributable to excess secretion draining into the respiratory tract; it occurs particularly when the patient is lying down or is trying to sleep. The cough associated with congestive heart failure also is likely to occur at night. Other coughs may be more troublesome in the morning because of accumulation of secretions, and still others may occur any time in the day. Treatment of the cough is, of course, secondary to treatment of the underlying disorder. Antitussives should not be given in situations in which retention of respiratory secretions or exudates may be harmful. Medications that may be used to relieve the cough include narcotic and nonnarcotic antitussives, demulcents, antiseptics, expectorants, and others.

Narcotic antitussives

Narcotics such as *morphine, dihydromorphinone,* and *Levo-Dromoran* are potent suppressants of the cough reflex, but their clinical usefulness is limited by their side effects. They inhibit the ciliary activity of the respiratory mucous membrane, depress respiration, and may cause bronchial constriction in allergic or asthmatic patients. In addition, they are habit-forming drugs.

Codeine and *dihydrocodeinone* (Hycodan) exhibit less pronounced antitussive effects but they also have fewer side effects. They have been widely used. Dihydrocodeinone is more active than codeine, but its addiction liability is also greater. The usual dose of Hycodan is 5 to 10 mg. three to four times a day.

Methadone is not an opiate but it resembles morphine in a number of respects. Its ability to suppress the cough reflex is similar to that of morphine. A dose of 1.5 to 2 mg. will effectively relieve a cough. Its main disadvantage as an antitussive agent lies in its habit-forming qualities.

Nonnarcotic antitussive agents

The instillation of a local anesthetic agent prior to procedures such as bronchoscopy is effective in suppressing the cough reflex. This has led to the investigation of other agents which exert a similar action. Benzonatate and carbetapentane are two such preparations.

*Benzonatate** (Tessalon). This preparation is chemically related to the local anesthetic tetracaine and is employed as a drug to relieve cough. It does not depress respirations. After oral administration its

---

*Described in annual publication of A. M. A. Council on Drugs, N.N.D., 1960.

effects are noticed within 15 to 20 minutes and they last for several hours. Side effects do not seem to be serious but may include drowsiness, nausea, tightness in the chest, dizziness, and nasal congestion. Side effects like those associated with the narcotic antitussives have not been reported. This preparation is administered orally. It is marketed in 50 and 100 mg. capsules, and the dosage is 100 mg. several times daily. The ultimate status of this agent will be determined by further study and observation.

*Carbetapentane Citrate** (Toclase). This is a synthetic preparation said to exhibit properties similar to atropine and certain local anesthetics. Its antitussive potency seems to be similar to that of codeine phosphate. It is marketed in 25 mg. tablets and as a syrup (1.45 mg. per milliliter) for oral administration. The proposed dosage for adults is 15 to 30 mg. three to four times a day.

*Noscapine** (Nectadon). This preparation is one of the isoquinoline alkaloids of opium, formerly known as narcotine. It resembles papaverine in its effects on smooth muscle, but its present use is based on its ability to depress the cough reflex. It resembles codeine in potency but produces no effects such as constipation, respiratory depression, constriction of the pupils, analgesia or sedation such as is associated with certain other opiates. Side effects after therapeutic dosage are minimal. Nausea occurs occasionally. It does not cause addiction. The usual dosage is 15 to 30 mg. administered orally three or four times daily.

*Dextromethorphan** (Romilar Hydrobromide). This drug is a synthetic derivative of morphine but is employed only as an agent to relieve cough. However, it possesses no significant analgesic properties, does not depress respiration, and does not cause addiction. Its toxicity is low and side effects appear to be negligible. Its antitussive effects appear to be well established by extensive experimental and clinical studies. It is administered orally. The usual adult dose is 10 to 20 mg. once to several times daily. It is available in 15 mg. tablets and as a syrup (3 mg. per milliliter).

Demulcents

Respiratory demulcents are sticky substances which protect the lining of the respiratory tract from the irritation of contact with air and thus check coughing. They are also used as vehicles for other drugs. The most common are syrups (tolu, citric acid, acacia, or glycyrrhiza).

Cough syrups are soothing partly because of their local effect in the throat; hence they should not be diluted and the patient should not drink water immediately after their administration.

Home remedies include simple syrup, honey, or a hard candy.

*Described in annual publication of A. M. A. Council on Drugs, N.N.D., 1960.

The soothing effect of steam inhalations upon irritated mucous membranes has a well-known demulcent effect. Plain or medicated steam may be administered with a special apparatus or by placing a basin of hot water over a hot plate so that resulting humidity of the room atmosphere is appreciably increased. There is little value, however, in administering steam when the doors or windows are open. Therefore, if the patient is to have the benefit of moisture-laden air which will in turn soothe the irritated respiratory tract, it is important to keep the patient's room warm and the doors and windows closed. The addition of some aromatic substance such as menthol or oil of pine may make the inhalation more pleasant or soothing.

Sprays or nebulae

The Council on Drugs has omitted from *New and Nonofficial Drugs* all brands of nasal inhalant preparations that contain liquid petrolatum because danger of lipid pneumonia attends their repeated use and other, safer vehicles are available. The Council has retained in *New and Nonofficial Drugs* only those oily inhalants that do not contain liquid petrolatum, pending the development of more positive evidence concerning undesirable properties of other kinds of oils.

Nasal sprays may contain epinephrine, ephedrine, isoproterenol (Isuprel), amphetamine, phenylephrine, naphazoline, and a number of other drugs (see sympathomimetic agents) for their effects on congested mucous membrane. Nasal douching and spraying are not approved by many physicians because of the danger of their overuse. Too frequent interference with the vasomotor mechanism in the nose may do more harm than good, and there is always the possibility of spreading the infection deeper into the sinuses or to the middle ear. Sprays and nose drops are of benefit when used judiciously under the advice of a physician.

Local anesthetics such as cocaine or its substitutes may be applied locally by spraying or swabbing on the mucous membrane.

Antiseptics

It is difficult to find an antiseptic for local use in the respiratory tract which is able to kill microorganisms without injuring the mucous membrane. Infections of the nose and throat are treated with antibiotics, either systemically or locally, in the form of sprays, or certain sulfonamide drugs, e.g., sulfadiazine.

Expectorants

Expectorants are drugs that increase or modify the secretion of mucus in the bronchi and facilitate the expulsion of sputum. They are therefore used in the treatment of coughs, bronchitis, and pneumonia. They are divided arbitrarily into stimulating and sedative or nauseating expectorants. The so-called stimulating expectorants are usually more or less volatile substances which are eliminated by the lungs and the respiratory mucous membranes, upon which they exert a stimulant action during their excretion.

It should be especially noted that the terms *stimulating* and *sedating* refer to the action of the drug on the patient and on the mucous membrane directly and are not judged by the amount of secretion produced. For example, the sedating expectorants—that is, those that depress and nauseate the patient—are usually the ones that cause the greatest amount of secretion. This is caused by a relaxation of the mucous membranes and a dilation of the vessels. The stimulating expectorants are those that tone up the patient or the mucous membranes and may diminish secretion.

The theory of the use of expectorants. Experimentally, little is known of their mode of action, but clinical experience attests their value. They are used empirically to modify the physiology of the respiratory passages. These passages are lined with ciliated epithelium which normally carries secretions of the tract toward the exterior. Mucus that becomes thick and tenacious probably interferes with these ciliated movements and coughing results. We do not know whether or not expectorants modify these movements.

Sedative expectorants

Sedative expectorants increase the secretion of mucus and thus protect the irritated mucous membrane and lessen the amount of coughing. A dry unproductive cough only wastes the patient's energy. An increased secretion of mucus may result in a productive cough and make the paroxysms of coughing less frequent. The value of adequate hydration of the patient, by oral intake of fluids as well as by inhalation of fully water-saturated vapors (steam), should be stressed as one of the most important means of producing increased amounts of mucus, as well as "thinning" such sputum.

Ammonium Chloride, U.S.P. This preparation is frequently administered in some vehicle such as Wild Cherry Syrup, Citric Acid Syrup, or Orange Syrup. Its exact method of action which results in increased mucus secretion is not agreed upon. Ammonium chloride is given in doses of 0.3 Gm. (5 gr.) four times a day in some suitable medium. It should be accompanied by a full glass of water because the increased fluid intake plays a part in the formation of increased mucus.

Ammonium Carbonate, U.S.P. This compound acts similarly to ammonium chloride, except that it causes gastric distress more easily. It is given in much the same manner and dosage as ammonium chloride. It is an alkaline salt and cannot be given in acid syrups. Usual dose is 0.3 Gm. (5 gr.).

Iodides (Sodium Iodide, U.S.P.; Potassium Iodide, U.S.P.; Hydriodic Acid Syrup, N.F.). Iodides are said to increase the bronchial secretion in subacute and chronic bronchitis. These preparations are too irritating to be used in acute inflammatory conditions of the respiratory tract. When sputum becomes particularly tenacious, they are given to fluidify the secretion or "loosen the cough." The average expectorant dose is 0.3 Gm. (5 gr.) three times a day, but quantities up to 2 Gm. (30 gr.) may be given. The salts may be administered in a saturated solution, or they may be administered in a cough mixture. If long continued, these drugs frequently produce symptoms of iodism. These are due to irritation of the nasal passage, bronchi, and skin, and include coryza and pain in the region of the frontal sinus and various skin eruptions, generally of a papular character. When such toxic symptoms occur, the drug should be discontinued, but it may be resumed in smaller doses after the disappearance of the symptoms.

Ipecac Syrup, U.S.P. This preparation is prescribed in doses of 1 to 8 ml. for adults and 5 minims for infants 1 year of age. A small increase of dosage is made for each additional year. In children, it is used to increase secretions and relieve bronchitis associated with croup.

Enzymes. Enzymes, namely desoxyribonucleases, are believed to be beneficial, if inhaled, in the liquefaction of viscid, tenacious mucus plugs in the tracheobronchial tree, thus producing increased amounts of thinner, more easily expectorated sputum. These agents are relatively irritating to the respiratory tree and must be used with care.

Detergents. Detergents such as Tergemist and Alevaire have been used in inhaled mixtures with the hope of liquefying secretions by altering surface tension. Their usefulness as such is questioned by some.

Stimulating expectorants

Stimulating expectorants tend to diminish secretions but they promote repair and healing in the bronchial mucosa. Some are aromatic substances, probably acting by their excretion via the respiratory tract and some are mild irritants.

Terpin Hydrate, N.F. This drug occurs as colorless, lustrous crystals, nearly odorless, having a slightly aromatic odor and somewhat bitter taste. Terpin hydrate is antiseptic, diaphoretic, and diuretic in action, but it is used chiefly to lessen secretion in bronchitis accompanied by free secretion. Usual dose of *Terpin Hydrate Elixir*, N.F., is 4 ml. (1 fluidram). Usual dose of *Terpin Hydrate and Codeine Elixir*, N.F. is

4 ml. (1 fluidram). The recommended dosage is usually too small to exert a significant effect and therefore it acts only as a vehicle.

Atropine. Atropine, although not classed as an expectorant, may be given cautiously to check secretion and excessive expectoration in certain forms of bronchitis.

Many of the remedies used to break up colds contain atropine. Morphine, codeine, and papaverine act not only as sedatives but also tend to dry the mucous membranes. In many cases the best treatment of a cold or inflammation of the respiratory mucous membranes consists of prescribing extra rest and the forcing of fluids and simple but nutritious food.

Antihistaminic agents for colds

Considerable difference of opinion exists at the present time as to the usefulness of the antihistamine drugs for the prevention or treatment of the common cold. These drugs include diphenhydramine hydrochloride (Benadryl) and tripelennamine hydrochloride (Pyribenzamine) as well as a number of others, further discussed in Chapter 12. Some investigators are of the opinion that if these drugs are taken early during the onset of a cold, the allergic manifestations of the disease are relieved; i.e., the patient experiences relief from the tickling sensation in the nose, sneezing, and the continuous irritating discharge from the nasal mucous membrane. The Council on Drugs warns that their indiscriminate use is not without harmful effects; e.g., people may become excessively drowsy and fall asleep while driving a car or operating power machinery. It is also possible that profound effects may occur in the central nervous system and the blood-forming tissues following prolonged use of these drugs.

Drugs used to relax bronchial spasm in asthma

Several drugs, which have been described elsewhere in the text under their chief therapeutic uses, are employed to relieve or prevent the paroxysms of asthma. They include preparations of ephedrine, epinephrine, isoproterenol, aminophylline, the nitrites, belladonna, and stramonium.

Steroids, by their anti-inflammatory action, may also afford dramatic relief from bronchial edema in asthma when used judiciously for short intervals. These drugs have been discussed elsewhere (see Index).

Oxygen and oxygen therapy

Oxygen is a gas which constitutes 20 per cent of ordinary air and is necessary to maintain life. Oxygen, U.S.P., is oxygen in a compressed state. It is a colorless, odorless, and tasteless gas. It is not flammable but it supports combustion much more vigorously than does air.

Oxygen is compressed and marketed in steel cylinders which are fitted with reducing valves for the delivery of the gas. Because it is under considerable pressure, the tanks must be handled carefully so as to prevent their falling or bumping into each other or into anything that may cause undue jarring.

Effects of oxygen deficiency in the body. Experiments in the use of oxygen in airplane travel at high altitudes have resulted in interesting observations of oxygen deficiency in otherwise normal individuals. It has long been known that deprivation of oxygen leads rapidly to death. Tissue cells must have a continuous supply since no provision is made for storage of oxygen in the body. Symptoms of anoxemia begin when the oxygen pressure of inspired air is 14 per cent of that at sea level.*

The individual may experience headache, excessive sleepiness, great lassitude, mental inefficiency, irritability, change in pulse and respiration, great fatigue, muscle incoordination, and finally unconsciousness. The cortical cells of the brain are the ones most sensitive to oxygen deficiency and the ones most likely to suffer irreparable damage. The depression of nerve tissue progresses downward as the oxygen deficiency continues until finally vital centers in the medulla are affected.

Effect of high concentrations of oxygen. Although high concentrations of oxygen may be breathed, the composition of the blood is changed relatively little. However, in conditions characterized by oxygen want, any increase in the oxygen content of the blood is certain to be beneficial. Inhalation of pure oxygen may bring about an increase of oxygen in the arterial blood to the extent of 15 per cent more than it usually carries. The beneficial effect is apparently due more to the increased oxygen pressure in the tissues than to the increased content of the blood. Although a difference of opinion exists as to the effect of high concentrations of oxygen upon body tissues, especially those of the lungs, there seems to be a growing belief that intermittent use of pure oxygen may not have an injurious effect in the human lung and that when conditions seem to warrant high concentrations they should be used.

Purposes for giving oxygen. Oxygen is used in medicine chiefly to treat hypoxia and hypoxemia (oxygen lack and diminished oxygen tension in the blood). It is indicated therefore in the following:

1. In conditions associated with inadequate oxygenation in the lungs such as pneumonia, both lobar and bronchopneumonia, pulmonary edema, and poisoning from gases such as carbon monoxide.

2. In severe asthma.

*Lovelace, W. R., Jr.: Oxygen for Therapy and Aviation, Proc. Staff Meet. Mayo Clin. 13: 647, 1938.

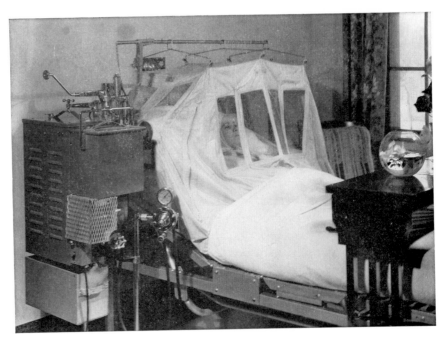

Fig. 36 Oxygen tent in position. Oxygen is introduced into the cabinet at a rate which provides for the desired concentration. The tent also serves as a small air-conditioning unit.

3. In cardiac failure or threatened cardiac decompensation and coronary occlusion.

4. In anesthesia to increase the safety of general anesthetics.

5. In treatment of abdominal distention due to intestinal ileus.

6. Also reported to have given satisfactory results in treatment of certain types of headache.

7. In certain conditions involving injury to the nervous system and threatened respiratory failure.

The gas causing gastrointestinal distention is mostly nitrogen. When the patient inhales pure oxygen or a high concentration of oxygen, the nitrogen which is dissolved in the blood gradually leaves by way of the lungs. The blood is then able to absorb the nitrogen from body cavities, such as the intestine, discharge it into the expired air, and thus relieve distention and gas pain.

Administration of oxygen. Oxygen is administered in a number of ways, including the oxygen tent, nasal catheter, face mask, head tent, and the oxygen chamber. It is often used under a regulated intermittent positive pressure during inspiration to produce deeper and more efficient breathing in patients who, for various reasons, cannot exchange

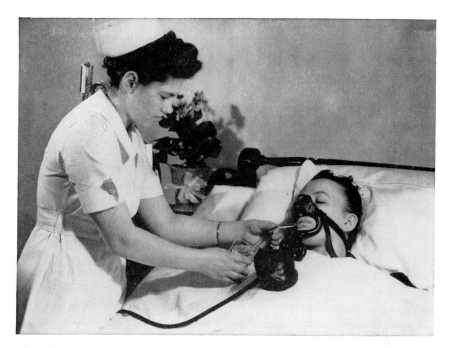

Fig. 37 Nasal type of B.L.B. oxygen inhalation apparatus in position. To keep the patient comfortable both the oronasal and the nasal type of apparatus should be removed at intervals of two hours, when the patient's face should be washed and the skin dried and powdered.

air efficiently. The problem of administering gas in a concentration high enough to be beneficial without excessive waste has not been easy, especially when the oxygen tent is used. A concentration of approximately 50 per cent is usually ordered, although higher concentrations are also used. The oxygen tent continues to be a favorite method of giving oxygen in many hospitals and for certain types of patients who are unable to tolerate a mask over the face. In the oxygen tent or room are special devices for regulating temperature and humidity. The nurse should plan her care of the patient so that the tent is removed or opened as little as possible. In addition, she should keep in mind two of the important properties of oxygen; first, that oxygen supports combustion and that any combustible material will burn with much greater ease and intensity when the oxygen content of the atmosphere is increased over and above the normal content. Visitors must be carefully instructed and watched to prevent any form of fire from entering the room where oxygen is being given. Hand bells are used in preference to an electric call signal. The application of lights to the wound, the use of an electric cautery, and a hot plate for steam inhalations are further examples of

Drugs that affect organs of respiratory system 489

situations to be avoided when there is a source of oxygen under pressure in the room.

Second, oxygen is heavier than air, and to prevent needless waste of oxygen a rubber plastic sheet should cover the entire mattress, and the canopy of the tent must be well tucked under the mattress and around the patient.

The mechanical simplicity and ease of operation make the face mask useful for oxygen administration in small hospitals, in the home, and also by pilots and passengers of airplanes. By this method oxygen of any desired concentration can be given economically and efficiently. Some patients, however, object to having the mask against the face for prolonged periods of time.

A word of extreme caution should be given regarding the use of oxygen in patients with severe respiratory disease who have become resistant to the usual respiratory stimulating effect of carbon dioxide and who are stimulated to breathe primarily by anoxemia. If one indescriminately administers nasal oxygen to these persons, their last stimulus to breathe is removed and death may ensue.

Helium

Helium-oxygen mixtures have been used for some time to treat obstructive types of dyspnea. Helium is an inert gas and so light that a mixture of 80 per cent helium and 20 per cent oxygen is only one third as heavy as air.* Helium is only slightly soluble in body fluids and has a high rate of diffusion. Its low specific gravity makes it possible for mixtures of this gas with oxygen to be breathed with less effort than either oxygen or air alone when there is obstruction in the air passages.

It is recommended for status asthmaticus, bronchiectasis, emphysema, and for anesthesia when dealing with a respiratory tract in which there is obstruction of some form.

*Goodman, L., and Gilman, A.: The Pharmacological Basis for Therapeutics, New York, 1955, The Macmillan Co., p. 922.

Questions
for review and study

1 Indicate two ways in which drugs affect the respiratory system.
2 Name several conditions during which coughing may be extremely harmful to a patient.
3 How many drugs act so as to produce relief from a cough?
4 Name several drugs illustrating the systemic action.
5 Define demulcent. Give some examples.
6 How do expectorants produce their effects? In what conditions are they useful?
7 Under what conditions is it preferable to stimulate expectoration?
8 Why does increased humidity of atmosphere in itself help to relieve coughing?
9 Mention several points that are essential in good nursing for a patient who is receiving steam inhalations.

490

10 How can a nurse help to minimize waste and expense in the administration of oxygen and carbon dioxide?
11 Why must a nurse exercise caution when giving advice about the free use of nose drops, nasal sprays, etc.?
12 What harmful effects may result from overmedication of the nasal mucous membranes?
13 Name several drugs given to relieve cough.
14 Give the action and uses of terpin hydrate.
15 Name several drugs that may be used to relieve the spasms of asthma.
16 State several therapeutic uses of oxygen.
17 Mention several precautions to be exercised in the administration of oxygen.

References

Text and reference books

A. M. A. Council on Drugs: New and Nonofficial Drugs, Philadelphia, 1960, J. B. Lippincott Co.

Bickerman, H. A.: The Choice of Antitussive Agents. In Modell, W. (editor): Choice of Drugs, 1960-1961, St. Louis, 1960, The C. V. Mosby Co.

Davison, F. R.: Handbook of Materia Medica, Toxicology, and Pharmacology, St. Louis, 1949, The C. V. Mosby Co.

Goodman, L., and Gilman, A.: The Pharmacological Basis of Therapeutics, New York, 1955, The Macmillan Co.

Sollmann, T.: A Manual of Pharmacology, Philadelphia, 1957, W. B. Saunders Co.

Original articles

Council on Pharmacy and Chemistry: Status Report on Antihistaminic Agents in the Prophylaxis and Treatment of the Common Cold, J. A. M. A. **142:** 566, 1950.

Editorial: Antihistaminics for Colds, J. A. M. A. **142:** 570, 1950.

Lovelace, W. R., Jr.: Oxygen Therapy and Aviation, Proc. Staff Meet. Mayo Clin. **13:** 647, 1938.

Chapter 16

Drugs that affect the skin
and mucous membranes
(dermatologic agents)

The skin is the largest organ of the body. It consists of two principal layers: (1) the epidermis, outer layer or cuticle, which is nonvascular, and (2) an inner layer of connective tissue containing blood vessels, nerves, and lymphatics. Four epidermal sublayers or strata are recognized as follows: (a) the stratum germinativum, the deepest layer where pigmentation occurs; (b) the stratum granulosum, a thin layer of cells; (c) the stratum lucidum, also very thin and not visible unless the skin is thick; and (d) the stratum corneum, or outermost layer, composed of flattened, dry, dead cells which gradually are exfoliated.

Absorption from the skin

Absorption from the skin is poor and uncertain. The flat cells of the outermost layer of the skin contain keratin, a substance that serves to waterproof the skin and to prevent the absorption of water and other substances. Absorption is affected, however, by the presence of sweat pores and of sebaceous glands which penetrate the epidermis from the deeper subcutaneous tissue and corium. Hair follicles, pigment cells, nerve endings, nerve networks, blood vessels, as well as collagen and elastic fibers, all contribute to the functions of the skin. Although the skin is not known for its powers of absorption, drugs that cannot penetrate the horny first layer are sometimes absorbed by way of the sebaceous glands. Absorption is increased if the skin is macerated either by water or perspiration. It is more likely to occur if the epidermis is thin, as it is in the axilla or in the skin of a child. From raw or denuded surfaces absorption will take place rapidly. The epithelium under the tongue is thin; hence sublingual medication is sometimes feasible. Methyl salicylate rubbed on the skin can be found in the urine in 30 minutes. Alcohol and volatile solvents promote absorption. The nature of the vehicle affects absorption; e.g., drugs that are fat soluble can be absorbed more rapidly than water-soluble drugs, and natural fats make a better vehicle by which to carry the drug into the skin than do substances such as petrolatum.

Symptoms associated with cutaneous disorders

The skin is capable of responding to stimuli by imparting to the sensorium many sensations, such as those of pain, smarting, itching, tingling, heat, cold, and a pricking sensation when the point of a pin is even lightly thrust against it. Reactions or disorders of the skin are made manifest by symptoms such as itching, pain, or tingling and by signs such as swelling, redness, papules, pustules, blisters, and hives.

The reaction of the skin which makes the patient uncomfortable or unsightly may be attributable to, or related to, many things, e.g., sensitivity to drugs, allergy, infection, emotional conflict, hormonal imbalance, or degenerative disease. Many times the cause of the skin disorder is unknown and the treatment may be empiric in the hope that the right remedy will be found.

Drugs excreted by way of the skin

Drugs may be excreted by the skin in small amounts. Silver, copper, arsenic, mercury, bromides, borates, phenol, salicylates, antipyrine, methylene blue, and phenolphthalein may be deposited in the skin and sweat glands, and this may explain the skin eruption sometimes caused. Many other drugs can be the cause of skin eruption.

Preparations that soothe

Emollients

Emollients are fatty or oily substances that may be used to soften or soothe irritated skin and mucous membrane. An emollient may also serve as a vehicle for application of other medicinal substances. Olive oil and liquid petrolatum frequently are used to cleanse dry areas which would be irritated by water.

Fixed Oils. These are used as emollients and include olive oil, flaxseed oil, and cottonseed oil.

Benzoinated Lard. This is made by incorporating 1 per cent benzoin with lard and then straining the preparation. The addition of the benzoin hinders the development of rancidity. The preparation is used as an ingredient of ointments.

Glycerin, U.S.P., B.P. (Glycerol). In pure form this tends to have a drying effect, but when diluted with water or rose water it is useful for application to irritated lips and skin.

Hydrous Wool Fat, U.S.P., B.P. (Lanolin). Hydrous wool fat is made by combining the purified fat of sheep's-wool with 25 to 30 per cent water. It is used as an ointment base. It does not become rancid, and as much as twice its weight of water can be incorporated with it. It has a somewhat unpleasant odor. It requires dilution for use in ointments, and from 20 to 100 per cent of petrolatum may be added for this purpose.

Hydrophilic Ointment, U.S.P. This is a type of ointment in which the oil in it is dispersed in the continuous water phase. It is an oil-in-water emulsion, and when medicaments are incorporated, the wetting agent in the emulsion enables the drugs to come in more direct contact with the skin and sebaceous glands. Among other advantages it is less greasy and more easily washed off. Inflamed or irritated skin is often intolerant of this kind of ointment.

Petrolatum, N.F. (Petroleum Jelly). This is a purified, semisolid mixture of hydrocarbons derived from petroleum. It is an important ointment base.

Liquid Petrolatum, N.F. This form is used as a vehicle for medicinal agents for local application. Light petrolatum can be employed as a spray.

Rose Water Ointment, N.F. (Cold Cream). This ointment is a pleasant-smelling water-in-oil emulsion of the cold cream type. It contains spermaceti and white wax as emulsifying agents in addition to expressed almond oil, sodium borate, rose water, oil of rose, and distilled water. Nonallergic cold creams do not contain perfume, to which some patients are intolerant.

Petrolatum Rose Water Ointment. This ointment is like Rose Water Ointment, U.S.P., except that liquid petrolatum is substituted for almond oil or persic oil.

Theobroma Oil, U.S.P., B.P. (Cacao or Cocoa Butter). This preparation is a fixed oil which is expressed from the roasted seeds of the *Theobromo cacao*. It is a yellowish white solid, having a faint, agreeable odor and a bland taste resembling chocolate. It is used chiefly for making suppositories and, to some extent, as a lubricant for massage and for application to sore nipples.

White Ointment. This is a mixture of white wax and white petrolatum. It is mostly petrolatum with a little white wax added to give it stiffness.

Yellow Ointment, N.F. This ointment contains yellow wax and petrolatum.

Zinc Oxide Ointment, U.S.P. This ointment contains 20 per cent zinc oxide in a base of liquid petrolatum and white ointment.

Zinc Ointment, B.P. This contains 15 per cent zinc oxide in a base of simple ointment.

Solutions and lotions

Soothing preparations may also be liquids, which carry an insoluble powder or suspension, or they may be mild acid or alkaline solutions, such as boric acid solution, limewater, or aluminum subacetate. The bismuth salts (the subcarbonate or the subnitrate) and starch are also commonly used for their soothing effect.

Aluminum Acetate Solution, U.S.P. (Burow's Solution). This contains, in 1,000 ml. of aqueous medium, 545 ml. of aluminum subacetate solution, and 15 ml. of glacial acetic acid. It is diluted with 10 to 40 parts of water before application.

Aluminum Subacetate Solution, U.S.P. This preparation contains, in 1,000 ml. of aqueous medium, 160 Gm. of aluminum sulfate, 160 ml. of acetic acid, and 70 Gm. of precipitated calcium carbonate. Applied topically after dilution with 20 to 40 parts of water as a wet dressing.

Calamine Lotion, U.S.P. Prepared calamine, zinc oxide, bentonite magma, glycerin, and calcium hydroxide solution are included in this lotion. It is a soothing lotion used for the dermatitis caused by poison ivy, insect bites, prickly heat, and so on. It is patted on the involved skin area.

Zinc Stearate, U.S.P. This is a compound of zinc and variable proportions of stearic and palmitic acids. It contains about 14 per cent zinc oxide and is similar to zinc oxide. It is used as a dusting powder, but caution should be observed with its use, particularly around infants, to prevent inhalation of the powder.

Antiseptics and parasiticides

It is generally agreed that thorough washing of the skin with warm water and a mild soap should precede the application of antiseptics to the skin. It is impossible to sterilize the skin, but adequate soaping and washing will do much to remove bacteria and the outer, loose epithelium. Strong antiseptics may do more harm than good by producing an irritation which will decrease the natural resistance of the skin to bacterial invasion. Antiseptics that are used to lower bacterial content are presented in Chapter 23.

A number of skin conditions for which antiseptics are used are caused by staphylococci and streptococci. Invasion by these organisms is likely to occur, especially when the normal protective mechanisms of the skin are broken down.

Drugs that affect skin and mucous membranes 495

Antibiotics

Although relatively costly, bacitracin and tyrothricin are very useful in the local treatment of infectious lesions. *Bacitracin* is most often used in an ointment, although it can be used to irrigate wet dressings or as a dusting powder. It is odorless and nonstaining and its use seldom results in sensitization. *Tyrothricin* is said to be more effective in wet dressings than in a cream or an ointment. Tyrothricin does not cause local irritation and its use rarely is attended by sensitization. *Neomycin* has been used successfully in the treatment of a number of infections of skin and mucous membrane. It is applied topically but occasionally it irritates the skin. An ointment combining neomycin, bacitracin, and polymyxin B may be more efficacious in mixed infections than when these agents are used singly. *Vioform* and *xeroform* are helpful in skin infections; there is seldom any irritation, but temporary discoloration of the skin and linens occurs. A number of antibiotics can be given orally or parenterally for treatment of infections of the skin (boils, carbuncles, etc.).

Ammoniated Mercury Ointment

Ammoniated Mercury Ointment, U.S.P., B.P. The U.S.P. preparation contains 5 Gm. of ammoniated mercury in each 100 Gm. of finished preparation, along with liquid petrolatum and white ointment. In this strength, local irritation seldom occurs. The preparation has no odor and it does not stain. It occasionally causes sensitization, particularly when combined with salicylic acid.

Nitrofurazone

Nitrofurazone, N.F. (Furacin). This is a synthetic, bright yellow, antibacterial substance which is inhibitory to bacteria in concentrations of 1:100,000 to 1:200,000 and bactericidal in concentrations of 1:50,000 to 1:75,000. It is effective against a variety of both gram-positive and gram-negative organisms. It is least effective against *Pseudomonas aeruginosa* and *Diplococcus pneumoniae*.

Nitrofurazone is useful for topical application in the treatment and prophylaxis of superficial mixed infections commonly found in contaminated wounds, burns, ulcerations, impetigo, and ecthyma. It is also said to be useful in the preparation of areas for skin grafting. Applications of nitrofurazone may produce a generalized allergic skin reaction in certain individuals. Its internal use for the present is not recommended, although it appears to have a low level of toxicity. Any systemic untoward effects due to absorption from dressings seem unlikely.

Nitrofurazone is applied locally in a 0.2 per cent ointment-like base or solution.* It is either applied directly to the area or applied to a dressing which is then applied to the infected area. Since the base is water soluble and softens at body temperature, special re-enforcement of the dressing may be required to maintain an effective contact with the area or to limit absorption into the dressing.

Antifungal agents

Coparaffinate† (Iso-Par). This compound is used in the treatment of mycotic infections of the hands and feet, for eczemas of the ear, and for certain skin conditions associated with allergic reactions. It is applied topically in a 17 per cent ointment. It should be applied with a rubber finger cot or a piece of absorbent cotton to avoid retention of an objectionable odor on the fingers. It is applied on the infected area in the evening before going to bed and again the next morning. Relief should be obtained within a week or two or some other form of treatment should be given.

Diamthazole Dihydrochloride† (Asterol Dihydrochloride). This preparation is effective for the treatment of fungous infections due to trichophytons, microsporons, and *Candida albicans*. It has been used especially for athlete's foot, ringworm of the scalp, and fungous infections around the nails. It is available as a 5 per cent ointment, powder, and tincture. It is applied topically. Its use for young children (under the age of 2 years) is not recommended because they may suck their fingers and develop untoward systemic effects.

Salicylanilide, N.F. (Ansadol, Salinidol). This antifungous preparation is used externally for the treatment of ringworm of the scalp. It is available as a 5 per cent ointment and is applied alone or along with less irritating fungistatics. The ointment is rubbed into the affected areas once or twice a day for 6 days of the week over a period of about 8 weeks.

Propionate Compound (Propion Gel). This is a mixture of calcium propionate and sodium propionate, in the form of a water-miscible jelly. It is used in the treatment of vulvovaginal moniliasis. It is placed, by means of an applicator, in the upper part of the vagina twice a day. A plain water douche is recommended before the first treatment, but no more douches are allowed as long as treatment continues.

Methylrosaniline Chloride, U.S.P. (Gentian Violet). For external application this is available in a solution containing 1 per cent of the dye in an alcohol-water solvent. Its principal disadvantage is that it stains clothing.

*N.N.R., 1960, p. 48.
†Described in annual publication of A. M. A. Council on Drugs, N.N.D., 1960.

Drugs that affect skin and mucous membranes 497

Potassium Permanganate Solution, U.S.P. (1:100 to 1:10,000). This solution is sometimes prescribed for foot soaks for epidermophytosis of the feet. It is inexpensive and odorless but leaves brown stains on fabrics, skin, and nails.

Sulfur Ointment, U.S.P.; *Sulphur Ointment,* B.P. Sulfur ointment contains about 10 per cent of the precipitated sulfur in a base of liquid petrolatum and white ointment and is used in the treatment of fungous infections (ringworm) and seborrhea. An ointment containing precipitated sulfur, salicylic acid, and resorcin may be more helpful than sulfur alone in the treatment of seborrheic dermatitis and fungous infections.

Benzoic and Salicylic Acid Ointment, U.S.P. (Whitfield's Ointment). This ointment contains salicylic acid, benzoic acid, and polyethylene glycol ointment. It is used for epidermophytosis of the feet (athlete's foot).

*Nystatin** (Mycostatin). This drug is an antibiotic substance used to treat infections of the skin and mucous membranes which are due to *Candida albicans.* Vaginal infections are treated with suppositories or tablets, each containing 100,000 units, once or twice daily. An ointment and cream are available (100,000 units per gram) for moniliasis of the skin and should be applied to the affected areas once to several times a day.

Griseofulvin. This preparation is a recent important addition to the treatment of superficial fungous infections, particularly those caused by the trichophyton and microsporon organisms. Given orally in a dosage of 1 Gm. per day (in children the dosage is decreased by one half), it has a fungistatic action by combining with the keratin of skin, hair, and nails. Topical therapy should be continued while the griseofulvin is ingested. It is available in 250 mg. tablets for oral administration.

Pediculicides

The following agents are used to kill lice.

Gamma Benzene Hexachloride, U.S.P., B.P. (Gexane, Kwell). This white, crystalline powder acts both as a pediculicide and scabicide. It is toxic and its use should be supervised by a physician. One application is sufficient to remove the active parasites. The preparation does not dissolve nits and, after 1 week, a second application may be given if necessary. Repeated use should be avoided because the substance tends to cause skin irritation. It should be kept away from the eyes, as it is irritating to mucous membranes. It is applied topically as a 1 per cent lotion or ointment. A small brush may be used to facilitate application to the scalp. All clothing and bed linen should be sterilized by boiling to prevent reinfection. Wool clothing should be dry cleaned. The patient should not bathe or wash the hair until 24 hours after the treatment. A 10 per cent solution of acetic acid or vinegar will help to remove nits from hairy regions but should be followed by a cleansing bath.

*Isobornyl Thiocyanoacetate-Technical** (Bornate). This preparation is one of the thiocyanates that kill lice. It may be mildly irritating to the skin of certain persons but it does not seem to act as a sensitizing agent. It should not be applied near the eyes or on mucous membranes.

An oil emulsion is used in amounts of 30 to 60 ml., depending on the site (amount of hair). It is applied and worked into a lather, after which it is allowed to remain for 10 minutes. In a scalp treatment, the hair is then combed with a fine-tooth comb and washed with a bland soap and water. The preparation should not remain on the skin too long. More than two applications should be avoided.

Scabicides

Scabicides are used in the treatment of scabies or of itch caused by the itch mite. The old-fashioned sulfur ointment is effective but frequently is overused and may produce a dermatitis which is as bad as the original trouble. The newer drugs do not necessarily do away with the need for bathing and sterilization of clothing and linen, but they act more rapidly, one or two applications usually being sufficient. Some of the preparations are effective for both lice and scabies.

*Gamma Benzene Hexachloride** (Gexane, Kwell). This agent is a scabicide and a pediculicide for topical use. Patients should not bathe for at least 24 hours after treatment. Clothing and bed linen should be sterilized to prevent reinfection.

Benzyl Benzoate Lotion, N.F. (Benylate, Albacide). Benzyl benzoate is applied in a 10 to 30 per cent lotion or emulsion. Application is sometimes followed by a slight, transient, burning sensation. In patients with sensitive skins, severe irritation sometimes develops. It should be kept away from the eyes.

The entire body should be bathed, and the lesions caused by the itch mite should be well scrubbed with soap and warm water. Then the entire body surface, except the face, should be covered with the drug in the form of the emulsion or lotion, the application being made with a swab or brush. Particular care should be given to the region of the nails. After the first application has dried, a second one should be made to the

*Described in annual publication of A. M. A. Council on Drugs, N.N.D., 1960.

most involved areas. Sterilization of clothing and bed linen is essential. Twenty-four hours later, clean clothing is put on after a warm, soaking bath. A second or third treatment should be given if the parasite has not been eradicated.

Benzyl Benzoate-Chlorophenothane-Ethyl Aminobenzoate Lotion. This mixture of drugs is used in the treatment of pediculosis and coexistent scabies. For treatment of scabies, the body first should have a warm, soapy bath. All soap should then be rinsed from the skin. An emulsion or an ointment of the mixture should then be rubbed over the entire body surface below the neck. Folds of skin and the nails should receive special attention. One application usually is sufficient, but it may be repeated in a week if necessary. Clothing and bed linen must be properly sterilized.

Stimulants and irritants

Stimulants

Stimulants are those substances that produce a mild irritation and in that way promote healing and the disappearance of inflammatory exudates. Most of the irritant drugs when applied in low concentrations exert a stimulating effect. Good examples of preparations that may have a stimulating effect are the tars obtained from the restructive distillation of wood and coal.

Tars when diluted act as antiseptics as well as irritants. Official preparations include *Juniper Tar*, U.S.P., *Cade Oil*, B.P., *Coal Tar*, U.S.P., and *Prepared Coal Tar*, B.P. The tars are sometimes prescribed in the treatment of psoriasis and chronic *eczematous* dermatitis. The official tars are seldom employed full strength. Coal tar is the most antiseptic but also the most irritant, and it has the most disagreeable odor. *Ichthammol*, N.F., B.P., derived from destructive distillation of coal, is used in the form of an ointment for eczema and seborrheic conditions of the skin.

Vulneraries are a form of tissue stimulant which are used to hasten the granulation of wounds or stimulate the growth of cells over a denuded area.

Compound Benzoin Tincture, U.S.P., B.P., is useful as a stimulant and protective for ulcers, bedsores, cracked nipples, and fissures of the lips, anus, etc.

Preparations made of red blood cells also have been used to stimulate healing of indolent wounds and ulcers.

Irritants

Irritants are agents that injure the skin and set up defense mechanisms which protect the tissues. The first response to local irritation is increased blood supply to the part, redness, and feeling of warmth. Drugs which when rubbed on the skin produce a hyperemia are called rubefacients. Turpentine, camphor, chloroform, ammonia, and methyl salicylate in the form of liniments all have a rubefacient action. Mustard and capsicum plasters are also rubefacient in effect, and if applied too long they may act as vesicants.

Vesicants are irritants that are capable of greater degree of irritation. They cause the capillaries to dilate widely and become permeable. This results in escape of plasma and the formation of blisters. Vesicants are little used today. Cantharides and ammonia are typical vesicant drugs. Many rubefacients are capable of acting as vesicants if used too strong or too long.

Escharotics, corrosives, or caustics are substances that cause necrosis or death of tissue. They act by combining with the tissue and precipitating it as a compound. The caustics are acids (glacial acetic or nitric), alkalies such as sodium or potassium hydroxide, metallic salts like silver nitrate or zinc chloride, or concentrated phenol. Carbon dioxide in either liquid or solid form is able to destroy tissue by freezing it. Corrosives or caustics are used to remove exuberant granulations, polyps, warts, and similar pathologic growths. They should not be used in the treatment of moles or precancerous skin conditions because of the danger of stimulating malignant degeneration.

Keratolytics

Keratolytics (horn dissolvers) are drugs that soften scales and loosen the outer horny layer of the skin. *Salicylic Acid*, U.S.P., B.P., and *Resorcinol*, U.S.P., B.P., are the drugs of choice. Their action makes possible the penetration of other medicinal substances by a cleaning of the lesions involved. *Salicylic acid* is particularly important for its keratolytic effect in local treatment of scalp conditions, warts, corns, fungous infections, and chronic types of dermatitis. It is used in ointments or plasters or in collodion up to 20 per cent for this purpose.

Antipruritics

Antipruritics are drugs given to allay itching of skin and mucous membranes. There is less need for these preparations as the constitutional treatment of patients with skin disorders is better understood. Dilute solutions containing phenol as well as tars have been widely used. They may be applied as lotions, pastes, or ointments. Dressings wet with potassium permanganate 1:4,000, aluminum subacetate 1:16, boric acid, or normal saline solution may cool and soothe and thus prevent itching. Lotions such as calamine or calamine with phenol (phenolated calamine,

U.S.P.) and cornstarch or oatmeal baths may also be employed to relieve itching.

Local anesthetics such as dibucaine and benzocaine may decrease pruritus, but their use is not recommended because of their high sensitizing and irritating effects. The application of hydrocortisone in a lotion or ointment in a strength of 0.5 to 1.0 per cent has proved to be one of the best methods of relieving pruritus and decreasing inflammation. It has the additional advantage of possessing a low sensitizing index. It may be necessary to administer sedatives which have a systemic effect. Chloral hydrate or one of the newer nonbarbiturate sedatives may prove valuable, e.g., *ethchlorvynol* (Placidyl). Some physicians prefer not to use barbiturates because they decrease cortical control of the scratch reflex. Ataractics such as *meprobamate* (Miltown) are usually effective and safe when given in small doses. *Trimeprazine* (Temaril), one of the phenothiazine derivatives, is said to be effective for the relief of itching.

In addition to the measures mentioned used to relieve itching, preparations of *ergotamine* are used to relieve the generalized itching associated with jaundice, cirrhosis of the liver, Hodgkin's disease, etc. Ergotamine Tartrate, U.S.P. (Gynergen), is one of the preparations, and there are others, one of which is dihydroergotamine. This preparation is said to relieve itching in a way similar to ergotamine tartrate without producing the common undesirable side effects of that preparation, i.e., nausea, vomiting, and cardiovascular reactions.

Other preparations to relieve itching related to allergic reactions are the antihistaminic drugs (see Index).

Protectives

Protectives are soothing, cooling preparations that form a film on the skin. Protectives to be useful must not macerate the skin, must prevent drying of the tissues, and must keep out light, air, and dust. Nonabsorbable powders are usually listed as protectives, but they are not particularly useful because they stick to wet surfaces and have to be scraped off and do not stick to dry surfaces at all.

Collodion, U.S.P. Collodion is a 4 per cent solution of pyroxylin, or guncotton, in a mixture of ether and alcohol. When collodion is applied to the skin, the ether and alcohol evaporate, leaving a transparent film which adheres to the skin and protects it.

Flexible Collodion, U.S.P., B.P. This is a mixture of collodion with 2 per cent of camphor and 3 per cent of castor oil. The addition of the latter makes the resulting film elastic and more tenacious. *Styptic* collodion contains 20 per cent of tannic acid and is, therefore, astringent as well as protective.

Adhesive Plaster. Adhesive plaster is a tenacious preparation which is solid at ordinary temperature but pliable and adhesive at the temperature of the body. It consists of rubber, lead plaster, and petrolatum spread on linen or muslin. Besides its use as a general protective agent, adhesive plaster is widely used to re-enforce weak muscles, cover ulcers, limit effusions, etc. and to keep dressings in place.

Nonabsorbable Powders. These include zinc stearate, zinc oxide, certain bismuth preparations, talcum powder, and aluminum silicate. The disadvantages associated with their use have been mentioned previously.

Although it is safe to say that no substances known at present can stimulate healing to take place at a more rapid rate than is normal under optimal conditions, nonetheless, preparations that act as bland protectives may help in the healing of wounds by prevention of crusting and trauma. In some instances they may reduce offensive odors.

*Water-Soluble Chlorophyll Derivatives** (Chloresium). A mixture of water-soluble derivatives of chlorophyll is employed topically to produce a bland, soothing effect, to deodorize, to promote tissue repair and to relieve itching in ulcers, burns, or wounds. It is applied in solution or as an ointment. These derivatives of chlorophyll may aid in producing a clean, granulating wound base suitable for the normal repair of tissues, but they do not take the place of anti-infective agents for the treatment of infection.

Solutions containing 0.2 per cent water-soluble chlorophyl derivatives are applied one or more times daily. A 0.5 per cent ointment may be spread over affected areas and covered with a fine mesh gauze or dressing.

Astringents

Astringents are drugs that tend to harden and contract tissues with which they come in contact. When applied to mucous membranes or to denuded or bleeding areas, they coagulate the albumins of the superficial layer of cells, thus hardening and contracting them. This action also forms a thin coating over the cells which protects them from irritation and promotes healing. They constrict the small blood vessels in the area of their application, thus relieving congestion; and they stop bleeding by coagulating the blood albumin at the point of rupture of the blood vessel.

Astringents may be divided into two groups: Mineral or Inorganic Astringents and Vegetable or Organic Astringents.

---

*Described in annual publication of A. M. A. Council on Drugs, N.N.D., 1960.

The mineral astringents are various salts of metals, the most important of which are the following:

Alum	Silver nitrate
Bismuth subnitrate	Zinc acetate
Bismuth subcarbonate	Zinc chloride
Ferric chloride	Zinc sulfate
Lead acetate	Zinc oxide
Potassium chlorate	

Vegetable astringents are vegetable substances which owe their power to contract tissues to the *tannic acid* which they contain. Tannic acid is used externally as an astringent and hemostatic.

Tannic Acid Glycerite, N.F. This is a 20 per cent solution of tannic acid in glycerin. It affords a convenient means for making dilute solutions for local application.

Burns

It is said that approximately 6,000 or more people die each year of burns in the United States alone. The chief cause of death is shock, a fact of considerable significance in any effective plan of treatment.

Consideration of what takes place in the damaged tissues clarifies many points of treatment. At first there is an altered capillary permeability in the local injured area. That is, the permeability is increased and a loss of plasma and weeping of the surface tissues result. If the burn is at all extensive, considerable amounts of plasma fluid may be lost in a relatively short time. This depletes the blood volume and causes a decreased cardiac output and diminished blood flow. Unless the situation is rapidly brought under control, irreparable damage may result from the rapidly developing tissue anoxia. Lack of sufficient oxygen and the accumulation of waste products from inadequate oxidation result in loss of tone in the minute blood vessels, and the increased capillary permeability then extends to tissues remote from those suffering the initial injury. Thus a generalized edema often develops and the vicious cycle once established tends to be self-perpetuating. One of the aims in the treatment of burns is therefore to stop the loss of plasma in so far as possible and replenish that which is lost as quickly as possible.

Second or third degree burns must be thought of as open wounds with the accompanying danger of infection. Another aim must be to prevent or treat infection. The treatment, however, must be such that it will not bring about any further destruction of tissue or of the small islands of remaining epithelium from which growth and regeneration can take place.

Local treatment. Sometimes the best local first-aid treatment is to cover the burned area with as clean a towel or dressing as may be obtained until the part can be treated aseptically in a hospital. A sterile dressing or towel would be preferable, but these may not be available. The first impulse of many well-intentioned persons to apply some greasy ointment such as lard or butter is often a bad one, for such a measure may be the means of infecting the wound. Furthermore, the chances are that all of the grease or ointment will have to be removed later if the burn is anything more than a superficial first degree burn.

The local treatment of burns usually consists merely of exposing the part or parts to air. Foreign particles may be removed and the patient is placed on sterile sheets and covered with a cradle, over which clean sheets are placed. Tracheotomy is frequently done early if respiratory difficulty is observed. No immediate cleansing, washing, or débridement is done.

General treatment. This includes supportive measures to treat shock and relieve pain and restlessness, as well as the treatment or prevention of infection.

Measures to relieve shock due to the loss of circulating fluids. It has long been recognized that persons who have been severely burned will die of shock from loss of blood and circulating fluids unless the shock can be adequately treated. This can usually be accomplished by the oral and intravenous administration of salt solutions which resemble the ionic composition of the extracellular fluids of the body.

Recent studies seem to indicate that immediate or very early administration of whole blood or plasma is unnecessary and in some instances may be harmful.* An exception to the early use of plasma is said to exist in the case of burned infants and the malnourished infants whose blood was deficient in protein prior to the burn.

The amount of salt solution administered varies with the extent of the burn and the size of the patient. Fluid replacement is in certain instances achieved by oral administration of hypotonic salt solution. Fluid containing approximately 3 Gm. of sodium chloride and 1.5 Gm. of sodium bicarbonate per liter has been found suitable for oral administration in the early treatment of shock.

Later control of anemia and malnutrition may include transfusions of whole blood, plasma, and/or amino acids.

Relief of pain. The intravenous administration of morphine sulfate or meperidine hydrochloride is usually effective for the relief of pain. The dosage recommended is 8 to 10 mg. and administration is discontinued as soon as possible. Analgesia rather than sedation is sought. It is probable that the burned patient suffers less pain than is frequently

*Wilson, B. J., and Stirman, J. A.: Initial Treatment of Burns, J. A. M. A. **173**: 509, 1960.

supposed. The restlessness frequently observed may be due to anoxia rather than to pain. Large doses of analgesics are avoided because of the danger of respiratory depression, since patients in shock are particularly sensitive to depressant drugs. The anoxia is relieved by the replacement of lost fluid volume and the administration of oxygen. Respiratory insufficiency may require that an early tracheotomy be performed.

Prevention and treatment of infection. Penicillin and streptomycin are frequently used for the early treatment of burned patients other than those with a first degree burn and an intact skin. These agents are given parenterally during the first few days and are then discontinued until débridement has been performed or until there is evidence of infection.

A booster dose of tetanus toxoid is given to the patient who has been previously immunized, and active immunization is started for those not previously immunized. Passive immunization is not always indicated because of the incidence of severe allergic manifestations, unless there is marked contamination with material likely to contain the tetanus organisms.

Sunburn

Sunburn is an acute erythema caused by too long an exposure to the rays of the sun. In some cases, especially if a large area is involved, it may be serious, and the skin surface should be treated as any serious burn. Exposure to the sun is preferably done gradually a few minutes each day when a general tan is desired. As would be true for any first degree burn when the epithelium is intact and remains so, ordinary protective demulcents or emollients are sufficient to allay irritation. A good cold cream, acacia mucilage, or olive oil may be used.

Butesin Picrate. This preparation is both antiseptic and anesthetic and is used in a 1 per cent ointment for burns. It may be useful to relieve the pain but often acts as an irritant, so that bland applications are preferable.

Baths

Baths may be employed to cleanse the skin, to medicate it, or to reduce temperature. The usual method of cleansing the skin is by the use of soap and water, but this may not be tolerated in skin diseases. In some cases even water is not tolerated and inert oils must be substituted. Persons with dry skin should bathe less frequently than those with oily skin.

It is possible to keep the skin clean without a daily bath. Nurses are sometimes accused of overbathing hospital patients, causing the patient's skin to become dry and itchy. An oily lotion is preferable to alcohol for the dry skin.

To render baths soothing in irritative conditions, bran, starch, gelatin, etc. may be added in the proportion of about 1 to 2 ounces to the gallon. Oils such as Alpha-Keri, lubath, and oilated oatmeal in a proportion of 1 ounce to the tub of water decrease the drying effect of water and thus help to relieve the itching of a sensitive, xerotic skin.

Soaps

Ordinary soap is the sodium salt of palmitic, oleic, or stearic acids or mixtures of these. They are prepared by saponifying fats or oils with the alkalies. The fats or oils that are used vary considerably. The oil used for castile soap is supposed to be olive oil. Some soaps are made with coconut oil to which the skin of some persons is sensitive. Soaps contain glycerin unless it has been removed from the preparation. The consistency of the soap depends upon the predominating acid and alkali that is used.

Although all soaps are alkaline, the presence of an excess of free alkali or acid will constitute a potential source of skin irritation. The best soaps are only slightly alkaline, and they are likely to be found among the inexpensive soaps rather than in the highly scented, highly colored, and expensive varieties.

Medicated soaps contain antiseptics and other added substances, such as cresol, thymol, sulfur, etc.; but soaps per se are antiseptic only in so far as they favor the mechanical cleansing of the skin.

The belief that soap and water are bad for the complexion is erroneous for the most part. A clean skin helps to promote a healthy skin. The soap used in maintaining a clean skin should be mild and contain a minimum of irritating materials.

Soaps are irritant to mucous membranes, and their use in enemas is due mainly to this action. They are used in the manufacture of pills, liniments, and tooth powders. If soaps contain much free alkali their use on the skin may cause eczema. One of the mildest soaps is shaving soap.

Bromidrosis (Osmidrosis)

Bromidrosis is a condition in which the sweat of the body is fetid. It may be attributable to functional disturbances or to decomposition of the sweat after it has been secreted. The axillae, genitocrural regions, and feet are the portions of the body especially involved. The secretion may be excessive, although not necessarily so. The condition often is associated with nervousness and also with the presence of odoriferous substances in the sweat, such as asafetida, garlic, onion, and musk. Patients who have been taking certain medicines, such as sodium salicylate, will perspire more than usual, and their perspiration is likely to have a strong odor.

Treatment. Absolute cleanliness is essential, although bathing alone often does not protect against offensive perspiration for more than a relatively short time. Some of the well-known deodorants on the market owe their efficacy to benzoic acid and zinc oxide, zinc oxide alone, or boric acid. Deodorants that suppress the flow of perspiration usually contain aluminum chloride in varying strengths. The feet may be bathed in weak antiseptic solutions such as 1:1,000 potassium permanganate, solution of cresol, 2 to 3 teaspoonfuls in a gallon of water, 2 per cent formaldehyde solution, or alum in 1 per cent solution. Daily change of underclothing, hose, and so forth is important.

Questions
for review and study

1 What are some of the nursing problems peculiar to the care of patients with disorders of the skin?
2 What are some of the points for or against giving a hospital patient a daily, complete bath with soap and water?
3 What information or help would you try to give a patient who complains of a dry, itchy skin?
4 What can be done for the patient who has an offensive body odor? What are some of the conditions under which bromidrosis is likely to be present?
5 What constitutes a good soap? What can and cannot be expected from a soap?
6 Why is an extensive burn of the skin likely to be dangerous? What are some of the main points in treatment of burns? How are patients with burns treated in your hospital?
7 What precautions must be observed by the patient being treated for scabies in order to prevent reinfection?

References
Text and reference books

A. M. A. Council on Drugs: New and Non-official Drugs, Philadelphia, 1960, J. B. Lippincott Co.

Davison, F. R.: Handbook of Materia Medica, Toxicology, and Pharmacology, St. Louis, 1949, The C. V. Mosby Co.

Goodman, L., and Gilman, A.: The Pharmacological Basis of Therapeutics, New York, 1955, The Macmillan Co.

Military Surgical Manuals V, National Research Council: Burns, Shock, Wound Healing and Vascular Disease, Philadelphia, 1943, W. B. Saunders Co.

Salter, W. T.: A Textbook of Pharmacology, Philadelphia, 1952, W. B. Saunders Co.

Journal articles

Baker, T. J.: Open Technique in the Management of Burns, Am. J. Nursing **59:** 1262, 1959.

Cope, Oliver: The Chemical Aspects of Burn Treatment, J. A. M. A. **125:** 536, 1944.

Council on Pharmacy and Chemistry: Pharmacologic and Toxicologic Aspects of DDT (Chlorophenothane, U.S.P.), J. A. M. A. **145:** 728, 1951.

Evans, E. I.: The Burn Problem in Atomic Warfare, J. A. M. A. **143:** 1143, 1950.

Federal Civil Defense Administration: Health Services and Special Weapons Defense, Washington, D. C., 1950, U. S. Government Printing Office.

Gallagher, John L.: Compression Therapy, Am. J. Nursing **44**: 423, 1944.

Kierland, R. R.: Use of Sedatives and Tranquilizers, Minnesota Med. **41**: 539, 1959.

Lam, Conrad R.: The General Care of the Burned Patient, J. A. M. A. **125**: 543, 1944.

Lee, Walter E., and Rhoads, Jonathan E.: The Present Status of the Tannic Acid Method in the Treatment of Burns, J. A. M. A. **125**: 610, 1944.

Pendleton, Ralph C.: The Paraffin Wax Open Air Treatment of Burns, J. A. M. A. **122**: 414, 1943.

Wilson, B. J., and Stirman, J. A.: Initial Treatment of Burns, J. A. M. A. **173**: 509, 1960.

Chapter 17

Drugs that affect the kidney
and organs of
the urinary tract

Functions of the kidneys

The kidneys are the chief organs that excrete nonvolatile, water-soluble substances from the body. These substances include products of metabolism, e.g., urea, uric acid, and creatinine, as well as electrolytes such as sodium chloride and potassium salts, along with foreign substances that may have gained entrance into the blood.

The normal kidney does not excrete colloids, such as plasma proteins, or large molecular-weight colloids introduced into the blood stream, such as gelatin or gum acacia. The kidney plays an important part in maintaining the osmotic pressure of the blood. It also acts to maintain optimum concentrations of the individual constituents of the plasma. This is accomplished by the excretion of water and specific solutes in carefully regulated amounts. It is largely the responsibility of the renal tubules to effect this precise regulation of the substances excreted into the urine. The tubules accomplish this function in a number of ways. Some substances are completely reabsorbed from the tubular urine and are returned to the blood quantitatively, e.g., glucose and amino acids. Others, such as sodium and chloride, are partially reabsorbed; whereas some substances, e.g., inulin and creatinine, are not reabsorbed at all and are excreted quantitatively. The renal tubules also add some substances to the urine by a process of secretion. Potassium and hydrogen ions are secreted by the cells of the renal tubule.

Histology of the kidney

The kidney is composed of many functional units called nephrons, each of which begins as a dilated ovoid-shaped structure known as Bowman's capsule. Into Bowman's capsule is invaginated a tuft of capillary vessels, the glomerulus, through which blood flows which orig-

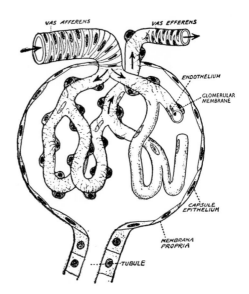

Fig. 38 Diagram of a *malpighian body.* This consists of a tuft of capillaries, the glomerulus, within an invaginated membrane, *Bowman's capsule,* which forms the head of the *tubule.* Note that the capsule epithelium is reflected over the outside of the capillaries of the glomerular tuft. There are in reality many more capillary loops than are shown. Blood enters the glomerulus from the *vas afferens* and leaves it by the *vas efferens.* The former is definitely larger than the latter. (After v. Möllendorff, from Winton, F. R., and Bayliss, L. E.: Human Physiology, London, J. & A. Churchill, Ltd.)

inally came from the renal artery. The glomerulus is connected to a long tortuous tubule which is divided into several segments. The first part is termed the proximal convoluted tubule.

This is followed by a narrowed hairpin-shaped structure called Henle's loop. The initial part of Henle's loop descends toward the pelvis of the kidney and is the descending limb, which is lined with flattened squamous cells. This is followed by the ascending limb, which is lined with cuboidal epithelium. The next part of the tubule is the distal convoluted tubule, also lined with cuboidal epithelium. The distal part of the tubule empties into the collecting tubule, which eventually terminates in the renal pyramid and pelvis of the kidney. The collecting tubule is also lined with cuboidal epithelium. The number of glomeruli in the kidney of man is estimated to be 1,000,000 in each kidney. The total length of the tubules of both kidneys is estimated to be approximately 75 miles.*

In general, the excretion of urine is attuned to the needs of the body. For most substances the kidney serves to maintain constant amounts and concentrations in the body fluids. This is accomplished by excreting the same amounts of solutes and water as are acquired each day (minus the amounts lost through sweat, feces, and other extrarenal routes). In physiologic terms, the kidney acts to preserve *balance* of most major constituents of body fluids.

Factors that influence the volume and composition of urine

Factors that most affect the formation of urine include the following:
1. *Glomerular filtration.* The force needed for filtration through the

*Greisheimer, E. M.: Physiology and Anatomy, Philadelphia, 1955, J. B. Lippincott Co., p. 664.

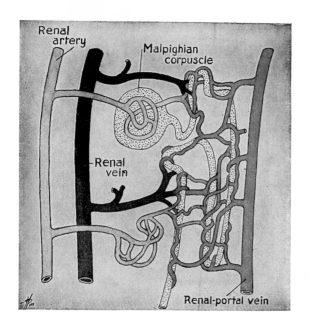

Fig. 39 Diagram of blood supply of malpighian corpuscle and of convoluted tubules in amphibian kidney. (Redrawn from Cushny.) The discoverer of these corpuscles was Marcello Malpighi (1628-1694), an Italian anatomist.

glomerular capillaries and into the glomerular capsule is derived from the force of the blood (blood pressure). It is sometimes referred to as hydrostatic pressure. The osmotic pressure of the plasma proteins represents an opposing force to hold fluid in the blood. Various constituents dissolved in the plasma filter through the glomerulus and are found in the filtrate in about the same concentration as they are found in the blood. Blood cells, plasma proteins, and lipids do not diffuse through the capillary walls and are not found in the glomerular filtrate if the kidney is functioning normally. Increased glomerular filtration caused by dilution of the plasma or by increased intraglomerular pressure usually achieves a moderately increased formation of urine.

2. *Tubular reabsorption.* The cells lining the renal tubules exhibit a high level of metabolic activity and expend considerable energy in transporting electrolytes, water, etc., back into the extracellular fluid (blood, lymph, and interstitial fluid) of the body. Because they tend to be active cells they are also the cells that are most easily injured when renal damage occurs. For every 100 ml. of fluid filtered through the glomerulus, approximately 99 ml. are reabsorbed in the tubule. Most diuretics used clinically act by interference with tubular reabsorption (water and electrolyte reabsorption). The activity of the tubule cells is greatly affected by pituitary hormone (antidiuretic hormone, A.D.H.) and certain adrenal hormones. Reabsorption of water is also affected by the amount of nonreabsorbable substances in the blood, which in turn enter the tubule and obligate the excretion of water.

512

3. *Tubular secretion.* It has been found that the tubule cells actively secrete certain substances into the urine as well as absorb certain other substances from the urine. Penicillin is an example of a drug that is excreted this way.

The secretion of hydrogen ions by the tubule cells is an effective way whereby the kidney helps to maintain acid-base equilibrium. The hydrogen ions in the tubular cells are exchanged for the sodium ions in the urine. The rate of this exchange can be greatly affected by drugs and constitutes a basis of diuresis.

Diuretics

Diuretics are drugs given to increase the flow of urine. They are not all equally effective in removing fluid of edema. They will be presented under the following headings: (1) water, (2) osmotic diuretics, (3) acid-forming salts, (4) xanthine diuretics, (5) mercurial diuretics, (6) nonmercurial diuretics, (7) carbonic anhydrase inhibitors, and (8) anti-aldosterone compounds.

Water

Water is a physiologic diuretic but is seldom considered a drug. Fluid intake is frequently forced to increase the urine output. The mechanism of water diuresis has been explained on the basis of decreased diffusion of water back to the blood, across the tubular cells, and out of the urine. The result may be that water intake stimulates a greater loss of water than that ingested so water can be considered a true diuretic. The barrier to water diffusion presented by the tubule cells appears to be related to the concentration of the posterior pituitary secretion in the blood. When the fluid intake is increased, the posterior pituitary activity is decreased, less water is removed from the urine, and diuresis results. Water is not a diuretic in the sense that it causes the excretion of edema fluid from the tissues. It frequently is considered unnecessary to restrict fluids for edematous patients, provided there is a restriction placed on the intake of sodium.

Osmotic diuretics
Sodium Chloride

Sodium chloride is occasionally administered for a diuretic effect in the form of either an isotonic or hypertonic solution. However, it is relatively ineffective in man, and under certain circumstances it may be dangerous. Isotonic salt solution increases the volume of the extracellular fluids much more than plain water because its retention in extracellular fluids prevents passage of water into the cells, due to its osmotic pressure, i.e., equal concentrations of solute exist on both sides of the cell membrane and sodium and chloride remain almost exclusively in the extracellular fluid. The blood volume is therefore increased and this rarely promotes greater glomerular filtration, which in turn would induce diuresis. However, under most conditions, when diuresis occurs it is slow and ineffectual.

Hypertonic solutions of sodium chloride increase the blood volume by the amount of fluid injected and also draw fluid from the body cells. As a result, the glomerular filtration may increase and tubular reabsorption decrease. Hypertonic solutions are potentially dangerous and should be used only under conditions of strict medical supervision. The use of hypertonic solutions of sodium chloride is generally contraindicated in cases of clinical edema.

Potassium Salts

Potassium salts possess weak diuretic properties and are of little clinical value for diuresis. They should be administered only when the renal function is normal. Potassium salts can produce toxic effects if the function of the kidney is impaired.

Potassium Chloride and Potassium Nitrate

Potassium Chloride, U.S.P., B.P., and *Potassium Nitrate*, N.F., B.P. These are the preparations used, although the bicarbonate, citrate, and acetate salts of potassium are also used. The usual dosage is 1 Gm. several times a day, given orally during or just after meals. Larger doses (5 to 10 Gm.) are not considered unusual. Enteric-coated tablets or capsules decrease the incidence of gastric irritation.

Urea

Urea, N.F., B.P. (Carbamide). Urea, though normally present in body fluids, serves as an osmotic diuretic when given in sufficiently large amounts. In a person with normal kidneys it is rapidly eliminated and is not toxic. It should not be administered when there is renal disease characterized by retention of nitrogen. Since a large amount of it is not reabsorbed by the tubular cells it presents the reabsorption of a proportional amount of water.

Urea is administered orally and the usual dose is 8 to 20 Gm. taken three times a day, preferably after meals to minimize gastric irritation. Although all patients do not respond satisfactorily, it has been used successfully in the treatment of cardiac and nephrotic edema.

Glucose and Sucrose

Glucose, when given in quantity sufficient to exceed the renal threshold for this substance, is excreted into the urine and results in increased excretion of water and, to a lesser degree, sodium and chloride. To bring about this effect, the glucose in the blood must be increased markedly and, in general, the avenue of administration must be intravenous. The usual dose is 50 ml. of a 50 per cent solution.

Sucrose solution likewise acts as an osmotic diuretic, and in some ways it is more efficient than glucose. When given directly into the blood stream its form is too complex to be utilized by the tissues and the kidney excretes it as a foreign substance with little or no reabsorption in the tubule. It exerts osmotic effects similar to those produced by glucose. Since so little is reabsorbed in the tubule, its effects are more marked than those of glucose. Large or repeated doses of sucrose may produce renal damage, and hence its use as a diuretic is rarely justified. Hypertonic solutions of glucose and sucrose are marketed in ampules containing varying concentrations up to 50 per cent. They are used, at times, for the treatment of cerebral edema and shock.

Acid-forming salts

The acidifying diuretics are chiefly ammonium chloride, ammonium nitrate, and calcium chloride. Of these, only ammonium chloride continues to be used with any regularity. The acidifying salts bring about a disturbance in blood chemistry to the extent that acidosis may result. The kidney, in its effort to maintain constancy of body fluids, excretes the acid-forming radicals (i.e., the hydrogen ions), and some increase in the excretion of sodium and water may follow. The mechanism of diuresis is not completely understood. Ammonium chloride is available in 0.5 Gm. enteric-coated tablets or capsules for oral administration. The dose varies, although 8 to 12 Gm. are sometimes given daily in divided doses. It may cause gastric irritation, nausea, and vomiting. It should not be used if renal function is seriously impaired, because of the danger of causing uncompensated acidosis. The chief value of ammonium chloride is observed when it is used in combination with the mercurial diuretics.

Xanthine diuretics

Xanthine diuretics include caffeine, theobromine, and theophylline, all of which exert similar actions in the body but differ in degree of effect upon various tissues and organs. Caffeine exerts a marked action on the central nervous system but is relatively weak in its action on the kidney, whereas theobromine and theophylline are weak in their action on the nervous system but have a somewhat greater effect on the kidney and cardiovascular system.

Action and result. The action of this group of drugs on the nervous system, heart, and blood vessels has been presented in previous chapters.

Drugs that affect kidney and organs of urinary tract 515

Theophylline is the more effective diuretic but its action is of short duration. Theobromine is somewhat less active but its effects last longer. The mechanism of their diuretic action is somewhat obscure and has been the subject of controversy. There now seems to be general agreement that the chief diuretic action is produced by depression of the tubular epithelium, causing decreased reabsorption of water and salt (sodium chloride).

Uses. The effects of the xanthine diuretics are inferior to those that can be obtained from the organic mercurials. When used, aminophylline, a preparation of theophylline and ethylenediamine, is the preparation of choice. For the patient with cardiac edema, especially the patient who has become refractory to other forms of treatment, theophylline compounds are sometimes used to supplement therapy with digitalis and the mercurials. The oral forms of the xanthines are little used as diuretics since more effective drugs are available.

Aminophylline is also used in the treatment of bronchial asthma to relax constricted bronchial musculature. In addition it is sometimes administered to patients in cardiac failure who have paroxysmal dyspnea.

Preparation, dosage, and administration.

Aminophylline, U.S.P., B.P. This is a mixture of theophylline and ethylenediamine. It is available in plain or enteric-coated tablets containing 100 or 200 mg. of aminophylline, for oral administration. It is also available in solution for injection (vials containing 250 or 500 mg. of aminophylline). The solution may be injected intramuscularly or intravenously. Caution is recommended when the drug is given intravenously. It should be injected *slowly* and this method of administration reserved for emergencies. Aminophylline is also marketed in suppositories (125, 250, and 500 mg.). All the above preparations are official in both the U.S.P. and the B.P. The dose is 100 to 500 mg. several times daily.

There are a number of other preparations of theobromine and theophylline listed in the *National Formulary.*

Side effects and toxic effects. Although the xanthines have a low level of toxicity, when given orally they are likely to cause gastric discomfort, nausea, and vomiting. They therefore should be administered after meals or with food. Stimulation of the central nervous system often occurs after large doses or when idiosyncrasy is present. This may produce symptoms such as headache, restlessness, dizziness, anxiety, delirium, and convulsions. Aminophylline, when given intravenously, can cause cardiac arrest or ventricular fibrillation. This is why it must be administered slowly. Repeated administration results in the development of tolerance in man. Xanthines could therefore be expected to be less effective in persons who habitually drink tea and coffee.

Mercurial diuretics

The organic mercurial diuretics are considered to be among the more potent drugs that are given to increase the output of urine.

Action and result. These compounds are believed to enter the tubular cells where they interfere with enzyme systems which function in the reabsorption of chloride ions. If the chloride ion is not reabsorbed, an equivalent amount of cation such as the sodium ion will not be reabsorbed either. This results in an increased excretion of sodium chloride along with a certain amount of water. This type of interference with enzymes can occur elsewhere in the body and is said to account for the toxic effect of these compounds on the heart when they are given intravenously.[*]

After parenteral administration of an average dose, the diuretic effect of the organic mercurials can be expected to appear within 1 to 3 hours and to reach a peak effect in 6 to 8 or 9 hours. The diuretic effect can be expected to end within 12 to 24 hours. As much as 8 or 9 liters of urine may be excreted the first day by a markedly edematous patient.

Uses. The organic mercurial diuretics are used chiefly to relieve cardiac edema or the edema associated with nephrosis, cirrhotic conditions of the liver, or portal obstruction. They may be administered alone or combined with theophylline or their administration may be preceded by large doses of an acidifying salt such as ammonium chloride. The latter substance enhances the diuretic effect of the mercurials.

Preparation, dosage, and administration.

Meralluride Injection, U.S.P. (Mercuhydrin Injection). This preparation is available in 1 and 2 ml. ampules and in 10 ml. vials. Each milliliter contains 39 mg. of organically combined mercury and 48 mg. of theophylline. It is usually administered intramuscularly or intravenously. The range of dosage is 1 to 2 ml.

Mercaptomerin Sodium, U.S.P. (Thiomerin Sodium). This is a mercurial diuretic which has the advantage of being less irritating at the site of injection than is true of a number of the other organic mercurial diuretics. However, it has been found to produce local reactions. It is less toxic to the heart. In other respects, it resembles the older mercurials. It is sensitive to heat and should be kept in the refrigerator.

Mercaptomerin sodium can be administered subcutaneously with safety, although care should be taken to make the injection beneath the subcutaneous fat and to avoid edematous areas. The usual dose is 0.5 to 2 ml. of a 13 per cent solution, depending on the individual needs of the patient. It is marketed as a powder for injection, 1.4 and 4.2 Gm.; as a solution for injection, 280 mg. in 2 ml. and 1.4 Gm. in 10 ml.; and

[*]Beckman, H.: Drugs, Their Nature, Action and Use, Philadelphia, 1958, W. B. Saunders Co., p. 410.

Drugs that affect kidney and organs of urinary tract 517

also as suppositories containing 500 mg. of the drug. The rectal dose is 1 suppository daily after the rectum has been emptied.*

Chlormerodrin† (Neohydrin). This agent has the advantage that it can be administered orally. It is available in 18.3 mg. tablets. Average dose for adults is 55 to 110 mg. daily, depending on severity of the edema.

Mercumatilin† (Cumertilin). This mercurial is available in tablets containing 67 mg. of the drug. The average daily dose is 1 to 2 tablets. It is usually given orally along with parenteral therapy with the sodium salt of this drug.

Mercumatilin Sodium† (Cumertilin Sodium). This preparation is available in solution for injection (132 mg. per milliliter) and is administered intramuscularly or intravenously. It produces the same diuretic effect as other combinations of mercury and theophylline.

A number of other organic mercurials are listed in the *National Formulary* and include *mersalyl, mersalyl* and *theophylline* (tablets and injection), and *mercurophylline* (tablets and injection). *Mersalyl* and *Mersalyl and Theophylline Injection* are also listed in B.P.

With the present preparations available it is said that satisfactory control of edema can be attained after oral administration if adequate amounts of the mercurial are administered. The disappearance of the edema is less marked and dramatic as compared to results after parenteral administration, but diuresis may be gradual and continuous. If the edema is severe, oral administration may need to be supplemented by parenteral administration, at least occasionally. Intramuscular administration is the preferred channel of administration if oral therapy does not prove adequate. Rectal administration is not reliable and may cause local irritation. Certain preparations may be administered intravenously, but they should be given slowly and only under the most carefully controlled conditions. Injections, as a rule, should not be repeated more often than every 3 or 4 days. The drug should preferably be given in the morning, so that the major effects occur during the day.

Side effects and toxic effects. The signs of toxic reactions are the same as those for other mercurials. Stomatitis, gingivitis, increased salivation, diarrhea, albuminuria, hematuria, circulatory collapse, flushing, febrile reactions, and skin eruptions may occur. Severe reactions are characterized by sudden fall in blood pressure, cardiac irregularity, cyanosis, severe dyspnea. Renal damage may result from prolonged usage.

Contraindication and precautions. Mercurials are contraindicated in acute nephritis and in advanced chronic kidney disease. Patients who are sensitive to one mercurial may, however, tolerate another satisfactorily. Caution needs to be exercised when mercurials are given intra-

---

*N.N.D., 1960, p. 667.
†Described in annual publication of A. M. A. Council on Drugs, N.N.D., 1960.

venously, because sudden fatalities have occurred which are thought to be due to ventricular arrhythmia. Patients therefore who have frequent ventricular beats or myocardial infarction or who have been heavily digitalized may react to mercurials unfavorably. Patients who received mercurials are carefully selected and initial tests for sensitivity are given. When it is necessary to give these drugs repeatedly, the urine should be examined periodically for blood cells, albumin, and casts.

The addition of theophylline to the mercurial preparations increases their diuretic effects by improving absorption. At present most mercury preparations are available in this combination.

Nonmercurial diuretic

Amisometradine (Rolicton)

Action. Amisometradine is a nonmercurial diuretic which is related to another and similar diuretic, aminometradine (Mincard). Amisometradine has the advantage of producing fewer symptoms of gastrointestinal irritation. The clinical effectiveness of the two drugs is said to be about the same. The mode of their action is not clear, but they are believed to inhibit the reabsorption of sodium ions by the tubular cells of the kidney.

Uses. Amisometradine is used to bring about gradual mobilization of edematous fluid in selected patients with congestive heart failure (mild to moderate in severity), cirrhosis of the liver, and nephrosis. It is also used in the management of water and electrolyte retention during pregnancy and in the premenstrual phase of the menstrual cycle.

Preparation, dosage, and administration.

Amisometradine* (Rolicton). It is available in 400 mg. tablets for oral administration, four times (with food) on the first day and twice daily thereafter.

Side effects and toxic effects. Serious toxic effects have not been observed, but prolonged administration and large doses increase the possibility that untoward effects will develop.

Carbonic anhydrase inhibitors

It has been found that various anions (chloride, phosphate, bicarbonate) are returned to the extracellular fluids (blood, etc.), from the urine by specific transport mechanisms, i.e., activities that take place through the cellular membranes of the tubule cells. Chloride and bicarbonate are two important anions that are reabsorbed by active processes that are believed to be enzymatic. Any interference with the reabsorption of these anions results in a change in acid-base equilibrium and diuresis.

*Described in annual publication of A. M. A. Council on Drugs, N.N.D., 1960.

Normally, hydrogen ions (H⁺) are excreted by the tubular cell into the tubular urine, and, in exchange for them, sodium ions (Na⁺) are reabsorbed from the urine by the tubular cell. This process of ion exchange provides a way both of excreting acid (H⁺) and of conserving basic components (Na⁺). The source of much of the hydrogen ions so excreted is from carbonic acid (H_2CO_3), which in turn is formed from carbon dioxide and water.

$$H_2O + CO_2 \rightleftharpoons H_2CO_3 \rightleftharpoons H^+ + HCO_3^-$$

The conversion of water and carbon dioxide to carbonic acid is greatly speeded up by the enzyme carbonic anhydrase (so named because it removes water from carbonic acid). A deficiency of this enzyme reduces the rate of carbonic acid formation, and this in turn reduces the availability of hydrogen ions (H⁺) from carbonic acid (H_2CO_3). With diminished hydrogen ions to be excreted, less sodium ions can be reabsorbed and thus more stay in the urine. With an increased amount of sodium ions in the tubular urine there is an accompanying increase of bicarbonate ions (HCO_3^-), the chief anions of the plasma and the tubular urine. The greater ionic concentration of the tubular urine therefore obligates holding more water in the urine and eliminating it.

Any drug that seriously inhibits the enzyme carbonic anhydrase may then be expected to increase the excretion of both sodium and bicarbonate ions with a related excretion of water.

The carbonic anhydrase inhibitors therefore act as *diuretics* by increasing the excretion of water indirectly through reduced reabsorption of sodium and bicarbonate ions and also by acting as acidosis-producing drugs, i.e., by increasing the excretion of the base (HCO_3^-). These drugs make the urine alkaline and contribute to metabolic acidosis.

Acetazolamide (Diamox)

Acetazolamide is a relatively new diuretic which is one of the carbonic anhydrase inhibitors. It is a synthetic preparation chemically related to the sulfonamides.

Action and result. It exerts a type of depressant action on the tubule cells and promotes the excretion of bicarbonate ions, causing the kidney to elaborate an increased volume of alkaline urine. The excretion of chloride may not be significantly altered. It produces a mild degree of metabolic acidosis. Effects last about 8 to 12 hours after a single dose.

Uses. Acetazolamide is used to mobilize fluid of edema in the body and also to prevent the accumulation of such fluid. A single dose every other day can maintain an occasional cardiac patient in an edema-free condition. It is not useful in the treatment of patients with nephritis. It has also been used to relieve fluid retention in patients prior to menstruation or for toxemia of pregnancy. It depresses the formation of aqueous humor and has been used in the treatment of glaucoma. Its status in this type of therapy is not fully established.

Preparation, dosage, and administration.

Acetazolamide, U.S.P. (Diamox). This drug is available in 250 mg. tablets and as a syrup, 50 mg. per milliliter, for oral administration. It is well absorbed from the gastrointestinal tract and readily excreted via the kidney. When given once daily it is active over a period of 6 to 8 hours. It may be combined with a mercurial, each drug being given on alternate days. The usual daily dose is 250 mg.

Acetazolamide Sodium, U.S.P. (Diamox Sodium). This form is available in vials containing 500 mg. of powder for injection. It is more soluble than plain acetazolamide and therefore better suited for parenteral administration (intramuscular and intravenous). Usual dose is 275 mg.

Side effects and toxic effects. Side effects are frequently encountered but they are not serious usually and they disappear when the administration of the drug is discontinued. Drowsiness and paresthesias of the face and extremities are the symptoms most frequently noted. Thirst, fatigue, and gastrointestinal disturbances have also been reported.

Chlorothiazide (Diuril)

Chlorothiazide is also a synthetic drug chemically related to the sulfonamides.

Action and result. Although included with the carbonic anhydrase inhibitors, this does not apparently explain the primary mechanism whereby chlorathiazide produces diuresis, at least after ordinary therapeutic doses. Diuretic doses bring about diminished reabsorption of sodium and chloride ions, which result in an increased urine output. Potassium is also excreted after diuretic doses of the drug. This may necessitate the administration of a preparation such as potassium chloride to avoid serious depletion of potassium (hypokalemia). At higher dose levels, inhibition of carbonic anhydrase causes excretion of bicarbonate.

Uses. Chlorothiazide is effective in relieving edema associated with congestive heart failure and cirrhosis of the liver. It is said to be much less effective when there is a reduction of glomerular filtration in the kidney. It is also used to diminish fluid retention in toxemia of pregnancy and in the management of hypertension. It is reported that chlorothiazide alone as well as when given with other antihypertensive drugs is capable of exerting a hypotensive effect. Part of the action is related to its diuretic effect and part is thought to be due to other inherent properties of the drug.*

---

*Wilkins, R. W.: New Drugs for Hypertension, With Special Reference to Chlorothiazide, New England J. Med. **257:** 1030, 1957.

Preparation, dosage, and administration.

Chlorothiazide, U.S.P. (Diuril). This drug is available in 250 and 500 mg. tablets for oral administration. The usual diuretic dose for adults is from 500 mg. to 1 Gm. daily or twice daily. When used for its hypertensive effects the dose may vary from 250 to 500 mg. one to three times daily.

Chlorothiazide Sodium° (Lyovac Diuril). This is the sodium salt of chlorothiazide which is more soluble than chlorothiazide and is therefore better suited to parenteral administration. It is available in vials which contain 500 mg. of the drug in the form of a powder.

Side effects and toxic effects. Side effects include allergic reactions, skin eruptions, nausea, epigastric discomfort, weakness, dizziness, and paresthesias. A lowering of the number of leukocytes and thrombocytes, as well as agranulocytosis, has occurred, but the incidence is said to be low. When large doses are administered, bicarbonate is excreted and this can cause acidosis.

Chlorothiazide may be contraindicated for patients with severe hepatic or renal dysfunction.

Ethoxzolamide (Cardrase)

Ethoxzolamide° is chemically similar to acetazolamide, but is about twice as active. Both diuretics have about the same duration of action, 8 to 12 hours after a single dose. It is administered orally in doses of 62.5 to 125 mg. on three consecutive days of the week or on alternate days. It is available in 125 mg. tablets.

Antialdosterone compounds

A new type of diuretic is being subjected to study and investigation at the present time. These compounds act by blocking certain effects of aldosterone, one of the hormones produced by the cortex of the adrenal gland. Patients with edema have been found to excrete unusually large amounts of this hormone in the urine. Aldosterone is known to promote the retention of sodium and the excretion of potassium. One of these new diuretics, a derivative of 17-spironolactone, is known also as *Aldactone*. It is administered orally. It apparently blocks the sodium-retaining and potassium-excreting properties of aldosterone. It may prove useful in treatment of edema associated with conditions such as hepatic cirrhosis, nephrosis, congestive heart failure, and other edematous conditions.

Cation exchange resins

These drugs are occasionally used in the management of sodium retention associated with chronic heart failure, cirrhosis of the liver, and

°Described in annual publication of A. M. A. Council on Drugs, N.N.D., 1960.

nephrosis. They are used to remove sodium from food, and they cause sodium to be eliminated from the gastrointestinal tract, thus preventing its absorption. Use of these exchange resins appeals to patients whose diet must be low in salt or salt free. Prevention of absorption of sodium can result in considerable loss of edema fluid. Unfortunately, potassium and calcium ions may be removed as well as sodium. This can result in potassium and calcium deficiencies unless suitable precautions are taken. The patients who receive these drugs should be watched for constipation. Some will object to the disagreeable texture of these substances or to the gastric distress which may follow the taking of large doses. These resins may supplement the action of mercurial diuretics in the treatment of recurring edema but they are not intended to supplant the use of them.

Carbacrylamine Resins (Carbo-Resin)

Carbacrylamine resins contain 87.5 per cent cation exchangers, carbacrylic resin and potassium carbacrylic resin, and 12.5 per cent of the anion exchanger, polyamine-methylene resin. The cation exchange resin, being of the carboxylic acid type, gives up its hydrogen ions for cations (potassium, sodium, or calcium) in accordance with the valence or the concentration of the latter. Because the concentration of sodium in the intestinal tract tends to be relatively high, it is chiefly sodium that is fixed by the resin. One third of the resin is present as a potassium salt to prevent serum deficiency of that important substance. The presence of the anion exchange resin helps to reduce the chances of acidosis in the patient with severe renal impairment.

Preparation, dosage, and administration.

*Carbacrylic Resins** (Carbo-Resin). These resins are given orally, as a powder stirred into water or fruit juices and swallowed at once. The usual initial dose is 16 Gm. The mouth may be rinsed free of particles after each dose. Maintenance dosage is adjusted on the basis of constant body weight and the requirements of each individual patient.

Antidiuretics

In diabetes insipidus, the amount of urine is greatly increased. The abnormality is due to a lack of hormone elaborated by the posterior lobe of the pituitary gland. This hormone (the antidiuretic hormone) normally acts upon the renal tubule and promotes the diffusion of water out of the urine and back into the blood. Drugs that aid this disease serve as replacement therapy for the missing hormone and may properly be called antidiuretics. Hypodermic injection or application to the nasal mem-

*Described in annual publication of A. M. A. Council on Drugs, N.N.D., 1960.

branes of extract of the posterior lobe of the pituitary gland greatly diminishes the volume of urine in diabetes insipidus.

Drugs that act on the bladder

Disturbance of bladder function as seen in hospitalized patients is frequently due to one of two causes: either the patient's bladder has too much muscle tone or too little. If the bladder is hypertonic and irritable, the emptying reflex is stimulated very easily and the bladder feels full although it really has not filled to anywhere near its normal capacity. The patient then has symptoms of frequency, and voiding may be accompanied by painful contractions. In such instances derivatives of belladonna are more effective than the opiates. Hyoscyamus tincture is sometimes the preparation of choice. It acts like other belladonna derivatives to relax the hypertonic muscle of the bladder. When the bladder is lacking in muscle tone, the patient is often unable to empty the organ completely, and this condition may predispose the patient to the development of infection, particularly when he is catheterized. The following drugs have been used to improve the atonic condition, encourage micturition, and eliminate the need for catheterization: neostigmine and bethanechol chloride (Urecholine Chloride) (see cholinergic drugs).

Urinary antiseptics

Urinary antiseptics are substances which, when given by mouth or by some other suitable channel, are excreted and concentrated in the urine in sufficient amounts to have an antiseptic effect on the urine and the urinary passages. Present-day urinary antiseptics of choice include some of the older drugs such as methenamine and mandelic acid, either alone or in combination, as well as a number of the sulfonamides and a number of the antibiotics. The selection of one of these preparations in preference to another is made on the basis of identification of the pathogens by Gram stain or by urine culture in the severe, recurrent, or chronic infections. The relative costs of antibacterial agents, too, is worthy of consideration, especially when the infection is mild. The cost of a sulfonamide is much less than that for treatment of a patient with tetracycline, penicillin, or nitrofurantoin (Furadantin). Many physicians advocate the treatment of a urinary infection for at least a week after symptoms have subsided or the results of cultures have become negative. No available drug will inhibit or destroy all the organisms causing urinary infections. Each of the agents used has its own bacterial spectrum against which it is effective. Some infections subside without specific therapy.

524

General measures such as rest and fluid intake to produce at least 2,000 ml. daily output are important.

Specific organisms that may be found in the urinary tract

The most common organisms found in the urinary tract are gram-negative bacilli, and of this group *Escherichia coli* is found to be responsible for many of the infections. *Aerobacter aerogenes* is also frequently found, as well as the organisms of the species of Proteus and Pseudomonas.* Since these are often regarded as contaminants, strict aseptic technic assumes a role of major importance in the examination or treatment of disorders of the urinary tract. The most commonly found coccus in urinary tract infections is the *Streptococcus faecalis*, which is an enterococcus commonly found in the large bowel. *Staphylococcus aureus* is the next most commonly found coccus, hemolytic streptococci being found only occasionally.

There appears to have been a decided change in the bacterial flora of urinary tract infections since the introduction of some of the newer antiseptics. *Aerobacter aerogenes* and *Pseudomonas aeruginosa* seem to be isolated with greater frequency. As the surviving strains, they may be responsible for a higher percentage of infections as the more susceptible strains are destroyed.

Sulfonamides

Sulfonamides are often effective against gram-negative bacilli which infect the urinary tract, although the incidence of resistant strains has increased markedly in recent years. Sulfonamides may also be effective against gram-positive cocci such as *Staphylococcus aureus* but are usually ineffective against *Streptococcus faecalis*. Sulfonamides are easily administered since they can be given orally. In a small percentage of patients this route of administration may not be possible, in which case the sodium salt of a sulfonamide may be given intravenously. The sulfonamides are discussed in greater detail in Chapter 20.

Sulfisoxazole, U.S.P. (Gantrisin). This is an effective chemotherapeutic agent which, because of its high solubility in body fluids (including acid urine), is less likely to cause crystalluria and renal blocking than some of the less-soluble sulfonamides employed singly. In other respects it is potentially as toxic as other drugs of this group. When used as a urinary antiseptic, forcing of fluids or alkalinization of the urine is not thought to be essential, although the output of fluid should be within the normal range. The dosage is the same as that for other sulfona-

*Martin, W. J., Nichols, D. R., and Cook, E. N.: Current Practices in General Medicine. 3. Infections of the Urinary Tract, Proc. Staff Meet. Mayo Clin. 34: 189, 1959.

mides which are given as urinary antiseptics. The initial dose may be as high as 4 Gm. followed by 0.5 to 1 Gm. every 4 to 6 hours.

Sulfamethoxypyridazine, U.S.P. (Kynex, Midicel). This agent is readily absorbed after oral administration but it is eliminated slowly. It is available in 500 mg. tablets and as a syrup (250 mg. per 5 ml.). The usual adult dose is 0.5 Gm. daily.

Sulfacetamide, N.F. (Sulamyd). This compound has the advantage of a high degree of solubility in urine, even when it is acid in reaction. The likelihood of crystalluria is therefore reduced to a minimum. Sulfacetamide is excreted rapidly, exhibits good antibacterial activity, and is, in general, of a low level of toxicity. The dosage is the same as that for sulfisoxizole. This dosage rarely produces toxic symptoms.

Sulfonamide mixtures have been recommended for treatment of certain infections of the urinary tract, to reduce the danger of renal damage which must be taken into account when sulfonamides are used. Each member of the mixture is present in smaller concentration than when it is used alone. Renal excretion is on the basis of individual drugs, although therapeutic action of the mixture is on the basis of the sum total of all drugs present. Renal crystalluria is said to be reduced more by triple than by dual mixtures.

Sulfadiazine and Sulfamerazine Tablets, N.F. Usual dose is 2 Gm.

Sulfacetamide, Sulfadiazine, and Sulfamerazine Tablets, N.F.; *Sulfacetamide, Sulfadiazine and Sulfamerazine Suspension,* N.F. These preparations are mixtures containing equal amounts of the three sulfonamides mentioned. This mixture has been sold under a number of trade names. The tablets usually available contain 0.5 Gm. of the three sulfonamides. Usual daily dose is 2 Gm.

Trisulfapyrimidines Tablets, U.S.P. These tablets contain 0.5 Gm. of a mixture of equal weights of sulfadiazine, sulfamerazine, and sulfamethazine.

Trisulfapyrimidines Oral Suspension, U.S.P. This form contains a total of 100 mg. in 1 ml.

For further discussion of sulfonamides used for infections of urine and urinary tract, see p. 573.

Antibiotics

The antibiotics mentioned have been presented previously in Chapter 8.

Penicillin has not been found particularly effective for most bacillary infections of the urinary tract. It is not as useful as certain other antibiotics because the infecting organisms are so often gram-negative and not affected by penicillin. If the infection is due to staphylococci or other cocci which are sensitive to penicillin, oral preparations of penicillin V have been successfully used for mild infections. The dose of the oral preparation for urinary infections is twice the intramuscular dose and is given in divided portions.

Streptomycin, especially when combined with tetracycline therapy, is effective and preferable to penicillin for serious infections due to gram-negative bacilli. Bacteria rapidly become resistant to streptomycin if it is used alone. Combined *streptomycin and penicillin* therapy is sometimes used for treatment of infections due to enterococci such as *Streptococcus faecalis.* The dosage for streptomycin is 2 Gm. daily in 2 doses not to exceed two weeks or 1 Gm. daily in 2 doses not to exceed four weeks. Neurotoxic symptoms occur rarely with short-term therapy. The tetracyclines are given in doses of 500 to 750 mg. every 6 hours. The tetracyclines have the disadvantage of bringing about superimposed infections by organisms resistant to them.

Erythromycin, novobiocin, kanamycin, and *Vancomycin* are also available for use against urinary infections due to staphylococci. The latter two drugs, however, exhibit toxic potentialities and they must be given parenterally to obtain systemic effects. Novobiocin is sometimes effective for infections due to Proteus organisms.

Chloramphenicol is useful against certain strains of staphylococci, but its ability to depress the bone marrow is a disadvantage which must be considered. It is effective in the treatment of Salmonella infections.

Polymyxin B in doses of 25 to 50 mg. every 6 to 12 hours may be effective in treatment of infections due to Pseudomonas.

Bacitracin and *neomycin* both are nephrotoxic agents and can be given only for short periods of time in the treatment of staphylococcal infections. They may have value when combined with other agents. The dose of bacitracin is 10,000 to 25,000 units every 6 to 12 hours, and the dose of neomycin is 250 mg. every 6 hours. Both must be given intramuscularly for this purpose.

Methenamine (Urotropin)

Methenamine is a synthetic drug made by the action of ammonia on formaldehyde. It occurs in the form of colorless, lustrous, odorless crystals which are freely soluble in water. Methenamine owes its antiseptic effects to the formaldehyde which it yields in the presence of free acid. Methenamine is excreted chiefly in the urine; and when the urine is acid, the drug is decomposed, liberating small amounts of formaldehyde, which exerts an antiseptic action in the urine and on the surface of the mucous membrane of the genitourinary tract. When the urine is alkaline, methenamine is not decomposed and is then ineffective.

Uses. Methenamine is used chiefly as a urinary antiseptic, in an attempt to free the urine from microorganisms. Usually, an acid salt such as ammonium chloride or sodium acid phosphate are given at the same time to ensure adequate acidity in the urine.

Preparation, dosage, and administration.

Methenamine (Urotropin). The drug is available in 500 mg. tablets for oral administration. The average dose for adults is 500 mg. every 4 hours, but in current medical practice this preparation has been largely discarded for newer forms of therapy.

Methenamine Mandelate (Mandelamine)

Methenamine mandelate combines the action of methenamine and mandelic acid and is used for treatment of infections of the urinary tract due to most of the common urinary tract pathogens. This antiseptic is sometimes effective against organisms that have developed resistance to other agents to which they are ordinarily susceptible.

Uses. It is useful in the treatment of pyelitis, pyelonephritis, and cystitis.

Preparation, dosage, and administration.

Methenamine Mandelate, U.S.P. (Mandelamine). This drug is available in 250 and 500 mg. tablets and as a suspension, 50 mg. per milliliter, for oral administration. The average initial dose is 1 to 1.5 Gm. four times a day.

Side effects and toxic effects. When the drug is given in therapeutic amounts, gastric disturbance and other toxic effects occur rarely.

Contraindications. It is contraindicated for patients with renal insufficiency. Microorganisms do not acquire resistance to this antiseptic.

Calcium Mandelate

Calcium mandelate is a salt of mandelic acid and is conveniently administered in tablet form. It is sometimes prescribed for enterococcal infections of the urinary tract. The dose is 3 Gm. four times daily. Acidification of the urine may be necessary. For this purpose, *methionine* (D-L) is available in capsule or tablet form. It may be administered in doses up to 3 and 4 Gm. or more daily.

Nitrofurantoin (Furadantin)

Nitrofurantoin is a nitrofuran derivative and is chemically related to nitrofurazone (Furacin). It is a yellow, bitter-tasting powder.

Action and result. Nitrofurantoin exhibits antibacterial activity against a wide range of both gram-negative and gram-positive microorganisms. It is both bacteriostatic and bactericidal to many strains of *Staphylococcus* (*albus* and *aureus*), *Streptococcus pyogenes, Escherichia coli, Aerobacter aerogenes,* and Paracolobactrum species. It is less effective against *Proteus vulgaris, Alcaligenes faecalis, Pseudomonas aeruginosa,* and

Corynebacterium species. It has no effect on viruses and fungi.

Uses. Nitrofurantoin is used in the treatment of bacterial infections of the urinary tract caused by microorganisms sensitive to the drug. It is rapidly and completely absorbed from the intestinal tract and hence has little effect on the intestinal flora. About 40 to 50 per cent of the drug is excreted unchanged in the urine and with sufficient rapidity to require administration at intervals of 4 to 6 hours. Much of the remainder of the drug is changed in the body tissues to inactive compounds which have a brownish color. These compounds may cause the urine to be tinted.

Preparation, dosage, and administration.

Nitrofurantoin, U.S.P. (Furadantin). This drug is available in 50 and 100 mg. tablets and as a suspension, 5 mg. per milliliter, for oral administration. The average total daily dose is 5 to 8 mg. per kilogram of body weight. The total daily dose should be divided into four equal doses and given after meals and at bedtime with some food to minimize the possibility of nausea. Some physicians prescribe this drug in doses of 100 mg. four times a day (adults). Administration of the drug should be continued at least 3 days after the urine has become sterile. Larger doses may be required for refractory infections.

Side effects and toxic effects. Nitrofurantoin has a low level of toxicity. It occasionally causes nausea and vomiting, and an occasional case of sensitization has been observed. The low dosage required for an effective urinary concentration is not associated with a noticeable amount of the drug in the blood. The two advantages of the drug as a urinary antiseptic are (1) its high solubility in urine even when the urine is acid and (2) the small dosage required. Both of these factors operate to minimize the likelihood that the drug will precipitate out of solution and cause crystalluria in the kidney.

Contraindications. It is not recommended for patients having anuria, oliguria, or severe renal damage.

Phenylazo-diamino-pyridine Hydrochloride (Pyridium)

Pyridium is a brand of phenylazo-diamino-pyridine hydrochloride. It is an azo dye which occurs as a fine crystalline red powder. It is slowly soluble in cold water but is readily soluble in hot water, in alcohol, and in glycerin. It was used at one time as a urinary antiseptic, but now it is used more for the analgesic effect which it produces on the urinary mucosa. It is used to bring about relief of symptoms such as urgency and frequency of micturition. It is also used to achieve preoperative and postoperative surface analgesia in urologic surgical procedures and after diagnostic tests in which instrumentation has been necessary. It is sometimes given to patients who experience discomfort due to the presence of a retention catheter.

Preparation, dosage, and administration.

Phenylazo-diamino-pyridine Hydrochloride (Pyridium). This preparation is available in 100 mg. tablets for oral administration. The usual adult dose is 1 to 2 tablets three times a day before meals. It is marketed in combination with sulfonamide drugs, e.g., Azo-Gantrisin, which is available in tablets containing 500 mg. of sulfisoxizole (Gantrisin) and 50 mg. of Pyridium in each tablet.

Side effects and toxic effects. Patients occasionally exhibit symptoms of sensitivity.

Contraindications. Its use for patients with diminished renal function or severe hepatitis is not recommended.

Questions
for review and study

1 Which of the following reasons *best* explains why ammonium chloride is given in the form of enteric-coated tablets?
a. to promote absorption
b. to lessen nausea and vomiting
c. to increase solubility
d. to decrease the taste of the drug
2 Which of the following represents a disadvantage of urea when it is given orally for its diuretic effect?
a. toxicity
b. disagreeable taste
c. low solubility
d. instability
3 Which of the following xanthine diuretics is given parenterally as well as orally?
a. theophylline
b. theobromine
c. aminophylline
d. caffeine, citrated
4 In selected cases the mercurial diuretics may be very effective because they promote elimination of both water *and* which of the following?
a. urea
b. purine wastes
c. sodium chloride
d. potassium
5 The mercurial diuretics promote diuresis in which of the following ways?
a. by depressing certain activities in tubule cells in the nephron of the kidney
b. by increasing the secretory activity of the tubule cells
c. by increasing the circulation of blood through the kidney
d. by increasing glomerular filtration

6 Which of the following mercurial diuretics is given subcutaneously?
a. meralluride
b. mercumatilin
c. mercaptomerin sodium (Thiomerin Sodium)
d. chlormerodrin (Neohydrin)
7 Which of the following characteristics of sulfisoxizole best explains its popularity as a urinary antiseptic?
a. has a high antibacterial index
b. is highly soluble in body fluids
c. is rapidly excreted
d. can be given by mouth
8 After parenteral administration of an organic mercurial diuretic to an edematous patient, peak effects can be expected in:
a. 1 to 2 hours
b. 3 to 4 hours
c. 6 to 8 hours
d. 12 to 18 hours
9 Which of the following factors is likely to receive priority in selecting a drug for a severe urinary infection?
a. cost of the urinary antiseptic
b. sensitivity of infecting organism to the drug
c. ease of administration
d. side effects
10 Gantrisin is a proprietary name for which of the following sulfonamide drugs?
a. sulfadiazine   c. sulfisoxazole
b. sulfacetamide   d. sulfamerazine

References

A. M. A. Council on Drugs: New and Nonofficial Drugs, Philadelphia, 1960, J. B. Lippincott Co.

Beckman, H.: Drugs, Their Nature, Action and Use, Philadelphia, 1958, W. B. Saunders Co.

Burdon, K. L.: Textbook of Microbiology, New York, 1958, The Macmillan Co.

Carroll, G., Allen, H. N., and Flynn, H.: Gantrisin in the Treatment of Urinary Infections, J. A. M. A. **142:** 85, 1950.

Cook, E. N.: Symptoms, Diagnosis and Treatment of Infections of the Urinary Tract, M. Clin. North America **33:** 1071, 1949.

Goodman, L., and Gilman, A.: The Pharmacological Basis of Therapeutics, New York, 1955, The Macmillan Co.

Herrell, W. E.: Observations on the Clinical Use of Aureomycin, Proc. Staff Meet. Mayo Clin. **24:** 612, 1949.

Herrell, W. E.: Newer Antibiotics, Ann. Rev. Microbiol. **4:** 101, 1950.

Herrold, R. D., and Karabatsos, N.: Current Status of Anti-infective Therapy in Urology, J. A. M. A. **172:** 771-773, 1960.

Kirby, W. M.: Recent Trends in Antibiotic Therapy, J. A. M. A. **144:** 233-236, 1950.

Martin, W. J., Nichols, D. R., and Cook, E. N.: Current Practices in General Medicine: Infections of the Urinary Tract, Proc. Staff Meet. Mayo Clin. **34:** 187, 1959.

Modell, W. (editor): Drugs of Choice, 1960-1961, St. Louis, 1960, The C. V. Mosby Co.

Sollmann, T.: A Manual of Pharmacology, Philadelphia, 1957, W. B. Saunders Co.

Stein, I. F., and Meyer, K. A.: The Effect of Urecholine on the Stomach, Intestine and Urinary Bladder, J. A. M. A. **140:** 522, 1949.

Walder, H. J.: Office Treatment of Urinary Tract Infections, Minnesota Med. **34:** 26, 1951.

Wilson, C. O., and Gisvold, O.: Textbook of Organic Medicinal and Pharmaceutical Chemistry, Philadelphia, 1949, J. B. Lippincott Co.

Witton, C. J.: Microbiology With Applications to Nursing, New York, 1950, McGraw-Hill Book Co., Inc.

Chapter 18

Drugs that affect the eye

Anatomy and physiology

The eye is the receptor organ for one of our most delicate and valuable senses, vision; as such, it demands only the most thoughtful and expert care.

The eyeball itself has three layers or coats: the protective external (corneoscleral) coat, the nutritive middle vascular (uveal) coat, and the light-sensitive inner neural receptor (the retinal) layer.

The anterior segment of the eye serves as an optical system to focus images upon the retina (Fig. 40). This system is composed of the cornea, the iris, and the lens. The lens is capable of changing its shape in response to contraction or relaxation of the ciliary muscle, and hence can bring into sharp focus objects at various distances from the eye. Strong contraction of the ciliary muscle is necessary to allow the lens to bring nearby objects into focus (accommodation) and relaxation is necessary to focus objects at a distance. Drug-induced paralysis of the ciliary body so that it is incapable of contraction is called cycloplegia. The iris forms the pupillary opening, and in response to strong light or accommodation it contracts to make this opening smaller (miosis), whereas in dim light or in cases in which the eye is focusing an object at a distance the iris relaxes and allows the pupil to become larger (mydriasis). Miosis and mydriasis may also be induced by appropriate drugs.

The eyeball is protected in a deep depression of the skull, the orbit, and is moved in the orbit by six small extraocular muscles. The retina is connected to the brain by the optic nerve which leaves the orbit through a bony canal in the posterior wall. The anterior surface of the eye is kept moist by the tears, which then drain away into the nose through two small ducts (the lacrimal canaliculi) at the inner corners of the eyelids.

Autonomic drugs

The muscles of the ciliary body and the iris receive both parasympathetic and sympathetic innervation and respond to drugs which affect these systems.

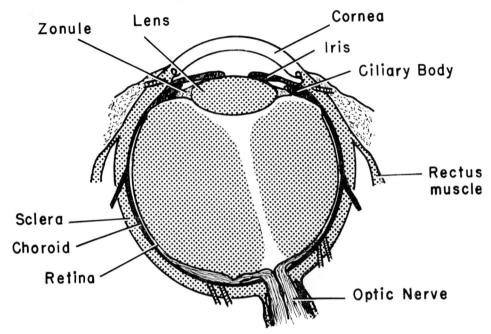

Fig. 40 Some of the main structures of the eye are labeled in this diagram of a section of the eyeball.

Parasympathomimetic drugs

Drugs in this category produce strong contractions of the iris (miosis) and ciliary body musculature (accommodation). These drugs have been found to lower the intraocular pressure in patients with glaucoma and are also used to treat patients with certain types of strabismus (crossed eyes).

Clinical toxicity from overdosage or unusual sensitivity to these drugs is manifested by headache, salivation, sweating, abdominal discomfort, diarrhea, asthmatic attacks, and a fall in blood pressure.

Pilocarpine Nitrate, U.S.P., B.P., or *Pilocarpine Hydrochloride,* U.S.P. This drug is used in 0.25 to 4 per cent solution. One drop into the eye will cause miosis and spasm of accommodation in 15 minutes. The pupillary effect lasts for as long as 24 hours, but the fixation of the lens for near-vision disappears in about 2 hours.

Carbachol, U.S.P. (Carcholin). Used as a topical solution or ointment it is available in concentrations up to 3 per cent. Its effects are similar to those of pilocarpine.

Physostigmine Salicylate, U.S.P., B.P. (Eserine Salicylate). This drug is used in solutions as strong as 0.5 per cent. The aqueous solutions of this compound tend to oxidize on exposure to light and air and turn pink or brown. Such colored solutions should never be used. Maximum effect of topical application is reached in 30 minutes and may last as long as 2 days.

Neostigmine Bromide, U.S.P., B.P. (Prostigmin Bromide). This drug is used in ophthalmology as a 5 per cent solution.

Demecarium Bromide (Humorsol). This is prepared as a 0.25 per cent solution. It is an extremely powerful agent and one drop will produce miosis and ciliary muscle contraction for as long as 5 to 12 days. Care must be taken to prevent general systemic absorption.

Phospholine Iodide (Echothiophate). This drug is used as a 0.1 to 0.25 per cent solution and is another very potent agent with prolonged effects similar to those of demecarium bromide.

Isoflurophate (Diisopropyl Fluorophosphate or DFP, Floropryl). The effects of this drug are similar to those of physostigmine, but it is more powerful. It is used as a 0.1 per cent solution in peanut oil since it is rapidly hydrolyzed in water. Care must be taken to prevent tears or other moisture from contaminating the solution. *Isoflurophate Ophthalmic Solution* and *Isoflurophate Ophthalmic Ointment* are preparations listed in the U.S.P.

Parasympatholytic drugs

Parasympatholytic drugs cause the smooth muscle of the ciliary body and iris to relax, thus producing mydriasis and cycloplegia. Ophthalmologists take advantage of these effects to examine the interior of the eye, measure the proper strength of lenses for spectacles (refraction), and also to put the eye at rest in inflammatory conditions. Systemic absorption of these drugs can result in serious side effects such as dryness of the mouth, inhibition of sweating, flushing, tachycardia, fever, delirium, and coma. Pupillary dilatation from either local or systemic administration can precipitate acute glaucoma in predisposed persons, which, if unrecognized or untreated, can result in blindness.

Atropine Sulfate, U.S.P., B.P. This is used in 0.5, 1, and 3 per cent aqueous solutions. Note that one drop of a 3 per cent solution contains more than 1 mg. of atropine sulfate. *If all of this is absorbed it will have the same effect as twice the usual adult subcutaneous dose and could result in atropine poisoning.* The ocular mydriasis and cycloplegia produced by local application can persist as long as 7 to 12 days. The patient must be aware that during this time he may be unable to focus on nearby objects and will be unusually sensitive to light.

Scopolamine Hydrobromide, U.S.P.; *Hyoscine Hydrobromide*, B.P. This drug in aqueous solutions of 0.25 to 0.5 per cent has actions and side effects similar to those of atropine.

Homatropine Hydrobromide, U.S.P., B.P., or *Homatropine Hydrochloride*. These preparations are available in 2 to 5 per cent solutions.

The effects are similar to those of atropine, but the duration of action is only 24 hours.

Eucatropine Hydrochloride, U.S.P. (Euphthalmine Hydrochloride). This agent is administered locally as a 2 per cent solution and produces pupillary dilatation that persists for only a few hours. It has little effect on the power of accommodation.

Cyclopentolate Hydrochloride, U.S.P. (Cyclogyl Hydrochloride). This drug in 0.5 to 2 per cent solution produces rapid and brief mydriasis and cycloplegia. It finds its greatest use as an aid to eye examination and refraction.

Sympathomimetic drugs

Stimulation of the sympathetic end organs in the iris results in vascular constriction and mydriasis. Serious systemic side effects with these drugs are unusual, but care must be taken in patients with cardiovascular disease. The cautionary comments concerning mydriasis and glaucoma apply here just as well as with the parasympatholytic drugs.

Epinephrine Hydrochloride, U.S.P.; *Adrenaline,* B.P. This agent has several uses in ophthalmology. Dilute solutions are employed at times in treating local allergies and superficial hyperemia. It is mixed with other agents for injection because its vasoconstrictive effects prevent too rapid absorption of the other drugs. Concentrated preparations such as 2 per cent Epitrate is used in lowering intraocular pressure in certain types of glaucoma in which pupillary dilatation is not harmful.

Phenylephrine Hydrochloride, U.S.P., B.P. (Neo-Synephrine). This preparation is commonly used in 2.5 to 10 per cent solutions to produce mydriasis for ocular examination. *Care must be taken to prevent systemic absorption since one drop of a 10 per cent solution contains about 5 mg.* This is equal to the usual subcutaneous dose and can produce a considerable rise in blood pressure.

Cocaine. Cocaine is a powerful local anesthetic and is generally used only for this property, but it also has indirect sympathomimetic effects and will produce mydriasis if applied topically to the eye.

Anesthetics

Local anesthetics, both topical and for injection, are used to prevent pain during certain surgical procedures and examinations. Unfortunately all of the topical anesthetic drugs interfere with healing of epithelial defects, particularly those of the cornea. The practice of repeatedly applying such an anesthetic to an eye after removal of a foreign body is to be condemned.

Cocaine Hydrochloride, U.S.P., B.P. Solutions of 1 to 4 per cent are used for deep topical anesthesia of the eye. The drug has both anesthetizing and sympathomimetic effects. Local administration may rarely produce an acute cocaine poisoning with sudden severe confusion, delirium, and convulsions. Short-acting barbiturates must be given at once to prevent a fatal termination.

Procaine Hydrochloride, U.S.P., B.P. Injections of 1 to 2 per cent solutions are used for local nerve block or regional anesthesia.

Lidocaine Hydrochloride Injection, U.S.P. (Xylocaine Hydrochloride). This drug in 1 to 2 per cent solution has more rapid onset of action and produces deeper anesthesia than equal quantities of procaine hydrochloride.

Tetracaine Hydrochloride, U.S.P. (Pontocaine Hydrochloride). This preparation is used topically in 0.5 per cent solution for rapid, brief, superficial anesthesia.

*Proparacaine Hydrochloride** (Ophthaine). This drug is similar to tetracaine. A 0.5 per cent solution is administered by topical instillation.

Chemotherapy of ocular infection

The basic principles guiding the use of chemotherapy are the same in all branches of medicine. The drug of choice and the dose required must be established by adequate laboratory isolation of the offending organism; the initial culture from the infected area must be obtained before any chemotherapeutic agent is applied. Prophylactic use of antibiotic agents in general is useless as well as wasteful and potentially dangerous. A large proportion of the inflammatory diseases seen in ophthalmology are caused by viruses or other agents that are not susceptible to any currently available antibiotic; obviously the use of antibiotics in such situations is unwarranted.

Antibiotics

All known systemically administered antibiotics are available and used at indicated times to treat ocular infections. In addition, frequent use is made of topical ointments and solutions to treat superficial infections. Care must be taken to use an antibiotic that will not cause local or general sensitivity and to use drugs that are unlikely to ever be used systemically. Solutions are preferred since ointment bases often tend to interfere with healing.

Penicillin. This antibiotic is never used topically. Local sensitivity reactions are very common and unfortunately the patient may develop a generalized sensitivity which will forever prohibit the use of penicillin in any form.

*Described in annual publication of A. M. A. Council on Drugs, N.N.D., 1960.

The Tetracyclines (Chlortetracycline, Oxytetracycline, and Tetracycline), *Chloramphenicol, Erythromycin,* and *Streptomycin.* These drugs are all used topically as ointments, suspensions, or solutions in 0.5 to 1 per cent preparations. They are commonly used systemically and therefore are not employed topically without positive indication.

Bacitracin, U.S.P., B.P. Bacitracin is rarely used systemically because of its nephrotoxic effects. Ophthalmic ointments contain 500 units per gram of suitable base and are particularly useful in treating superficial infections due to gram-positive bacteria.

Neomycin Sulfate, U.S.P., B.P. This drug is available as an ointment containing 5 mg. per gram of base or as 0.5 per cent solution. It has a broad antibacterial spectrum and a low index of allergenicity. Because of auditory and renal toxicity it is generally not used parenterally.

Polymyxin B Sulfate, U.S.P., B.P. This agent is used largely for its activity against gram-negative bacteria. Hypersensitivity reaction to the 0.25 per cent topical solution is practically unknown.

Tyrothricin, N.F. Tyrothricin has a low rate of hypersensitivity reactions and is effective over a fairly large bacterial spectrum. It contains both gramicidin and tyrocidine. The usual concentration employed is 0.5 mg. per milliliter or gram of vehicle.

Nitrofurazone (Furacin)

Nitrofurazone, N.F. (Furacin). This highly bacteriostatic agent has a fairly broad spectrum. Unfortunately the rate of patient sensitization is high.

Sulfonamides

Sulfacetamide Sodium, U.S.P., B.P. (Sodium Sulamyd). Used in a 10 per cent ointment or a 30 per cent solution, this preparation provides high local concentrations that are relatively nonirritating.

Sulfisoxazole Diethanolamine, U.S.P. (Gantrisin Diethanolamine). The sulfonamide is available in a 4 per cent ophthalmic solution and a 4 per cent ophthalmic ointment. It is applied topically to the conjunctiva.

Antiseptics

The use of antiseptic agents for anything except the mechanical cleansing and sterilization of instruments and surface tissues is largely obsolete. Solutions are employed in ophthalmology for irrigation, dissolution of secretions, and precipitation of mucus and in certain instances in which specific antimicrobial agents cannot be used.

Silver Nitrate, U.S.P., B.P. A solution of 1 or 2 per cent is routinely employed as a prophylaxis against ophthalmia neonatorum in newborn infants. The gonococci are particularly susceptible to silver salts, and effective antibiotic agents may sensitize the patient. *Silver Nitrate Ophthalmic Solution*, U.S.P., is available in collapsible capsules containing about 5 drops of a 1 per cent solution.

Mercury Compounds. Inorganic mercuric salts such as *Yellow Mercuric Oxide Ointment*, N.F., *Mercuric Oxide Eye Ointment*, B.P., *Ammoniated Mercury*, U.S.P., B.P., and *Mercury Bichloride Ophthalmic Ointment*, N.F., formerly served as bacteriostatic agents. Today they are seldom used.

Organic mercurials such as *Metaphen* and *Thimerosal*, N.F. (Merthiolate), are used in 1:5,000 solution and, in general, are less irritating and more bacteriostatic than the inorganic salts.

Zinc Sulfate, U.S.P., B.P. An aqueous solution of 0.1 to 1.0 per cent is used as an astringent and mildly antiseptic eyewash in conjunctivitis caused by the Morax-Axenfeld bacillus.

Iodine Tincture, U.S.P. This preparation contains 2 per cent iodine and 2 per cent sodium iodide in dilute alcohol. Its only ophthalmologic use is for the chemical cautery of corneal lesions produced by the herpes simplex virus.

Steroids

The natural and synthetic adrenal steroids and corticotropin (ACTH) have been widely employed in ophthalmology to suppress inflammatory reactions of many etiologies. They are particularly valuable in allergic and hypersensitivity reactions in any part of the eye or its adnexa. They do not cure any disease and indeed may mask and aid the onset and spread of infection due to viruses, bacteria, and fungi. The combination of antibiotic agents with steroids does not prevent this effect unless the causative organism is specifically sensitive to the particular antibiotic used.

The following topical preparations are commonly employed:

Cortisone and Hydrocortisone Acetate Ophthalmic Suspensions. Available in 0.5 to 2.5 per cent concentrations.

Prednisone and Prednisolone Acetate Suspensions. Available in 0.5 per cent concentrations.

*Triamcinolone** (Aristocort, Kenacort). Used in 0.1 per cent ointment.

Dexamethasone (Decadron). Available as 0.1 per cent solution and 0.5 per cent ointment.

Carbonic anhydrase inhibitors

The intraocular pressure is maintained by the production of an aqueous humor inside the eye. It has been found that one of the substances necessary for the production of this fluid is the enzyme carbonic an-

*Described in annual publication of A. M. A. Council on Drugs, N.N.D., 1960.

hydrase. In glaucoma, where the intraocular pressure is abnormally high, it is desirable to slow the production of this fluid and thus decrease the pressure. The specific drugs used to inhibit carbonic anhydrase are quite effective when taken orally. Side reactions are not usually severe and consist of lethargy, anorexia, numbness, and tingling of the face and extremities. A diuresis is produced and potassium depletion can occur. The duration of action of a single oral therapeutic dose is 6 to 8 hours.

The commonly used preparations are as follows:

Acetazolamide, U.S.P., B.P. (Diamox). Available in 250 mg. tablets.

Ethoxzolamide* (Cardrase). Available in 125 mg. tablets.

Methazolamide (Neptazane). Available in 50 mg. tablets.

Dichlorphenamide (Daranide). Available in 50 mg. tablets.

Enzymatic preparations

Hyaluronidase for Injection, U.S.P.; *Hyaluronidase*, B.P. This enzyme is available in ampules containing 150 turbidity reducing units. It is employed in local nerve block anesthesia to increase the dispersal of the local anesthetic. Seven and one-half turbidity units are mixed with each milliliter of the anesthetic.

Alpha-Chymotrypsin. This enzyme is used in selected cases to facilitate cataract extraction. It is irrigated into the open eye and loosens the attachment of the lens. It is available in ampules containing 750 units of lyophilized enzyme which is to be dissolved in 10 ml. of diluent.

Miscellaneous materials

Sodium Chloride Ointment. This 5 per cent ointment is employed to reduce the corneal edema that occurs in certain corneal dystrophies.

Methylcellulose, U.S.P. A preparation of methylcellulose is used as a 0.5 to 1.0 per cent solution to provide moisture and lubrication in diseases in which tear production is deficient.

Benzalkonium Chloride, U.S.P., 1:5,000. This is a cationic surface-active wetting agent which has several applications in ophthalmology. Its antiseptic properties make it useful in the preservation of other solutions and the sterilization of small instruments. It is also used in balanced salt solutions to aid in the cleansing and application of contact lenses.

Fluorescein Sodium, U.S.P., B.P. This is a dye that is used as a diagnostic aid. When applied to the cornea, only areas denuded of epithelium are stained. Solutions of this dye are easily contaminated by *Pseudomonas aeruginosa*, a bacterium that produces intense corneal ulceration. For this reason prepared solutions are never used but strips of filter paper impregnated with the dry dye are moistened just before use.

*Described in annual publication of A. M. A. Council on Drugs, N.N.D., 1960.

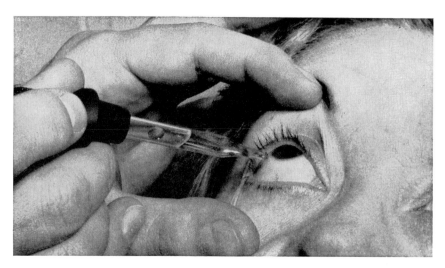

Fig. 41 Instillation of drops in the eye.

Instillation of topical preparations

The patient's head is placed on a suitable rest so that his face is directed upward. He is then instructed to fix his gaze on a point above his head. Gentle traction with the clean fingertips is applied to the lid bases at the bony rim of the orbit; *care is taken not to apply any pressure to the eyeball itself.* The dropper or ointment tube approaches the eye from below, outside the patient's field of vision, with due care to avoid contact with the eye. The drop is applied gently and not allowed to fall more than one inch before it strikes the eye (Fig. 41).

Many of the solutions employed in ophthalmology are extremely potent and care must be taken to prevent their systemic absorption. Gentle pressure is applied for two minutes to the lacrimal canaliculi at the inner corner of the eyelids and is directed inward and downward against the bones of the nose. This will prevent the solution from entering the nasal cavity and being absorbed through its highly vascular mucosa.

References

A. M. A. Council on Drugs, New and Nonofficial Drugs, Philadelphia, 1960, J. B. Lippincott Co.

Beckman, H.: Drugs, Their Nature, Action and Uses, Philadelphia, 1958, W. B. Saunders Co.

Lerman, S.: Glaucoma, Scient. Am. **201**: 110, Aug., 1959.

Modell, W. (editor): Drugs of Choice, 1960-1961, St. Louis, 1960, The C. V. Mosby Co.

Chapter 19

Drugs that act on

organs

of the reproductive system

The reproductive system of the female consists of the ovaries, the uterine (fallopian) tubes, the uterus, and the vagina; in the male, it consists of the testes, the seminal vesicles, the prostate gland, the bulbourethral glands, and the penis. The reproductive organs of both the male and the female are largely under the control of the endocrine glands, especially the pituitary gland. The ovaries and testes are known as gonads and not only produce ova and sperm cells but also form endocrine secretions which initiate and maintain the secondary sexual characteristics in men and women. When gonadal function diminishes and finally ceases, the secondary sexual characteristics gradually change and reproductive function ceases. The period of change is marked in women by the cessation of menses and is known as the menopause. In men, diminution of output of the sex hormone also occurs in later life, but it is less clearly definable and is sometimes called the male climacteric.

Action of drugs on the myometrium

The uterus is a highly muscular organ which exhibits a number of characteristic properties and activities. The smooth muscle fibers extend longitudinally, circularly, and obliquely in the organ. The uterus has a rich blood supply, but when the uterine muscle contracts, blood flow is diminished. Profound changes occur in the uterus during pregnancy. The uterus of women increases in weight during pregnancy from about 50 grams to approximately 1,000 grams. Its capacity increases tenfold in length, and new muscle fibers may be formed. These changes are accompanied by changes in response to drugs. Since the uterine smooth muscle responds sensitively to many drugs, the uterus of virgin guinea pigs or rabbits is used in standardizing a number of drugs that have a stimulating action on smooth muscle.

Drugs that act on organs of reproductive system 541

The uterus, both in situ and when excised, contracts rhythmically. Both pendular and peristaltic movements may be seen. In nongravid animals, peristaltic movements are relatively slight and, just as in the intestine, pauses occur between peristaltic contractions. These vary greatly with the condition of sexual activity. Movements are depressed early in pregnancy but increase later. Parturition is accomplished by powerful peristaltic waves, which cause labor pains.

Drugs that act upon the uterus include (1) those that increase the motility of the uterus, (2) those that decrease uterine motility, and (3) the sex hormones.

Oxytocics

In the human being, stimulation of either the sympathetic or the parasympathetic division of the autonomic nervous system may bring about increased uterine contractions. However, the response of the human uterus to cholinergic or adrenergic drugs is not dependable. There are drugs that exert a selective action on the smooth muscle of the uterus and these drugs are known as oxytocics. The ones used most are alkaloids of ergot and extracts from the secretion of the posterior pituitary gland, although there are many other drugs that may exhibit some effect on uterine motility.

Ergot

Ergot is the dried sclerotium (mycelium) of the parasitic fungus *Claviceps purpurea* which grows on many species of grain but especially on rye, where it forms long black bodies on the ears of the rye. It is especially prevalent when the weather is moist and warm. It grows in the grain fields of North America and Europe. Ergot was known as an "obstetrical herb" to midwives long before it was recognized by the medical profession.

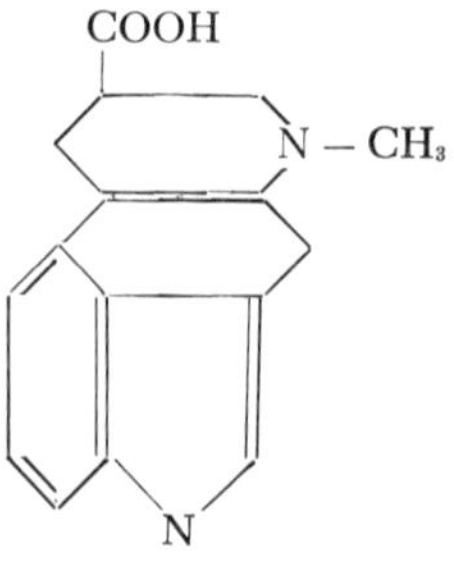

Lysergic acid

Active constituents. Both levorotatory and dextrorotatory alkaloids have been isolated from ergot, but only the levorotatory compounds are

542

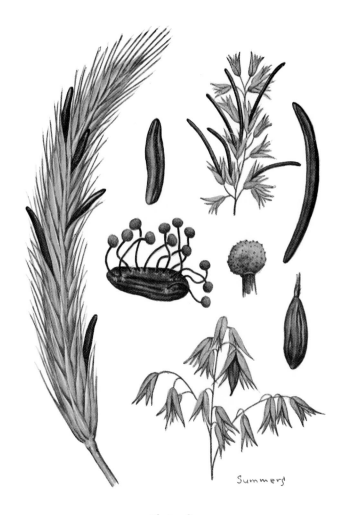

Plate 8

Claviceps purpurea (rye ergot). (From Jackson, D. E.: Experimental Pharmacology and Materia Medica, St. Louis, The C. V. Mosby Co.)

pharmacologically significant. These are derivatives of a substance called lysergic acid. The basic structure of the diverse and complex group of alkaloids of ergot is that of the substance lysergic acid (see accompanying structural formula). The individual ergot alkaloids all are compounds in which substitutions have been made at the carboxyl group.

The entire large group of individual alkaloids derived from ergot can be further divided into three groups: the *ergotamine group,* the *ergotoxine group,* and the *ergobasine group.* Members of each group have certain common chemical features and certain common pharmacologic actions. The first two have a peptide chain substituted at the carboxyl group of lysergic acid, whereas alkaloids of the ergobasine group are chemically simpler and contain a relatively small side chain, that of an amino alcohol, e.g., *ergonovine* in which alaninol is linked to lysergic acid (see structural formula).

Ergonovine

Action and result. All three groups of the alkaloids of ergot act on uterine muscle. Some of them also have other pharmacologic actions, which are referred to elsewhere under appropriate headings (see Index for uses of ergotamine). For convenience the other effects will be classified here.

Ergotamine and ergotoxine groups. The major groups of alkaloids of ergot are contrasted and compared as follows.

ON UTERUS. Ergotoxine* and ergotamine exert their most powerful effect on the uterus. The mechanism of action is a direct muscular stimulation since it occurs in the uterus after removal as well as when it is in the body.† Small doses produce normal uterine contractions which may be spastic in nature. A gravid uterus is more sensitive to the alkaloids of

*When the term ergotoxine is used, reference is being made to the alkaloids ergocristine, ergocornine, and ergokryptine.

†Goodman, L., and Gilman, A.: The Pharmacological Basis of Therapeutics, New York, 1955, The Macmillan Co., p. 891.

ergot than a nongravid or immature uterus. Ordinary therapeutic doses of the alkaloids produce an effect in the gravid or parturient uterus that is unaccompanied by side actions.

IN CIRCULATORY SYSTEM. The action on blood vessels is a direct muscular constriction particularly of the smaller vessels. This effect is of value in reducing uterine hemorrhage after childbirth. When ergotamine and related alkaloids are administered in large doses, there follows a definite rise in blood pressure. The effect on blood pressure is less powerful than that of epinephrine, but it lasts longer.

Both ergotamine and ergotoxine are capable of damaging the capillary epithelium, which in turn may give rise to thrombosis and possible gangrene. Man is particularly sensitive to this toxic effect of the alkaloids of ergot.

ON SYMPATHETIC NERVOUS SYSTEM. Ergotamine and ergotoxine act as autonomic blocking agents to paralyze the effector cells and make them nonresponsive to epinephrine. This action is not significant in man, provided the dosage remains within therapeutic limits.

Ergobasine group—ergonovine. Ergonovine resembles ergotamine and ergotoxine in its effect upon the uterus, although it appears to have a greater selective action on uterine muscle and produces its effects more rapidly. Ergotamine and ergotoxine are poorly and irregularly absorbed from the gastrointestinal tract, whereas oral doses of ergonovine are readily absorbed; it is therefore effective in smaller doses and weaker concentrations than the other alkaloids. Because small doses are effective and because the parturient uterus is especially sensitive to ergonovine, side actions rarely accompany its use in obstetrics. Its duration of action is thought to be somewhat less than that of the other two alkaloids.

Ergonovine differs from ergotoxine and ergotamine in that it appears to stimulate the effector cells connected with adrenergic nerves rather than paralyze them. It produces little or no rise in blood pressure, and although it shares with the other alkaloids the ability to cause gangrene, it appears to be definitely less toxic than ergotamine and ergotoxine. Ergonovine is the preparation of ergot most used in obstetrics.

Uses. Preparations of ergot, especially ergonovine and methylergonovine, are used primarily to promote involution of the uterus and to prevent or control post-partum hemorrhage. Routine use of oxytocics during the first and second stages of labor is not recommended. The contractions which these drugs produce are such that the life of the mother and the fetus may be endangered by their use.

Ergotamine tartrate has been advocated for the relief of certain types of headache and for relief of excessive itching associated with jaundiced conditions (see Chapter 14).

Preparation, dosage, and administration (used in obstetrics).

Ergonovine Maleate, U.S.P. (Ergotrate Maleate); *Ergometrine Maleate,* B.P. This drug is available in 0.2 mg. tablets for oral administration and in solution for intramuscular or subcutaneous injection, 0.2 mg. per milliliter. The usual oral dose is 0.2 to 0.4 mg. repeated two or three times daily for a period of 2 to 3 days. Some physicians prescribe 0.2 mg. every 4 hours for 6 doses, starting immediately after delivery. The usual dose for parenteral administration is also 0.2 to 0.4 mg. Prolonged therapy should be avoided.

*Methylergonovine Maleate** (Methergine Maleate); *Methylergometrine Maleate,* B.P. This agent is a synthetic oxytocic and is available in 0.2 mg. tablets for oral administration and in solution for parenteral administration, 0.2 mg. per milliliter. The usual dose is 0.2 mg. This preparation is chemically related to ergonovine, but it is more potent and its action is said to be more prolonged. It has less tendency to cause an elevation of blood pressure and is preferred for patients who are threatened with eclampsia or in cases in which the condition is actually present. Although toxic effects are not ordinarily encountered they can occur.

Ergot Fluidextract, N.F. Dosage is 2 ml. orally. This preparation, although official, is seldom used.

Side effects and toxic effects. Toxic symptoms of acute poisoning seen after the administration of ergonovine and similar alkaloids usually result from stimulation of the central nervous system and include nausea and vomiting, tremor, weakness, excitement, convulsive seizures, dilated pupils, and rapid pulse.

The ergotamine and ergotoxine alkaloids usually produce symptoms of circulatory disturbance before they produce effects in the nervous system. Such symptoms include tingling, itching, coldness of the skin, and rapid weak pulse. Other symptoms are thirst, headache, nausea, vomiting, dizziness, and diarrhea and abdominal cramps. They may develop after ingesting large doses in an attempt to induce abortion. It has been observed that increased sensitivity to alkaloids of ergot seems to accompany hepatic disease and febrile and septic states.

Chronic ergotism, *ergotismus chronicus,* is now of rare occurrence where modern milling methods are used, but before the cause was known, it was frequent in wet seasons and times of poor harvest, due to the ergot in the grain.

Chronic ergotism may occur in two forms: gangrenous and convulsive. Gangrene results from prolonged constriction of the blood vessels, which at the same time fill with a hyaline substance that blocks the circulation. Prolonged constriction of cerebral blood vessels results

*Described in annual publication of A. M. A. Council on Drugs, N.N.D., 1960.

in degenerative changes in the brain. Constriction in retinal vessels may cause blindness. The most striking symptom of ergotism is the dry, painless gangrene of some part of the body such as fingers or toes. The part affected first becomes cold, numb and dark in color, and then shrivels up and drops off without pain or bleeding. These symptoms are due to the fact that the blood supply to the part is shut off by the constriction of the vessels. The disease was called "St. Anthony's fire," or "hell fire." The cure at that time was a pilgrimage to the shrine of St. Anthony, hence the name.

Treatment of ergot poisoning requires complete withdrawal of the medication and the use of symptomatic measures such as the use of vasodilator drugs and sedatives and sometimes the injection of calcium gluconate to relieve muscular pain.

Posterior pituitary hormone

The pituitary gland is a small ductless gland situated in a small cup-shaped depression in the sphenoid bone at the base of the brain and consists of two lobes, the anterior and the posterior, and an intermediate portion called the *pars intermedia*. Extracts are obtained from the posterior lobe of the pituitary glands of cattle and sheep, and when injected they produce the following effects: (1) stimulation of uterine muscle (oxytocic effect), (2) promotion of water absorption in the tubules of the kidney (antidiuretic effect), and (3) constriction of peripheral blood vessels (pressor effect).

A great advance in the pharmacology of the posterior lobe has been the recent identification and chemical analysis of the two major hormones obtained from the gland in pure form. These compounds, oxytocin and vasopressin, are both peptides, each containing eight amino acids. After their isolation and determination it proved possible to synthesize them chemically. Availability of the only oxytocic and vasopressor pituitary hormones in pure form have cleared up a number of uncertainties about their action and has also opened the door to their better-controlled therapeutic use. It is now known, for example, that there is a certain overlap of pharmacologic action in the pure preparations: pure oxytocin has some vasopressor activity and vice versa. Vasopressin is also the antidiuretic hormone, its antidiuretic potency being much more marked than its pressor potency. Although clinicians still use mainly the cruder preparations of oxytocic and vasopressor activity, it may be expected that eventually the pure compounds will replace the present extracts.

Action and result. Posterior pituitary injection and particularly oxytocin stimulate the uterine muscle and produce rhythmic contractions. The action in the human being is modified by the pregnant or nonpregnant state as well as by the stage of pregnancy. Sensitivity to the extract increases as the pregnancy progresses. The effects of the pituitary preparation are produced rapidly as compared to ergot, which acts more slowly.

Posterior pituitary preparations stimulate certain contractile tissues in the mammary gland and promote the emptying of the milk into the larger ducts and reservoirs and contribute to milk ejection. They do not affect the total amount of milk formed over a period of time.

A transient fall in blood pressure is sometimes observed after the administration of oxytocin, which is thought to be due to myocardial depression. Fortunately it does not last long.

Uses. Posterior pituitary injection and oxytocin injection are used to increase contractions of the uterus at the time of childbirth. They may be used in a long labor when normal contractions do not bring about expulsion of the fetus or to constrict the uterus and decrease hemorrhage after delivery of the placenta. Their use should be attended with caution and avoided when the cervix is not thoroughly effaced and easily dilatable. Their use is usually contraindicated during the first stage of labor. If used when the cervix is undilated and rigid, severe laceration and excessive trauma are likely to result. Ill-advised use of oxytocics is thought to explain high maternal and infant mortality rates.

Oxytocin is sometimes used to induce labor, although this needs to be done under careful medical supervision.

Preparation, dosage, and administration.

Posterior Pituitary Injection, U.S.P. This preparation is available in ampules containing 0.5 and 1 ml. of sterile aqueous solution prepared from the pituitary glands of domestic animals. The official preparation possesses in each milliliter the activity equivalent to 10 U.S.P. units. This preparation contains a mixture of hormones. The usual dose is 0.3 to 1 ml. This preparation is sometimes known as obstetrical Pituitrin. It is administered subcutaneously.

Oxytocin Injection, U.S.P., B.P. (Pitocin). This solution is available in 0.5 and 1 ml. ampules. It is a sterile aqueous solution of the oxytocic principle, which is the preparation of choice when an oxytocic effect rather than a pressor effect is desired. Dosage depends upon the stage of labor. The usual intramuscular postpartum dose is 0.5 to 1 ml. Each milliliter of this preparation contains the equivalent of 10 U.S.P. units. When used to induce labor, 1 ml. in 1,000 ml. of 5 per cent dextrose in water may be given slowly by intravenous drip. This method of administration must be used cautiously.

Oxytocin (Syntocinon). This is a preparation of synthetic oxytocin. It is available in 0.5 and 1 ml. ampules. Dosage and administration are the same as those for oxytocin injection.

Drugs that act on organs of reproductive system 547

Preparations of *vasopressin* are presented in Chapter 24.

Side effects and toxic effects. In the human being, the response of the myometrium to posterior pituitary extracts is variable and is influenced by many factors. Overdosage may produce uterine tetany followed by increasing clonic contractions. Uterine rupture and fetal death can result. These preparations are therefore contraindicated or given with great caution to patients with cardiovascular disease or those who have previously had a cesarean section or when there is a malpresentation of the fetus or rupture of the uterus threatens for any reason at all.

Patients receiving oxytocin or related drugs during labor should be under constant observation. This means the blood pressure should be taken frequently, careful and periodic check on the fetal heart tones should be made, and the strength and duration of the uterine contractions should be noted. Prolonged contractions of the uterus result in diminished blood flow and decreased oxygen for the fetus.

Drugs that decrease uterine motility

There are times when the inhibition of uterine contractions are indicated. One time is when the patient is going into premature labor and another may be when the uterine tone is high and contractions are unusually frequent and uncoordinated. Drugs that combat these conditions include certain depressants of the central nervous system and antispasmodics.

Analgesics and sedatives

Large doses of opiates, general anesthetics, and barbiturates tend to decrease uterine motility. Average doses of barbiturates probably have little or no effect. Morphine is effective because it not only relieves pain but it also alters the patient's emotional reaction to pain, allaying fear and anxiety. Methadone is excellent to relieve pain, but it has no effect on fear and anxiety. Demerol as compared to morphine has much less effect on respiration. Its analgesic potency is somewhere between that of morphine and codeine. Codeine, especially when combined with aspirin, is useful to relieve the discomfort associated with repair work on the perineum, but it has little use during the course of labor. Promethazine hydrochloride (Phenergan Hydrochloride) is utilized clinically for obstetric sedation. It relieves apprehension and potentiates the action of drugs such as morphine sulfate and meperidine hydrochloride (Demerol Hydrochloride), permitting a reduction in their dosage.

Antispasmodics

Antispasmodics reduce muscle spasm or relax muscles. They include drugs that exhibit various mechanisms of action and include a number of depressants of the nervous system which act by decreasing reflex hyperactivity. In addition, several other agents are herein mentioned.

Relaxin (Releasin)

Relaxin is a naturally occurring substance which for commercial purposes is extracted from the ovaries of pregnant sows. It exhibits an ability to inhibit uterine contractions. Its use as an agent to prevent the onset of premature labor has been recommended but its true status for this form of therapy has not been established. The results of a number of experiments on animals led to its clinical trial as a drug to soften and relax the cervix and thus shorten the course of labor. Differences of opinion exist about its merits as such an agent. It has also been proposed for the relief of dysmenorrhea. Only time and careful research studies can determine the true worth of this preparation.

Preparation, dosage, and administration.

*Relaxin*** (Releasin). This drug is available in solution, 20 mg. per milliliter, for intramuscular and intravenous injection. It is given in doses of 20 to 40 mg. When administered intravenously it is given slowly by intravenous drip in 250 to 500 ml. of sterile diluent.

Side effects and toxic effects. Relaxin contains a pork protein and may induce sensitivity in patients, which may range in severity from chills to acute anaphylaxis after intravenous administration.

Lututrin (Lutrexin)

Lututrin is a protein-like substance which is extracted from the corpus luteum of the ovaries of the sow.

Action. It produces relaxation of the symphysis pubis in the guinea pig and in some respects resembles the action of relaxin. It decreases the muscular contraction of the human uterus.

Uses. It is used in the treatment of severe functional dysmenorrhea. Its value in the treatment of premature labor and threatened abortion is uncertain.

Preparation, dosage, and administration.

*Lututrin*** (Lutrexin). This is available in tablets containing 2,000 units each, the units being determined by the assay of the relaxing effect on the uterus of the guinea pig. For dysmenorrhea, initial doses of 4,000 to 6,000 units are given prior to the onset of symptoms and followed by 4,000 to 6,000 units every 3 to 4 hours as needed. As much as 50,000 units have been administered without observable untoward effects.

*Described in annual publication of A. M. A. Council on Drugs, N.N.D., 1960.

Clearly defined dosage schedules for prevention of premature labor and abortion have not been agreed upon.

Magnesium Sulfate

Many students will think of magnesium sulfate as a saline cathartic only. The fact of the matter is that when this salt is administered parenterally it not only will depress the central nervous system but it will also depress all forms of muscular tissue (smooth, skeletal, and cardiac).

Uses. It is effective to counteract uterine tetany such as may occur after large doses of oxytocin or when the myometrium is for some reason contracting abnormally. Because of its depressant effect on skeletal muscle it is employed in the treatment of eclampsia when patients are threatened with convulsive seizures. Another reason for its use for eclamptic patients is because of its depressant action on the central nervous system.

Preparation, dosage, and administration.

Magnesium Sulfate, U.S.P., B.P. It is administered intramuscularly and sometimes intravenously. For rapid effect an intravenous dose of 20 ml. of a 20 per cent solution may be given. Effects last approximately 30 minutes. It is poorly absorbed after oral administration.

Side effects and toxic effects. Parenteral administration of magnesium sulfate is not without attendant danger. Respiratory depression and failure can occur. Abrupt injection of large doses can cause cardiac arrest. The patient receiving magnesium sulfate parenterally should never be left alone. An injection of calcium gluconate (10 per cent solution) is an effective antidote since it counteracts the effect of magnesium sulfate on muscle tissue. Artificial respiration may also be indicated.

Sex hormones

The hormones concerned with ovarian function include the *anterior pituitary hormones,* which are required for the normal development and function of the gonads, the *gonadotropic hormones* of *placental* origin, and the *ovarian hormones* themselves. As we shall see, the ovarian hormones include the naturally occurring steroids, the synthetic and partly synthetic steroids, and the nonsteroid compounds, such as stilbestrol, which have ovarian hormonelike function.

A similar group of hormones play corresponding roles in regulating gonadal growth and function in the male.

Pituitary gonadotropic hormones

The endocrine gland which exerts the chief gonadotropic influence in the body is the anterior lobe of the pituitary gland. How many hormones are made by this gland is somewhat uncertain, but three are believed to have an effect on the ovary. One stimulates the development of the graafian follicle and is known as the follicle-stimulating hormone (FSH). Another, the luteinizing hormone (LH) or interstitial cell stimulating hormone (ICSH), promotes the growth of the interstitial cells in the follicle and the formation of the corpus luteum. A third hormone is known as the luteotropic hormone (LTH). It is probably identical with the lactogenic hormone. The follicle-stimulating hormone initiates the cycle of events in the ovary. Under the influence of both FSH and LH the graafian follicle grows, matures, secretes estrogen, ovulates, and forms the corpus luteum. The LTH promotes the secretory activity of the corpus luteum and the formation of progesterone. In the absence of LTH the corpus luteum undergoes regressive changes and fails to make progesterone.

In the male, FSH acts only on the seminiferous tubules and promotes the formation of sperm cells. ICSH stimulates the interstitial cells in the testes and promotes the formation of androgen.

The clinical use of the pituitary gonadotropic hormones has been handicapped by the lack of sufficiently refined preparations. Commercial preparations often contain other proteins and inert substances which make injections painful and make allergic reactions possible.

Some degree of success has accompanied the use of these gonadotropic extracts when used in the treatment of amenorrhea, Fröhlich's syndrome, sterility, undescended testicle (cryptorchidism), and hypogenitalism. Lack of success in treatment can sometimes be attributed to the fact that when a deficiency of one of the pituitary hormones exists, it is more than likely that there is a deficiency in a number of others which may not be of a direct gonadotropic nature.

There are no official gonadotropic preparations from the anterior pituitary gland.

Gonadotropic hormones of placental origin

Gonadotropic substances are formed by the placenta during pregnancy in the human being and in certain animals. Human chorionic gonadotropic hormone differs from pituitary gonadotropins, both biologically and chemically. It produces little of the follicle-stimulating effect but affects principally the growth of the interstitial cells and the secretion of luteal hormone. In women, it is capable of prolonging the luteal phase of the menstrual cycle. Its normal role seems to be to enhance and prolong the secretion of the corpus luteum during early pregnancy. It does not initiate the formation of corpus luteum, however.

In the male, it stimulates the interstitial cells of the testes, causing them to increase production of androgens, which in turn promotes the growth and development of accessory sex organs.

Chorionic gonadotropin has also been found in the blood of pregnant mares, but only the human chorionic gonadotropin is used therapeutically because it does not induce the formation of antihormones in the patient since it is of human origin. It is believed to be the substance that forms the basis of pregnancy tests (Friedman and Aschheim-Zondek). This substance was originally thought to come from the anterior pituitary gland, but it is now recognized as coming from the placenta. The reason that the urine of pregnancy can be used to test for the gravid state is that the laboratory animal used for this test is usually a rodent, and in these animals the chorionic gonadotropic factor stimulates growth of the follicle as well as the corpus luteum.

Uses. Gonadotropic hormones are used in the treatment of cryptorchidism (undescended testicle) when there is no anatomic obstruction to prevent testicular descent. It is being used experimentally in the treatment of hypogonadism and functional uterine bleeding, but there is considerable difference of opinion about its value.

Preparation, dosage, and administration.

Chorionic Gonadotropin,* B.P. (Follutein, Entromone). A water-soluble gonadotropic substance obtained from the urine of pregnant women. It is a glycoprotein containing about 12 per cent galactose. The dosage used in treating cryptorchidism is 500 to 1,000 international units two or three times a week. Therapy should be discontinued if there are signs of precocious maturity.

Ovarian hormones

The ovaries are the female sex glands which are situated on either side of the uterus. They not only develop and periodically discharge the ripened ova but also secrete the ovarian hormones.

One of the ovarian hormones is made by the cells of the graafian follicle and is referred to as the follicular hormone. The other is the luteal hormone made by the cells of the corpus luteum. Normal development and activity of the reproductive organs are dependent in part on the right state of balance between these hormones. They are secreted in sequence under the influence of the gonadotropins of the anterior pituitary gland.

Estrogens

The follicular hormone is responsible for the development of the sex organs at puberty and for the secondary sex characteristics such as the growth and distribution of hair, texture of skin, distribution of body fat,

*Described in annual publication of A. M. A. Council on Drugs, N.N.D., 1960.

growth of the breasts, and character of the voice and the maintenance of these characteristics throughout adult life. The follicular hormone apparently exists not as an entity but as a number of related polymorphic forms which differ in their activity. This group of substances which exhibits similar estrogenic activity is called estrogens. The group includes both the natural estrogens and the synthetic substances which have similar effects in the body.

Chemistry. The naturally occurring estrogens are steroids in which ring "A" (ring at the lower left of the accompanying formula) is a benzene (aromatic ring) in place of the saturated ring of the other major steroids. Compare formulas with those of the adrenal steroids in Chapter 24. The primary natural estrogen believed to be secreted by the follicle is estradiol (estrin), so named for the two hydroxyl groups.

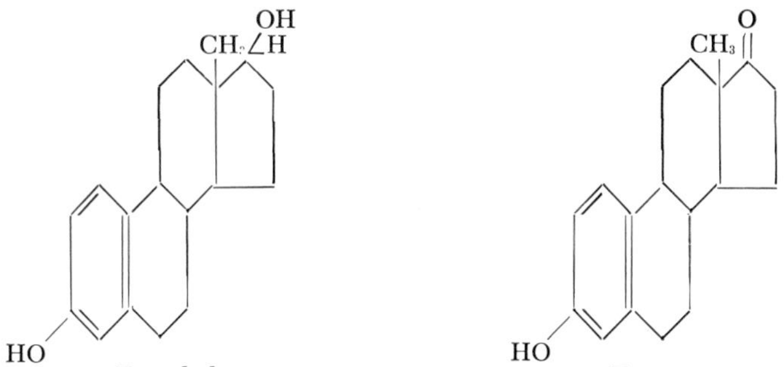

Estradiol

Estrone

Both estrone (Theelin) and estradiol are naturally occurring estrogens. In the body, estrone can be converted into estradiol and vice versa. There are a number of other naturally occurring estrogens.

The synthetic estrogens include both *steroid* and *nonsteroid* forms. The steroid forms include modifications of the naturally occurring steroid estrogens so as to increase potency (ethinyl estrogens). The more important group, however, are the nonsteroid synthetic estrogen compounds which do not closely resemble the natural estrogens, chemically, yet have remarkably similar pharmacologic action. A typical member of this group is diethylstilbestrol.

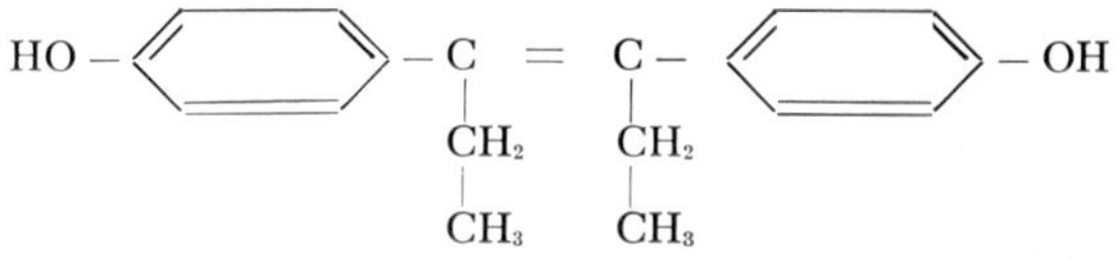

Diethylstilbestrol

Natural estrogenic substances are found in a variety of places in both plants and animals. They are found in the blood of both sexes, in testicu-

Drugs that act on organs of reproductive system 553

lar fluid, feces, bile, and in the urine of both pregnant women and mares. Estrogens have also been found and isolated from the adrenal gland. These substances vary somewhat chemically in accordance with the source from which they are obtained.

Pharmacologic action and result. When estrogenic substances (natural or synthetic) are injected into immature animals such as rats they are capable of hastening sexual maturity and producing estrus. In these animals the vaginal epithelium changes after the administration of estrogens and appears as it does in mature animals. This is the basis of bioassay and standardization of preparations of these substances.

When estrogens are administered in doses which compare favorably with the amount normally secreted by the ovaries, the effect is like that produced by the natural secretion of these glands. When estrogens are administered in larger amounts than these, however, other effects may be produced.

One effect is that of inhibiting hyperactivity of the pituitary gland. Increased activity of the pituitary gland is believed to occur at menopause or after surgical removal of the ovaries. This may cause symptoms such as flushing, sweating, hot flashes, etc. The administration of estrogen prevents hyperactivity of the pituitary gland at least temporarily or while the estrogen continues to be given.

The same changes occur in the myometrium and endometrium when estrogens are administered as occur naturally, i.e., the myometrium and endometrium proliferate (cells reproduce rapidly). When the estrogen is withdrawn, uterine bleeding frequently occurs. It sometimes occurs even with continued administration of the estrogen.

Estrogens naturally stimulate the development of the breasts, that is, the development of the ducts in the gland and possibly both the ducts and the alveoli. Whether this occurs as a direct action on the mammary gland or because of indirect effect on the pituitary gland is not clear. Estrogens are known to inhibit the secretion of milk.

Estrogens exhibit effects in other parts of the body, e.g., on the skeletal system. Large doses inhibit the development of the long bones by causing premature closure of the epiphyses and by preventing the formation of bone from cartilage (endochondral bone formation). On the other hand, some aspects of bone formation are augmented by the presence of estrogens, and when these substances are lacking, osteoporosis may develop such as is seen in women after menopause.

Estrogens resemble the hormones made in the adrenal cortex in that large doses affect water and electrolyte balance and are prone to cause retention of sodium and development of edema. Their ability to do this is much less marked than that of the adrenal steroid hormones, however. It is known that the estrogen level in the blood is high just prior to menstruation, and at this time retention of water and electrolyte is recognized as a cause of gain in weight.

Some of the responses to estrogens in the body can be antagonized by the administration of androgens (male hormones), and the reverse is also true.

Uses. Estrogens are used for a variety of conditions in which there is a deficiency of these substances, e.g., to relieve certain symptoms associated with menopause. At the time of menopause the normal endocrine balance is disturbed by the gradual cessation of ovarian function. The pituitary gland apparently attempts to compensate for the lack of ovarian activity by temporary hyperfunction. Symptoms caused by this compensatory reaction respond well to estrogenic therapy. This is due to the fact that large doses of ovarian hormones depress the secretion of the gonadotropic hormones of the anterior pituitary. Vasomotor disturbances and headache can often be relieved. Symptoms which are of psychic origin do not respond to this type of therapy as a rule. The estrogenic substances may be administered orally, intravaginally, or parenterally. Both the dosage and the method of administration must be decided in relation to each individual patient.

Vaginitis in children has been satisfactorily and successfully treated with estrogens, but with the advent of successful antibiotics the use of estrogens is no longer indicated.

They are used to relieve engorgement of the breast in a post-partum patient when lactation is to be suppressed. Administration of estrogens is believed to suppress the formation of the lactogenic hormone made by the pituitary gland.

Limited palliative effect is also produced in women past menopause who have inoperable breast cancer with metastases of the soft tissues.[*]

Estrogenic material may serve as a substitute for castration for the relief of discomfort associated with prostatic carcinoma and its metastases.

Suppositories containing estrogenic substances are also used in the treatment of senile vaginitis and pruritus vulvae.

Postmenopausal osteoporosis is frequently successfully treated with estrogens.

Natural estrogens—preparation, dosage, and administration.

Estrone, U.S.P. (Theelin); *Oestrone,* B.P. Estrone is a crystalline estrogenic substance which is marketed in 1 ml. ampules or 10 ml. vials containing estrone in oil or aqueous suspension. The concentration varies from 0.2 to 1 mg. per milliliter for the preparation in oil and from 1 to 5 mg. per milliliter for the aqueous suspension. Estrone is also available in vaginal suppositories containing 0.2 mg. of the drug. For menopausal

[*]N.N.D., 1960, p. 557.

symptoms the drug is usually administered intramuscularly in doses of 0.2 to 1 mg. once or twice weekly.

Estradiol, N.F. (Diogyn, Progynon). This drug is marketed as an aqueous suspension and in pellets, tablets, and suppositories. Preparations for injection contain 0.1 to 5 mg. per milliliter. It is administered topically, orally, or parenterally.

Estradiol Benzoate, U.S.P. (Diogyn B, Dimenformon Benzoate); Oestradiol Benzoate, B.P. This form is less subject to destruction in the tissues than the parent substance and hence is suitable for parenteral administration (intramuscularly). Dosage varies from 0.1 to 5 mg., depending on the condition for which it is given and the severity of the symptoms.

Estradiol Dipropionate, U.S.P. (Ovocylin Dipropionate). This preparation is absorbed more slowly and excreted more slowly than estradiol, but in other respects its effects are similar to other estradiol compounds. It is administered intramuscularly as a solution in oil and is available in 1 ml. ampules containing 1, 2.5 and 5 mg. of the drug or in 10 ml. ampules containing 10 or 50 mg. of the drug. Dosage ranges from 1 to 5 mg. given weekly or biweekly.

Estradiol Cyclopentylpropionate, N.F. (Depo-Estradiol Cyclopentylpropionate). This preparation may produce more prolonged effects than the estradiol compounds mentioned previously. It is available as an oil solution (10 mg. per 1 ml. or 25 mg. in 5 ml.). It is administered by intramuscular injection. One to 5 mg. may be administered weekly for 2 to 3 weeks and then every 3 or 4 weeks to produce maintenance effects.

Ethinyl Estradiol, U.S.P. (Diogyn E, Estinyl); *Ethinyl Oestradiol,* B.P. This preparation is a potent estrogen which is made suitable for oral administration. It is available in tablets, 0.01, 0.02, 0.05, and 0.5 mg., and as an elixir, 0.006 to 0.03 mg. per milliliter. Dosage varies greatly with the condition treated. For control of menopausal symptoms 0.02 to 0.05 mg. is given once to three times a day.

Conjugated estrogens—preparation, dosage, and administration.

Estrogenic Substances, Conjugated, U.S.P.* (Premarin). This preparation contains water-soluble, conjugated forms of mixed estrogens from the urine of pregnant mares. The principal estrogen present is sodium estrone sulfate. This preparation is available in tablets and in solution for oral administration. It is also available in the form of topical creams and lotions, as well as in powder form for injection (intramuscular or intravenous). The action and uses of this preparation are similar to those of other estrogens. Dosage of 1.25 mg. daily is usually sufficient to control menopausal symptoms. Senile vaginitis and pruritus vulvae are usually

°U.S.P. XVI Interim Admission.

relieved with doses of between 1.25 and 3.75 mg. For palliation of breast cancer, a daily oral dose of 30 mg. is recommended.*

Piperazine Estrone Sulfate† (Sulestrex Piperazine). This preparation has the same actions and uses as the naturally occurring conjugated estrogens. It is administered orally. For the control of menopausal symptoms the dosage is usually 1.5 mg.; for the treatment of senile vaginitis and pruritus vulvae, 1.5 to 4.5 mg.; for breast engorgement, 4.5 mg. at intervals of 4 hours for 5 doses.

Synthetic estrogens—preparation, dosage, and administration.

Diethylstilbestrol, U.S.P.; Stilboestrol, B.P. This drug is a relatively cheap synthetic estrogenic substance which duplicates practically all known actions of the natural estrogens. It is relatively active when given by mouth as well as when given parenterally. It is not significantly more toxic than the natural estrogens. It is available in plain tablets, enteric-coated tablets, and capsules for oral administration, in solution for injection, and in the form of vaginal suppositories. These dosage forms are available in a wide range of concentrations. The average oral dose for treatment of menopausal symptoms is 0.5 to 1 mg. daily. The dosage should be reduced if discomfort results. For the suppression of lactation, 5 mg. once or twice daily for 2 to 4 days are considered sufficient; for prostatic cancer, 3 mg. daily (intramuscularly) reduced to 1 mg. daily or 0.5 mg. three times a day (orally); and for the palliation of mammary cancer, 15 mg. is the daily oral dose recommended.‡ Dosage of all preparations should be kept at the minimum necessary for the relief of symptoms.

Diethylstilbestrol Dipropionate.† This form is used for the same conditions for which other estrogenic substances are used. It is given intramuscularly in oil and is said to have a rather prolonged effect; hence reactions such as nausea, vomiting, headache, and dizziness occur less frequently than with free diethylstilbestrol. It is also administered orally (tablets). Dosage for the relief of menopausal symptoms is 0.5 to 2 mg. two or three times a week; larger doses are required for suppression of lactation and for the treatment of prostatic cancer.

Dienestrol, U.S.P. (Restrol, Synestrol). This is a nonsteroid estrogen which can be administered orally. It is said to cause fewer side effects than diethylstilbestrol. It is also less potent. Dosage for the relief of menopausal symptoms is 0.1 to 1.5 mg. daily. Larger doses may be ordered for the patient with mammary cancer. Dienestrol also can be given subcutaneously and intramuscularly. It is available in 0.1, 0.5, and 10 mg. tablets for oral administration; in a suspension for injection, 50 mg. in 10 ml.; and as a vaginal cream, 0.1 mg. per gram.

*N.N.D., 1960, p. 572.
†Described in annual publication of A. M. A. Council on Drugs, N.N.D., 1960.
‡N.N.D., 1960, p. 577.

*Chlorotrianisene** (Tace). This drug in general shares the actions and uses of other estrogenic substances, although it exhibits some points of difference. The compound is stored in body fat, from which it is slowly released. Therefore its action extends beyond the time when administration of the drug has been discontinued. It is effective in the relief of mammary engorgement, but its use in large amounts is not recommended for cancer of the breast of patients beyond the age of menopause because it may induce uterine bleeding. Average oral dose for relief of menopausal symptoms is 12 to 24 mg. daily; in cases of prostatic cancer, 24 mg. daily; for relief of mammary engorgement, 48 mg. daily. The last-mentioned dosage is to be continued only for 1 week. It is available in 12 and 25 mg. capsules for oral administration.

Hexestrol, N.F. This is a compound that is less potent and less toxic than diethylstilbestrol. It is used for many of the same conditions for which the latter estrogen is used. It is available in 1 and 3 mg. tablets for oral administration. The dosage recommended for the control of menopausal symptoms is 2 to 3 mg., which is reduced as the symptoms are brought under control.

*Methallenestril** (Vallestril), *benzestrol** (Benzestrol), and *promethestrol dipropionate** (Meprane Dipropionate). These are additional synthetic estrogens listed in N.N.D. They produce effects similar to those produced by diethylstilbestrol.

The synthetic estrogens offer the advantage of ease of administration since they can be given orally, and they are also relatively inexpensive.

Side effects and toxic effects. Side effects seen in connection with estrogen therapy frequently include nausea and vomiting, diarrhea, and skin rash. The symptoms are usually mild and are usually related to dosage, potency of the compound, and route of administration. Other symptoms include edema and an increased amount of calcium in the blood of patients who have been given prolonged therapy. Adjustment of dosage, substitutions of another estrogen, and perhaps parenteral administration rather than oral may relieve the gastrointestinal symptoms. Periodic tests of the blood and renal function tests are recommended.

Estrogens are carcinogenic when administered experimentally in animals that have inherited sensitivity to certain types of carcinoma.[†] Many clinicians believe that estrogens are therefore contraindicated for women who have a personal or family history of malignancy of the reproductive system. Estrogens are used, however, for inoperable breast cancer.

*Described in annual publication of A. M. A. Council on Drugs, N.N.D., 1960.
†Goodman, L., and Gilman, A.: Pharmaceutical Basis of Therapeutics, New York, 1955, The Macmillan Co., p. 1594.

Luteal hormone

The secretion of progesterone by the corpus luteum is under the influence of one of the pituitary hormones, luteotropin (LTH). The chemical structure of progesterone resembles that of the estrogens and also the androgens.

Progesterone

The chemistry of progesterone and related compounds differ from the estrogens in that ring "A" (ring at the lower left of the accompanying structural formula) is not aromatic and they also have a 2 carbon side chain at the 17 position (upper right). Chemically they are closely related to the adrenal steroids (see Chapter 24).

The luteal hormone functions in the preparation and maintenance of the lining of the uterus for the implantation and nourishment of the embryo. It supplements the action of the follicular hormone in the action on the uterus and also in the mammary glands. It suppresses ovulation during pregnancy and keeps the uterus in a quiescent state by decreasing the irritability of the uterine muscle. After the third month of pregnancy its production is taken over by the placenta.

Progesterone was formerly obtained from the corpus luteum but it is now prepared synthetically.

Uses. It was thought at one time that progesterone had therapeutic usefulness in the treatment of dysmenorrhea, menorrhagia, and habitual abortion, but positive evidence is insufficient to support this conclusion. It is said to be of value in the treatment of functional uterine bleeding. After the endometrium is primed with estrogen, progesterone may be used in the treatment of amenorrhea. Some of the newer preparations are given to promote fertility when failure to conceive is due to a luteal phase defect. Some have been reported to be helpful in cases of habitual abortion.

Preparation, dosage, and administration.

Progesterone, U.S.P., B.P. (Corlutone, Lipo-Lutin, Progestin, Proluton). This preparation is available in an oil solution or aqueous suspension for injection. It is ineffective when given orally. The solution in oil is administered intramuscularly and the suspension may be administered

Drugs that act on organs of reproductive system 559

subcutaneously. It is given in doses up to 25 mg. or more daily. Tablets of 10 and 25 mg. are available for sublingual administration up to four times a day.

Ethisterone, U.S.P., B.P. (Anhydrohydroxyprogesterone) (Lutocyclol, Pranone). Ethisterone is a derivative of progesterone which can be given orally. It is available in 5, 10 and 25 mg. tablets. The usual dose is 25 mg. up to 4 times a day.

Norethindrone* (Norlutin). This is a synthetic compound chemically related to ethisterone. It produces effects similar to those produced by progesterone. It is being used for the treatment of patients who have amenorrhea, menstrual irregularity, and infertility. It is available in 5 mg. tablets and is administered orally in doses of 10 to 20 mg.

Hydroxyprogesterone Acetate* (Prodox). This synthetic substance differs from progesterone mainly in that it is active after oral administration. It can be used for all conditions for which progesterone is indicated. It is available in 25 and 50 mg. tablets. The usual dose is 25 to 50 mg. daily.

Hydroxyprogesterone Caproate* (Delalutin). A synthetic derivative of progesterone, it is a great deal like progesterone except that it has a longer duration of action. It is available in oil solution, 250 mg. in 2 ml., for intramuscular injection. The usual single dose is 125 to 250 mg., and one dose every 4 weeks may be sufficient in treatment of menstrual disorders and ovarian and uterine dysfunction.

Side effects and toxic effects. Preparations of luteal hormone or related compounds appear to have a low order of toxicity. Patients occasionally have gastrointestinal symptoms, headache, dizziness, and allergic manifestations. Cases have been reported in which masculinization of female infants occurred in connection with the administration of progesterone to the mothers during pregnancy.

Androgens

Normal development and maintenance of male sex characteristics depend on adequate amounts of the male sex hormones, which are called androgens. All androgenic compounds have, in common, a steroid nucleus. In fact, natural estrogens, androgens, and some of the hormones of the adrenal cortex all exhibit an interesting similarity in their structural formulas.

Testosterone is believed to be the true testicular hormone and it is chemically similar to progesterone. Androgens chemically similar to testosterone are excreted in the urine and are usually referred to as 17-ketosteroids because there is a ketone group attached to carbon 17 of the steroid structure (see androsterone). It should be remembered, how-

*Described in annual publication of A. M. A. Council on Drugs, N.N.D., 1960.

ever, that the urinary 17-ketosteroids are also products of the adrenal cortex in both men and women. Androsterone is one of the 17-ketosteroids found in the urine. Testosterone is not excreted, as such, in the urine.

CH₃

OH
CH₃ — H

CH₃

O

CH₃
C=O
CH₃

CH₃

O

O
CH₃ — Carbon 17

CH

OH
H

Testosterone
(male sex hormone)

Progesterone
(female sex hormone)

Androsterone
(one of 17-ketosteroids
found in urine of
both sexes)

Action and result. The androgens function in the development and maintenance of normal states in the sex organs. Administration to immature males causes growth of the sex organs and the appearance of secondary sex characteristics. When administered for therapeutic purposes they therefore simply replace the missing hormone. When a high concentration of androgenic substances is maintained in the circulation, anterior pituitary secretion is inhibited and spermatogenesis is retarded.

In mammals, both sexes form both the male and female hormones, although they are antagonistic to each other. The administration of testosterone can suppress menstruation and cause atrophy of the endometrium.

Another effect produced by androgens is concerned with anabolism, i.e., the formation as well as the maintenance of muscular and skeletal protein. The administration of androgenic substances is associated with an increase in muscular development and weight. They bring about retention of nitrogen (essential to the formation of protein in the body) and also affect the storage of inorganic phosphorus, sulfate, sodium, and potassium.

The retention of nitrogen, prevention of atrophy in bones from disuse, and promotion of the healing of wounds are effects of testosterone and related compounds which have been reported.* These effects are of particular significance in patients who are paraplegic after trauma to the spinal cord because in these patients the maintenance of adequate nutrition, prevention of atrophy in muscles and bones, and prevention as well as treatment of decubitus ulcers constitute serious problems. Similar

*Cooper, I. S., and others: Testosterone Preparations as a Nitrogen Sparing Agent After Spinal Cord Injury, J. A. M. A. 145: 552, 1951.

problems are encountered in the care of patients who are chronically ill, malnourished, or have a wasting disease such as carcinoma.

Uses. Androgens have been used in replacement therapy for patients with hypogonadism and eunuchoidism (castrates). They produce marked changes in sex organs, body contour, and voice, provided the deficiency state has not been present too long. Androgens have little effect on senile men and on patients with psychogenic impotence.

Alone or with gonadotropic substances, androgens have been employed in the treatment of cryptorchidism (undescended testicle).

Androgens have also been used in the treatment of dysmenorrhea, menopausal states, and for the suppression of lactation and breast engorgement. Favorable results are sometimes obtained from their use to relieve subjective symptoms associated with the male climacteric just as estrogens are of value in relieving symptoms of similar origin in women.

Androgens have been employed for palliative relief of advanced inoperable cancer of the breast. Their mechanism of action is not clear. Subjective improvement (improved appetite, gain in weight, and relief of pain) seems to be more marked than objective improvement. Improvement is temporary and seldom exceeds a period of one year. Androgens are preferred for patients with this condition prior to or during menopause since estrogens may promote the development of the cancer at this time.

Preparation, dosage, and administration.

Testosterone, N.F., B.P. Testosterone produces effects similar to testosterone propionate. When given in aqueous suspension its duration of androgenic effects is slightly longer than those of testosterone propionate. It is available in 75 mg. pellets; as an aqueous injectable suspension, 25 mg. per milliliter; and tablets for oral and sublingual administration. For dosage, see testosterone propionate.

Testosterone Propionate, U.S.P., B.P. (Oreton, Andronate). This form is available in 5 and 10 mg. buccal tablets and as a solution for intramuscular injection. Dosage ranges from 10 to 60 mg. two to six times weekly, depending upon the response obtained and the effect desired. Five to 10 mg. daily may be sufficient as maintenance doses for therapy in men. For relief of symptoms of breast cancer, 150 to 300 mg. weekly (in several doses) may be administered. This preparation is synthesized from cholesterol or extracted from bull testes.

Testosterone Enanthate, U.S.P. (Delatestryl). This preparation is administered as a solution in oil and provides a prolonged effect of 3 weeks or more. The usual intramuscular dose is 200 mg. every 2 to 4 weeks.

Methyltestosterone, U.S.P., B.P. (Oreton M, Metandren). This preparation is available in 5, 10, and 25 mg. tablets for oral administration, in 10 mg. buccal tablets (these are held in the space between the teeth and cheek), and in 5 and 10 mg. tablets for sublingual administration. The indications and actions of this compound are essentially the same as those for testosterone propionate. The usual oral dose is 10 mg. three times a day. Doses for the suppression of lactation are larger. Dosage is adjusted according to the needs and response of the patient.

Testosterone Cyclopentylpropionate, U.S.P. Although highly similar to testosterone propionate, it exhibits the advantage of more prolonged androgenic effects. It is available in solution, 100 mg. per 1 ml. and 500 mg. and 1 Gm. in 10 ml. It is administered intramuscularly in doses from 10 to 50 mg. at intervals of 1 or 2 weeks.

*Stanolone** (Neodrol). Stanolone is an androgen that has the same action and uses as testosterone and related compounds. It is used clinically for its anabolic effects and for its effects on inoperable or metastatic carcinoma of the breast. For cancer of the breast the average effective dose is 100 mg. daily, which is given intramuscularly as long as the patient shows improvement or is able to tolerate the metabolic and masculinizing effects.

*Norethandrolone** (Nilevar). This is a synthetic androgen which is chemically and pharmacologically related to testosterone. It is not used as an androgen since its androgenic properties are less significant than its ability to affect protein anabolism (see action of androgens). It is administered orally and intramuscularly in amounts that range from 30 to 50 mg. daily in divided doses. It is available as a solution, 8.3 mg. per milliliter, and in 10 mg. tablets for oral administration. Large doses can produce androgenic effects like those encountered with the other androgens.

*Fluoxymesterone** (Halotestin, Ultandren). This compound is a synthetic halogenated derivative of methyltestosterone. It is available in 2 and 5 mg. tablets for oral administration. It is several times more potent than methyltestosterone, both from the standpoint of androgenic and anabolic activity. Dosage for anabolic effects ranges from 4 to 10 mg., and for palliation of breast cancer, 6 to 20 mg. daily have been used. Dosage varies greatly with the condition being treated, response of the patient, etc. The daily dose is given at one time or divided into three or more portions.

Side effects and toxic effects. Effects which are regarded as untoward effects in the female include deepening of the voice, hirsutism (excessive growth of hair), flushing, acne, regression of the breasts, enlargement of the clitoris, and general masculinization. Less prominent effects, but probably more serious, are the retention of sodium, potassium, water, and chloride, which can contribute to heart failure. Jaundice has occasionally been observed after the administration of methyltestosterone

*Described in annual publication of A. M. A. Council on Drugs, N.N.D., 1960.

and norethandrolone and means that administration of the androgen should be discontinued. Nausea and gastrointestinal upsets occur occasionally. Patients receiving androgens should be observed carefully for elevation of blood calcium, acceleration of the disease being treated, and the appearance of edema. Edema is sometimes controlled with the use of diuretics and a diet low in salt.

Contraindications. Androgens are contraindicated for patients with prostatic cancer.

Questions
for study and review

1 Diethystilbestrol belongs to which of the following groups?
   a. gonadotropins
   b. androgens
   c. estrogens
2 A drug which is a male sex hormone is said to be a (an):
   a. estrogen
   b. androgen
   c. gonadotropin
3 Which of the following preparations is sometimes used to relieve symptoms associated with menopause?
   a. progesterone
   b. methyl testosterone
   c. diethylstilbestrol
   d. ergonovine maleate
4 Meperidine (Demerol) may be preferred to morphine for the obstetric patient for which of the following reasons? It:
   a. is a more potent analgesic
   b. produces less respiratory depression
   c. acts more quickly
   d. does not affect the bowel
5 All central nervous system depressants tend to be used in small doses for the patient in labor to avoid:
   a. prolongation of labor
   b. excessive response on the part of the mother
   c. respiratory depression in the fetus
6 Which of the following reasons may explain why estrogens are sometimes used in treatment of mammary cancer (in patients past menopause) in preference to androgens?
   a. are less expensive
   b. produce relief of symptoms more quickly
   c. produce no side effects
   d. can be administered orally

7 Which of the following preparations might you expect to see ordered for the suppression of lactation?
   a. Chlorotrianisene (Tace)
   b. Oxytocin (Pitocin)
   c. Lututrin (Lutrexin)
   d. Methylergonovine maleate (Methergine Maleate)
8 Patients receiving oxytocin (Pitocin) to induce labor must be watched especially for:
   a. tetanic contractions of the uterus
   b. maternal exhaustion
   c. drop in blood pressure
   d. prolapse of the umbilical cord
9 The main reason for giving promethazine hydrochloride (Phenergan Hydrochloride) to a patient in labor is likely to be for which of the following reasons?
   a. to relieve pain
   b. to reduce the amount of post-partum nausea
   c. to reduce the amount of narcotic needed by the mother
   d. to produce sleep
10 Which of the following preparations might you expect to see ordered for a patient who is inactive and whose muscular and osseous tissues seem to be wasting away?
   a. diethylstilbestrol
   b. chlorotrianisene (Tace)
   c. lututrin (Lutrexin)
   d. norethandrolone (Nilevar)
11 Which of the following is a synthetic estrogen that is stored in body fat from which it is slowly released?
   a. testosterone propionate
   b. chlorotrianisene
   c. estradiol benzoate
   d. relaxin
12 Which of the following preparations might you expect to see used to produce central nervous system depression and re-

lief of edema in an obstetric patient with toxemia?

a. morphine sulfate
b. phenobarbital
c. magnesium sulfate
d. promethazine hydrochloride

References

A. M. A. Council of Pharmacy and Chemistry: New and Nonofficial Drugs, Philadelphia, 1960, J. B. Lippincott Co.

Barger, G.: Ergot and Ergotism, London, 1931, Gurney and Jackson.

Beckman, H.: Drugs, Their Nature, Action, and Uses, Philadelphia, 1958, W. B. Saunders Co.

Cooper, I. S., Rynearson, E. H., MacCarty, C. S., and Power, M. H.: Testosterone Preparations as a Nitrogen Sparing Agent After Spinal Cord Injury, J. A. M. A. 145: 549, 1951.

Dill, L. V., and Chanatry, J.: Effect of Relaxin in Normal Labor, J. A. M. A. 167: 1910, 1958.

Garland, L. H., Baker, M., Picard, W. H., and Sisson, M. A.: Roentgen and Steroid Hormone Therapy in Mammary Cancer Metastatic to Bone, J. A. M. A. 144: 997, 1950.

Goodman, L., and Gilman, A.: The Pharmacological Basis of Therapeutics, New York, 1955, The Macmillan Co.

Hayles, A. B., and Nolan, R. B.: Masculinization of Female Fetus, Possibly Related to Administration of Progesterone During Pregnancy, Proc. Staff Meet. Mayo Clin. 33: 200, 1958.

MacBryde, C. M., Castrodale, D., Loeffel, E., and Freedman, H.: The Synthetic Estrogen Diethylstilbestrol, J. A. M. A. 117: 1240, 1941.

McLennon, C. E.: Reflections on the Physiology of Menstruation, J. A. M. A. 156: 578, 1954.

Moir, J. Chassar: The History and Present-Day Use of Ergot, Canad. M. A. J. 72: 727, 1955.

Novak, E. R.: The Menopause, J. A. M. A. 156: 575, 1954.

Salter, W. T.: Textbook of Pharmacology, Philadelphia, 1952, W. B. Saunders Co.

Thompson, W. O.: Uses and Abuses of the Male Sex Hormone, J. A. M. A. 132: 185, 1946.

Tyler, E. T., and Olson, H. J.: Fertility Promoting and Inhibiting Effects of New Steroid Hormonal Substances, J. A. M. A. 169: 1843, 1959.

Wilkins, L.: Masculinization of Female Fetus Due to Use of Orally Given Progestins, J. A. M. A. 172: 1028, 1960.

Williams, R. H.: Textbook of Endocrinology, Philadelphia, 1955, W. B. Saunders Co.

Chapter 20

Anti-infectives other than antibiotics–sulfonamides

Since 1935, when Domagk discovered the antibacterial action of prontosil in mice infected with fatal doses of hemolytic streptococci, the treatment of infectious diseases with specific agents has developed to an amazing degree. Millions of people are the recipients of anti-infective agents which are either prepared synthetically or are obtained from microbial growth.

The following two chapters deal with antibacterial chemotherapeutic agents other than antibiotics. A few words of explanation about these two commonly used words, "chemotherapeutic" and "antibiotic," are in order. *Chemotherapeutic* agent has been generally used to mean a antimicrobial compound that is made synthetically and is sufficiently selective (relatively harmless to the patient) so as to be useful in the treatment of infectious disease. *Antibiotic,* on the other hand, generally refers to a substance produced by a given microbial form which is active in killing or inhibiting the growth of other microbes. It should be noted that all antibiotics are not medically useful; many have been too toxic to the mammalian host to employ in killing the parasite. These words, however, have undergone some shift in meaning. Some antibiotics have been chemically synthesized, so that the distinction in natural versus synthetic origin has been partly lost. In addition, "chemotherapeutic" has been broadened to include the chemical therapy of diseases other than infections, e.g., "antimalignant chemotherapy." Here we shall use the term to include those important antimicrobial drugs that were originally obtained by chemical synthesis and are not derived from nature, so far as we know. The antibiotics as another broad group of anti-infective agents are dealt with in a previous chapter (see Chapter 8).

Sulfonamide compounds

The rapid expansion of penicillin therapy, at a time when the sulfonamide drugs were just coming into their own, sidetracked many studies which would have increased knowledge of these compounds. Some authorities are of the opinion that the sulfonamides in one form or another again will assume importance in spite of the fact that they tend to be much more toxic to human tissues than are penicillin and certain other antibiotics. The sulfonamides all are prepared synthetically.

Chemistry. All of the sulfonamides used therapeutically contain the para-amino-benzene-sulfonamido group ($H_2N-C_6H_4-SO_2NH-$) which gives them their common characteristics. To this group is attached hydrogen or another group which gives each compound its individually characteristic features.

Some 5,000 sulfonamides have been made and tested since Domagk's discovery of the antibacterial action of prontosil. Of these, 20 to 30 are clinically useful. Except under unusual circumstances, all of these are *bacteriostatic* (in clinically achieved concentrations) rather than *bactericidal.* All act basically in the same general way. The chemical differences among the various sulfonamides largely determine factors such as the quantitative aspect of antibacterial potency and the distribution, excretion, and toxicity of the drug in the tissues of the patient. Most of the sulfonamides are white, crystalline powders which are relatively insoluble in water. Their sodium salts are readily soluble.

Sulfanilamide
Shows H attached to p-amino-benzene-sulfonamido group

Sulfadiazine
Shows pyrimidine ring attached to p-amino-benzene-sulfonamido group

Although sulfanilamide was not the first of these compounds to be synthesized, it is considered the parent substance of most other sulfonamides. All active members contain a free NH_2 group.

Action and result. The sulfonamides apparently act as bacteriostatic agents and inhibit or weaken susceptible bacteria and make them more vulnerable to the action of the phagocytes in the blood stream of the host. The biochemical mechanism of the sulfonamides in selectively inhibiting the growth of certain bacteria is relatively well understood. It is believed that para-aminobenzoic acid (PABA) is essential to the formation of an important group of coenzymes, of which folic acid is an active constituent. The sulfonamides interfere with the incorporation of PABA into the folic acid molecule; and since PABA and, ultimately, folic acid

Anti-infectives other than antibiotics 567

are essential to the growth of certain bacteria, the microorganisms are inhibited by the sulfonamides because the drugs resemble PABA in chemical structure and compete with it in an enzyme system of the microorganism. Bacteriostasis is achieved, however, only in bacteria that must synthesize their own folic acid. Organisms that must utilize preformed folic acid are not affected by sulfonamides.

NH₂ ... R — SO₂ ... NH₂ ... COOH

The sulfonamide drugs   Para-aminobenzoic acid (PABA)
R = a variety of nitrogen-containing groups

The chemical similarity of a sulfonamide and para-aminobenzoic acid is thought to explain why certain microorganisms take in the sulfonamide even though they cannot utilize it as they would PABA.

Although all the biochemical details of this metabolic antagonism are still not understood, the general picture is consistent with the most important known facts of sulfonamide bacteriostasis.

Bactericidal effects of the sulfonamides are known to occur in the urine where the drug becomes concentrated and the organisms are at a disadvantage because urine is naturally a poor culture medium.

Absorption, diffusion, and excretion. Many of the commonly used sulfonamides (sulfadiazine, sulfamerazine, sulfamethazine, and sulfisoxazole) are well absorbed from the gastrointestinal tract and can therefore be administered orally. Some of the sulfonamides, such as succinylsulfathiazole and phthalylsulfathiazole, are rather poorly absorbed and are used therefore to reduce bacterial growth in the colon itself.

One of the outstanding features about the sulfonamides is the ease with which many of them diffuse into all body fluids. This constitutes an advantage over the antibiotics in the treatment of such conditions as empyema and meningitis. A number of sulfonamides, when given orally, are soon found in the cerebrospinal fluid and in the peritoneal and synovial fluids and are present in concentrations which are therapeutically significant. Obviously the amount of drug present at any one time depends on how rapidly it is absorbed and how rapidly it is excreted, as well as on certain other factors such as the degree to which it is bound by protein and the extent of acetylation.

Acetylation is the major process by which the sulfonamides are metabolically inactivated. This change is probably due to the action of the liver. Acetylation is important to the physician when choosing a drug

568

because the acetylated forms are believed to be nontherapeutic but they may produce toxic symptoms. A sulfonamide with a low percentage of acetylation in the tissues could be given in smaller doses than one that undergoes greater acetylation, other factors being equal.

Excretion of the sulfonamides is chiefly by way of the kidney where both the free and the acetylated forms of the drug are filtered through the glomerulus. Most sulfonamides are reabsorbed to some extent in the kidney. Some of the sulfonamides are relatively insoluble in neutral or acid media, and as the kidney concentrates the urine and it becomes acid in reaction, there is some danger that the sulfonamide will precipitate out of solution. Forcing of fluids to keep the urine dilute and administration of an alkaline substance such as sodium bicarbonate help to keep a number of the sulfonamides in solution in the urine. However, this is no longer a clinical problem. Sulfonamides are now available, such as sulfisoxazole and sulfacetamide, which are quite soluble even at the acid conditions of urine. The problem of solubility in the urine can also be dealt with by using combinations of small doses of two or three different sulfonamides. The saturation point of each is not reached in this way and each drug remains in solution. Sulfonamides are also excreted by way of milk, bile, saliva, tears, sweat, and various other body fluids. Sulfamethazine and sulfamerazine are excreted more slowly than sulfadiazine.

Uses. The choice of sulfonamide to be used depends upon the organism causing the infection, the clinical efficacy of the drug, and the variety, frequency, and severity of the toxic reactions which may be produced. They have the advantage of low cost and ease of administration. Many infections which were formerly treated with one of the sulfonamides are now treated with an antibiotic or with a sulfonamide and an antibiotic. New sulfonamides continue to be synthesized and some may take the place of drugs used in present-day therapy. Rational therapy is directed toward the identification of the organism causing the infection and the use of the drug to which the infecting agent is susceptible. Sulfonamides continue to be useful for a number of infections, including the following:

Meningococcic meningitis. The sulfonamides continue to be drugs of choice for this disease. Sulfadiazine is especially effective since it diffuses well into the cerebrospinal fluid and has a low level of acetylation. Therapy with penicillin may be combined advantageously with that of a sulfonamide in the treatment of this condition. Sulfadiazine may also be employed along with penicillin or one of the broad-spectrum antibiotics in the treatment of other types of meningitis, i.e., meningitis due to other organisms which are sensitive to sulfadiazine.

Intestinal infections. Sulfonamides are especially effective for acute

Anti-infectives other than antibiotics 569

bacillary dysentery due to Shigella organisms. Sulfadiazine is considered the drug of choice because it is well absorbed and because it has been found that the infecting organisms often invade the wall of the bowel.

Sulfonamides are also used in the treatment of chronic ulcerative colitis. For this condition some clinicians prefer salicylazosulfapyridine (Azulfidine). Sulfadiazine is the sulfonamide of choice in the treatment of cholera, along with various supportive measures, e.g., intravenous infusions. Sulfonamides are also employed to lower the bacterial count in the bowel prior to surgery on the intestine.

Urinary tract infections. Sulfonamides are used extensively for bacterial infections of the urinary tract. They are especially effective against *Escherichia coli* and less effective for infections due to *Proteus vulgaris, Pseudomonas aeruginosa,* and *Streptococcus faecalis.* Sulfisoxazole (Gantrisin), sulfamethoxypyridazine (Kynex), triple sulfonamides, as well as sulfadiazine have been used successfully.

Other infections for which the sulfonamides are valuable either alone or combined with antibiotic therapy include plague, actinomycosis, brucellosis, psittacosis, lymphogranuloma venereum, and trachoma. Although once used for many other infections, they are no longer used as drugs of choice, having been supplanted by the antibiotics. However, the use of sulfonamides may be resorted to in the event that antibiotics cannot be used. Infections due to organisms such as the hemolytic streptococci, pneumococci, *Hemophilus influenzae,* and certain strains of staphylococci may respond satisfactorily to sulfonamide therapy.

Dermatitis herpetiformis has been successfully treated with sulfapyridine and more recently with sulfamethoxypyridazine. Sulfonamides are sometimes prescribed for prophylactic purposes, e.g., to prevent rheumatic fever or for persons who have had rheumatic fever and appear to be susceptible to streptococcic infections. Penicillin is usually the drug of choice for this purpose nonetheless.

Sulfonamides are of no value in the treatment of tuberculosis, malaria, leprosy, typhoid fever, tetanus, syphilis, most viral diseases such as measles and the common cold, and rickettsial diseases.

Resistance. It was early noted that a number of kinds of microorganisms were able to develop resistance to the effects of the sulfonamides. Some organisms seem to develop an ability to circumvent the interference of the sulfonamide molecule in their enzyme systems. This type of resistance may develop rapidly but seemingly is also rapidly lost. Another type of resistance which develops more slowly is due to the emergence of a few resistant organisms which then increase in number. Although the latter type of resistance may disappear after a period of time, it tends to be permanent.

The problem of resistance necessitates the maintenance of adequate dosage at all times since it is believed that inadequate dosage fosters the development of resistant strains. It also emphasizes the hazards associated with indiscriminate and unnecessary use of these compounds.

Preparation, dosage, and administration. The sulfonamides are usually administered orally. When, for some reason, a patient is unable to take the drug by mouth, sodium salts of a number of the sulfonamides are available for parenteral administration. Topical application of sulfonamides for the treatment of superficial infections, burns, or wounds is contraindicated except for certain ophthalmic conditions for which the use of sodium sulfacetamide or sulfisoxazole diethanolamine is recommended.* Most sulfonamides when applied topically have proved to be relatively ineffective in dealing with the infection, and, furthermore, hypersensitivity is more likely to develop. For the treatment of systemic infections the initial dose is frequently 0.1 Gm. per kilogram of body weight (usually about 4 Gm.) and then 1 Gm. every 4 hours (day and night) until the temperature has been normal for 72 hours. If the dosage differs from this it has been so indicated for individual preparations. Patients with minor infections may be given correspondingly smaller doses. A concentration of 15 mg. of the drug in 100 ml. of blood is thought to be desirable when severe infection is present, and 5 to 10 mg. per 100 ml. is usually satisfactory for less severe infections.

The frequent determination of concentrations of the sulfonamides in the blood previously has been accepted as an important measure to prevent overdosage of the patient, on the one hand, and, on the other, to ensure adequate dosage. This is now thought to be essential only in special cases. Experience seems to indicate that when a standard course of therapy is followed, it produces, in most instances, an adequate concentration of the drug in the blood and tissue fluids.

Sulfacetamide, N.F. This preparation is marketed in 500 mg. tablets for oral administration.

Sulfacetamide Sodium, U.S.P., B.P.† (Sodium Sulamyd). Official preparations of this sulfonamide are available as a 10 per cent ophthalmic ointment (the ointment listed in B.P. is 6 per cent) and a 30 per cent ophthalmic solution for topical application to the eyes. It has been widely used for certain infections of the eye because it rarely produces sensitivity.

Sulfadiazine, U.S.P., B.P.† This is marketed in 300 and 500 mg. tablets for oral administration. *Sulfadiazine Tablets,* U.S.P., contain 500 mg. each.

Sulfadiazine Sodium, U.S.P. This form is highly soluble in water and is suited for intravenous administration.

---

*N.N.D., 1960, p. 51.

†The sulfonamides listed in the *British Pharmacopoeia* are spelled sulpha, e.g., sulphacetamide.

Sulfadiazine Sodium Injection, U.S.P. This form is a solution available in concentrations of 2.5 Gm. in 10 and 50 ml.

Sulfamerazine, U.S.P., B.P.*; *Sulfamerazine Tablets,* N.F., B.P.* Official tablets contain 500 mg. each.

Sulfamerazine Sodium Injection, N.F. This form is suitable for intravenous administration. As is true of other sodium salts of sulfonamide compounds, the preferred method of administration is as a 5 per cent solution in distilled water or isotonic sodium chloride solution.

Sulfamethazine, U.S.P. This preparation is available in 500 mg. tablets for oral administration. Since it is excreted slowly it is recommended that the maintenance dose be administered every 6 hours instead of every 4 hours. It is a constituent of preparations of trisulfapyrimidines.

Sulfapyridine, U.S.P. The N.F. official tablet contains 500 mg. of sulfapyridine and is given orally. Although this is one of the more toxic sulfonamides it is one of the preparations of choice for *dermatitis herpetiformis.* The usual dose is 0.5 to 1 Gm. three times a day.

Sulfisoxazole, U.S.P. (Gantrisin). Sulfisoxazole is similar to many of the other sulfonamides in effectiveness and uses. It is highly soluble in body fluids; crystals are less likely to be precipitated in the urine, and renal blocking is less likely to occur since both the free and the acetylated forms of the drug are more soluble in the urine than is true for a number of these drugs. In other respects, however, sulfisoxazole is capable of producing toxic effects similar to those produced by other sulfonamides. The initial dose for a systemic infection is similar to that of other compounds of this group of drugs—4 Gm. followed by 1 Gm. every 4 hours until the temperature is normal for 48 hours; for infections of the urinary tract the dosage is usually less since urine is a poor culture medium for microorganisms and the kidney concentrates the urine as it excretes it. *Sulfisoxazole Tablets,* U.S.P., each contains 500 mg. of drug.

Acetyl Sulfisoxazole, U.S.P. (Gantrisin Acetyl). This form is available as an emulsion, 200 mg. per milliliter, and as a suspension and a syrup, 100 mg. per milliliter for oral administration. It is tasteless, and in the intestine it is changed into sulfisoxazole; hence its properties and dosage are comparable to those of the parent drug. The suspension is official (U.S.P.).

Sulfisoxazole Diethanolamine, U.S.P. (Gantrisin Diethanolamine). This is a preparation which can be given parenterally (intravenously, intramuscularly, and subcutaneously) when the parent drug cannot be administered adequately by the oral route. Official preparations are available as a solution for injection, 2 Gm. in 5 ml.; as a solution (4 per cent) for instillation in the eye; or as a 4 per cent ophthalmic ointment. The ophthalmic preparations must be used cautiously for patients who

*Spelled sulphamerazine in *British Pharmacopoeia.*

have previously exhibited sensitivity to any of the sulfonamides.

Sulfamethoxypyridazine, U.S.P. (Kynex, Midicel). This is one of the newer sulfonamides. It is readily absorbed from the digestive tract after oral administration but it is slowly excreted. Because it is slowly eliminated in the urine, concentrations which could cause renal damage are seldom achieved. Diffusion into the cerebral spinal fluid is said to be greater than that of other sulfonamides commonly employed. It is capable of causing many of the same side effects as other sulfonamides (nausea, drug fever, dermatitis, destruction of blood cells, etc.). The initial oral dose is 2 Gm. for the first day; after that, 1 Gm. daily. Some physicians prefer to give 1 Gm. every other day or 0.5 Gm. daily for infections of the urinary tract. This preparation is available in 500 mg. tablets (peach colored) and as a syrup in which each teaspoon (5 ml.) contains 250 mg. of the drug. The tablet is an official preparation.

*Sulfisomidine** (Elkosin); *Sulphadimidine,* B.P. This preparation is available in 500 mg. tablets and as a syrup, 62.5 mg. per milliliter, for oral administration. This drug is chemically related to sulfamethazine and is used for the treatment of both systemic and urinary tract infections. Renal toxicity is rarely encountered. Although it can be used for systemic infections it is usually prescribed for infections of the urinary tract.

*Sulfamethizole** (Thiosulfil). This drug is highly similar to other sulfonamides. It is readily soluble in the urine and hence is useful for infections of the urinary tract. It is available in 250 mg. tablets and as a suspension, 50 mg. per milliliter, for oral administration. The usual adult dose is 250 to 500 mg. four times a day. The dosage for children is less.

Sulfaethidole, N.F. (Sul-Spansion, Sul-Spantab). This preparation is highly similar to sulfamethizole except that it is longer acting. It is prepared as a sustained release suspension, in which each milliliter contains 130 mg. of the drug, and in sustained release tablets, 650 mg., for oral administration. The average adult maintenance dose is 1.3 Gm. every 12 hours. The initial dose is twice this amount. Dosage may be greater for severe infections or less when given for prophylaxis.

Sulfaguanidine, succinylsulfathiazole, and *phthalylsulfathiazole* are relatively insoluble compounds, which are poorly absorbed from the gastrointestinal tract. They rarely achieve significant concentrations in the blood and therefore rarely cause symptoms of toxicity after therapeutic doses. Some of these drugs have been used to suppress the growth of bacteria in the large bowel because high concentrations of drug are achieved in the intestine. They have been employed both before and

*Described in annual publication of A. M. A. Council on Drugs, N.N.D., 1960.

Anti-infectives other than antibiotics 573

after surgery on the bowel, for bacillary dysentery (sulfaguanidine) and for ulcerative colitis (salicylazosulfapyridine).

Sulfaguanidine, N.F., B.P. This drug is available in 500 mg. tablets for oral administration. It has been employed in the treatment of bacillary dysentery and as an intestinal antiseptic, but sulfadiazine is considered to be a superior preparation.

Succinylsulfathiazole, N.F., B.P. (Sulfasuxidine). This compound is available in 500 mg. tablets. The usual dose is 250 mg. per kilogram of body weight, divided into 6 doses which are given every 4 hours.

Phthalylsulfathiazole, B.P. (Sulfathalidine). This preparation is available in 500 mg. tablets. The initial dose as an intestinal antiseptic is 125 mg. per kilogram of body weight, followed by the same amount daily in several evenly divided doses for a period of several days (3 to 5).

p-Nitrosulfathiazole, N.F. (Nisulfazole). This drug is administered rectally in the form of a 10 per cent stabilized suspension to patients with ulcerative colitis. Ten to 60 ml. of the 10 per cent suspension are given after each stool and at bedtime. The preparation is rarely absorbed.

*Salicylazosulfapyridine** (Azulfidine). This is available in 500 mg. tablets (brownish yellow color) for oral administration. It is an azo compound of salicylic acid and sulfapyridine. In the body it is broken down to aminosalicylic acid and sulfapyridine. Its affinity for connective tissue has been noted, and because of this, its use for chronic ulcerative colitis was proposed. Although difference of opinion exists about its value in the treatment of this disease, the drug apparently is not superior to other sulfonamides in the management of this condition. The drug colors the urine orange-yellow if it is alkaline in reaction but causes no color change in acid urine. The average adult dose is 1 Gm. four to six times daily. For children over 7 years of age, the dose is 0.5 to 1 Gm. three to six times daily. Periodic blood counts and careful medical supervision of the patient is essential because of the comparative toxicity of sulfapyridine.

Sulfonamide mixtures

A number of preparations have been marketed which are composed of two or more sulfonamides. Their introduction was a major step in solving the problem of renal complications associated with therapy with the sulfonamides. The decreased danger of crystalluria is explained by the distinct urinary solubility which characterizes each member of the mixture.

Triple mixtures have been found to reduce the incidence of renal complications even more than dual mixtures. Other untoward effects, however, are not affected by combining the drugs. On the other hand, it is possible to obtain approximately the same therapeutic activity and the

*Described in annual publication of A. M. A. Council on Drugs, N.N.D., 1960.

same total sulfonamide level in the blood as can be obtained when each drug is used alone but in larger dosage.

It is believed that the incidence of sensitization is directly related to dosage; hence a decreased dose of each drug in the mixture is believed to reduce the danger of sensitization of the patient. Sulfamerazine, sulfadiazine, and sulfacetamide have been combined, but currently available mixtures also contain sulfadiazine, sulfamerazine, and sulfamethazine or only sulfadiazine and sulfamerazine. These are available in suitable dosage forms. *Trisulfapyrimidines Oral Suspension*, U.S.P., and *Trisulfapyrimidines Tablets*, U.S.P., are official preparations of sulfadiazine, sulfamerazine, and sulfamethazine.

Side effects and toxic effects. A number of toxic effects have already been mentioned. Some of the effects seen formerly when sulfanilamide, sulfathiazole, and sulfapyridine were extensively used are now seen much less often since these preparations are seldom used. With the preparations employed at the present time, the incidence of toxicity is relatively rare; however, when toxicity does occur it is likely to be due to the development of hypersensitivity, renal disturbance, or a personal idiosyncrasy on the part of the patient. On the other hand, toxic effects can result from the administration of any sulfonamide that is capable of exerting systemic effects. Those that are poorly absorbed are naturally unlikely to cause symptoms of toxicity. When renal function is impaired the incidence of toxicity is increased. Although the incidence of toxic effects is lower with the newer sulfonamides, they must be administered with the same precautions as used with the older preparations. Some reactions are relatively mild and more of a nuisance than a real threat to the welfare of the patient. Toxic and side effects include the following:

1. Nausea and vomiting, which occur less often than formerly, but still occur in as many as 5 per cent of the patients.* Stopping administration of the drug is not usually indicated.

2. Other undesirable reactions include dizziness, headache, mental depression, restlessness and irritability, drug, fever, and dermatitis.

3. Among the more severe reactions are granulocytopenia, agranulocytosis, hemolytic anemia, and jaundice. The development of symptoms associated with these conditions mean that administration of the drug must cease immediately. However, it is felt that the occasional severe toxic effect on the blood should not exclude the use of sulfonamides when they are clinically indicated.

4. Symptoms associated with renal damage include oliguria, crystalluria, and anuria. These may result from precipitation of the drug in the

*Bass, A. D.: Chemotherapy of Bacterial Infections. II. Sulfonamides. In Drill, V. A. (editor): Pharmacology in Medicine, New York, 1958, McGraw-Hill Book Co., Inc., p. 1110.

renal tubules and happens when a sulfonamide that is not very soluble in urine is administered or when the fluid intake is inadequate.

A number of the toxic effects of the sulfonamides are more easily prevented than treated. It is important for the nurse to remember that damage to the kidneys can be minimized by making certain that the patient has an adequate fluid intake. Although this is not the problem that it was with the older compounds, it is still believed to be advisable to regulate the fluid intake so that there will be an output of at least 1,500 ml. daily. Preparations such as sulfadiazine are made more soluble in the urine if the urine is kept alkaline, and for that reason sodium bicarbonate is sometimes prescribed to be given with it. This precaution is not considered necessary when the more soluble (soluble in urine) preparations are used.

Physicians frequently like their patients to know that if at any time they develop a sore throat, fever, rash, or hematuria during treatment with these drugs, they should stop taking the drug immediately and contact their doctor.

References

A. M. A. Council on Drugs: New and Non-official Drugs, Philadelphia, 1960, J. B. Lippincott Co.

Beckman, Harry: Drugs, Their Nature, Action and Use, Philadelphia, 1958, W. B. Saunders Co.

Dowling, H. F., Dumoff, S. E., Lepper, M. H., and Sweet, L. K.: Relative Toxicity of Sulfamerazine and Sulfadiazine, J. A. M. A. **125:** 103, 1944.

Editorial: The Mode of Action of the Sulfonamides, J. A. M. A. **126:** 31, 1944.

Feldman, W. H.: Modern Chemotherapy of Infectious Diseases; Implications and Significance, Dis. Chest **26:** 1, 1954.

Hageman, P. O., Harford, C. G., Sobin, S. S., and Aherns, R. E.: Sulfamerazine, J. A. M. A. **123:** 125, 1943.

Holsinger, D. R., Hanlon, D. G., and Welch, J. S.: Fatal Aplastic Anemia Following Sulfamethoxypyridazine Therapy, Proc. Staff Meet. Mayo Clin. **33:** 679, 1958.

Janovsky, R. C.: Fatal Thrombocytopenic Purpura After Administration of Sulfamethoxypyridazine, J. A. M. A. **172:** 155, 1960.

Perry, H. O., and Winkelmann, R. K.: Dermatitis Herpetiformis Treated With Sulfamethoxypyridazine, Proc. Staff Meet. Mayo Clin. **33:** 164, 1958.

Price, A. H., and Pedulla, J. C.: The Effect of Sulfadiazine on the Coordination and Reaction Time of Young Men, J. A. M. A. **125:** 105, 1944.

Ritz, N. D., and Fisher, M. J.: Agranulocytosis Due to Administration of Salicylazosulfapyridine (Azulfadine), J. A. M. A. **172:** 237, 1960.

Schwartz, M. J., and Norton, W. S., II: Thrombocytopenia and Leukopenia Associated With the Use of Sulfamethoxypyridazine, J. A. M. A. **167:** 457, 1958.

Terrell, W., Yow, E. M., and Daeschner, W.: The Newer Sulfonamides, Medical Clinics of North America, Philadelphia, 1957, W. B. Saunders Co., pp. 539-551.

Chapter 21

Systemic anti-infectives—drugs used in the treatment of tuberculosis, leprosy, syphilis, and certain protozoan diseases

Chemotherapy, as noted in the last chapter, originally meant the treatment of infectious diseases by the use of chemicals which killed the causative organisms but produced little or no effect on the patient. In this chapter, certain chemotherapeutic agents (other than antibiotics and sulfonamides) that act systemically will be discussed.

Until recently, chemicals used to kill pathogenic protozoa and closely related organisms were much more successful than the chemicals used against bacteria. Thus we find that for many years systemic chemotherapy has been used against the organisms causing malaria, syphilis, and amebiasis. Not until sulfanilamide was introduced in 1935 was there really an effective chemical against the pneumococcus, meningococcus, and many other bacteria. A major chemotherapeutic problem still facing medicine is that of finding effective agents to control the majority of diseases caused by viruses.

Drugs used in treatment of tuberculosis

The important problem of antimicrobial therapy for tuberculous infections has already been introduced in the discussion of streptomycin in Chapter 8. More recently a number of synthetic chemotherapeutic agents have been found useful in treating tuberculosis. A variety of agents now exists for the chemical control of the disease; the availability of a number of different drugs has been particularly advantageous because of the liability of the organism to develop resistance.

A rather large number of drugs exhibit tuberculostatic effects, but their usefulness is limited by the toxic effects they produce or by their lack of therapeutic potency. The drugs that seem to be of greatest value in the treatment of tuberculosis are the streptomycins, para-aminosalicylic acid (PAS), and the isonicotinic acid derivatives. Antituberculosis drugs act chiefly by preventing the tubercle bacilli from multiplying. The ultimate defeat of the organisms is due to the immunity which the human body develops against the infection. As mentioned previously, one of the greatest problems encountered in the chemotherapy of this disease is how to prevent the emergence of resistant tubercle bacilli. The administration of two or more of these drugs, at the same time, has been reasonably successful in delaying the development of resistance. Once chemotherapy has been started it should be continued without interruption until the physician decides to stop the treatment. Interruptions in drug therapy encourage the development of resistant organisms.

The aim of chemotherapy in tuberculosis is to arrest the disease. To do this, drugs must be combined with adequate medical and sometimes surgical procedures.

Para-aminosalicylic acid (PAS)

Para-aminosalicylic acid is a synthetic, white, crystalline powder with a faint fruity odor. It is only slightly soluble in water, but its sodium salt is much more soluble.

Action and result. This drug inhibits the action of virulent tubercle bacilli but it is less potent than the streptomycins or isoniazid. It has little or no effect on other microorganisms. The precise mechanism of its action seems to be controversial. Some authorities contend that an antagonism exists between PAS and PABA (para-aminobenzoic acid) similar to the competition that exists between the sulfonamides and PABA.

PAS, as well as its salts, is well absorbed from the gastrointestinal tract following oral administration. The drug diffuses rapidly into pleural fluids and into various tissues, although its diffusion into cerebrospinal fluid is erratic and not dependable. It is excreted chiefly by way of the kidneys, although it is not effective for tuberculosis of the urinary tract since it is subject to change in the liver and the resulting metabolic products are therapeutically inactive.

Resistance. The tubercle bacilli develop resistance to PAS slowly. Several months of treatment may elapse before the organisms are insensitive to the drug.

Uses. Para-aminosalicylic acid is not very effective when used alone, but when combined with streptomycin or isoniazid it delays the emergence of resistant tubercle bacilli and also increases the effectiveness of the drug with which it is combined. This sometimes makes it possible to reduce the dosage and decrease the chances of toxic reactions to the companion drug.

Preparation, dosage, and administration.

Aminosalicylic Acid (PAS), U.S.P. (Para-Pas, *p*-Aminosalicylic Acid). This preparation is available in 300 and 500 mg. and 1 Gm. tablets for oral administration. The recommended daily dose is 8 to 16 Gm. Some physicians recommend dosage up to 20 Gm. daily. The drug may be given as a single dose or in four or more doses with or after meals. It is also available as a powder from which 2 to 5 per cent solutions can be made for use in cavities and sinuses.

Calcium Aminosalicylate, N.F. This form is available in 500 mg. tablets and capsules for oral administration. It has no advantages over the sodium salt except that it may be given to patients whose dietary intake of sodium is restricted. The dosage is similar to that for PAS.

*Potassium Aminosalicylate** (Parasal Potassium). This form is available in 500 mg. tablets. It is also given orally. The average adult dose is 12 Gm. daily. It may cause fewer symptoms of gastric irritation than the acid or the sodium salt.

Sodium Aminosalicylate, U.S.P. (Sodium Para-Aminosalicylate). This form is marketed in 500 mg. capsules and in tablets containing 500 and 690 mg. of the drug. The sodium salt is said to produce less gastrointestinal irritation than the parent drug. Usual dose is 3 Gm. five times a day.

Side effects and toxic effects. Gastrointestinal irritation, allergic reactions, and the need for a large daily dosage are the chief disadvantages encountered in connection with PAS therapy. Gastrointestinal symptoms are said to develop in approximately 10 to 15 per cent of the patients.† Such symptoms include nausea and vomiting, loss of appetite, loose stools, and sometimes diarrhea. Allergic reactions are shown by the development of skin eruption, fever, painful joints, and occasionally localized pulmonary edema, with an increase in the number of eosinophils. In addition, patients occasionally develop hepatitis, renal failure, hemolytic anemia, and leukopenia. After therapy has continued for some time the clotting time of the blood is likely to be prolonged. This can be prevented by the administration of vitamin K. Other salicylates such as sodium salicylate and aspirin should be avoided, if possible, during therapy with PAS because of the possibility of producing severe salicylate poisoning.

Isoniazid (INH)

Isoniazid is a synthetic substance derived from isonicotinic acid. It is a white, crystalline, odorless compound. It is freely soluble in water.

---

*Described in annual publication of A.M.A. Council on Drugs, N.N.D., 1960.

†Weiss, M.: Chemotherapy and Tuberculosis, Am. J. Nursing **59:** 1713, 1959.

Action and result. Isoniazid is a tuberculostatic agent similar to streptomycin. It exerts a selective action against the *Mycobacterium tuberculosis* and produces a bacteriostatic effect. Little is known about the mechanism of its action, but it has been suggested that it probably interferes with the formation of some substance essential to the metabolism of the tubercle bacilli.

Therapeutic effects are manifested by reduction of fever, improvement in the patient's appetite, and a gain in weight. The patient may feel so much better his mental reactions at times may approach a state of euphoria. Coughing is diminished, and the number of acid-fast organisms in the sputum may diminish in number or disappear altogether.

The drug is readily absorbed from the gastrointestinal tract and it diffuses readily into the various body tissues and fluids. It passes into the cerebrospinal fluid in amounts sufficient to produce a therapeutic concentration. It is excreted chiefly by way of the kidney. It is inexpensive and relatively nontoxic when dosage is kept within the usual therapeutic range.

Uses. Isoniazid is used alone or concurrently with PAS or streptomycin or occasionally with both. Any regimen that includes isoniazid is considered superior to any drug or combination of drugs that does not contain it. Isoniazid-PAS and isoniazid-streptomycin are at present considered especially effective combinations. The isoniazid-PAS combination is the most convenient regimen since both drugs can be given orally. Therapy for at least 1 year is considered advisable for minimal tuberculosis and for a longer period (2 to 3 years) when the disease is advanced or cavitation has occurred.

Preparation, dosage, and administration.

Isoniazid, U.S.P., B.P. (Isonicotinic Acid Hydrazide, INH). This drug is available in 50 and 100 mg. tablets and as a syrup, 10 mg. per milliliter for oral administration, also as a solution, 1 Gm. in 10 ml., for intramuscular injection.

The usual adult dose is 3 to 5 mg. per kilogram of body weight divided into two or three portions. A patient may receive as much as 300 mg. daily along with 8 to 16 Gm. of PAS. Higher dosage is sometimes employed. It is believed that isoniazid is inactivated faster in some patients than in others.

A dosage form is now available that contains isoniazid and streptomycin in combination. It is marketed under the trade name of *Streptohydrazide*. It is available as a vial of dry powder to which water for injection is added prior to intramuscular administration. The vial contains the equivalent of 1 Gm. of streptomycin and 236 mg. of isoniazid.

Side effects and toxic effects. Isoniazid resembles streptomycin in that tubercle bacilli readily become resistant to it. Undesirable side effects are more likely to occur when the dosage is elevated. The less serious effects include constipation, dryness of the mouth, headache, visual disturbances, insomnia, orthostatic hypotension, slight anemia, and occasionally albuminuria. With elevated doses, convulsive seizures and peripheral neuritis may develop. The disturbance of the peripheral nerves can be prevented by the administration of pyridoxine (vitamin B$_6$), and the administration of 300 mg. daily reduces the incidence of neurotoxicity following large doses of isoniazid.[*]

The drug is used with caution for patients with epilepsy or for those with a history of convulsive seizures.

Other drugs used in treatment of tuberculosis

Since isoniazid, streptomycin, and PAS cannot always be prescribed for the treatment of tuberculosis for reasons such as (1) the organisms have become resistant, (2) the patient has become hypersensitive to the drug or drugs, (3) toxic effects have been produced, or (4) the drugs have failed to be effective, secondary drugs may therefore be valuable as reserve agents to be used individually or, more often, in combination with one of the older drugs.

Pyrazinamide.[†] This is a synthetic drug made from nicotinamide. It is considered an effective drug, especially when given with isoniazid for short-term therapy, such as that which precedes surgery of patients in whom the causative organism is resistant to other drugs. It is prone to cause liver damage, and the tubercle bacilli develop resistance to the drug relatively fast. It is available in 500 mg. tablets for oral administration. A dose of 1.5 to 2 Gm. daily (after meals) in two or three equally divided portions is recommended.[‡] Jaundice is occasionally observed in patients; hence it should be used only when regular tests of liver function, e.g., the transaminase test, can be performed to detect a developing toxic reaction.

Viomycin Sulfate.[†] This preparation is said to possess definite although limited value as a tuberculostatic agent. It is given in doses of 2 Gm. twice weekly (intramuscularly) along with a more potent agent such as isoniazid, streptomycin, or PAS. In large doses it may cause renal damage.

Cycloserine[†] (Seromycin). This agent exhibits some activity against the organisms causing human tuberculosis, especially when administered in combination with other drugs (isoniazid). Its chief disadvantage is that it can be highly toxic to the nervous system and can cause convulsive disorders. Other toxic effects include headache, visual disturbances, skin lesions, and mental symptoms which may progress to psychosis. It

[*]Weiss, M.: Chemotherapy and Tuberculosis, Am. J. Nursing **59:** 1713, 1959.
[†]Described in annual publication of A. M. A. Council on Drugs, N.N.D., 1960.
[‡]Badger, T. L.: Medical Progress—Tuberculosis, New England J. Med. **261:** 77, 1959.

is usually administered in doses of 0.5 Gm. daily per os. The initial dose is less and then gradually increased.

Several other antibiotics have been undergoing study and investigation. These include *streptovaracin, thiocarbanidin,* and *kanamycin.* The first two drugs are thought to have minor value as drugs in the treatment of tuberculosis. Kanamycin has moderate antituberculosis activity, and it has been found to be toxic to the eighth cranial nerve, causing loss of hearing. Its use (as a last resort) is likely to be restricted to short periods of therapy.

Drugs used in treatment of leprosy

Leprosy is a chronic disease caused by the acid-fast bacillus *Mycobacterium leprae.* For many years chaulmoogra oil or one of its derivatives was used in the treatment of leprosy, but since it is no longer believed that either the oil or its derivatives have any therapeutic significance, they are no longer official preparations in the United States.

Sulfones

The sulfones in current use are synthetic compounds chemically related to the parent drug, diaminodiphenylsulfone. The latter substance was found to be an effective antibacterial agent, but because it was used in doses which produced toxic reactions it was soon replaced by less toxic sulfones. The members of this group of drugs which have been studied most extensively are sulfoxone sodium (Sodium Diasone), glucosulfone sodium (Sodium Promin), and thiazolsulfone (Promizole).

Action and results. To be effective, the more complicated derivatives apparently are changed into the parent compound prior to or after absorption. Although the sulfones have an antibacterial spectrum similar to that of the sulfonamides, their chief usefulness is in the treatment of leprosy. They exert a bacteriostatic rather than a bactericidal effect on the *Mycobacterium leprae.* This is evidenced by the slow disappearance of the organisms from the leprous lesions. They bring about a suppression of the disease, prevent new lesions from appearing, promote the healing of many lesions, and allow the defense mechanisms of the body to keep the disease inactive. Their action is slow; improvement may not be seen for several months. The most encouraging feature about their use is that they almost universally bring about improvement to the extent that many patients may become presentable members of society again. However, even though the disease apparently becomes inactive, maintenance doses should be continued indefinitely to prevent relapses.*

*Johansen, F. A., and Erickson, P. T.: Current Status of Therapy in Leprosy, J.A.M.A. 144: 988, 1950.

The sulfones are excreted mainly by the kidneys. The body tissues retain considerable amounts of the drug and release it slowly for some time after administration is discontinued.

Preparation, dosage, and administration.

Sodium Sulfoxone, U.S.P. (Sodium Diasone). This compound is available in 330 mg. enteric-coated tablets for oral administration. The usual adult dose is 300 mg. daily which is gradually increased to 900 mg. unless toxic symptoms occur. Periodic rest periods are advocated. At least 6 months of treatment are required to evaluate therapeutic effects.

Sodium Glucosulfone Injection, U.S.P. (Sodium Promin). This drug is available as a solution for intravenous injection (5 Gm. in 12.5 ml.). The intravenous dose is 2 to 5 Gm. given 6 days of each week. Periodic rest periods are recommended, but the treatment may continue over many months.

*Thiazolsulfone** (Promizole). This sulfone is available in 500 mg. tablets for oral administration. It is said to be less valuable than the other sulfones used in the treatment of leprosy. The usual daily adult dose should not exceed 4 to 6 Gm., which is given in divided doses.

Diaminodiphenylsulfone (DDS). The official preparation in the British Pharmacopoeia is *Dapsone.* It is not commercially available in the United States. It is used in parts of the world where leprosy is prevalent. The initial dosage is 25 to 50 mg. twice weekly, increasing by 50 to 100 mg. every month until 200 to 400 mg. are given twice weekly.

Side effects and toxic effects. The administration of the sulfones is not recommended unless there is adequate medical supervision and access to adequate laboratory facilities. Toxic effects include nausea and vomiting, anemia, dermatitis, hepatitis, glandular enlargement, and occasionally liver damage and psychosis. Toxic reactions are associated with increased concentrations of the drug in the blood. If the sulfones are employed in minimum effective doses with rest periods interspersed between courses of therapy, serious reactions tend to be rare and the patient may be able to tolerate the medication for years.

Drugs used in treatment of syphilis

Syphilis is an infectious disease caused by the *Treponema pallidum.* Syphilis is also a systemic disease which has been endemic in man for over 400 years. Inadequate treatment or the absence of treatment may result in the formation of destructive lesions in the skin, bone, and cardiovascular system and irreversible changes in the nervous system. In the absence of treatment, death results in approximately 10 per cent of the persons infected. Early diagnosis and treatment have always been,

*Described in annual publication of A. M. A. Council on Drugs, N.N.D., 1960.

and continue to be, important factors in successful control of the disease.

Trends in the treatment of syphilis have undergone very definite changes in the past 20 years. Penicillin is now the chief agent employed in the treatment of all forms of syphilis, in this part of the world at least.

Drugs formerly used in the treatment of syphilis included mercury, organic arsenicals such as arsphenamine, neoarsphenamine, oxophenarsine, and sulfarsphenamine. Treatment with the arsphenamines was frequently interspersed with the administration of a preparation of bismuth. Treatment was long and expensive, and numerous unpleasant side effects were encountered. As a result, many patients failed to complete a full course of treatment.

Penicillin

Penicillin acts directly on the causative organism of syphilis and kills it, i.e., it is treponemicidal. The exact mechanism of action is unknown but within a few days after the administration of this antibiotic the lesions begin to heal. This does not mean that the patient is cured. The drug is effective in relatively low plasma concentrations, but its action on the treponema is slow (as compared to its bactericidal effects on certain other microorganisms) and successful therapy can be accomplished with relatively low concentrations of the drug but a period of time is required. Penicillin is said to kill the *Treponema pallidum* at a concentration of 0.002 mcg. per milliliter, but its optimum effects are secured when the concentration of the drug is 0.1 mcg. per milliliter.[*] And it does not follow that huge concentrations over a short period of time are more effective, since time is such an important factor in eradication of the organisms.

The incidence of cure of primary syphilis is often better than 98 per cent for patients in whom treatment is given early, before the patient becomes seropositive. After the patient is seropositive, the incidence of complete cure is not as good, and from 2 to 10 per cent of such patients are said to have relapse.

Penicillin is also effective for the treatment of cardiovascular syphilis, neurosyphilis, congenital syphilis, and latent syphilis. The latter condition is one in which the serum tests are positive but clinical symptoms are not apparent. Penicillin is the drug of choice in the treatment of a pregnant woman who is syphilitic. Adequate treatment of the mother greatly reduces the incidence of a syphilitic baby (2 per cent or less).[†]

Difference of opinion exists as to the preparation of penicillin which should be used for primary and secondary syphilis and the dosage sched-

[*]Eagle, H., and Magnusen, H. J.: Chemotherapy of the Treponematoses. In Drill, V. A. (editor): Pharmacology in Medicine, New York, 1958, McGraw-Hill Book Co., Inc., p. 1174.
[†]Ibid., p. 1178.

ule which should be followed. Both the rapidly absorbed and the more slowly absorbed preparations of penicillin are employed.

Sterile Procaine Penicillin G with Aluminum Stearate Suspension, U.S.P. This preparation of penicillin is absorbed slowly and has proved effective for syphilis when given intramuscularly in doses of 600,000 to 1,200,000 units twice weekly for 2 weeks or until a total of 5 to 6 million units has been given.

Sterile Procaine Penicillin G Suspension, U.S.P. This aqueous suspension may be injected intramuscularly in doses of 300,000 to 600,000 units once or twice daily for 8 to 16 injections.

Benzathine Penicillin G, U.S.P., B.P. This preparation has a low level of solubility and is slowly absorbed. A single injection of 1,000,000 to 2,500,000 units (intramuscular) is said to provide a therapeutic level over a period of a week or more. Some authorities recommend dividing the dose into two or four intramuscular sites of injection.

Buffered Penicillin G for Injection, U.S.P.; *Benzyl Penicillin,* B.P. These solutions may be injected intramuscularly in doses of 20,000 to 60,000 units every 4 to 6 hours over a period of 4 to 8 days.

For late syphilis, some physicians prefer to give somewhat larger total doses, which are also given over a longer period of time.

The Jarisch-Herxheimer reaction. This is a reaction due to the rapid destruction of a large number of treponemas and to the liberation and absorption of their proteins. The patient has chills, malaise, fever, and aching. The syphilitic lesions are temporarily activated. This can be serious when it involves gummatous lesions of the larynx, heart, or brain. Some physicians therefore prefer to use a preparation of bismuth for several weeks before using penicillin. This reaction can usually be ignored, especially in the treatment of early syphilis, although the reaction should be explained to the patient in order to avoid needless anxiety.

Other antibiotics

Occasionally patients are so sensitive to penicillin that it cannot be employed, or its administration must be discontinued. It is considered preferable to use one of the other antibiotics which are treponemicidal than to revert to the use of arsenicals and bismuth. *Chlortetracycline* (Aureomycin), when administered orally in a total dosage of 70 Gm., has proved effective. An initial dose of 2 Gm. may be given followed in 4 hours with another 2 Gm. and thereafter 1 Gm. every 4 hours (around the clock) until 70 Gm. have been given. *Oxytetracycline* (Terramycin) or *chloramphenicol* (Chloromycetin), given in a dosage of 60 mg. per kilogram of body weight (daily) for 6 to 8 days, is said to be effective. Other antibiotics that have been reported to exhibit some therapeutic effectiveness include *carbomycin* and *erythromycin*.

Bismuth compounds

Bismuth compounds were once used in the treatment of syphilis, but they have been, for the most part, discarded in favor of penicillin. They are occasionally used in the plan of treatment of syphilitic patients with gummatous laryngitis. The preliminary use of bismuth is believed to decrease the likelihood of intensifying a local inflammatory reaction in the larynx which otherwise might occur when penicillin is used first. An activation of the lesions with swelling or edema in the larynx could cause death.

Preparation, dosage, and administration.

Bismuth Sodium Triglycollamate, U.S.P. (Bistrimate). This compound is available in 400 mg. tablets for oral administration. It is given in doses of 1 tablet two or three times daily after meals. It is not recommended for the treatment of an early or active syphilitic infection. It is indicated primarily when the patient exhibits intolerance to other drugs or other forms of bismuth ordinarily used for the same purpose.

Sterile Bismuth Subsalicylate Suspension, U.S.P. This is a 10 per cent suspension of bismuth in oil. It is administered by deep intramuscular injection. Absorption is slow. The average dose is 1 ml. once a week.

Side effects and toxic effects. Toxic effects are uncommon, although the following symptoms may be encountered: stomatitis, a blue line along the gums, albumin in the urine, and dermatitis.

Antiprotozoan agents

Antimalarial drugs

Malaria is the most prevalent of all diseases in spite of efforts to control the causative organisms and their insect vectors. The organisms that cause this disease are protozoa called *Plasmodium vivax* or tertian parasite, *Plasmodium malariae* or quartan parasite, and *Plasmodium falciparum* or estivo-autumnal parasite. Each of these causes a different type of malaria. Each species is made up of several strains, each with idiosyncrasies that modify response to treatment.

Plasmodium falciparum is thought to be the most recently acquired malarial infection of man. It causes the highest mortality and has the simplest life cycle. Eradication of the blood forms of this species is relatively easy. *Plasmodium vivax* is better adapted to the tissues of the human host and is more difficult to eradicate. The malarial parasites undergo two phases of development: the sexual cycle, which takes place in the mosquito, and the asexual cycle, which occurs in the human body. The mosquito which bites an infected human being ingests the asexual forms known as schizonts and the sexual forms known as gametocytes. In the mosquito the asexual forms are destroyed, but the female gametocytes are fertilized by the male gametocytes and development into asexual forms results. These are introduced into the blood of human beings by the bite of the Anopheles mosquitoes.

The parasites when injected into man by the bite of the mosquito are known as sporozoites. Shortly after their introduction into the blood of man they disappear and enter fixed tissue cells (reticulo-endothelial cells of the liver and possibly certain other organs) where development and multiplication takes place. For a period of time, which varies with the different plasmodia (6 to 14 days or sometimes longer), the patient exhibits no symptoms, no parasites are found in the erythrocytes, and the blood is noninfective. This is known as the prepatent period, or tissue phase. The parasites are called primary tissue schizonts or pre-erythrocytic forms. After the prepatent period the parasites burst from the tissue cells as merozoites, enter the blood stream and penetrate erythrocytes, and begin the erythrocytic phase of their existence. In the case of *P. vivax* (but not *P. falciparum*) some of the merozoites invade other tissue cells to form secondary exo-erythrocytic forms. The relapses in *P. vivax* malaria are believed to be due to the successive formations of merozoites produced by various secondary exo-erythrocytic forms of the parasite. Drugs that affect malarial parasites in the blood stream do not necessarily destroy those in the exo-erythrocytic or tissue stage.

The erythrocytic phase of development refers to the activity of the parasite within the red blood cell. The merozoites bore into the cell, undergo development and multiplication, and finally cause rupture of the red cell to set free many more merozoites. Some of the merozoites may be destroyed in the plasma of the blood by leukocytes and other agents, but many more enter other erythrocytes to repeat the cycle. The recurring chills, fever, and prostration which are prominent clinical symptoms of malaria occur when the red cells rupture and release the young parasites. In malaria due to *P. falciparum*, this process takes place particularly in the capillaries of internal organs and explains the pernicious nature of this kind of malaria, e.g., the comatose type in which the parasites accumulate in the capillaries of the brain.

After a few cycles some of the asexual forms of the malarial parasites develop into sexual forms called gametocytes (the female form is called a macrogamete and the male is a microgamete). When the mosquito bites a person infected with malarial parasites and ingests the sexual forms, a rather complicated phase of sexual development takes place in the stomach of the mosquito. The female parasite is fertilized by the male, enters the wall of the stomach where it becomes encysted, and forms many spindle-shaped forms known as sporozoites. After a time the cyst ruptures and the sporozoites find their way into the saliva of the mosquito and are thus transferred to the next victim of its bite.

Persons who harbor the sexual forms of the plasmodia are called carriers, since it is from carriers that mosquitoes receive the forms of the parasite which perpetuate the disease. The asexual forms cause the clinical symptoms of malaria.

The life cycle of the *P. malariae* is similar to that of *P. vivax*.

The control of malaria is one of the major health problems of the world. Today there are still many millions of people who are exposed to the disease. The World Health Organization has changed its policy from that of malarial control to that of world-wide eradication. This involves many complex problems. Both insecticides to kill the mosquitoes and drugs for the protection of human beings will continue to play important roles. A number of new antimalarial drugs has been studied, and although no perfect drug has been found, the combined use of certain drugs now available makes possible complete suppression and radical cure of all malarial infections in the human being.*

A number of terms are used in relation to the drug therapy for malarial infections:

suppressants drugs that prevent the development of clinical symptoms by action on the asexual forms of the parasite (action against the schizonts).
radical cure complete eradication of the parasite from the body either naturally or as a result of treatment.
suppressive cure radical cure which has been accomplished while the patient has received a suppressive drug; possible because the gametocytes eventually disappear after the sexual forms of the parasite have been destroyed by the suppressive drug.
prophylaxis when used in connection with chemotherapy refers to the destruction of the sporozoites or other pre-erythrocytic forms of the parasite.†

Characteristics of a good antimalarial drug

The ideal antimalarial drug should be effective in the treatment of all forms of malaria, effective both as a prophylactic agent to destroy the exo-erythrocytic forms and as a suppressive agent to prevent the development of clinical symptoms. It should also bring about a rapid curative action, and it should not create parasitic resistance. It should be excreted slowly so that the drug need not be given often. It should be palatable and inexpensive and readily available. No drug is known which combines all these qualities, but research continues. Quinine is of historical importance and will be presented first, although it is now one of the least important of the drugs used for malaria.

Quinine

Cinchona bark is the source of quinine, the alkaloid which was long considered a specific in the treatment of malaria. The cinchona trees

*WHO Chronicle 13: 360, Sept.-Oct., 1959.
†N.N.D., 1960, p. 150.

are indigenous to South America, but because of the great demand for quinine they were introduced into the East Indies, Jamaica, Java, and other countries.

The most important alkaloids belonging to the cinchona group are quinine and quinidine. The latter is discussed in Chapter 14, under heart depressants.

Action and result. Quinine acts as a selective parasiticide. In sufficient concentration it is fatal to all cells. It affects protozoa more than it affects bacteria. In therapeutic doses it is effective against the plasmodia causing malaria. Adequate doses promptly suppress the symptoms of the disease, killing the asexual forms of all types of malaria. It kills the sexual forms of both *P. vivax* and *P. malariae* but not of *P. falciparum*. It is not effective against the pre-erythrocytic forms of the parasite; hence relapse is likely to occur when treatment is discontinued for infection due to *P. vivax* or *P. malariae*.

Quinine acts as an antipyretic and analgesic. It acts as an antipyretic by resetting the hypothalamus for normal temperature. It acts as an analgesic by depressing the optic thalami. These actions are similar to those of the salicylates, but compared with the salicylates the antipyretic action is slower and the analgesic action is not as effective.

Quinine is irritating locally. When taken orally, large doses cause nausea, vomiting, and diarrhea. When injected intramuscularly, it is likely to cause abscesses. When injected intravenously, it causes irritation of the intima, which may result in thrombosis.

Quinine stimulates contractions of uterine muscles. Its action is not as reliable as other uterine stimulants such as ergot and oxytocin.

Uses. Quinine is used in some parts of the world when other antimalarials are not available or are too expensive. It has a number of disadvantages among which are the following: the inconvenience of daily administration (doses should not be missed), ineffectiveness against *P. falciparum*, bitter taste, and the likelihood of side effects associated with therapeutic dosage. However, it can be used to cure vivax malaria when combined with a drug such as primaquine.

It has sometimes been used alone or in combination with other drugs to a lower fever. Occasionally it is used as an analgesic for relief of headache and pain in muscles and joints. Quinine dihydrochloride and urethane, 5 to 10 per cent solutions, are used as a sclerosing agent in the treatment of varicose veins. It causes a slough if the solution gets outside the vein. Other drugs such as sodium morrhuate, which do not cause sloughing when they get outside the veins, are preferred as sclerosing agents. It may also be given at bedtime to prevent muscular cramps, e.g., cramps in the muscles of the legs and back.

Preparation, dosage, and administration. When used in the treatment of malaria the oral route of administration is preferred. When oral administration is not feasible, certain salts of quinine may be given intravenously, but this method should be used only in emergencies, and the injection should be made slowly, for a dangerous lowering of blood pressure usually occurs.

Quinine Sulfate, N.F. Usual oral dose is 1 Gm. daily for 2 days; then 600 mg. for 5 days. Quinine sulfate is available in tablets and capsules.

Quinine Bisulfate, N.F. Dose is 1 Gm.

Quinine Hydrochloride, N.F. The usual dose, given intravenously, is 600 mg. in 200 ml. of water.

Quinine Dihydrochloride, N.F. Dose is 1 Gm.

Quinine Dihydrochloride Injection, N.F. Dose is 500 mg. Quinine dihydrochloride is more soluble in water than is quinine. It is used when aqueous solutions of quinine are desired for intravenous injection in cases of severe malaria in which oral administration is not feasible.

Side effects and toxic effects. Quinine has the disadvantage of a bitter taste, and it must be taken daily when used for malaria. Serious consequences can develop when doses are omitted for the malarial patient. When the maximum therapeutic dosage is administered, symptoms of cinchonism are likely to occur. Such symptoms include ringing in the ears, headache, nausea, dizziness, and disturbance of vision. More severe poisoning may be indicated by the following: renal damage, acute hemolytic anemia, and involvement of the central nervous system which includes first a stimulation of the respiratory center and eventually respiratory arrest.

Quinacrine (Atabrine)

Atabrine is the trade name for the synthetic drug of the acridine dye series which is used in treatment of malaria. It is yellow in color. Available evidence indicates that Atabrine is more effective than quinine, both for suppression of symptoms and for treatment of clinical attacks.

Action and result. The action of quinacrine resembles that of quinine; it is effective against the asexual forms of all types of malarial parasites. It is more effective than quinine against infections due to the malignant subtertian *(P. falciparum)* malaria, although it will not kill the gametocytes (sexual forms) of this organism. If taken faithfully, it is thought to lengthen the intervals between relapses in benign and quartan malaria. This is probably due to the fact that it is eliminated slowly.

It is not, however, considered a perfect suppressive drug, and neither quinine nor quinacrine when used therapeutically is capable of completely eradicating the infection. It is of value chiefly in suppressive therapy. It has been replaced to a great extent by chloroquine and amodiaquin. Quinacrine has an advantage over quinine in that it can be rapidly manufactured in large quantities. It does not stimulate uterine muscle, so it can be used during pregnancy. Quinacrine is also used as an anthelmintic (500 mg. with 500 mg. sodium bicarbonate).

Preparation, dosage, and administration.

Quinacrine Hydrochloride, U.S.P. (Atabrine Hydrochloride); *Mepacrine Hydrochloride*, B.P. This preparation is available in 100 mg. tablets for oral administration. To suppress symptoms, the dose for adults is 100 mg. daily for 6 days a week. For treatment of a clinical attack, 200 mg. of quinacrine with 1 Gm. of sodium bicarbonate are administered every 6 hours for 5 doses and then 100 mg. three times daily for 6 days. All doses of the drug should be accompanied by a full glass of water and taken after meals. Quinacrine hydrochloride can also be administered parenterally (preferably intramuscularly).

Side effects and toxic effects. The untoward effects are usually mild and consist of nausea, headache, vomiting, and diarrhea. Discoloration (yellow color) of the skin occurs, and the urine becomes yellow. This color change usually disappears a few weeks after the drug is discontinued. The drug is not toxic to the liver and kidneys. Toxic psychosis and aplastic anemia have been known to occur after long periods of suppressive therapy.

The treatment must suit the symptoms. Mild poisoning usually subsides when the medication is discontinued. In the more severe forms body temperature must be maintained, respiratory stimulants given as indicated, and a stomach lavage performed if the fairly insoluble salts have been ingested.

Other antimalarial drugs

Today, more important than quinine are a series of synthetic drugs which are active antimalarials and which share certain chemical features with the naturally occurring cinchona alkaloids. The structural similarities can be seen by studying the accompanying formulas. It should be noted that many of these drugs contain the quinoline nucleus and also share certain general types of side chains.

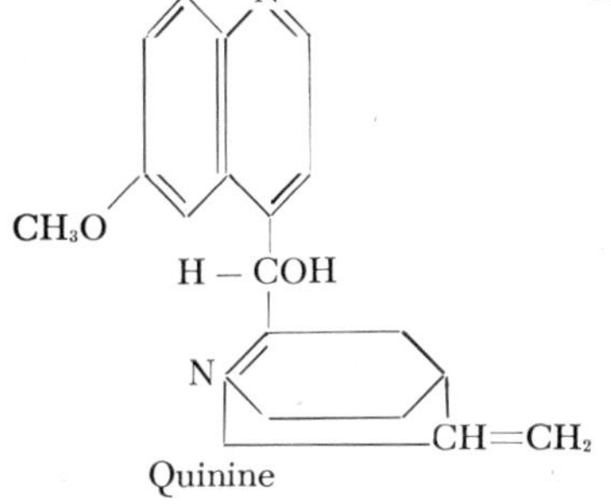

Quinine

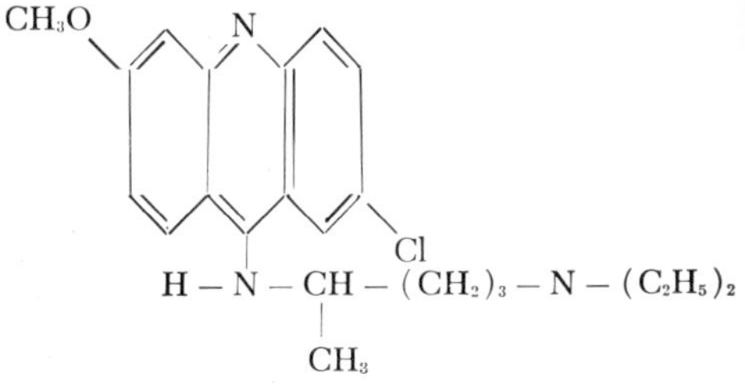

Quinacrine

Primaquine

$$\text{H}-\text{N}-\overset{\overset{\textstyle CH_3}{|}}{\text{CH}}-(CH_2)_3-NH_2$$

H₃CO (quinoline ring system)

Primaquine

Chloroquine

Cl (quinoline ring system)

$$\text{H}-\text{N}-\text{CH}-(CH_2)_3-\text{N}-(C_2H_5)_2$$
$$\overset{|}{CH_3}$$

Chloroquine

Pyrimethamine

$$Cl-\underset{}{\bigcirc}-\underset{\underset{\textstyle NH_2}{|}}{\overset{\overset{\textstyle C_2H_5}{|}}{\bigcirc}}-NH_2$$

Pyrimethamine

Chloroguanide

$$Cl-\bigcirc-NH-\overset{\overset{\textstyle NH}{||}}{C}-NH-\overset{\overset{\textstyle NH}{||}}{C}-NH-CH(CH_3)_2$$

Chloroguanide

Chloroquine (Aralen)

Chloroquine is a synthetic antimalarial drug chemically related to amodiaquin. It was synthesized in Germany and introduced for the treatment of malaria in 1944. It is considered superior to both quinacrine and quinine. The mechanism of its action against the plasmodia of malaria is not known, although it is known to have a strong affinity for nucleoproteins. It had been suggested that this may explain why the drug accumulates in the liver, spleen, and blood and in the cells which contain parasites. It is effective against the asexual forms of all plasmodia causing human malaria. It abolishes acute attacks of falciparum malaria and brings about complete cure of the infection (suppressive cure). However, it does not kill the sexual forms, and hence patients continue to be infective to mosquitoes for a period of time. It does not cure malaria due to *P. vivax*, but it is an effective suppressive agent, terminates attacks, and delays relapse. Neither chloroquine nor amodiaquin is effective against the pre-erythrocytic forms of the plasmodia (tissue phase). Only falciparum infections, in which there are no persistent tissue forms, are radically cured by these drugs.

Chloroquine also possesses amebicidal properties and is sometimes effective in the treatment of chronic lupus erythematosus.

Chloroquine is rapidly and almost completely absorbed from the gastrointestinal tract, and a portion of it is slowly eliminated in the urine.

Preparation, dosage, and administration.

Chloroquine Phosphate, U.S.P., B.P. (Aralen Phosphate). This drug is available in 125 and 250 mg. tablets for oral administration, before or after meals. For acute attacks, an initial dose of 1 Gm. is followed by 500 mg. after 6 or 8 hours and by 500 mg. on each of two successive days. This is sufficient to eradicate most infections due to *P. falciparum* and to terminate an acute attack due to *P. vivax.* Suppressive doses of 500 mg. every 7 days prevent clinical attacks of vivax malaria.[*]

Chloroquine Phosphate Injection, B.P. This form, is available for parenteral (intramuscular or intravenous) use. The B.P. also lists *Chloroquine Sulfate* and *Chloroquine Sulfate Injection* for oral and parenteral administration, respectively.

Side effects and toxic effects. When given in therapeutic doses the drug is well tolerated. However, mild headache, itching, gastrointestinal disorders, and visual disturbances are sometimes observed even with therapeutic doses. These symptoms disappear when administration is discontinued. When given intravenously, chloroquine may produce effects on the heart similar to quinidine.

Chloroquine and amodiaquin have the advantage of low toxicity and rapid action which makes possible a short course of treatment.

Amodiaquin (Camoquin)

Amodiaquin is a synthetic antimalarial drug which greatly resembles chloroquine both in its effectiveness for treatment of malaria and in its level of toxicity. Like chloroquine, it is effective only in the erythrocytic stages of malaria. It is capable of producing a radical cure only when the infection is due to *P. falciparum.* It does not effect a similar cure for other forms of malaria but it is effective in the treatment of an acute attack, relieves symptoms, and delays relapse. It is therefore an effective suppressive agent in areas of the world where malaria is endemic.

Like chloroquine, amodiaquin is rapidly absorbed from the gastrointestinal tract and is concentrated in the liver, spleen, kidney, and blood cells. It is said to be concentrated slightly less than is chloroquine.

Preparation, dosage, and administration.

Amodiaquin Hydrochloride, U.S.P. (Camoquin Hydrochloride); *Amodiaquine Hydrochloride,* B.P. This drug is available in 200 mg. tablets for oral administration. The usual single dose for adults in an acute attack of the disease (in term of the base) is 400 to 600 mg. For suppression of endemic malaria the usual dose is 400 to 600 mg. administered once every two weeks. The dosage for children is reduced in accordance with the age of the child.

Side effects and toxic effects. Side effects include nausea and vomiting, increased flow of saliva, and diarrhea. Large doses may produce

[*]N.N.D., 1960, p. 153.

spasticity, incoordination of movement, and convulsions, but these are seldom encountered. It does not discolor the skin.

Primaquine

Primaquine, pamaquine, and pentaquine are all synthetic antimalarial drugs which belong to the same chemical group of drugs (8-aminoquinolines). The latter two members are more toxic and less potent than primaquine and hence will be omitted from this edition.

Primaquine exerts a distinctive action on all gametocytes (sexual forms), especially those of *P. falciparum*. The gametocytes cause no clinical symptoms, but they are responsible for the transmission of malaria to the mosquito and thus keep the mosquito effective in the malarial cycle. The drug is ineffective or only slightly effective against asexual forms of the parasites (*P. falciparum*); hence effective treatment of acute attacks of malaria is dependent on simultaneous administration of another antimalarial such as chloroquine. Its greatest value lies in its ability to destroy the late tissue forms (which can cause secondary erythrocytic parasites) and thus treat relapses of vivax malaria. If it is administered during the latent period (period between the time the person is bitten by an infected mosquito and the time that the parasites enter the red blood cells), radical cure of vivax malaria can be secured by this drug alone.

Preparation, dosage, and administration.

Primaquine Phosphate, U.S.P., B.P. This compound is available in tablets containing 26.3 mg. of the drug for oral administration. For the treatment of relapsing vivax infections, 1 tablet each day for 14 days is considered adequate to produce a radical cure. If the patient has symptoms of an attack or a relapse, primaquine phosphate is supplemented with chloroquine or amodiaquin.

Side effects and toxic effects. When given in the dosage recommended primaquine exhibits a low level of toxicity, but it can cause all the toxic effects associated with pamaquine (depression of the bone marrow, hemolytic anemia, and agranulocytosis). Epigastric distress, nausea and vomiting, and abdominal pains occur occasionally. Large doses result in hemolytic effects, particularly in persons belonging to the deeply pigmented races. Its main disadvantages are its narrow margin of safety between the therapeutic and toxic dose and its ineffectiveness against asexual forms of *P. falciparum*.

Pyrimethamine (Daraprim)

Pyrimethamine is a potent antimalarial agent especially valuable as a suppressive agent. It therefore prevents the clinical attacks of all forms of malaria, and it interrupts the malarial cycle by preventing the formation of sporozoites in the mosquito. If suppressive therapy is continued long enough, "suppressive cure" of vivax infections may occur. Its use as a suppressive agent for falciparum infections results in a radical cure in most cases. This is due to the fact that the gametocytes eventually disappear spontaneously after the asexual blood forms are eliminated by the suppressive drug. Pyrimethamine acts slowly and should not be used in the treatment of acute primary attacks.

Preparation, dosage, and administration.

Pyrimethamine, U.S.P., B.P. (Daraprim). This agent is available in 25 mg. tablets for oral administration. The usual suppressive dose is 25 mg. per week. It is recommended that this dosage is continued indefinitely in areas where malaria is endemic. The dosage is 12.5 mg. for children under the age of 15 years. Therapeutic dosage (adults) is 25 mg. daily for 2 days.

Side effects and toxic effects. Pyrimethamine has a wide margin of safety, and toxic effects are seldom encountered, although overdosage can result in anemia and leukopenia. Plasmodia which are resistant to chloroguanide may develop resistance to pyrimethamine. Therefore its use is not recommended in areas of the world where it is known that the plasmodia have developed a resistance to chloroguanide.

Chloroguanide (Proguanil)

Chloroguanide (Proguanil, B.P.) has been used as an antimalarial agent but it is no longer official in the U.S.P. Its chief disadvantage is that it has resulted in the development of resistant strains of plasmodia.

Choice of antimalarial drugs

Chloroquine, amodiaquin, pyrimethamine, and primaquine are among the drugs most often employed in programs for eradication of malaria, according to the World Health Organization.*

Chloroquine and amodiaquin are especially useful in the treatment of acute malaria. They are also effective for suppressive therapy for all kinds of human malaria. But since they do not affect the primary or secondary tissue forms of the parasites they do not prevent infection or relapse.

Pyrimethamine is said to be the most effective single suppressive agent. Single weekly doses will prevent clinical attacks of malaria associated with all species of the malarial plasmodia. Furthermore, it affects the gametocytes of all species of human malarial parasites so that the mosquito is unable to transmit the disease after feeding on persons taking the drug. Primaquine and related members of this group of drugs also

*WHO Chronicle 13: 360, 1959.

have the advantage of destroying persistent exo-erythrocytic parasites in the liver which are known to cause relapses of vivax and malariae infections.

In some parts of the world antimalarial drugs such as chloroquine are added to salt (sodium chloride) in much the same way that iodine is added to salt to prevent goiter in certain areas of the world. This would appear to be a useful way of dealing with malaria in places where difficulties are encountered in using other methods of eradication.

Other antiprotozoan agents

Antimony

Preparations of antimony are used in the treatment of certain parasitic infestations. Their use in the treatment of schistomiasis (fluke infestation) is mentioned in Chapter 23. Antimonials have also been used in the treatment of filariasis but are no longer the preparations of choice. Leishmaniasis is a protozoan disease which occurs in two forms: visceral leishmania (kala-azar) and cutaneous leishmania (Oriental sore). It is seen in the Orient, India, and the Mediterranean countries. The pentavalent compounds of antimony are the drugs of choice for this condition.

Antimony is not used widely in the United States but it is used a great deal in tropical countries. The official trivalent preparations of antimony are mentioned in Chapter 23.

Pentavalent preparation, dosage, and administration.

Stibamine Glucoside (Neostam Stibamine Glucoside). This drug is available as a 4 per cent solution. It is administered both intramuscularly and intravenously. The adult dose is usually 100 mg. per 100 pounds of body weight and is gradually increased to 200 or 300 mg. and up to 3 Gm. per 100 pounds.

Ethylstibamine (Neostibosan). This preparation is also administered intramuscularly or by intravenous injection cautiously. It is given in a 5 per cent solution. The dosage is similar to that of stibamine glucoside. The solution must be freshly prepared.

Side effects and toxic effects. Unpleasant side effects include nausea and vomiting during or after injections of these compounds, acute sensitivity reactions, dermatitis, and lowering of the blood pressure. Liver and kidney damage has been known to occur and these drugs are therefore contraindicated when these organs are impaired.

Suramin (Naphuride)

Suramin is a nonmetallic dye which is used both as a prophylactic and as a therapeutic agent for trypanosomiasis. This disease is due to a parasitic protozoan organism which is spread by the bite of the tsetse fly. The disease is also known as African sleeping sickness. There is more than one species of the parasite and they are not equally virulent. Therapy in which suramin is given with an arsenical (tryparsamide) or alternated with it is particularly successful. This drug is excreted slowly and tends to persist in the tissues for some time after administration is discontinued.

Preparation, dosage, and administration.

Suramin Sodium, U.S.P., B.P. (Naphuride Sodium). This drug is not manufactured in the United States since it is used very little in this part of the world. The usual single dose is 1 Gm. given intravenously. A course of treatment consists of 5 to 10 weekly injections.

Side effects and toxic effects. The drug is said to be somewhat toxic to the kidney, causing albumin, casts, and sometimes red blood cells to appear in the urine. It occasionally produces hemolytic reactions. Periodic urine and blood examinations are therefore recommended. In addition, the following symptoms may be seen: headache, chills, fever, itching, and dermatitis.

Tryparsamide

Tryparsamide is an organic arsenical which was originally introduced into medicine for the treatment of neurosyphilis. As mentioned previously, the arsenicals have been replaced to a great extent by penicillin for the treatment of syphilis. It is now used in combination or alternately with a drug such as suramin in the early treatment of trypanosomiasis or alone in the advanced stages of certain cases of trypanosomiasis.

Preparation, dosage, and administration.

Tryparsamide, U.S.P., B.P. This drug is administered intravenously or occasionally intramuscularly. Dosage ranges from 1 to 3 Gm. weekly for several weeks (10 to 12). Freshly prepared solutions are given each time.

Side effects and toxic effects. Like other arsenicals, tryparsamide is capable of producing toxic effects. Changes in the optic nerve and retina of the eye, blindness, jaundice, and dermatitis have been known to occur and mean that administration of the drug should be discontinued when early symptoms of the toxicity are detected.

Stilbamidine

Stilbamidine belongs to the diamidine group of drugs and is used in the treatment of trypanosomiasis, leishmaniasis, and certain systemic fungal infections. It has also been recommended for the treatment of multiple myeloma, but results are not always good and relapse is prone to occur. Results from its use in the treatment of blastomycosis appear to be good.

Preparation, dosage, and administration.

Stilbamidine Isethionate. This agent is marketed in ampules containing 150 mg. of the drug. It is administered intravenously. The dosage is gradually increased from 50 to 150 mg., given on alternate days.

Side effects and toxic effects. Side effects which may be observed when the rate of administration is too rapid include a fall in blood pressure, flushing, rapid pulse, dizziness, headache, nausea and vomiting, salivation, sweating, lethargy, and muscle twitching. A late toxic reaction may occur which consists of progressive sensory changes along the distribution of the trigeminal nerve.

Hydroxystilbamidine Isethionate

This drug is a derivative of stilbamidine and has the same type of effect on fungal and protozoan infections as the latter preparation. It is effective in the treatment of certain types of leishmaniasis, especially for patients who do not respond favorably to treatment with a preparation of antimony. It is also said to be useful in the treatment of actinomycosis, although the antibiotics are drugs of choice for this condition. It appears to be useful in the treatment of North American blastomycosis. It is of no value for histoplasmosis.

It has been suggested that it may prove of value in the treatment of African trypanosomiasis since it bears a close similarity to stilbamidine.

Hydroxystilbamidine differs from the parent drug stilbamidine, mainly in that it produces less effect on the trigeminal nerve.

Preparation, dosage, and administration.

Hydroxystilbamidine Isethionate, U.S.P. This preparation is available in ampules containing 225 mg. of sterile powder suitable for slow intravenous injection. It is occasionally given by intramuscular injection, but this is likely to cause pain at the site of injection. Solutions of the powder are made by dissolving the drug in 5 per cent dextrose in water or isotonic solution of sodium chloride prior to injection. The suggested dosage for susceptible fungal or protozoan infections is 150 to 225 mg. daily for a week to 10 days, or in cases of severe infection the treatment may be extended much longer.

Side effects and toxic effects. With the exception of the toxic effects on the fifth cranial nerve, the other side effects are highly similar to those seen after the administration of stilbamidine. They tend to disappear within a relatively short time after injection. Slow administration and dilute solutions help to minimize the unpleasant effects.

References

Antituberculosis drugs

Badger, T. L.: Medical Progress—Tuberculosis, New England J. Med. **261**: 30, 74, 131, 1959.

D'Esopo, N. D.: Drugs That Fight TB, National Tuberculosis Association.

D'Esopo, N. D.: Chemotherapy of Tuberculosis, Progress and Promise, Pub. Health Rep. **72**: 412, 1957.

Douglass, B. E.: Treatment of Tuberculous Meningitis, Proc. Staff Meet. Mayo Clin. **28**: 381, 1953.

Tebrock, H. E., Fisher, M. M., and Mamlock, M. M.: The New Drug—Isoniazid, Am. J. Nursing **52**: 1342, 1952.

Weiss, Moe: Chemotherapy and Tuberculosis, Am. J. Nursing **59**: 1711, 1959.

Leprosy

Bass, A. D.: Chemotherapy of Bacterial Infections. III. Sulfones. In Drill, V. A. (editor): Pharmacology in Medicine, New York, 1958, McGraw-Hill Book Co., Inc., pp. 1115-1118.

Doull, J. A.: Current Status of the Therapy of Leprosy, J. A. M. A. **173**: 363, 1960.

Faget, G. H., and Erickson, Paul T.: Chemotherapy of Leprosy, J. A. M. A. **136**: 451, 1948.

Johansen, F. A.: Advances in the Treatment of Leprosy, Am. J. Nursing **51**: 445, 1951.

Johansen, F. A., and Erickson, P. T.: Current Status of Therapy in Leprosy, J. A. M. A. **144**: 985, 1950.

Antimalarial drugs

Alving, A. S., Arnold, J., and Robinson, D. H.: Status of Primaquine Mass Therapy of Subclinical Vivax Malaria With Primaquine, J. A. M. A. **149**: 1558, 1952.

Coggeshall, L. T.: Malaria as a World Menace, J. A. M. A. **122**: 8, 1943.

Committee on Malaria: Chronicle of the World Health Organization, Malaria, Antimalarial Drugs **3**: 256, 1949.

Cooper, W. C.: Summary of Antimalarial Drugs, Pub. Health Rep. **64**: 717, 1949.

Editorial: Primaquine for Vivax Malaria, J. A. M. A. **149**: 1572, 1952.

Office of the Surgeon General, U. S. Army: The Drug Material of Malaria, Suppressive and Clinical, Circular Letter No. 153, J. A. M. A. **123**: 205, 1943.

Todd, J. C., and Sanford, A. H.: Clinical Diagnosis by Laboratory Methods, Philadelphia, 1953, W. B. Saunders Co.

World Health Organization: WHO Chronicle **13**: 341-389, Sept.-Oct., 1959

Antisyphilitic drugs

Bloomfield, A. L.: The Clinical Use of Penicillin, J. A. M. A. **124**: 627, 1944.

Blumberg, M. L., and Gleich, M.: The Simplified Treatment of Gonococcic Ophthalmia Neonatorum With Chemotherapy, J. A. M. A. **123**: 132, 1943.

Council of Pharmacy and Chemistry Report: Penicillin in the Treatment of Syphilis, J. A. M. A. **136**: 873, 1948.

Kierland, R. R., Herrell, W. E., and O'Leary, Paul A.: The Treatment of Syphilis With Aureomycin Administered by Mouth, Collected Papers of the Mayo Clinic and the Mayo Foundation **41**: 307, 1949.

Mahoney, J. F., and others: Penicillin Treatment of Early Syphilis, J. A. M. A. **126**: 63, 1944.

Moore, J. E., and others: The Treatment of Early Syphilis With Penicillin, J. A. M. A. **126**: 67, 1944.

O'Leary, Paul A.: The Changed Trends in the Treatment of Syphilis, Collected Papers of the Mayo Clinic and the Mayo Foundation **41**: 304, 1949.

O'Leary, P. A., Kierland, R. R., and Herrell, W. E.: The Oral Administration of Aureomycin (Duomycin) and Its Effects on Treponema Pallidum in Man, Proc. Staff Meet. Mayo Clin. **23**: 574, 1948.

Smadel, J. E.: Clinical Use of Chloramphenicol, J. A. M. A. **142**: 315, 1950.

Stokes, J. H., and others: The Action of Penicillin in Late Syphilis, J. A. M. A. **126**: 73, 1944.

Stokes, J. H., and Taylor, J. B.: Dermatology and Venereology for Nurses, Philadelphia, 1948, W. B. Saunders Co.

Struble, G. C., and Bellows, J. G.: Studies on the Distribution of Penicillin in the Eye and Its Clinical Application, J. A. M. A. **125**: 685, 1944.

Top, F. H.: Newer Drugs in the Treatment of Communicable Diseases, Am. J. Nursing **49**: 700, 1950.

Perry, H. O., Kierland, R. R., and Magath, T. B.: The Clinical Problem of Syphilis Today, Minnesota Med. **39**: 717, 736, 1956.

Chapter 22

Local anti-infectives—antiseptics
and
disinfectants

Early in the history of mankind it was found that certain gums, balsams, and resins had the power to prevent decay in the bodies of the dead, and today the Egyptian mummy is an evidence of the efficiency of the materials used. Some of these substances were also used for healing wounds, but it was not until the latter part of the nineteenth century when Pasteur made his astounding discoveries regarding the germ theory and Lister, in consequence, began the systematic use of carbolic acid in his surgical work that antiseptics came into general use.

Local anti-infectives now include a wide variety of agents used for many purposes. A number of the older agents continue to be used for such purposes as the preparation of the skin prior to surgical incision or parenteral administration of drugs, the disinfection of thermometers, and the treatment of contaminated clothing, infected human excreta, etc. Local anti-infectives are used in the home for the treatment of minor wounds and abrasions, and in the community at large they play a role in the safe handling of sewage, in the purification of water supplies, and in the preservation of food supplies.

Definitions

There continues to be some misunderstanding about the terms used when speaking about groups of anti-infective agents. An *antiseptic* is a chemical agent that inhibits the growth and development of microorganisms but does not necessarily kill them. It is synonymous with the term *bacteriostatic*. It means against sepsis or, more literally, "against putrefaction or decay." This term was used long before bacteria were known to exist. It is now used especially to mean agents applied to living tissues, e.g., an antiseptic for the skin.

Disinfectants, germicides, or bactericides are agents that produce rapid death of harmful microorganisms, and the terms are used synonymously. There is a trend to use the word disinfectant to refer to germicides used on inanimate objects. Whether a given agent kills microorganisms or inhibits their growth may depend upon a number of factors such as the mechanism of action, the length of time the organisms are subjected to the agent, the number of microorganisms present, the concentration of the chemical agent, the temperature, and the presence and amount of organic matter.

The older disinfectants were used for killing harmful microorganisms on dishes, instruments, or on the surface of the skin, but they were generally found to be too poisonous for man to be used internally. The introduction of antibiotics, however, changed this concept of bactericidal agents, since antibiotics include many effective bactericidal agents which are quite nontoxic for man. Although theoretically antibiotics could also be used topically like the older disinfectants, they are generally too costly to be used for instruments, etc. and their topical use on the skin is often objectionable because of their capacity to induce allergic reactions in the individual. Exceptions are found in the use of bacitracin and neomycin which exhibit a low incidence of sensitivity reactions when applied topically or when they act locally. Agents used to treat local fungal, viral, or parasitic infections may also be thought of as local anti-infectives.

Mechanisms of action

Anti-infectives may act in three ways: (1) By bringing about a change in the structure of the protein of the microbial cell (denaturation) which often proceeds to coagulation of protein with increased concentration of the chemical agent. (2) By lowering the surface tension of the aqueous medium of the parasitic cell. This increases the permeability of the plasma membrane and the cellular constituents are destroyed by lysis. The cell is unable to maintain its equilibrium in its environment. (The surface-active agents are thought to act this way.) (3) By interfering with some metabolic processes of the microbial cells in such ways as to interfere with the cell's ability to survive and multiply.

Concern about the effectiveness of disinfectants has been heightened by the problem of hospital-acquired infections due to antibiotic-resistant staphylococci. On the other hand, these microorganisms are apparently no more resistant to the usual chemical disinfectants than they ever were. A good anti-infective must be more effective against the parasitic cells than against the cells of the host. Many good anti-infectives are so toxic to all cells that they cannot be used except for inanimate objects, and they constitute a hazard around a home or anywhere that individuals may be accidentally poisoned. Both physical and chemical agents are used in disinfection, but in this chapter emphasis is given to chemical agents. There is no ideal chemical agent suitable for all purposes for which these agents are needed.

Criteria for evaluating disinfectants

An ideal disinfectant may never be found, but if it is, it would need to be able to destroy all forms of infectious agents without being toxic to the cells of human tissues and it should not induce sensitization. In present-day practice what constitutes a satisfactory germicide for a given article depends on whether vegetative organisms only must be destroyed or whether fungi, tubercle bacilli, viruses, and spores also must be killed, since the latter are generally more resistant to germicides. It is important to select the best anti-infective to accomplish the results desired. All germicides and disinfectants recommended for hospital use must be effective against gram-negative enteric organisms and gram-positive pyogenic organisms when used as directed. The demands made of a good disinfectant have gradually become greater as better disinfectants have been developed. Some authorities now say that we should expect a solution of a disinfectant to kill within 10 minutes all vegetative bacteria and fungi, tubercle bacilli, animal parasites, and all viruses with the possible exception of the one causing infectious hepatitis.[*] They cannot be expected to kill spores. Not all disinfectants in present-day use will do this, at least not in a few minutes. Some may do so when several hours of exposure to the disinfectant are provided. The ideal disinfectant should not only kill all of the organisms mentioned but should also act in the presence of organic material and be stable, noncorrosive, and inexpensive.

It should never be overlooked that heat, and particularly moist heat under pressure (autoclaving), is the method of choice for killing all forms of living organisms, but since all things which require disinfection cannot be autoclaved, there continues to be a need for satisfactory chemical disinfectants.

Phenol and related compounds

Within this group of compounds a relationship between chemical structure and antimicrobial activity has been noted. For this reason the chemical formulas have been included. This relationship has not been observed for all chemical agents.

Phenol (Carbolic Acid)

Phenol is a crystalline compound with a characteristic odor. The needle-shaped crystals may become pinkish upon standing. Phenol was

[*]Spaulding, E. H., and Emmons, E. K.: Chemical Disinfection, Am. J. Nursing **58:** 1240, 1958.

introduced into medicine as an antiseptic by Sir Joseph Lister in 1867. Its use was so firmly established that it has been employed as a standard against which the antibacterial activity of other similar compounds (particularly other phenols) is measured. The relative power of a disinfectant as compared to phenol is known as the phenol coefficient (P/C). A disinfectant 30 times as efficient as phenol (i.e., producing the same killing effect at one-thirtieth the concentration) is said to have a phenol coefficient of 30.

Solutions of phenol are antiseptic, germicidal, or escharotic (scarring to tissue), depending upon the concentration used. Antiseptic solutions are irritating or toxic to tissues, and concentrated solutions may produce death when taken internally or when applied topically to abraded surfaces of the skin. When applied locally, phenol penetrates the skin and exerts a local anesthetic effect on sensory nerve endings. This explains its presence in certain lotions or ointments used to relieve itching (antipruritic).

Phenol is believed to exert its germicidal action by altering the structure of the protein in the parasitic cells (denaturation). In high concentrations it precipitates cellular protein. It is not affected much by the presence of organic matter or by high concentrations of bacteria. The use of phenol has declined because better disinfectants have been found, i.e., disinfectants that are less irritating and less toxic to human tissues and more efficient in killing microorganisms. Bacterial spores and viruses tend to be resistant to phenol. Phenol is occasionally used in full strength (88 per cent aqueous solution) to cauterize small wounds such as snake bites, in 5 per cent strength to disinfect sinks, toilets, and excreta, and in dilute solutions (0.5 to 1 per cent) to relieve itching.

Preparation.

Phenol, U.S.P., B.P.

Liquefied Phenol, U.S.P., B.P. This is an 88 per cent aqueous solution of phenol (80 per cent, B.P.).

Phenol Glycerin, B.P. This is a preparation of 16 per cent phenol and 84 per cent glycerin.

Phenolated Calamine Lotion, U.S.P. This is 1 per cent phenol in calamine lotion.

Cresol

Cresol is made available as a mixture of the ortho, meta, and para methyl phenols and is derived from coal tar. Cresols are phenols in which one of the hydrogen atoms in the benzene ring has been replaced by a methyl group (CH_3).

o-cresol   m-cresol   p-cresol

Cresol is a thick, heavy, straw-colored liquid with a phenol-like odor. It is 2 to 5 times as active as phenol but no more toxic. It is only slightly soluble in water but is soluble in liquid soap. Preparations of cresol are used for disinfecting excreta, sinks, bedpans, toilets, etc. All are poisonous and should be used for external purposes only or as mentioned.

Preparation.

Saponated Cresol Solution, N.F. This is a 50 per cent solution of cresol in vegetable oil (saponified). This is also known as Lysol.

Cresol and Soap Solution, B.P. This is essentially the same as the Saponated Cresol Solution.

Lysol forms a milky emulsion in water, but it is more soluble than pure cresol. Its action is not hampered by the presence of organic material. It is used in a 2 to 5 per cent strength to disinfect excreta, sinks, toilets, bedpans, and similar utensils. It is like the other cresols and phenol in that it is poisonous.

Hexachlorophene (Gamophen, Hex-O-San, pHisoHex, Surgi-Cen)

Hexachlorophene is a chlorinated diphenol. It is a white to light tan powder relatively insoluble in water but soluble in alcohol, fats, and soaps. It is incorporated into detergent creams, oils, soaps (e.g., Dial soap), and other media for topical application to reduce numbers of pathogenic bacteria on the skin and to reduce the incidence of pyogenic skin infections. It is much more effective against gram-positive than gram-negative bacteria. Optimum effects are secured only when regular and repeated applications are made. If other cleansing agents are substituted, a rapid increase of organisms normally found on the skin may be observed.

Hexachlorophene should not be looked upon as a substitute for mechanical cleansing of the skin, although products containing this substance are used for preoperative preparation of the skin. It is also used by food handlers and dentists. Its activity is reduced by the presence of organic material and blood serum. Alcohol and other organic solvents should be avoided when hexachlorophene is used. Hexachlorophene is an active ingredient in a number of deodorants.

Preparation.

Hexachlorophene, U.S.P.

Hexachlorophene Liquid Soap, U.S.P. The soap contains between 225 and 260 mg. of hexachlorophene in each 100 ml. of 10 to 13 per cent potassium soap base.

Resorcinol

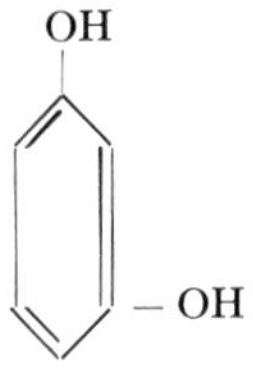

OH

— OH

Resorcinol resembles phenol in effectiveness, but it is less toxic, irritating, and caustic. It is used chiefly as an antiseptic and keratolytic (softening or dissolving the keratin-containing epidermis) in the treatment of various diseases of the skin. It is used in strengths that vary from 2 to 20 per cent. It acts by precipitating proteins of the cells.

Preparation.

Resorcinol, U.S.P., B.P. This compound occurs as colorless needle-shaped crystals with a faint aromatic odor. It is applied topically as an ointment or paste.

Compound Resorcinol Ointment, N.F. This contains 6 per cent resorcinol in a number of media to make a suitable ointment.

Hexylresorcinol

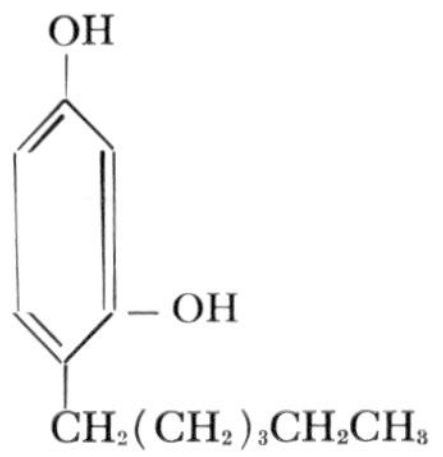

OH

— OH

$CH_2(CH_2)_3CH_2CH_3$

Hexylresorcinol was first introduced as a urinary antiseptic. Much of its efficiency is due to its low surface tension which accounts for the name "ST 37," which is used for a 1:1,000 solution of hexylresorcinol in glycerin and water.

Hexylresorcinol is stainless and odorless, but it may be irritating to tissues; some persons who become sensitive to it may exhibit allergic reactions. One of its more important uses is the treatment of patients with worm infestations. Its use as an anthelmintic will be discussed later.

Thymol

$$\text{OH} \quad C_3H_7 \quad CH_3$$

Thymol, N.F., B.P., is a colorless crystalline solid with an aromatic odor and taste. Chemically it is related to one of the cresols and is more effective than phenol. It possesses fungicidal properties, and it is an effective anthelmintic (hookworm). Because of its pleasant odor and taste it is an ingredient of many gargles and mouthwashes, e.g., Listerine.

Selected phenol derivatives

A combination of *o*-phenyl phenol and potassium resinoleate furnishes the active ingredient of O-syl. A similar type of compound is marketed under the name of Amphyl. These compounds do not have the typical odor of phenolic compounds. When used in 3 per cent concentrations they are said to be effective against vegetative forms of microorganisms but they do not kill spores. They are moderately active against tubercle bacilli and viruses. They are suitable as germicidal solutions to be used for cleaning of walls, furniture, and floors.

Dyes

Certain dyes are used as antiseptics and antiprotozoal agents, as well as to promote the healing of wounds. Because they are rapidly adsorbed on proteins, they exhibit limited ability to penetrate tissues, and their germicidal action tends to be slow.

Triphenylmethane dyes (rosaniline dyes)

Triphenylmethane dyes are a group of basic dyes which include crystal violet, gentian violet, methyl violet, brilliant green, and fuchsin. Solutions of these dyes are used in the form of antiseptic dressings on wounds, serous surfaces, and mucous membranes, or they are applied topically for the treatment of superficial fungous infections of the skin

606

and mucous membranes. Gentian violet is also used in the treatment of certain types of worm infestation.

Preparation.

Methylrosaniline Chloride, U.S.P., B.P. This dye is available in bulk powder and in tablet form, 10, 15, and 30 mg.

Methylrosaniline Chloride Solution, U.S.P. The solution consists mainly of gentian violet with some admixture of the other two violet compounds. It is a 1 per cent solution of the dyes in 10 per cent alcohol.

Carbol-Fuchsin Solution, N.F. (Castellani's Paint). This preparation contains fuchsin, phenol, resorcinol, and boric acid in an acetone-alcohol-water solution. It is used in the treatment of fungous infection. Fuchsin is *p*-rosaniline chloride and is a red dye.

Azo dyes

The azo dyes are more effective as agents which promote the healing of wounds than they are as antiseptics. They appear to stimulate the growth of epithelium and are sometimes used in the treatment of burns, chronic ulcers, and bedsores. Difference of opinion, howexer, exists regarding their effectiveness.

Preparation.

Scarlet Red Ointment. This preparation contains 5 per cent scarlet red in olive oil, wool fat, and petrolatum.

Pyridium (phenyl-azo-diamino pyridine hydrochloride). It is used for its analgesic action on irritated mucous membrane of the urinary tract. It is for this reason that it is found in combination with urinary antiseptics, e.g., Azo-Gantrisin.

Acridine dyes

Acridine dyes have been called "flavines" because of their yellow color. They are applied to open wounds in 0.1 to 1 per cent solutions or ointments. In this strength they are relatively nonirritating and they do not retard the healing of wounds.

Preparation.

Acriflavine; Proflavine Hemisulfate, B.P. Both of these preparations are used in solution or ointment in above-mentioned strengths.

Salts of heavy metals

Mercury compounds

Inorganic compounds of mercury were among the earliest antiseptics to be used, and they long were regarded as potent germicides. Investigation has shown that their action, in many instances, is bacteriostatic rather than bactericidal, since their effects can be reversed under some conditions and microorganisms revived that were previously considered dead.[*] Although the mercuric ion brings about the precipitation of cellular proteins, its bacteriostatic action is said to be due to inhibition of specific enzymes of bacterial cells. Mercurial antiseptics may also exert toxic effects on the tissue cells of the host when taken internally. The mercurials fall far short of being ideal antiseptics or germicides. The inorganic compounds are irritating to tissues, penetrate poorly, are toxic systemically, are adversely affected by the presence of organic materials, have little or no action on spores, and are corrosive to metals. However, they are effective bacteriostatic agents for certain uses. Some of the organic compounds are more potent than the inorganic ones, especially if they are in alcoholic solution. Some authorities believe that certain organic mercurials are useful antiseptics if used appropriately in proper concentration.

Preparation.

Mercury Bichloride, N.F.; *Mercuric Chloride*, B.P. (Corrosive Sublimate). This is the oldest of the mercurial antiseptics. Tablets of mercury bichloride are coffin shaped and are stamped with a skull and crossbones and the word "Poison." They are colored blue to prevent their solutions from being mistaken for water. Mercuric chloride is available in 0.5 and 0.12 Gm. tablets. It is occasionally used in a 1:1,000 concentration to disinfect objects that would be harmed by heat or to disinfect hands that have previously been scrubbed with soap and water.

Mercurial ointments

A number of compounds of mercury and metallic mercury are incorporated into ointments for use as antiseptics. The drug slowly dissolves in the tissues to release a low concentration of mercuric ions and thus exerts a prolonged effect. A number of such ointments are listed in the *National Formulary*. Two official ointments are included here.

Preparation.

Ammoniated Mercury Ointment, U.S.P., B.P. (White Precipitate Ointment). The U.S.P. preparation contains 5 per cent ammoniated mercury; the B.P. preparation, 2.5 per cent. The U.S.P. preparation has a base of white ointment and liquid petrolatum. The B.P. preparation is made with simple ointment. Ammoniated mercury is also used in ointments of 2 to 10 per cent concentrations as antiseptics and local stimulants in cases of suppurating dermatitis and eczematous and parasitic skin diseases.

Ammoniated Mercury Ophthalmic Ointment, U.S.P. This contains 3

---

*Giarman, N. J.: Chemotherapy of Bacterial Infections. In Drill, V. A. (editor): Pharmacology in Medicine, New York, 1958, McGraw-Hill Book Co., Inc., p. 1096.

per cent ammoniated mercury and is applied as an antiseptic to the eyelids.

Organic mercurial preparations

These compounds are less toxic and less irritating than the inorganic mercurial antiseptics.

Preparation.

Merbromin, N.F. (Mercurochrome). Although widely used at one time merbromin has been supplanted by more effective agents. It was the first organic mercurial to be used.

Thimerosal, N.F. (Merthiolate). This compound is a light cream-colored, crystalline powder. It contains about 50 per cent mercury. It can be used safely as a skin antiseptic on abraded skin in concentrations of 1:1,000, and aqueous solutions can be used on mucous membranes. *Thimerosal Solution*, N.F., is an alcohol-acetone-water solution which has been colored red by a suitable coal-tar color. Thimerosal solutions are incompatible with acids, salts of heavy metals, and iodine. *Thimerosal Tincture* and *Thimerosal Ointment* are also listed in N.F.

Nitromersol, N.F. (Metaphen); *Nitromersol Tincture*, N.F. This is a 0.5 per cent solution of nitromersol in acetone, alcohol, and water. It is used chiefly as a skin disinfectant. *Nitromersol Solution*, N.F., is an aqueous solution sometimes used to disinfect instruments in concentrations of 1:1,000 to 1:5,000; for the skin, 1:1,000 to 1:5,000; and for irrigation of mucous membranes (eye and urethra), 1:5,000 to 1:10,000.

Acetomeroctol* (Merbak). This is an organic mercurial applied topically as an antiseptic. Its activity and effectiveness are similar to those of other organic mercurials. A 1:1,000 concentration contains 50 per cent alcohol and 10 per cent acetone, to which part of its activity is due.

Phenylmercuric compounds

Phenylmercuric compounds are active against a variety of pathogenic bacteria and exhibit a low level of toxicity in human tissue. Like other mercurial antiseptics they cannot be depended upon to kill spores. These compounds occasionally cause irritation and poisoning in persons of undue sensitivity. Buffered solutions are odorless, colorless, and stainless and do not react with body proteins. They are noncorrosive to metals with the exception of aluminum, and they do not destroy rubber.

Preparation.

Phenyl Mercuric Nitrate, N.F., B.P. (Merphenyl Nitrate Basic). This drug is applied topically, 1:1,500 solutions for prophylactic disinfection of intact skin and minor injuries, 1:15,000 to 1:2,400 for mucous membranes and wet dressings.

*Described in annual publication of A. M. A. Council on Drugs, N.N.D., 1960.

Silver and silver compounds

Silver compounds

Silver compounds are used in medicine for their antiseptic, caustic, and astringent effects, which in turn are due to the release of free silver ions. The soluble salts of silver ionize readily in solution, whereas the colloidal silver compounds dissociate only slightly. Silver ions will precipitate cellular protein; hence the inorganic salts of silver are germicidal in solution, but the colloidal preparations are bacteriostatic even in very dilute solutions. It is thought that silver, like mercury, is capable of interfering with important metabolic activities of microbial cells.[*]

Preparation.

Silver Nitrate, U.S.P., B.P. This compound occurs as flat, transparent crystals which become grayish black on exposure to light and in the presence of organic material. It is odorless and has a bitter, strongly metallic taste. It is freely soluble in water, ionizes readily, and hence is germicidal. Silver nitrate reacts with soluble chlorides, iodides, and bromides to form in soluble salts; hence the action of silver salts can be stopped by washing with a solution of sodium chloride. This chemical property also explains why solutions of silver salts penetrate tissues slowly due to the precipitation of silver ions in the tissues as chlorides or phosphates. A 1:1,000 solution is antiseptic. Weak solutions are astringent on mucous membranes, and strong solutions are caustic when applied to mucous membranes or the skin. Silver salts stain tissues black, due to the deposit of silver.

Silver nitrate is used on inflamed mucous membranes and ulcerated surfaces. For diseases of the conjunctiva, solutions varying in strength from 0.2 to 2 per cent may be used. To prevent the development of gonorrheal conjunctivitis in the newborn infant, a drop or two of 1 per cent solution is instilled into each eye as soon as possible after delivery. A stronger solution has been used, but it is dangerous, because strong solutions will kill tissue in a short time and may thus permit the gonococcus to enter and spread into deeper tissues. Blindness has been caused in this way. To stop the action if too much has been used, wash with physiologic saline solution. Even a 1 per cent silver nitrate solution produces a chemical conjunctivitis in a rather large number of cases. For this reason, some physicians are advocating the use of penicillin ointment. Solutions of silver nitrate which vary in concentration from 1:1,000 to 1:10,000 are used for irrigation of the bladder and urethra. A 1:1,000 solution is germicidal but irritating. Long-continued use of any silver preparation may produce permanent discoloration of the skin and mucous membranes, a condition known as argyria.

[*]Goodman, L. S., and Gilman, A.: The Pharmacological Basis of Therapeutics, New York, 1955, The Macmillan Co., p. 1105.

Toughened Silver Nitrate, U.S.P., B.P. (Lunar Caustic). This form is a white solid generally used in the form of pencils or cones. It is applied as a mild caustic to wounds, ulcers, and granulation tissue. It should be moistened before use and, to avoid blackening the fingers, should be held with forceps. It may be fused on a probe for application to parts that are difficult of access. The mucous membranes to which solutions of silver nitrate are applied should receive a preliminary cleansing to remove mucous, pus, food, etc., which would interfere with the action of the drug.

Colloidal silver preparations

Colloidal silver preparations do not ionize readily and do not act as corrosives, irritants, and astringents. They penetrate tissue more readily than do the solutions of simple salts of silver. They exert a bacteriostatic effect, due to the concentration of silver ions which gradually is produced.

The terms *strong* and *mild* refer to the relative antiseptic values and not to the amount of silver they contain, for the strong contains about 8 per cent silver and the weak contains about 20 per cent. The antiseptic value depends on the extent of ionization in any given liquid. Mild silver protein preparations should be freshly made and dispensed in amber-colored bottles.

Preparation.

Strong Silver Protein (Protargol); *Silver Protein*, B.P. This compound contains not less than 7.5 per cent and not more than 8.5 per cent of silver.

Mild Silver Protein, N.F. (Argyn, Silvol). The mild form contains from 19 to 23 per cent silver. It is entirely nonirritating but also has less antiseptic action than the strong silver protein. It is usually employed in concentrations of 5 to 25 per cent. A concentration of 5 per cent is commonly used for bladder irrigation, 10 to 15 per cent in the nose, and 20 to 25 per cent in the eye.

The colloidal preparations of silver are used as antiseptics, particularly on mucous membranes of the nose and throat, the urinary bladder, the urethra, and the conjunctiva. Gonococci are particularly susceptible to the action of compounds of silver.

The halogens

Chlorine

Chlorine is a nonmetallic element which occurs in the form of a greenish yellow gas. It has an intensely disagreeable odor. One part of chlorine in 10,000 parts of air causes irritation of the respiratory tract and exposure to a 1:1,000 concentration is fatal after 5 minutes.[*] It causes spasm and pain of the muscles of the larynx and bronchial tubes, coughing, a burning sensation, fainting, unconsciousness, and death. Its extensive use for the purification of water, however, makes it one of the most widely used disinfectants. One part of chlorine in 1,000,000 parts of water will destroy most bacteria in a few minutes. Acid-fast organisms such as the *Mycobacterium tuberculosis* are unusually resistant to it. Chlorine is also effective against amebas, viruses, organisms of the colon-typhoid group, and many of the spore-forming pathogens. The antibacterial action of chlorine is said to be due to the formation of hypochlorous acid which results when chlorine reacts with water. Hypochlorous acid is a rapidly acting bactericidal agent. Its effect is partly due to its oxidizing action and partly to its effect on microbial enzymes which are concerned with the metabolism of glucose.[†]

The activity of chlorine and chlorine-releasing compounds is influenced by a number of factors such as the presence of organic material, the pH of the solution, and the temperature. Chlorine is more effective when there is a minimum of organic matter, when the medium is acid in reaction, and when the temperature is elevated. Chlorine is an efficient deodorant and a strong bleaching agent, and it corrodes many metals.

Gaseous chlorine has limited usefulness because it is difficult to handle. There are a number of compounds which yield hypochlorous acid and which are useful for certain kinds of disinfection.

Preparation.

Sodium Hypochlorite Solution, N.F. This is a 5 per cent solution of sodium hypochlorite. This concentration is too great to be used on living tissues.

Diluted Sodium Hypochlorite Solution, Modified Dakin's Solution, N.F.; *Surgical Chlorinated Soda Solution,* B.P. This preparation is a 0.5 per cent aqueous solution of sodium hypochlorite. It was once used extensively in the treatment of suppurating wounds. Although it is useful to cleanse wounds it also interferes with the formation of thrombin, delays clotting of blood, and is irritating to the skin. Dilute solutions have been used to prevent the development of athlete's foot (epidermophytosis). A 0.5 per cent solution of sodium hypochlorite is also used to disinfect walls, furniture, and especially floors. Preparations of sodium hypochlorite are unstable and need to be freshly prepared.

[*]Goodman, L. S., and Gilman, A.: The Pharmacological Basis of Therapeutics, New York, 1955, The Macmillan Co., p. 1096.

[†]Giarman, N. J.: Chemotherapy of Bacterial Infections. In Drill, V. A. (editor): Pharmacology in Medicine, New York, 1958, McGraw-Hill Book Co., Inc., p. 1094.

Chloramines

Several compounds are available in which chlorine is linked with nitrogen. The chloramines exert their effects by the release of chlorine to form hypochlorous acid and also by direct action of the parent compound. The chloramines are more stable, less irritating, and slower acting than the hypochlorites. However, their action is more prolonged and they are less readily affected by the presence of organic material.

Preparation.

Chloramine-T; Chloramine, B.P. This compound is used in 0.1 to 2 per cent aqueous solutions for irrigations of wounds or for dressings.

Halazone, N.F. Halazone is a chloramine. It is available in 4 mg. tablets and is employed for the sterilization of drinking water. One to 2 tablets (4 to 8 mg.) per liter of water will kill all pathogens usually found in water, in 30 to 60 minutes.

Iodine

Iodine is a heavy, bluish black, crystalline solid having a metallic luster and a characteristic odor. It is slightly soluble in water but is soluble in alcohol and in aqueous solutions of sodium and potassium iodide. Iodine is volatile, and its solutions should not be exposed to the air except during immediate use. The mechanism of disinfectant action is not entirely known. The concentration at which iodine acts as a disinfectant is similar for all bacteria. Iodine is thought to be one of the more efficient chemical disinfectants in present-day usage. Its activity does not vary greatly for vegetative pathogens; it is effective over a wide pH range, and it is effective against spores, viruses, and fungi. It is not affected by the presence of organic material found in body fluids and exudates. In combination with alcohol, iodine in 0.5 to 1 per cent solution will kill tubercle bacilli. However, iodine does not kill spores readily, and it has the disadvantage of staining skin, clothing, etc. In rare instances, individuals exhibit hypersensitivity reactions to iodine when it is applied to the skin. Toxic effects on tissues are said to be low. Iodine is used chiefly for disinfection of small wounds, abraded surfaces, and in the preoperative preparation of skin surfaces. A fact often overlooked is that aqueous solutions as well as alcoholic solutions of iodine are germicidal. Aqueous solutions are less irritating and are best used on abraded areas of the skin. Iodine penetrates the skin and slight amounts are absorbed.

Another use which may be made of iodine tincture is for emergency disinfection of water which is suspected of harboring pathogenic amebas. One drop of iodine tincture to a quart of water will kill the amebas and also bacteria in 15 minutes without making the water unpalatable.[*]

[*]Goodman, L. S., and Gilman, A.: The Pharmacological Basis of Therapeutics, New York, 1955, The Macmillan Co., p. 1095.

Iodine stains the skin and linens a brown color. These stains can be removed from the skin with alcohol or ammonia and from fabrics with boiling water.

Preparation.

Iodine Tincture, U.S.P. This preparation contains 2 per cent iodine and 2.4 per cent sodium iodide in 46 per cent ethyl alcohol. It has to a great extent replaced the Strong Iodine Tincture. *Weak Iodine Solution,* B.P., contains approximately the same amount of iodine along with potassium iodide and 90 per cent ethyl alcohol.

Strong Iodine Tincture, N.F. This form is an alcoholic solution containing 7 per cent iodine and 5 per cent potassium iodide in 83 per cent ethyl alcohol. *Strong Iodine Solution,* B.P., is a similar preparation.

Strong Iodine Solution, U.S.P. (Lugol's Solution). This aqueous solution contains 5 per cent iodine and 10 per cent potassium iodide. It is given (orally) for the treatment of goiter rather than for its antiseptic effect.

Iodine Solution, N.F. This aqueous solution contains 2 per cent iodine and 2.4 per cent sodium iodide.

Iodophors

Iodophors are complex combinations of iodine and a carrier or agent which increases the water solubility of iodine. The word literally means "iodine carrier." The combination contains and slowly releases iodine as it is needed but does not stain as aqueous solutions of iodine do. As used today, it frequently means a combination of iodine and a detergent. *Wescodyne* is one which is said to kill tubercle bacilli as well as other organisms sensitive to iodine. *Undecoylium Chloride-Iodine** (Virac) is a combination of iodine and a cationic detergent which is said to make a useful surface-acting agent. Polyvinylpyrrolidone iodine, known as PVP iodine or Povidone-Iodine,* is a stable, nonirritating compound which, when dissolved in water slowly, liberates iodine. It is claimed to be as effective and less irritating than aqueous solutions of free iodine. It is marketed as an antiseptic for external use under the name *Betadine.* It contains 1 per cent available iodine.

Oxidizing agents

Certain oxidizing agents are destructive to pathogenic organisms but mild enough to be used on living tissues. Their activity is due to the oxygen which they liberate. Oxygen combines readily with organic matter, and once combined, it is inert. Oxygen is especially harmful to

*Described in annual publication of A. M. A. Council on Drugs, N.N.D., 1960.

anaerobic organisms. On the whole, microorganisms vary considerably in their sensitivity to oxygen.

Preparation.

Hydrogen Peroxide Solution, U.S.P., B.P. The U.S.P. preparation is a 3 per cent solution of hydrogen peroxide in water.* It is a colorless, odorless liquid which deteriorates upon standing. It should be kept in a cool, dark place and should be well stoppered. Hydrogen peroxide decomposes to water and oxygen. This reaction occurs rapidly when the solution is in contact with organic matter. It is an active germicide only while it is actively releasing oxygen. Solutions have a high surface tension and do not penetrate readily. The effervescence (due to rapid formation of oxygen bubbles) which accompanies decomposition helps to clean suppurating wounds, but it should not be injected into closed body cavities or into abscesses from which the newly formed gas cannot easily escape. The official solution is usually diluted with 1 to 4 parts of water before it is used. It is used for the cleansing of wounds and for the treatment of Vincent's infection (trench mouth). In the latter case it is employed full strength for a limited period of time.

Medicinal Zinc Peroxide, U.S.P. This preparation consists of zinc peroxide, zinc carbonate, and zinc hydroxide. Upon hydrolysis it yields hydrogen peroxide. It has some value in the disinfection and deodorization of wounds, especially those infected with anaerobic organisms. It leaves a residue of zinc oxide which is slightly astringent in effect.

Potassium Permanganate, U.S.P., B.P. This agent occurs as dark purple crystals which are soluble in water (1:15). It decomposes in contact with organic matter and liberates oxygen, which combines with bacteria and inhibits their growth or destroys them. The bactericidal efficiency of solutions of potassium permanganate vary with the type of organism and the amount of organic material present. Solutions stronger than 1:5,000 may be irritating to tissues. It is used in vaginal douches in concentrations of 1:1,000 to 1:5,000 and is applied topically 1:500 to 1:10,000. After potassium permanganate solutions have lost oxygen they appear brown and are inert. Stains may be removed with dilute acids (lemon juice, oxalic acid, or dilute hydrochloric acid).

Potassium permanganate solutions produce irritant, astringent, deodorant, as well as germicidal effects. It is used much less now than formerly.

Sodium Perborate, N.F. This is a white powder soluble in water. In solution it forms hydrogen peroxide. It is used as a dusting powder or in 2 per cent solution as an oral antiseptic. Its chief use is in the treatment of Vincent's infection.

*The preparation described in B.P. is approximately a 6 per cent solution.

Surface-active agents

Surface-active agents are also known as wetting agents, emulsifiers, and detergents. In some respects, certain of these agents are considered superior to ordinary soap because they can be used in hard water, are stable in both acid and alkaline solutions, decrease surface tension more effectively, and are less irritating to the skin than ordinary soaps. They all lower surface tension, and when used to cleanse the skin they are useful in much the same way that soap is useful, i.e., they aid in the mechanical removal of bacteria, soil, etc. Many also exert a bactericidal action, although it is not apparently related entirely to their ability to lower surface tension, because while they all lower surface tension they all do not have germicidal properties. Many are believed to depress metabolic activities of bacteria, but how is not fully known. They have a weak antibacterial action against fungi, acid-fast organisms, spores, and viruses.* Their activity is reduced greatly by the presence of organic matter. If the active portion of the surface-active agent (surfactant) carries a negative electric charge, it is known as an anionic compound; if the active portion carries a positive charge, it is known as a cationic surfactant or surface-active agent.

Cationic agents

The most effective agents of this group of compounds have been the quaternary ammonium compounds (sometimes referred to as "quats"). These compounds combine a detergent and antiseptic action. In general, they are more effective antiseptics than the anionic group of compounds. They inhibit both gram-positive and gram-negative organisms. Soap inactivates cationic detergents and hence it must be removed before the detergent is used. Hard water also inactivates these agents and causes precipitation. Although they are recommended in the final rinse of laundry materials, they are often ineffective because conditions are not ideal for their use; e.g., there remain traces of soap or hard water. Cationic detergents cannot be relied upon to sterilize instruments and articles that cannot be subjected to heat but are sometimes used to preserve sterility of stored materials. They have also been used in aerosols to increase the penetrating power of antibiotics.

Preparation.

Benzalkonium Chloride, U.S.P., B.P. (Zephiran Chloride). When employed in proper concentration, benzalkonium chloride is an effective, relatively noninjurious surface disinfectant. It is germicidal for a number of pathogenic nonspore-forming pathogens, including fungi after several minutes of exposure. However, it has no effect on tubercle bacilli. Its viricidal activity is said to be limited. Benzalkonium chloride solu-

*N.N.D., 1960, p. 180.

616

tions have a low surface tension and possess keratolytic, detergent, and emulsifying properties. Solutions of soap reduce its germicidal activity unless well rinsed from the area to be disinfected. Seventy per cent alcohol serves to diminish the reaction of soap and the disinfectant and may well follow the use of soap and water preparation of the skin before the application of the disinfectant.

Solutions of benzalkonium chloride have a relatively low level of toxicity under conditions of use for which they are recommended.

It is suitable for prophylactic disinfection of the intact skin and in the treatment of superficial injuries when used in 1:1,000 concentration (tincture).

Solutions of 1:1,000 are used for preservation of metallic instruments and rubber articles. For disinfection of operating room equipment, 1:5,000 may be used.*

Benzethonium Chloride, U.S.P. (Phemerol Chloride). Is a detergent which exerts an inhibitory effect on the growth activities of commonly occurring bacteria and fungi. *Tincture of Phemerol Chloride* 1:500 and *Benzethonium Chloride Solution,* U.S.P., 1:1,000 are used full strength as general germicides and antiseptics except for use in the nose and eye. For the latter, the aqueous solution is used and diluted with four parts of water.

Cetyl Pyridinium Chloride.† (Ceepryn Chloride). This agent is used for preoperative disinfection of intact skin, in the treatment of minor wounds, and for the therapeutic disinfection of mucous membranes. Its effectiveness is reduced by detergents such as ordinary soap and by serums and tissue fluids, and it is ineffective against clostridial spores. Strengths used vary from 1:100 for skin preparations and 1:1,000 for minor abrasions to 1:5,000 and 1:10,000 for mucous membranes.

Methylbenzethonium Chloride.† (Diaparene Chloride). This preparation produces bacteriostasis of urea-splitting organisms. It is used for disinfecting babies' diapers; they should be free of soap, however, before being rinsed in this disinfectant. It is available in 0.09 Gm. tablets, and the solution is made by dissolving 1 tablet in 2,000 ml. of warm water. This amount is sufficient for rinsing six diapers. They should remain immersed in the disinfectant for 3 minutes.

Anionic surface agents

Anionic surface agents are the neutral or faintly alkaline salts of acids of high molecular weights exemplified by common soaps and a number of other compounds. They are incompatible with the cationic com-

*N.N.D., 1960, p. 183.
†Described in annual publication of A. M. A. Council on Drugs, N.N.D., 1960.

pounds. They act best in an acid medium and are most effective against gram-positive organisms.

Preparation.

Medicinal Soft Soap Liniment, U.S.P. (Tincture of Green Soap). This preparation is an alcoholic solution containing about 65 per cent of soft soap perfumed with oil of lavender. It is called green because it was first made from oils that contained chlorophyl-like coloring matter. Modern "green soap" may be colorless.

Medicinal Soft Soap, Green Soap, U.S.P.; *Soft Soap,* B.P. This is a potassium soap made by the saponification of vegetable oils without the removal of glycerin. Soft soap has little antiseptic value but is used as a cleansing agent.

Hard Soap, N.F. This is a sodium soap.

Hexachlorophene Liquid Soap, U.S.P. This is a potassium soap to which hexachlorophene has been added.

Other anionic surface agents include *pHisoderm,* which is a synthetic compound sometimes used as a substitute for soap. It is available as a cream or creamy emulsion. It is sometimes used for certain dermatologic conditions when soap is contraindicated. *pHisoHex* is pHisoderm to which 3 per cent hexachlorophene has been added. It exerts a prolonged antiseptic as well as emollient effect when used routinely.

Sodium Tetradecyl Sulfate* (Sodium Sotradecol). This is an anionic surface-acting agent which lowers surface tension of certain antiseptic solutions to which it may be added. It is also used as a sclerosing agent in the treatment of varicose veins and internal hemorrhoids.

Miscellaneous agents

Alcohols

Alcohols are one of the oldest and most widely used of the skin disinfectants. Both ethyl alcohol and isopropyl alcohol are used as disinfectants and their germicidal power is said to be underrated. They are used extensively to prepare the skin prior to the injection with a needle, e.g., for venepuncture, subcutaneous and intramuscular injection, ear or finger pricks for samples of blood, etc. Ethyl alcohol is reported to be most effective in concentrations of 50 to 70 per cent. The growth of some organisms is said to be inhibited by a 1 per cent solution, although the bactericidal action is unreliable when the concentration falls below 20 per cent or is above 95 per cent.†

*Described in annual publication of A. M. A. Council on Drugs, N.N.D., 1960.
†Giarman, N. J.: Chemotherapy of Bacterial Infections. In Drill, V. A. (editor): Pharmacology in Medicine, New York, 1958, McGraw-Hill Book Co., Inc., p. 1093.

Preparation.

Alcohol, Ethyl Alcohol, U.S.P., B.P.

Isopropyl Alcohol. This form is slightly more antiseptic than ethyl alcohol. It is employed full strength (99 per cent) or as *Alcohol Rubbing Compound,* N.F., which is a 70 per cent aqueous solution. It is also used extensively as a 75 per cent aqueous solution for the disinfection and storage of oral thermometers. It can be combined with other disinfectants such as formaldehyde solution to make an effective germicide.

Formaldehyde

Formaldehyde in a gaseous form is a powerful parasiticide because of its penetrating power but is active only in the presence of abundant moisture. It was used formerly for the fumigation of rooms.

Preparation.

Formaldehyde Solution, U.S.P., B.P. This is a 37 per cent solution of formaldehyde (by weight) known as formalin. It is a clear, colorless liquid which, on exposure to air, liberates a pungent, irritating gas. In proper concentration formaldehyde solution is germicidal against all forms of microorganisms. A 0.5 per cent solution will kill all organisms, including spores, in 6 to 12 hours. Higher concentrations are effective in less time. It is not affected by organic matter, and it is effective against viruses. It acts as a precipitant of protein.

Formaldehyde solution hardens tissues, and for this reason it is used as a preservative for specimens and as an astringent. When it is combined with isopropyl alcohol or hexachlorophene, it is probably the most powerful germicidal solution available at the present time. Various modifications of the Bard-Parker germicidal solution are made with formaldehyde solution, isopropyl alcohol, and antirust agents for the disinfection of instruments and articles that cannot be subjected to heat. These solutions are sometimes called "cold sterilization solutions."

The chief disadvantage encountered in using solutions of formaldehyde is that it is irritating to tissues and mucous membranes and has an unpleasant odor.

Boric Acid

Boric acid is a mild antiseptic and astringent. Dilute solutions of boric acid are nonirritating and therefore suitable for use on delicate structures such as the eye. Boric acid is an ingredient of many antiseptic solutions used as washes and gargles. It is still widely used for conditions of the skin in the form of wet dressings, dusting powders, and ointments. It is also used in solution form for irrigations of mucous membranes, e.g., irrigation of the urinary bladder.

Although boric acid is not customarily considered a toxic substance, since it is used externally, serious poisoning and deaths have resulted from its ingestion. Solutions of boric acid should be colored to help prevent accidents. Toxic reactions have occurred from topical application to large denuded areas, because of the absorption which took place.

Preparation.

Boric Acid, U.S.P., B.P.

Boric Acid Ointment, N.F. This preparation contains 10 per cent boric acid in liquid petrolatum and white ointment.

Boric Acid Solution, N.F. This is a 5 per cent aqueous solution of boric acid.

Boroglycerin Glycerite, N.F. This is a solution of boric acid in glycerin.

Ethylene Oxide

Ethylene oxide has come to be used for gaseous sterilization of materials that cannot be subjected to heat or liquid chemical agents, e.g., certain plastic parts of machines and optical instruments. It may come to be used for the disinfection of blankets, pillows, etc., which is a problem when dealing with such articles after they have been contaminated with staphylococci.

Ethylene oxide is a colorless gas at ordinary temperatures; it has a rather pleasant ethereal odor, and its toxicity when inhaled is said to compare with ammonia gas. It is flammable and when confined is capable of explosive violence. This agent is therefore used in small cabinets or in a mixture of ethylene oxide with carbon dioxide so that the flammable point is not reached. A preparation of 10 per cent ethylene oxide and 90 per cent carbon dioxide is on the market under the name of *Carboxide.*

Ethylene oxide is apparently effective against all types of microorganisms, including viruses and tubercle bacilli. It is also effective against spores. Its action is bactericidal rather than bacteriostatic. It is a more expensive form of sterilization than that achieved with heat or other chemical agents, but it has good penetrating power and can be used for many things that would be injured by heat or chemicals. In fact, it is the only chemical agent that has been accepted for registration under the law as a sterilizing agent for hospital use when used as directed in specially constructed chambers or autoclaves.*

*Stuart, L. S.: How Effective Are Chemical Germicides in Maintaining Hospital Antisepsis? J. A. H. A. Hosp. 33: 46, May 16, 1959.

References

A. M. A. Council on Drugs: New and Non-official Drugs, Philadelphia, 1960, J. B. Lippincott Co.

Bogash, R. C.: Polyvinylpyrrolidine Iodine, Bull. Am. Soc. Hosp. Pharm. **13**: 226, 1956.

Caswell, H. T.: Staphylococcal Infections Among Hospital Personnel, Am. J. Nursing **58**: 822, 1958.

Drill, V. A. (editor): Pharmacology in Medicine, New York, 1958, McGraw-Hill Book Co., Inc.

Engley, F. B., Jr.: Evaluation of Mercurial Compounds as Antiseptics, Ann. New York Acad. Sc. **53**: 197, 1950.

Goodman, L., and Gilman, A.: The Pharmacological Basis of Therapeutics, New York, 1955, The Macmillan Co.

Hugo, W. B.: The Mode of Action of Antiseptics, J. Pharm. & Pharmacol. **9**: 145, 1957.

Reddish, G. F. (editor): Antiseptics, Disinfectants, Fungicides and Chemical and Physical Sterilization, Philadelphia, 1957, Lea & Febiger.

Spaulding, E. H., and Emmons, E. K.: Chemical Disinfection, Am. J. Nursing **58**: 1238, 1958.

Spaulding, E. H., Emmons, E. K., and Guzara, M. H.: Ethylene Oxide Sterilization, Am. J. Nursing **58**: 1530, 1958.

Stuart, L. S.: How Effective Are Chemical Germicides in Maintaining Hospital Antisepsis? J. A. H. A. Hosp. **33**: 46, 1959.

Chapter 23

Anti-infectives—anthelmintics
and
amebicides

Anthelmintics

Anthelmintics are drugs used to rid the body of worms (helminths). The use of anthelmintics (*anti*, against; *helminthos*, worms) is among the most primitive types of chemotherapy. Millions of people over the world are infested with these parasites.

Helminths may be present in the gastrointestinal tract, but several types also penetrate the tissues and some undergo developmental changes, during which they wander extensively in the host. Diagnosis of helminthiasis is often made by finding the worm or eggs of the worm in the stool.

Undesirable effects that may result from helminthiasis

Parasitic infestations do not necessarily cause clinical manifestations, although they may be injurious for a number of reasons:

1. Worms may cause mechanical injury to the tissues and organs; e.g., roundworms in large numbers may cause obstruction in the intestine; filariae may block lymphatic channels and cause massive edema; and hookworms often cause extensive damage to the wall of the intestine and cause considerable loss of blood.

2. Toxic substances made by the parasite may be absorbed by the host.

3. The tissues of the host may be traumatized by the presence of the parasite and thus made more susceptible to bacterial infections.

4. Heavy infestation with worms will rob the host of food. This is particularly significant in children.

Classification of helminths

Worms that are parasitic to man may be classified as cestodes, nematodes, and trematodes. The *cestodes* are the tapeworms, of which there are four varieties: (1) *Taenia saginata* (beef tapeworm), (2) *Taenia solium* (pork tapeworm), (3) *Diphyllobothrium latum* (fishworm), and (4) *Hymenolepis nana* (dwarf tapeworm). As indicated by the name of the worm, the parasite enters the intestine by way of improperly cooked beef, pork, or fish or from contaminated food, as in the case of the dwarf tapeworm.

The cestodes are segmented flatworms, having a head and a number of segments or proglottids which in some cases may extend for 20 or 30 feet in the bowel. The tapeworms, with the exception of the dwarf tapeworm, spend part of their life cycle in a host other than man, e.g., the pig, fish, or cattle. The dwarf tapeworm does not require an intermediate host.

The nematodes are round, unsegmented worms which vary in length from a fraction of an inch to a foot or more. They include *Ascaris lumbricoides* (roundworm), *Necator americanus* and *Ancylostoma duodenale* (two species of hookworms), *Trichuris trichiura* (whipworm), *Trichinella spiralis* (which produces trichinosis and for which there is no effective anthelmintic), *Oxyuris (Enterobius) vermicularis* (pinworm), *Wuchereria bancrofti* (causing filariasis), and *Strongyloides stercoralis* (infestation with which is known as strongyloidiasis).

The trematodes are flukes, among which are several blood flukes, e.g., *Schistosoma mansoni, japonicum,* and *hematobium.* There are also other flukes which are parasitic to man. Schistosomiasis is a disease caused by blood flukes. They penetrate the skin of persons who bathe in contaminated waters or in some other way come in contact with the infected water in which snails serve as the intermediate host. The adult blood flukes live in the veins of the mesentery and pelvis of man and accumulate in the portal tube. The liver and spleen are the organs mainly involved.

Properties of a good anthelmintic

Anthelmintics should be relatively safe and at the same time sufficiently potent to achieve their purpose. Many anthelmintics are toxic to man as well as to the parasite. A good anthelmintic has a minimal toxic effect on the host and a maximal toxic effect on the parasite. Other desirable properties include easy administration and low cost.

Effective treatment of the patient demands that the type of worm or worms be known, as well as the best anthelmintic to use, and a method for determining whether or not the treatment was successful. Although the technic of treatment necessarily varies with the drug used, maximum effects are related in certain instances to how well the intestinal tract is emptied before the drug is administered and how well it is evacuated afterward. Some of the newer anthelmintics do not require that the patient be purged and starved to promote the effectiveness of the drug.

Drugs used against cestodes and nematodes

Aspidium (male fern)

The male fern is one of the oldest of the anthelmintic agents. The species from which the official drug is obtained is the *Dryopteris filix-mas*, a fern commonly found in England and Europe. The anthelmintic action is due to the presence of several closely related substances, i.e., filicic acid, filmaron, etc.

Action and result. Aspidium has a number of effects on the host which constitute side effects and toxic effects, but the action on the worm is an action on smooth muscle, i.e., the smooth muscle of the worm is paralyzed and thus it is possible to expel the worm by means of a cathartic. A certain amount of the drug is absorbed, although one of the aims in therapy is to avoid absorption as much as possible. This is accomplished by minimizing the amount of fat in the diet of the patient just prior to and during treatment. The part of the drug which is absorbed is later excreted in the urine.

Uses. Aspidium can be employed to rid the body of tapeworms, especially *Taenia solium* (pork tapeworm). It can also be used against *Diphyllobothrium latum* (fish tapeworm) and *Hymenolepis nana* (dwarf tapeworm). Its use against the beef tapeworm is not thought to be justifiable since other less toxic agents are available to use against the *Taenia saginata*.

Preparation, dosage, and administration.

Aspidium Oleoresin, U.S.P.; *Male Fern Extract*, B.P. This drug is a dark green liquid with an unpleasant taste. The usual total dose of the oleoresin is 3 to 5 Gm. The dose for children of school age is one half this amount. A fat-free diet for a day or two before the aspidium is given is recommended because the presence of fat in the intestine promotes the absorption of the drug. Lunch and supper are omitted the day before the treatment, and a saline cathartic (magnesium sulfate, 15 Gm., in water) is given the evening before the treatment. The aspidium is administered the next morning on an empty stomach in divided doses, 1 hour apart. Since the taste is bitter and difficult to disguise, it is best given in enteric-coated capsules. A saline cathartic is again administered

2 hours after the last dose, and 2 hours later a large soapsuds enema is given to ensure removal of all of the drug.

Another way the drug may be administered is by instilling the agent in the intestine by way of a duodenal tube. The aspidium is administered along with mucilage of acacia (30 ml.) or powdered acacia and is followed by a saline cathartic. Food is permitted only after the saline purgative has been effective. The saline purgative promotes the elimination of both the worm and the anthelmintic.

The nurse who is caring for the patient should make certain *that all parts of the stool are saved.* Failure to do this may mean that the treatment has been in vain, for unless the head of the worm is found, there is no immediate assurance that the treatment has been successful. If the head of the worm is retained it will develop again.

Side effects and toxic effects. Serious symptoms of poisoning follow the absorption of the active constituents of aspidium. Toxic symptoms may occur after moderate doses and large doses are often dangerous, although not uniformly so. The milder symptoms include headache, dizziness, diarrhea, and nausea. The more severe symptoms include blood diarrhea, colic, vomiting, albuminuria, jaundice, yellow vision, dyspnea, and convulsions. Death may result from respiratory failure, and if recovery occurs, the blindness in one or both eyes can be permanent.

Treatment must be symptomatic. Saline cathartics are given to help rid the bowel of the drug and decrease absorption; sedatives may be ordered to control convulsions, and respiratory stimulants are given if indicated.

Contraindications. Aspidium should be avoided for the patient who is pregnant, weak, or debilitated or who suffers from disease of the liver or kidney. Ulceration or inflammation of the gastrointestinal tract also contraindicates the use of aspidium. It should be avoided for children, if possible, since children seem to be especially susceptible to its toxic effects.

Quinacrine Hydrochloride (Atabrine Hydrochloride)

Quinacrine Hydrochloride, U.S.P.; Mepacaine Hydrochloride, B.P., is an antimalarial agent and, as such, is discussed in Chapter 21, p. 590. Quinacrine hydrochloride is usually effective against the beef tapeworm after a single dose. It is also effective against pork tapeworm and fish tapeworm. A saline purgative is given the evening before the administration of the drug. The next morning no food is allowed, but quinacrine hydrochloride may be given orally in divided doses along with sodium bicarbonate, or it may be given in solution through a duodenal tube. The usual adult dose is 0.5 to 1 Gm. together with 1 Gm. of sodium bicarbonate. The latter agent helps to prevent gastric irritation and vomiting.

Piperazine Salts

Piperazine compounds were introduced into medicine as agents for the treatment of gout. Although they proved to be ineffective for this condition, they have come to be considered drugs of choice for the treatment of roundworms and pinworms. They seem to induce a state of narcosis in the worms and are more effective on the mature than on the immature forms of the worm; hence the advisability of an interrupted treatment schedule. These drugs have the advantage of being low in toxicity. Furthermore, starvation and purgation need not accompany their administration as is true of a number of the other anthelmintics.

Preparation, dosage, and administration.

Piperazine Citrate, U.S.P. (Antepar Citrate). This agent is available in 250 and 500 mg. tablets and as a syrup, 100 mg. per milliliter, for oral administration. The daily dose is calculated on a basis of 50 mg. per kilogram of body weight, but a daily dose of 2 Gm. should not be exceeded. For pinworms, a single course of treatment (14 days) is recommended or 7 days with a rest period of one week and then 7 more days of treatment. For roundworms (ascaris), a single course of treatment of 5 to 7 days is usually satisfactory.

*Piperazine Tartrate** (Piperat Tartrate). This form is available in 250 and 500 mg. tablets and as an oral solution, 100 mg. per milliliter. Administration and dosage is the same as for piperazine citrate.

*Piperazine Calcium Edathamil** (Perin). This form is available in 500 mg. wafers and as a syrup, 100 mg. per milliliter, for oral administration. The proposed dosage is 75 mg. per kilogram of body weight (children and adults) for pinworms, administered as one dose or in two doses over a period of 15 days; for roundworms, 100 mg. per kilogram of body weight.

Piperazine Adipate and *Piperazine Phosphate.* Official in the B.P.

Side effects and toxic effects. As mentioned previously, these drugs are among the least toxic of the anthelmintics. Excessively large doses may produce urticaria, muscular weakness, blurred vision, and vomiting. The symptoms disappear when the drug is discontinued.

Diethylcarbamazine (Hetrazan)

Diethylcarbamazine is a piperazine derivative which has been used for a number of years in the treatment of filariasis, and more recently it has been found effective for the treatment of roundworms (ascariasis). Like the piperazine preparations, its use need not be accompanied by

*Described in annual publication of A. M. A. Council on Drugs, N.N.D., 1960.

purgation and starvation. It appears to offer no advantage over salts of piperazine in the treatment of ascariasis.

Preparation, dosage, and administration.

Diethylcarbamazine Citrate, U.S.P. (Hetrazan). This drug is available in 50 mg. tablets and as a syrup, 30 mg. per milliliter, for oral administration. The usual treatment for ascariasis consists of 13 mg. per kilogram of body weight daily for 4 days. For the treatment of filariasis, the dose is 2 mg. per kilogram of body weight three times daily after meals, for 7 to 21 days.

Side effects and toxic effects. Fever, leukocytosis, and swelling and tenderness of the lymphatic glands are frequently seen in patients treated for filariasis. Other symptoms include allergic manifestations, headache, nausea, and vomiting.

Hexylresorcinol

Hexylresorcinol is an effective anthelmintic against roundworm, hookworm, pinworm, and the dwarf tapeworm. It exerts a paralyzing effect on the muscle of the parasite. It is less potent than some of the other anthelmintics, but it has the advantages of low toxicity and mildness which permits it to be used for children and debilitated individuals for whom some of the other anthelmintics are contraindicated. It is useful when mixed infestations are present.

Preparation, dosage, and administration.

Hexylresorcinol, U.S.P., B.P. This drug is available in pills containing 100 and 200 mg. of the drug. These are coated with a tough gelatin covering. A single oral dose of 1 Gm. for adults and 0.1 to 0.6 Gm. for pre-school children may prove effective in a large number of infections. A saline purgative the evening before and also 2 to 4 hours after administration of the drug is recommended. Food is withheld during the treatment. The procedure may need to be repeated after 3 to 4 days.

When the capsules of hexylresorcinol are administered, it is important that they be swallowed intact. If broken in the mouth, extensive irritation may result.

Side effects and toxic effects. The main untoward effect of hexylresorcinol is that of local irritation. Therapeutic doses do not seem to cause systemic toxicity.

Tetrachloroethylene

Tetrachloroethylene is said to be the drug of choice against hookworm. It is especially effective against *Necator americanus*. It is not particularly effective against other intestinal parasites. It has, to a great extent, replaced carbon tetrachloride as an anthelmintic. It is relatively insoluble in water, and in the absence of alcohol and fat in the intestine, very little drug is absorbed after oral administration. This probably explains its low level of toxicity.

Tetrachloroethylene should not be used for ascariasis because it irritates the worms, and in their attempt to escape from the drug they may migrate into the bile ducts and liver or cause intestinal obstruction and perforation. In mixed infestations of both hookworm and ascaris (which often occurs) hexylresorcinol or piperazine should be administered first.

Preparation, dosage, and administration.

Tetrachloroethylene, U.S.P., B.P. Gelatin capsules in 0.5 and 1 ml. are available for oral administration. The adult dose is 3 ml., and the dose for children is 0.2 ml. for each year up to the age of 15 years.

The drug should be stored in a cool place to avoid the formation of the poisonous substance phosgene. The effectiveness of the drug is increased by a saline purge the evening before as well as after the administration of the drug. Food is withheld the morning of treatment, and fats, oils, and alcohol should be avoided throughout the treatment. One dose of the drug may prove sufficient unless ova are found in the stools after a period of 1 week.

Side effects and toxic effects. Dizziness, drowsiness, giddiness, nausea, and vomiting occur occasionally. It is as effective as carbon tetrachloride but much less toxic.

Methylrosaniline Chloride (Gentian Violet)

Methylrosaniline chloride is used in the treatment of strongyloides and pinworm infestation. It is more effective for the first type of parasite than for the second. Pinworms are probably best treated with one of the piperazine salts.

Preparation, dosage, and administration.

Methylrosaniline Chloride Tablets (Gentian Violet), U.S.P. This preparation is administered orally three times a day before meals for a period of 2 weeks. Enteric-coated tablets are used. The usual adult dose is 60 mg. (10 mg. for children) three times a day for 1 to 2 weeks. Patients who show a poor response after oral therapy may respond more satisfactorily after duodenal intubation with a 1 per cent solution of the drug.

Side effects. Side effects such as nausea, vomiting, abdominal cramps, and diarrhea may occur.

Dithiazanine Iodide (Delvex)

Dithiazanine is one of the cyanine dyes which exhibits anthelmintic properties. It is said to be effective against *Trichuris trichiura* (whipworm), *Strongyloides stercoralis* (threadworm), *Enterobius vermicularis* (pinworm), and *Ascaris lumbricoides* (roundworm). It is also said to be effective for hookworm (*Necator americanus*), especially if supplemented with other hookworm drug therapy. It is believed to be inferior to tetrachloroethylene for this purpose, however.

Preparation, dosage, and administration.

Dithiazanine Iodide (Delvex). This agent is available in 50, 100, and 200 mg. enteric-coated tablets. The tablets should be swallowed whole. The usual oral adult dose is 100 to 200 mg. three times a day for a period of 5 days or more. For children weighing 20 to 60 pounds, the total dose of 100 mg. for every 10 pounds of weight is administered in divided doses after meals for 5 to 10 days. Reduction of dosage is recommended if the drug is not well tolerated.

Side effects and toxic effects. The drug seems to have a low level of toxicity unless for some reason systemic absorption occurs. Side effects may include nausea and vomiting and diarrhea. It is administered after meals preferably. The medication will cause the stool to be blue colored. No dietary restrictions are necessary.

Drugs used in treatment of schistosomiasis (a trematode infestation)

Schistosomiasis is a disease caused by a parasite which burrows through the skin. The drugs used in treatment include antimony potassium tartrate, stibophen (Fuadin), and Miracil-D (Nilodin). These preparations are not equally effective for all types of blood flukes which may cause this disease.

Antimony Potassium Tartrate (Tartar Emetic)

Antimony Potassium Tartrate, U.S.P., B.P. (Tartar Emetic). This preparation is administered intravenously as a 0.5 per cent solution. The initial dose recommended is 40 mg. Dosage thereafter is gradually increased. The total dosage for a course of treatment is 1.5 to 2 Gm. Therapy with this drug has been known to result in changes in the heart and liver and sometimes in other organs.

Stibophen (Fuadin)

Stibophen, U.S.P., B.P. (Fuadin). This is an antimony compound which is considered the drug of choice of schistosomiasis. It is administered intramuscularly. It is available in a solution (300 mg. in 5 ml.). Small doses are given initially and gradually increased. Therapy is interspersed with rest periods. The initial dose is 100 mg., and this is increased to as much as 300 mg., up to a total dose of 2.5 Gm.

Miracil-D (Nilodin)

Miracil-D (Nilodin). This is a relatively new synthetic preparation. Its precise mode of action is unknown but it interferes with the reproductive function of the parasite (egg production) and eventually causes its death. It can be administered orally in enteric-coated tablets. Dosage is calculated on the basis of 10 mg. per kilogram of body weight. It is given in two divided doses daily for 10 days. Nausea, vomiting, and gastric distress are sometimes experienced. Toxic dosage is said to border closely on therapeutic dosage.

Other anthelmintics

Santonin, chenopodium, thymol, and carbon tetrachloride are older anthelmintics which have, to a great extent, been replaced by safer, less toxic but also effective agents.

Therapeutic résumé

The drugs of choice for the treatment of helminthiasis include the following:

1. Against tapeworms—quinacrine, aspidium, and hexylresorcinol.

2. Against roundworms and whipworms—piperazine salts, diethylcarbamazine, and dithiazanine.

3. Against pinworms—piperazine salts, dithiazanine, hexylresorcinol, and gentian violet. Pinworms do not cling to the intestinal wall and may also be expelled by the use of a cathartic or enema. The anal region must be kept clean, and scratching of the anal region must be avoided if reinfection is to be prevented. Underclothing, washcloths, etc. must be boiled to kill the eggs of the parasite. Reinfection is a major problem.

4. Against hookworms—tetrachloroethylene and hexylresorcinol.

5. For strongyloidiasis—diethylcarbamazine and diethiazanine.

6. For schistosomiasis—antimony compounds (antimony potassium tartrate and stibophen) and miracil-D.

7. For filariasis—diethylcarbamazine seems to be the drug of choice, especially for the removal of the microfilariae, although the adult form of the worm is not much affected.

Amebiasis and amebicides

Although a number of nonpathogenic amebas may be found in the human bowel, amebiasis or amebic dysentery is a disease caused by the *Entamoeba histolytica*. The disease has become world wide and is no longer limited to tropical regions. The parasite occurs in two forms: the active motile form, known as a trophozoite, and the cystic form, which is inactive, resistant to drugs, and present in the intestinal excretions. The cysts seem to form in the lumen of the intestine when living conditions, for some reason, become unfavorable. Outside the body the cyst becomes the source of infection to others when transmitted by flies or contaminated food and water. Only the cystic forms of the parasite can cause the disease because the motile forms are killed by gastric acid.

The initial infection of the bowel is known as intestinal amebiasis and is associated with diarrhea and the presence of the motile forms of the parasite in the stools. However, many persons exhibit few clinical symptoms of the disease, although they may carry the parasite.

Secondary amebiasis means that the parasites have migrated to other parts of the body such as the liver (where an amebic abscess may develop), spleen, lungs, etc. Only motile forms of the parasite invade the tissues. The amebas live at the expense of the host and always produce areas of tissue destruction in the bowel, although in certain individuals few symptoms of the disease may be noted. Apparently in these persons tissue repair keeps up with the tissue destruction.

Complete cure of the disease is difficult to attain because it is necessary to kill not the majority of the parasites but all of them, if relapse is to be avoided.

Drugs used in the treatment of amebiasis include those drugs used for extraintestinal amebic infection (emetine and chloroquine) and those used for intestinal amebiasis, which includes the organic arsenicals, halogenated oxyquinolines, and antibiotics. Many physicians are of the opinion that the disease is best treated by using a combination of several drugs.

Drugs used for extraintestinal amebiasis

Ipecac and emetine

Ipecac is the dried root of the *Cephaëlis ipecacuanha,* a perennial shrub growing in Brazil and other South American countries. It was long used by native people in the treatment of diarrhea. It contains two alkaloids, emetine and cephaeline, both of which are amebicidal, although emetine is the more potent agent. Emetine apparently has a direct lethal action on the *Entamoeba histolytica* when it is in a motile form, but it has little effect on amebic cysts. It is readily absorbed from parenteral sites of administration but is excreted rather slowly. It may therefore produce cumulative effects in the tissues.

Uses. The chief use of emetine is to control the symptoms of acute amebic dysentery or the symptoms which may suddenly develop during chronic phases of the disease. It has come to be regarded as second only to chloroquine for the treatment of amebic hepatitis and amebic abscess in the liver. It should not be used for the relief of mild symptoms or for the treatment of carriers. Preparations of ipecac are seldom used because of their tendency to cause gastrointestinal irritation.

Preparation, dosage, and administration.

Emetine Hydrochloride, U.S.P., B.P. This preparation is available in 1 ml. ampules containing 30 or 60 mg. of the drug in solution. The usual daily adult dose is 1 mg. per kilogram of body weight. The dosage range for adults may be from 30 to 60 mg. For children, the dose is 10 to 20 mg., depending on their weight and age. The drug is given both by deep subcutaneous and deep intramuscular injection, over a period of 5 to 10 days. Enteric-coated tablets have been given orally, but they are prone to cause irritation of the digestive tract.

Side effects and toxic effects. Emetine is a general protoplasmic poison and causes a variety of toxic reactions. Degenerative changes in the liver, heart, kidney, and muscles may occur. Cardiac changes may vary from disturbance in rhythm to acute myocarditis and heart failure. Other symptoms of poisoning include dizziness, nausea and vomiting, severe diarrhea, and albuminuria. Pain is often experienced at the site of injection. Emetine is contraindicated for patients with organic disease of the heart and kidneys. It should be avoided for the pregnant, the aged, and the debilitated.

Six weeks to 2 months should intervene between courses of treatment.

Chloroquine (Aralen)

Chloroquine is one of the antimalarial drugs which also has amebicidal activity. Because it reaches many parts of the body and localizes in organs such as the liver, it is highly effective for the treatment of extraintestinal amebiasis, particularly amebic hepatitis and amebic abscess. It is not recommended for intestinal forms of amebiasis, partly because it is well absorbed from the small bowel and partly because the tissue in the wall of the bowel fails to concentrate the drug as well as does the liver. Since hepatic involvement may occur early in amebiasis with few if any clinical signs, some physicians recommend early use of chloroquine or emetine along with a drug that is effective against the intestinal forms of the disease, such as one of the arsenicals or one of the oxyquinoline drugs.

Preparation, dosage, and administration.

Chloroquine Phosphate, U.S.P., B.P. (Aralen Phosphate). This drug is available in 125 and 250 mg. tablets. For extraintestinal amebiasis the usual oral dose for adults is 500 mg. three times daily for 2 weeks, followed by 750 mg. two times a week for several months. The course of treatment may be repeated or alternated with emetine therapy. To effect a cure it is necessary to administer a drug effective for intestinal amebiasis to all patients receiving this drug for extraintestinal amebiasis.

Side effects and toxic effects. Severe side effects or toxic effects are not associated with therapeutic doses of chloroquine phosphate. However, patients may complain of headache, itching, visual disturbances, and gastrointestinal upsets. These symptoms subside when the administration of the drug is stopped.

Drugs used for intestinal amebiasis

Organic arsenicals

Pentavalent arsenic compounds such as acetarsone and carbarsone, as well as trivalent compounds such as thioarsenites, are amebicidal. Some arsenicals which were first used for syphilis have been found effective for amebic dysentery. Acetarsone has been replaced by carbarsone because the latter agent is less toxic.

Carbarsone

Carbarsone is one of the organic arsenicals and contains 28.5 per cent arsenic. It is absorbed slowly after oral or rectal administration and is excreted rather slowly by the kidney.

It is especially effective for chronic intestinal amebiasis uncomplicated by hepatic involvement. It is not effective against amebas in abscesses of the liver or other organs. It is also used in treatment of trichomonal infections of the vagina.

Preparation, dosage, and administration.

Carbarsone, U.S.P., B.P. Carbarsone is available in tablets, 250 mg., for oral administration and as vaginal suppositories, 130 mg. The adult oral dose for amebiasis is 250 mg. two or three times daily for 7 to 10 days. For acute amebiasis, a retention enema (for adults) may be prepared by dissolving 2 Gm. of the drug in 200 ml. of a warm 2 per cent sodium bicarbonate solution. The enema may be repeated every other night for five times. A cleansing enema should preferably precede the treatment. For trichomonal infections the dose is 1 suppository daily.

Side effects and toxic effects. Although carbarsone is considered one of the least toxic of the arsenicals, overdosage can produce damage to the liver and kidneys. Serious toxic effects rarely occur, however, although cutaneous rash, loss of weight, abdominal distress, and diarrhea have been noted. Exfoliative dermatitis, encephalitis, and damage of the optic nerve are almost unknown, but such effects must be kept in mind when an arsenical drug is being administered. Since excretion of the drug is rather slow there is a tendency to develop cumulative effects. BAL is effective in the treatment of arsenical poisoning.

Carbarsone is contraindicated for patients who have renal or hepatic pathology.

Glycobiarsol (Milibis)

Glycobiarsol is a pentavalent arsenical combined with bismuth (15 per cent arsenic and 42 per cent bismuth). It is recommended for the treatment of intestinal amebiasis only. It exhibits low toxicity because it is not very soluble and is poorly absorbed. It needs to be supplemented with other therapy when amebic hepatitis or deep-seated infestation is present. This drug has also been used for monilial and trichomonal infections of the vagina.

Preparation, dosage, and administration.

Glycobiarsol, U.S.P. (Milibis). This agent is available in 500 mg. tablets and in vaginal suppositories, 250 mg. The usual adult dose for amebiasis is 500 mg. three times daily for 1 week. Larger doses are sometimes necessary when diarrhea is severe. Additional course of treatment is indicated if pathogenic amebas continue to be found in the stool.

Side effects and toxic effects. This drug is not very toxic, but the presence of arsenic in the compound necessitates caution in its use.

Arsthinol (Belarsen)

Arsthinol is an organic thio-arsenical compound which has been found effective for intestinal amebiasis and also for yaws.

Preparation, dosage, and administration.

Arsthinol* (Belarsen). This compound is available in 100 mg. tablets for oral administration. The daily oral dose is 10 mg. per kilogram of body weight, not to exceed 500 mg. daily. It is given over a period of 5 days.

Side effects and toxic effects. The side effects are said to be minor but the possibility of arsenic poisoning should not be overlooked. Rest periods between courses of treatment are recommended.

Iodohydroxyquinoline compounds

Included in this group of compounds is chiniofon, diiodohydroxyquin, and iodochlorhydroxyquin. The following formulas indicate why these compounds are also called halogenated hydroxyquinolines.

Chiniofon   Diiodohydroxyquin   Iodochlorhydroxyquin
             (Diodoquin)   (Vioform)

*Described in annual publication of A. M. A. Council on Drugs, N.N.D., 1960.

Chiniofon (Yatren)

Chiniofon is an oxyquinoline derivative which contains about 28 per cent iodine. The drug has a direct amebicidal action, although just how it kills the trophozoites is not known. It apparently is useful only for the intestinal form of the disease and is ineffective for amebic abscess and amebic hepatitis. It can be used for ambulatory patients and for carriers. It does not bring about a cure of the disease when given alone.

Preparation, dosage, and administration.

Chiniofon, N.F.; *Chiniofon Sodium,* B.P. This drug is marketed in enteric-coated tablets and in powder form. The official preparation contains sodium bicarbonate, the sodium salt as well as the acidic substance of chiniofon. The usual oral adult dose is 250 mg. three times a day with meals for 7 to 10 days. Several courses of treatment may be necessary.

Side effects and toxic effects. Chiniofon has been reported to cause diarrhea, but serious symptoms of toxicity do not seem to occur when dosage is kept within the therapeutic range. It should be used with caution for patients with liver damage. It should be avoided for patients sensitive to iodine.

Diiodohydroxyquin (Diodoquin)

Diiodohydroxyquin is an oxyquinoline derivative which contains about 62 per cent iodine. Like chiniofon, it is directly amebicidal, although the mechanism of its action is not known. It is useful for intestinal amebiasis but not for amebic abscess or amebic hepatitis. Difference of opinion exists about its value as an amebicide. Some authorities consider it a valuable amebicide, especially when given with emetine.

It is also used in the treatment of Trichomonas infections of the vagina.

Preparation, dosage, and administration.

Diiodohydroxyquin, U.S.P. (Diodoquin); *Di-iodohydroxyquinoline,* B.P. This preparation is available as a bulky powder and in tablets, 650 mg. (300 mg., B.P.). It is administered orally as an amebicide and by insufflation for vaginitis. The adult dose is 650 mg. (650 mg. to 1 Gm.) three times a day and is given preferably between meals.

Side effects and toxic effects. Diiodohydroxyquin exhibits a low level of toxicity, which is probably explained by the fact that it is not very soluble. Symptoms of iodism may develop (itching, dermatitis, abdominal discomfort, diarrhea, and headache). It is contraindicated for patients who have liver damage and for those who are sensitive to iodine.

Iodochlorhydroxyquin (Vioform)

Iodochlorhydroxyquin is also an oxyquinoline derivative which has an iodine content of approximately 40 per cent. It is poorly soluble, although some intestinal absorption does occur. Like the other drugs of this group of compounds, it is most effective for intestinal amebiasis and is ineffective for amebic abscesses or amebic hepatitis. It is inexpensive, and its administration does not require bed rest for the patient. It stains clothing and linens a yellow color. Some authorities consider this the least effective of the iodohydroxyquinolines, but differences of opinion exist about their relative values. It is also employed in treatment of Trichomonas infections of the vagina and for various types of dermatitis.

Preparation, dosage, and administration.

Iodochlorhydroxyquin, U.S.P. (Vioform). This drug is available as a powder, as tablets, 250 mg., and as an ointment. The powder is suitably buffered for use as a vaginal insufflate. The usual adult dose is 250 mg. three times a day for 10 days. The drug may be used alternately with carbarsone, i.e., courses of treatment with one drug may follow the use of the other drug.

Side effects and toxic effects. Toxic reactions are seldom encountered. Mild symptoms of iodism may occur and some patients experience a severe gastritis. Contraindications are the same as those for chiniofon.

Antibiotics for amebiasis

A number of antibiotics have been used in the treatment of amebiasis but only one, fumagillin, has thus far been found to be directly amebicidal. Other antibiotics such as erythromycin and oxytetracycline (Terramycin) are effective but act indirectly by decreasing the number of intestinal bacteria on which the *Entamoeba histolytica* depends for some essential factor or factors.

Intestinal amebiasis appears to be controlled only as long as the associated bacteria are held in check. The tetracyclines and erythromycin are discussed elsewhere (see Index). One of the disadvantages of drugs such as oxytetracycline is that while it may be effective for mild amebiasis, it may produce marked gastrointestinal symptoms (diarrhea) which may be more troublesome than the mild amebiasis.

Since antibiotics are not effective for extraintestinal amebiasis, the concomitant administration of a drug such as chloroquine is advocated.

Fumagillin (Fumidil)

Fumagillin is an antibiotic obtained from the culture of *Aspergillus fumigatus.* It is a crystalline compound, the chemical structure of which has not been determined. Fumagillin is highly active against the *Escherichia histolytica,* but it does not exert much effect on the bacterial flora of the bowel. The emergence of an overgrowth of fungi, yeasts, and resistant bacteria is therefore not likely to occur.

Fumagillin is recommended for the treatment of intestinal amebiasis. It is not useful for the extraintestinal manifestations of the disease. Fumagillin in combination with erythromycin or oxytetracycline may provide more effective control than any one of the antibiotics used alone.

Preparation, dosage, and administration.

Fumagillin (Fumidil). This antibiotic is available in 10 mg. tablets for oral administration. The usual adult dose is 40 mg. daily in divided doses over a period of 10 to 14 days. For debilitated persons and children, dosage is determined on a basis of age and weight.

Side effects and toxic effects. The side effects are seldom such that therapy must be discontinued, and symptoms usually disappear as soon as dosage is decreased or administration of the drug is discontinued. The following effects are encountered: epigastric distress, loss of appetite, nausea and vomiting, diarrhea, headache, dizziness, and dermatitis. Occasionally, the white blood cells are decreased and therefore periodic examinations of the patients' blood are recommended.

*Described in annual publication of A. M. A. Council on Drugs, N.N.D., 1960.

References

Beckman, H.: Drugs, Their Nature, Action, and Use, Philadelphia, 1958, W. B. Saunders Co.

Brown, H. W., Chan, K. F., and Hussey, K. L.: Treatment of Enterobiasis and Ascariasis With Piperazine, J. A. M. A. **161:** 515, 1956.

Bumbalo, T. S., and Plummer, L. J.: Piperazine (Antepar) in the Treatment of Pinworm and Roundworm Infections, Medical Clinics of North America, Philadelphia, 1957, W. B. Saunders Co., pp. 575-585.

Goodman, L., and Gilman, A.: The Pharmacological Basis of Therapeutics, New York, 1955, The Macmillan Co.

Jung, R. C., and Faust, E. C.: The Treatment of Intestinal Parasitic Infections, A. M. A. Arch. Int. Med. **98:** 494, 1956.

Kean, B. H., and Chowdhury, A. B.: The Choice of Drugs for Intestinal Parasitism. In Modell, W. (editor): Drugs of Choice, 1960-1961, St. Louis, 1960, The C. V. Mosby Co., pp. 379-391.

Salter, W. T.: A Textbook of Pharmacology, Philadelphia, 1952, W. B. Saunders Co.

Sodeman, W. A., and Jung, R. C.: Treatment of Teniasis With Quinacrine Hydrochloride, J. A. M. A. **148:** 285, 1952.

Sollmann, T.: A Manual of Pharmacology, Philadelphia, 1957, W. B. Saunders Co.

Swartzweider, J. C., and others: Dithiazanine, an Effective Broad Spectrum Anthelmintic, J. A. M. A. **165:** 2063, 1957.

Chapter 24

Minerals, vitamins,
and hormones
used as drugs

If the student stops to consider the place of certain drugs in the body economy, she will quickly recognize that, in some instances, substances given as medicaments are not foreign to the body but are provided as "replacement therapy." They stand in contrast to a large number of drugs, the "foreign" compounds such as the anesthetics, the antibiotics, the antihistaminics, etc. given to achieve a certain desirable pharmacologic effect. This "normal" group of drugs are, rather, natural constituents of the body or the diet which are required in certain quantities to preserve healthy function. When absent, as in the nutritional deficiency diseases, they must be replaced, and as a replacement the normal vitamin or mineral then becomes, in a sense, a drug having most dramatic effects in curing the symptoms of disease caused by its lack.

On the other hand, such normal components of the body can sometimes be given in excessive amounts, with deleterious effects on body functions. In the following pages some of the more important compounds of this group will be discussed, with particular attention to their "pharmacologic" action—their effects when they are given as drugs to remedy certain symptoms of deficiency. As will be noted, such substances are sometimes used not only as replacements but are also given occasionally in physiologically excessive amounts to produce desired effects in disease; for example, water may be given in large amounts, not only to make up a deficiency of water in a dehydrated patient but also to maintain active flow of urine to promote the excretion of a toxic chemical. Similarly, the corticosteroids are frequently given to persons with normal adrenal function for their anti-inflammatory action at (physiologically) high levels of dosage.

Inorganic needs

Water

Dehydration associated with disease, such as loss of fluid by disease, or in adrenal cortical insufficiency or diabetes, is usually associated with severe electrolyte disturbance and generally requires expert medical management in selecting the proper parenteral fluids and in following the electrolyte pattern. Simple dehydration involving water loss without electrolyte loss (as may be caused by insufficient water intake) can be remedied by restoration of water by mouth or parenterally by giving isotonic (5 per cent) glucose solution.

Excesses of water relative to salt produce the symptoms known as water intoxication or miner's cramps, with muscular pains, spasmodic movements, and convulsions. It is a moot question whether this condition should be regarded as water excess or salt lack.

The commonest form of water excess occurs after extensive losses of water and electrolytes by sweating, followed by drinking large amounts of plain water. Its prevention and treatment involve "normalizing" the tonicity of body water by increasing the intake of salt to balance the water ingested, often in the form of salt tablets.

Sodium and Potassium

These cations (positive ions) are the principal ones in the extracellular and intracellular spaces, respectively. Normally, their concentration is automatically regulated by renal excretion, but a number of disease states can produce serious alterations in their levels. In addition, the possibility of administering rather concentrated solutions of the electrolytes parenterally makes it possible to produce inadvertent sodium and, particularly, potassium poisoning during efforts to correct deficiencies.

Sodium loss tends to occur in a number of pathologic states such as loss of gastric secretions, in metabolic disorders such as Addison's disease, and in prolonged diuresis with some of the mercurial drugs. Replacement can be made by parenteral means, giving hypertonic solutions of sodium chloride intravenously if rapid restoration is necessary. Such correction of electrolyte disturbance requires considerable experience and care.

Sodium excess is believed typical of congestive heart failure with edema and in the edema of advanced kidney disease or cirrhosis of the liver. Withholding dietary sodium is frequently practiced in these conditions in order to promote gradual net loss of sodium from the body through excretion.

Potassium loss is also a consequence of certain metabolic diseases or kidney diseases or the loss of gastrointestinal secretions which are rich in this ion. Potassium deficit is believed to affect the functions of both skeletal and cardiac muscle. One hazard of the parenteral correction of potassium deficiency is the production of potassium poisoning, and the administration of potassium salts intravenously must be performed cautiously to avoid reaching a concentration which can stop the heart.

Preparation, dosage, and administration. The following preparations are used to treat deficiency states.

Potassium Chloride, U.S.P., B.P. This agent is available in 300 and 500 mg. tablets for oral administration and in solution for parenteral administration.

Potassium Citrate, N.F., B.P. This form is administered orally.

Potassium Triplex. This is a nonofficial preparation of potassium acetate, potassium bicarbonate, and potassium citrate in aqueous solution. It contains 0.5 Gm. of each of these salts in each 5 ml. of solution, which provides 15 mEq. of potassium. It is administered orally.

Calcium

Calcium is necessary to the body for the growth of bone, for the regulation of the activities of nerves, muscles, and glands, for the maintenance of cardiac and vascular tone, and for the normal coagulation of blood. The intake of calcium in a balanced diet is sufficient for normal needs of the body, but in diseased conditions associated with a deficiency of calcium, the drug is administered in the form of its soluble salts, usually the chloride or lactate. When the calcium concentration of the blood is below normal, the continued administration of soluble calcium salts, especially calcium lactate, increases the calcium content to some extent, but it falls rapidly when the drug is discontinued.

Deficiency in calcium salts affects the peripheral neuromuscular mechanism, resulting in twitching and spasms in the muscles involved. Either a deficiency or an excess of calcium salts alters the function of the heart muscle. The absence or deficiency of salts of calcium causes the potassium salts to be more prominent in their effect, resulting in undue relaxation of the heart and cessation of beating. An excess of salts of calcium produces a prolonged state of contraction known as "calcium rigor."

The absorption of calcium will depend upon how well it is kept in solution in the digestive tube. An acid reaction favors calcium solubility; hence calcium is absorbed mainly in the upper intestinal tract. Absorption is decreased by the presence of alkalies and large amounts of fatty acids with which the calcium forms insoluble soaps. Adequate intake of vitamin D appears to promote calcium absorption. A normal individual excretes calcium both in the feces and in the urine.

Daily requirements. The average adult needs approximately 0.8 Gm. of calcium daily, but pregnant women or lactating mothers as well as growing children frequently need at least twice this amount. (1.5 to 2 Gm.)*

Patients who are bedridden tend to develop a negative calcium balance because the ion is lost from the bones and is excreted. This is likely to be serious only when long immobilization of the patient is necessary or when diseases of the bone are present.

Uses. Calcium salts are used as a nutritional supplement, particularly during pregnancy and lactation. They are specific in the treatment of hypocalcemic tetany. They have also been used for their antispasmodic effects in cases of abdominal pain, tenesmus, and colic due to disease of the gallbladder or painful contractions of the ureters. The basic salts of calcium are used as antacids.

Preparation, dosage, and administration.

Calcium Chloride, U.S.P., B.P. This is a salt of calcium which is irritating to the tissues when given parenterally other than by intravenous injection. Care must be taken that the needle does not slip out of the vein and cause serious irritation of tissue. Calcium chloride may be given orally, but it tends to cause gastric disturbance. It is given best in capsules, when administered orally. It is an acidifying salt and for that reason promotes the absorption of calcium. The average adult dose for oral administration is 1 Gm. (15 gr.) four times a day. *Calcium Chloride Injection*, U.S.P., is given intravenously.

Calcium Gluconate, U.S.P., B.P. This preparation is a white, crystalline or granular powder which is odorless and tasteless. It has an advantage over calcium chloride in that it is more palatable for oral administration and also that it can be given parenterally. It should not be administered intramuscularly to children, however, since there is some danger of abscess formation and tissue slough. For severe hypocalcemic tetany, *Calcium Gluconate Injection*, U.S.P., B.P., is administered slowly in a 10 per cent solution, intravenously (5 to 30 ml.). For mild hypocalcemic tetany, calcium gluconate may be given orally, 5 Gm. three times a day after meals. It is available in tablet form for oral administration. One part of calcium gluconate is soluble in 30 parts of cold water or in 5 parts of boiling water. Hence the nurse may be expected to dissolve the preparation in hot water before giving it to the patient, unless oral solutions are available.

Calcium Lactate, N.F., B.P. This compound is given orally. Its physical properties are similar to those of calcium gluconate. The usual adult dose is 5 Gm., which may be repeated three or four times a day. It is

*National Research Council, Recommended Dietary Allowances, Bulletin 589, 1958, p. 18.

marketed in 0.5 and 1 Gm. tablets. Calcium lactate is also more soluble in hot water than in cold and preferably should be dissolved in hot water before giving it to the patient. Calcium lactate is not given parenterally.

Organic needs

Vitamins

The chief class of organic nutrients which are sometimes required for replacement therapy are the vitamins. These are essential dietary constituents. Because the body itself cannot synthesize them in adequate amounts and because they are necessary for normal metabolic processes, they must be supplied from outside the body in continuing adequate amounts or symptoms of disease or death will result.

As biochemistry and cellular physiology have progressed, it has been recognized that the vitamins are not only necessary to man and the mammals but are also required for normal function of most living cells, including bacteria and plants, as well as the invertebrates and other animals only distantly related to man. Thus these compounds serve functions common to most living cells, but they are required as *dietary* components only by those living organisms which cannot synthesize them.

Those vitamins whose functions have been classified have been found to act as *coenzymes* in chemical reactions essential to the maintenance of life. Certain vitamins such as biotin, ascorbic acid, and vitamin B_{12} have functions which are still not well understood in terms of a coenzyme function.

When the Polish chemist Casimer Funk isolated a substance from the coating of rice polishings, which he thought was the nature of an amine and essential to the preservation of life, he called it a "vitamine." Later discoveries showed that many of these important factors are not amines; therefore the letter "e" was dropped so that the name would not have chemical significance.

Although diseases directly attributed to vitamin deficiencies are rare in this country, with the possible exception of pellagra, deficiency states are encountered in persons who for one reason or another have been eating a restricted diet. Alcoholics frequently suffer a multiple vitamin deficiency, even though their caloric needs are met by alcohol. Sick persons may not absorb the vitamins in their food, due to some abnormality in the absorbing surface of the bowel or to excessive peristaltic action in that organ.

It has been suggested that vitamin deficiency may result from diets which are supposedly normal adequate diets. This may be likely to occur when individuals are living through periods of rapid growth, pregnancy, gastrointestinal upsets, and infections. Individuals exhibit differences in their ability to assimilate and metabolize vitamins and in their ability to store or destroy them.

Vitamin-deficient foods may be eaten because of lack of understanding of what constitutes a well-balanced diet, or because of poor preparation of food, or often because undesirable food habits have been developed. Poor preparation of food and undesirable food habits, although correctable, are changed, as a rule, with difficulty. This is particularly true of elderly persons, and for them it has been more satisfactory to add vitamins to certain of their foods than to attempt the formation of different habits of eating. The fact remains, however, that a properly selected diet ordinarily affords the adult an adequate supply of vitamins.

Present status of vitamins

Because potent vitamin concentrates are now available, it is possible to prescribe exact dosage of preparations in pure form rather than to rely entirely on foods rich in the required vitamins. This has materially enriched the clinical knowledge about vitamins by making possible specific therapy for deficiency conditions and a more accurate evaluation of the concentrate.

The rather easy availability of vitamin preparations has led to certain abuses. In many of the proprietary preparations there is no apparent relationship between the amount of vitamins present and the normal requirement represented by the average therapeutic dose.

Furthermore, there is no evidence that vitamins are of value for disease unless that disease is accompanied by some degree of vitamin deficiency. And although the individual suffering from malnutrition is more susceptible to certain infections than the normal person, the administration of excessive amounts of vitamins does not make the individual any more resistant to disease than does the administration of the amount just sufficient to meet normal metabolic requirements.

Despite this rational position which would indicate only a limited use of vitamins in medicine, it is well known that vitamins constitute a multimillion dollar annual expense to the American public. This excess has been condemned by many physicians, but it has continued, partly because of a successful public campaign that vitamins will improve even normal health and partly because this is one class of drugs that carries virtually no significant toxicity.

Because they are so widely, although sometimes unjustifiably, used and because of their essential biologic importance, they justify being given consideration as drugs.

Vitamin potency

The U.S.P units for vitamins A, B_1, C_{12}, D, and E are identical in value with the International Units. The Council on Drugs, formerly the Council on Pharmacy and Chemistry, decided some time ago that, when practicable, the vitamin content of preparations should be stated in milligrams in preference to micrograms or units. This is to help prevent the spread of misinformation about the potency of preparations. Since a milligram is equal to 1,000 micrograms, expression of vitamin content in terms of micrograms may be misleading.

The potency of vitamins A and D, when appearing on a label, must be in U.S.P. units, but the vitamin content of ascorbic acid, thiamine, riboflavin, nicotinic acid, nicotinamide, pyridoxine, menadione, and other vitamin K preparations, when expressed, must be in terms of milligrams.

The fat-soluble vitamins

The fat-soluble vitamins include vitamins A, D, E, and K. Since they are fat soluble, their absorption, assimilation, and metabolism in the body are influenced by the factors which affect absorption and metabolism of any fat. They are stored in the body in relatively large amounts.

Vitamin A

Vitamin A, the fat-soluble, growth-promoting vitamin, is essential for growth in the young and for the maintenance of health at all ages. The chemistry of this vitamin has been established. It is related to the carotenoid pigments of plants, especially carotene. In fact the term *vitamin A* may be applied to vitamin A, alpha-carotene, beta-carotene, gamma-carotene, and cryptoxanthin. The last four bodies are formed in plants and are precursors of vitamin A in the body.

Accompanying are the structural formulas for vitamin A and beta-carotene. Beta-carotene in the body is hydrolyzed to form two molecules of vitamin A.

Chemists have failed to discover vitamin A in any plant foodstuff. The carotene of plants, therefore, seems to supply the pro-vitamin from which the body tissues prepare vitamin A. The amount of chlorophyl in the plant is a rough indication of the amount of carotene present. Animal fats such as that found in butter, milk, eggs, and fish liver are also sources of the carotenoids; in this case they are originally also derived from plants and are simply stored in the animal tissues.

Vitamin A is essential in man to promote normal growth and development of bones and teeth and to maintain the health of epithelial tissues of the body. Its function in relation to normal vision and the prevention of night blindness has been carefully studied. Vitamin A actually makes

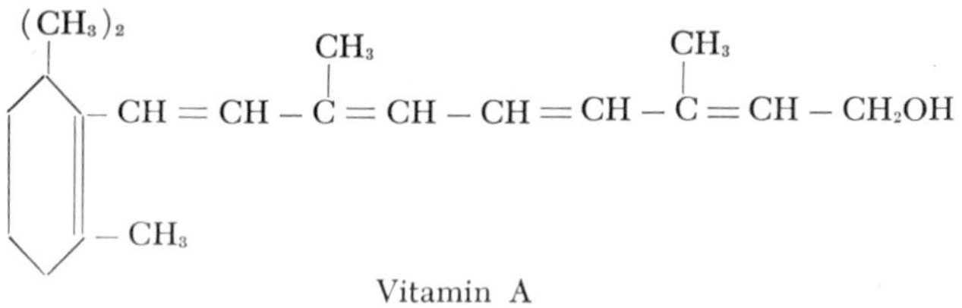

$$\text{Vitamin A structure}$$

(CH$_3$)$_2$ ... CH = CH – C = CH – CH = CH – C = CH – CH$_2$OH

with CH$_3$ groups

Vitamin A

$$\text{Beta-carotene structure}$$

(CH$_3$)$_2$ ... – CH = CH – C = CH – CH = CH – C = CH – CH

(CH$_3$)$_2$ ... – CH = CH – C = CH – CH = CH – C = CH – CH

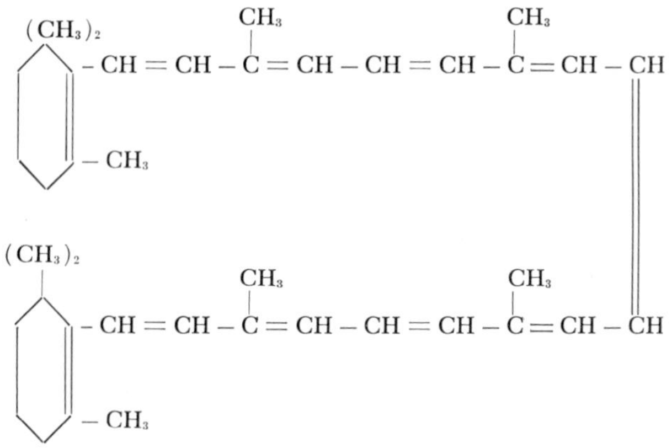

Beta-carotene (provitamin A)

up a portion of one of the major retinal pigments, rhodopsin, and is thus required for normal "rod vision" in the retina of man and many of the animals.

Absorption, storage, and excretion. Vitamin A and also carotene are readily absorbed from the normal gastrointestinal tract. Due to the fact that this vitamin and its precursors are fat soluble, their absorption is related to the ability of the body to absorb fat. Efficient absorption is therefore dependent on the presence of adequate bile salts in the intestine. Certain conditions such as obstructive jaundice, some infectious diseases, and the presence of mineral oil in the intestine may result in a definite deficiency of vitamin A in spite of the fact that the amount ingested was normal.

Vitamin A is stored in the liver to a greater extent than elsewhere. The liver also functions in changing carotene to vitamin A. This function is inhibited in certain diseases of the liver and also in diabetes. The amount of vitamin A stored in the liver depends upon the dietary intake. When the intake is high or even excessive, the stores formed in the liver may become sufficient to last for a long time. Vitamin A is lost chiefly by destruction. Little is lost through the ordinary channels of excretion.

Uses. Vitamin A is used to treat or relieve symptoms associated with a deficiency of vitamin A (avitaminosis), such as night blindness (nyctalopia), keratinization of epithelial cells, retarded growth, xerophthalmia, keratomalacia, weakness, and increased susceptibility of mucous membranes to infection.

The widespread use of vitamin A preparations to prevent upper respiratory infections in the winter is, however, open to question when they are given to a patient whose diet is adequate. The diet low in vitamin A should be corrected with foods rather than with drugs. On the other hand, it appears that large doses of vitamin A may be given with no apparent harm to the adult. On the other hand, excessive doses have been known to produce toxic effects in rats and in young children.

There are times when vitamin A concentrates have a legitimate use as supplements to the diet. Increased need occurs during pregnancy and lactation, in infancy and in conditions characterized by lack of normal absorption and storage of vitamin A.

Daily requirement. It has been conclusively established that the vitamin A daily requirement is a rather large one, if optimum conditions of nutrition are to be maintained. Vitamin A requirement is particularly high during periods of rapid growth, pregnancy, lactation, and also in certain disease conditions in which body capacity for adequate absorption and utilization is impaired.

The minimum daily requirements for vitamin A are 1,500 units for infants, 3,000 units for children, and 4,000 units for adults.* It is thought that the therapeutic dosages should be at least three times these amounts. Although larger doses have been used in experimental studies, there is no evidence that justifies the use of more than 25,000 units per day. It has not been shown that excess dosage over and above the daily requirement is of value in the prevention of colds, influenza, etc. Dosages in excess of 200,000 units are injurious to infants.*

When the vitamin A requirement is met in the form of carotene or the pro-vitamin A, twice as many units of the carotene are required to produce the same effect.

Vitamin A and vitamins A and D combined—preparation, dosage, and administration.

Oleovitamin A, U.S.P. This is either fish liver oil alone or fish liver oil diluted with vegetable oil, or a solution of vitamin A concentrate in fish liver oil or vegetable oil. *Oleovitamin A Capsules*, U.S.P., are available, containing 1.5, 7.5, and 15 mg. of vitamin A (5,000, 25,000, and 50,000 U.S.P. units). Usual therapeutic dose is 7.5 mg. (25,000 units) daily.

Oleovitamin A and D Capsules, N.F. These capsules contain 5,000 units of vitamin A and 100 units of vitamin D.

Water-Miscible Vitamin A Solution, U.S.P. This contains 7.5 and 15 mg. in 1 ml. Usual therapeutic dose is 7.5 mg. daily.

*N.N.R., 1960, p. 712.

Water-Miscible Vitamin A Capsules, U.S.P. (Aquasol A). These capsules contain a form of oleovitamin A, made water-miscible by the addition of a dispersing agent. Capsules available contain 25,000, 50,000 and 100,000 U.S.P. units of vitamin A. The dosage is the same as that for water-miscible vitamin A solution.

Concentrated Vitamin A Solution, B.P. This preparation contains not less than 45,000 units of vitamin A activity in each gram.

Cod Liver Oil, N.F., B.P. This is partially destearinated. Usual dosage is 4 ml. orally; 4 ml. of Cod Liver Oil, N.F., contains 3,000 U.S.P. units of vitamin A and 300 U.S.P. units of vitamin D. Cod liver oil is one of the cheapest sources of vitamin A and vitamin D.

Nondestearinated Cod Liver Oil, N.F. Dosage is 4 ml. orally. Each gram contains not less than 850 U.S.P. units of vitamin A and 85 U.S.P. units of vitamin D.

The above preparations are usually administered orally. Preparations of vitamin A for intramuscular injection are available but are seldom used.

Halibut Liver Oil, N.F., B.P. Usual daily prophylactic dose for infants and adults is 0.1 ml. (1½ minims). Halibut liver oil, N.F., contains in each gram not less than 60,000 units of vitamin A and not less than 600 units of vitamin D. In 0.1 ml. there are 5,000 units of vitamin A.

Halibut Liver Oil Capsules, N.F., B.P. The N.F. capsules contain either 5,000 or 25,000 units of vitamin A and 500 or 2,500 units of vitamin D, respectively. The dose is usually 0.2 to 0.6 ml. daily.

Vitamin D

Vitamin D is a term applied to two or more substances which affect the proper utilization of calcium and phosphorus in the body. Two forms of naturally occurring vitamin D have been isolated. One of these forms is obtained as one of the products of irradiated ergosterol and is known as D_2 or calciferol. Ergosterol has therefore been shown to be a precursor of vitamin D. Investigation has shown further that there are a number of precursors which by irradiation can be changed into compounds that have vitamin D activity. Irradiation of 7-dehydro-cholesterol results in the formation of vitamin D_3 and is the form of vitamin found in irradiated milk and in a number of fish oils. It is formed also in the skin when an individual is exposed to sunlight. Irradiated ergosterol (calciferol) is the active constituent in various vitamin preparations such as viosterol, irradiated yeast, etc.

Vitamin D_2 and vitamin D_3, as well as other products of irradiated ergosterol, are capable of antirachitic activity.

Although vitamin D is an essential vitamin, it is contained in only a few foods of the average American diet. Small amounts are present in

Minerals, vitamins, and hormones used as drugs   647

herring, sardines, salmon, tuna fish, and eggs. Butter contains only a small amount of vitamin D.[*] Vitamin D is found in high concentrations in a number of fish oils (cod, burbot, halibut, and percomorph).

At present, milk is the chief commercial food product enriched by the addition of vitamin D concentrate. By federal regulation, milk products are standardized at 400 international units per quart. This represents a day's requirement of vitamin D.

Action and result. The exact mechanism by which vitamin D functions in the metabolism of calcium and phosphorus is not known. It seems to be concerned directly with the absorption of calcium and phosphorus from the intestinal tract. In the absence of vitamin D, the amount of these substances absorbed from the bowel is diminished to such an extent that even though the calcium and phosphate intake is adequate, rickets results.

An enzyme called alkaline phosphatase exists in the body and is closely related to phosphorus metabolism. It is distributed widely in the animal body and is active particularly in ossifying cartilage. When rickets is present the value for the phosphatase in the blood serum is high. This is thought to be due to leakage from the diseased bone. Administration of vitamin D causes the enzyme to return to normal slowly.

Symptoms of deficiency. The chief indication of vitamin D deficiency is rickets, characterized by irritability, craniotabes. prominent frontal bosses, delayed closing of the fontanels, soft bones, pigeon breast, rachitic rosary, flaring ribs, epiphyseal enlargement at wrists and elbows, muscular weakness, protruding abdomen, bowed legs, delayed eruption of teeth, abnormal ratio of calcium and phosphorus in the blood, and perhaps infantile tetany. Adult rickets is known as osteomalacia.

Daily requirement. It is thought that either the human requirement of vitamin D is relatively low or else it is met by the action of sunlight on the skin. A daily intake of 400 units is considered adequate to meet the ordinary requirements of all age groups.[†]

Older children and adults who live in a climate where they do not have access to abundant sunshine need to supplement their vitamin D intake. The amount supplied probably should be up to the minimum requirements for the infant. To prevent the development of rickets, it is important to start the administration of vitamin D early in the infant's life, and full dosage should be given by the second month.

Uses. The prevention of rickets in young children is one of the most justified uses of vitamin D. The initial dose should be about 200 units daily, with an increase in dosage up to 800 units by the second month.

[*]American Medical Association Council on Foods and Nutrition, Handbook of Nutrition; A Symposium, Chicago, 1943, p. 197.

[†]National Research Council: Recommended Dietary Allowances, Bulletin 589, 1958, p. 18.

Premature infants or those who seem to be especially susceptible to the development of rickets need a larger intake (800 to 1,200 units usually). When children already have rickets the dosage is also greater. The average daily dose usually is about 1,200 to 1,500 units, but in some instances it may be increased to as much as 60,000 or more units daily. Vitamin D-resistant rickets is a condition which does not respond to usual doses of vitamin D but requires unusually large doses. If nausea or anorexia appears, the vitamin should be discontinued temporarily.

Adult rickets, or osteomalacia, also calls for large doses of vitamin D, along with improved dietary and living conditions (more exposure to sunlight).

Patients suffering from bone fractures, especially elderly individuals, may benefit from the administration of vitamin D, thus promoting optimum conditions for the healing of bone.

Vitamin D may be administered in a number of conditions, such as arthritis, psoriasis, diarrhea, steatorrhea, etc., if there is good evidence that a deficiency of this vitamin exists. Large doses of vitamin D are of value in the treatment of lupus vulgaris.

Preparation, dosage, and administration. Many of the official preparations containing vitamin A and vitamin D are listed under preparations of vitamin A. In addition, preparations of irradiated ergosterol are listed.

Calciferol, U.S.P., B.P. (Vitamin D_2, Drisdol). The U.S.P. official preparation of this vitamin is available in capsules, each containing 50,000 U.S.P. units (1.25 mg.) and in solution, 0.25 mg. (10,000 U.S.P. units) per 1 Gm., for oral administration. The average therapeutic dose for rickets is 5,000 U.S.P. units (125 mcg.). The normal daily intake for adults is 400 U.S.P. units (10 mcg.). This preparation is especially suitable for severe or refractory rickets. Therapeutic dosage varies from 125 mcg. to 5 mg.

Activated 7-Dehydrocholesterol, U.S.P. (Vitamin D_3). This is prepared by irradiating 7-dehydrocholesterol. It is contained in a number of commercially available oleovitamin preparations. The dosage is the same as that for calciferol.

Synthetic Oleovitamin D, U.S.P. (Viosterol in Oil). This is a solution of activated ergosterol or activated 7-dehydrocholesterol in edible vegetable oil. It is administered orally. Dosage is similar to that of calciferol.

Dehydrotachysterol* (Hytakerol). This product is chemically related to calciferol, although its antirachitic potency is much less. It is used to correct the low blood calcium associated with hypoparathyroidism and for the treatment of rickets which is resistant to the usual forms of therapy. It is administered orally either as an oil solution (1 ml. containing

*Described in annual publication of A. M. A. Council on Drugs, N.N.D., 1960.

1.25 mg. of the crystalline drug) or in capsules (0.5 ml. containing 0.625 mg. of dehydrotachysterol).

Side effects and toxic effects. Certain pathologic changes have been noted in animals after the administration of excessive doses of vitamin D, and this vitamin represents the exceptional case of a vitamin in which excessive dosage can cause disease. Doses greatly in excess of the usual therapeutic level can so increase the renal excretion of phosphate and calcium that these elements are withdrawn from bone, producing demineralization and sometimes calcium deposition in soft tissues. It is curious that both a lack and an excess of vitamin D may produce softening of the bones, although by different mechanisms. Elevation of serum calcium above 12 mg. per 100 ml. is considered a danger signal, and dosage should be reduced or temporarily discontinued.

Vitamin E

Vitamin E is known as the antisterility vitamin. It is a fat-soluble vitamin, and wheat germ oil is the richest source of it, although it occurs in other vegetable oils such as cottonseed oil and peanut oil. It is also found in green leafy vegetables.

A number of compounds have been found which exhibit vitamin E activity. The most active of these compounds are the tocopherols, of which three are naturally occurring compounds known as alpha, beta, and gamma tocopherol. The most potent of these compounds is said to be alpha tocopherol.

It has never been demonstrated that a deficiency of vitamin E occurs in man. In laboratory animals, a lack of vitamin E manifests itself by infertility or failure of the female to carry a pregnancy to term. Absence of vitamin E in the diet of rabbits and guinea pigs is followed by muscular dystrophy and paralysis of the hindquarters.

Although the role of vitamin E in human physiology has not been determined, it seems to have no value in the treatment of sterility or for the prevention of abortions.

Vitamin K is also a fat-soluble vitamin, but it has been presented in Chapter 14.

Water-soluble vitamins

Vitamin B complex

The vitamin B complex refers to a group of vitamins which are often found together in food although chemically dissimilar. They have different metabolic functions. Grouping them together is based largely on the historical basis of their having been discovered in a sequential order. They have little else in common other than their sources and the fact that they are water soluble. There is a sensible and increasingly popular trend to discard the names B_1, B_2, etc., and to refer to the individual vitamins as thiamine, riboflavin, etc. Vitamin B complex includes thiamine, riboflavin, nicotinic acid, pyridoxine, pantothenic acid, biotin, choline, inositol, and para-aminobenzoic acid.

Thiamine (Vitamin B₁)

Thiamine is also known as the antineuritic or the antiberiberi vitamin. It was first synthesized in 1937. It is found abundantly in yeast, in whole grain cereals, and in pork and liver.

Thiamine is believed to play an essential role in the intermediate steps of the metabolism of carbohydrates. Specifically, thiamine is a major portion of the coenzyme *cocarboxylase,* necessary for the normal metabolism of pyruvic acid, and certain other compounds as well. Thus it plays a part in the metabolism of all living cells.

Thiamine deficiency is recognized as being of fundamental importance in beriberi. This disease still is found in Asia but is seldom encountered in the United States and Europe except in persons whose dietary pattern is abnormal, such as that of the alcoholic. The symptoms of thiamine deficiency are particularly related to changes in the nervous and cardiovascular systems and include the following: muscular weakness, disturbances of sensation, tenderness over nerve trunks, polyneuritis, loss of appetite, dyspnea, epigastric disorders, and irregularities of heart action. Milder forms of deficiency may be seen when economic conditions are such that the thiamine intake cannot be sufficient or when food habits are such that individuals do not eat the right kind of food. Milder symptoms may consist of muscular aches and pains, anorexia, tachycardia, irritability, mental depression. Deficiency states in the United States are much less common since white flour has been enriched with thiamine.

Daily requirement. It has been estimated that adults require approximately 1 mg. of thiamine chloride daily, with an optimum intake of 1.5 to 2 mg., depending upon the degree of activity of the individual and the caloric intake. For the infant, 0.4 to 0.5 mg. is the optimum daily dose, increasing to 1.3 to 1.8 mg. between the ages of 13 and 20 years.[*] Requirements are increased during pregnancy and lactation and when the metabolic rate is increased or the body is unable to absorb or utilize the vitamin. Treatment of thiamine deficiency states requires several times the amount ordinarily needed. Thiamine is stored in the tissues to a limited extent, being found chiefly in the liver, brain, kidney, and heart. The amount that is stored is related directly to the amount of intake. Since the body stores are never large they are readily exhausted by febrile conditions, surgical operations, and other stress situations.

[*]National Academy of Sciences, National Research Council, Publication 589, 1958, p. 18.

Minerals, vitamins, and hormones used as drugs 651

Thiamine is found to some extent in all body tissues. It is absorbed from the gastrointestinal tract as well as from parenteral sites of administration.

Uses. The only therapeutic value of thiamine is for the treatment or prevention of thiamine deficiency. Since deficiency in one of the vitamin B factors may be accompanied by deficiency in others, some authorities prefer to give several components of the vitamin B complex. This is best accomplished by an adequate diet or preparations rich in the B factors, such as brewers' yeast. In other instances thiamine is indicated, as for the treatment of beriberi and polyneuritis and for the relief of symptoms that accompany the milder forms of thiamine deficiency.

Thiamine used to be given quite irrationally for the indiscriminate treatment of all types of pain of the back or extremities. In most of these cases any beneficial effects it may have had were probably of psychologic origin.

Preparation, dosage, and administration.

Thiamine Hydrochloride, U.S.P.; Aneurine Hydrochloride, B.P. This preparation is marketed in tablets for oral administration and in solution for injection. When injected, it is usually administered subcutaneously, or it may be added to intravenous fluids. The usual dosage of thiamine hydrochloride is 1 to 50 mg. daily. It is marketed under a number of trade names such as Berocca, Betalin, Betaxin, etc.

Thiamine Mononitrate, U.S.P. This form is available in 3, 5, 10, and 25 mg. tablets.

Dried Yeast, N.F. Dried yeast must contain in each gram not less than 0.12 mg. of thiamine hydrochloride, 0.04 mg. of riboflavin, and 30 mg. of nicotinic acid. The usual dose is 10 Gm. four times a day. *Dried Yeast Tablets, N.F.,* contain 500 mg. of dried yeast in each tablet.

Side effects and toxic effects. Large doses of thiamine, greatly in excess of therapeutic dosage, have been known to cause anaphylactic shock, probably because of allergic responses to the preparation. However, the incidence of toxicity is so low as to be almost nonexistent.

Riboflavin (Vitamin B₂)

Crystals of riboflavin are of an orange yellow color and are soluble in water. Thiamine contains sulfur; riboflavin does not. Riboflavin was identified first in milk. Later it was identified in other substances and was called lactoflavin because of its intense yellow color. Its relationship to the vitamin B complex was not appreciated until it was observed that concentrates of the vitamin B_2 (G) had a yellow color, the intensity of which was related to the potency of the concentrate. At present, the vitamin B_2 is synthesized and all doubt of its identity has been removed. It was named riboflavin because of the presence of ribose in its structure.

Metabolic function. Riboflavin seems to function in cellular respiration and is a constituent, apparently, of all cells. It is water soluble and heat stable. Many enzymes contain the riboflavin molecule as an essential portion of their molecule. These so-called flavo-enzymes include a number of oxidizing enzymes such as those which oxidize the common amino acids to keto-acids. In addition, flavo-enzymes form part of the chain of "electron-transport" by which the energy obtained from oxidizing foodstuffs is stored as chemical energy in the form of adenosine-triphosphate (ATP). The flavo-enzymes can carry out their function because the riboflavin molecule can be easily oxidized and reduced (loss and gain of electrons) so that it can act as a link in the bridge by which electrons are removed from organic compounds and transferred to oxygen.

The functions of flavo-enzymes are therefore so extensive and important that it becomes difficult to pinpoint single specific reactions which suffer from a riboflavin deficiency.

Symptoms of deficiency. Deficiency in human beings is associated with superficial fissures about the angles of the mouth (cheilosis) and nose at the junction between the mucous membrane and the skin, visual disturbances, glossitis (atrophic), and a peculiar red color of the tongue. Actual tissue changes in the eye may occur. Riboflavin deficiency is likely to occur along with a deficiency of other members of the B complex.

Milk is one of the most important sources of riboflavin. Other sources include yeast, liver, kidney, eggs, lean meat, and leafy vegetables. The addition of riboflavin to white flour has helped to increase the intake of this vitamin for many persons.

Daily requirement. The requirement of riboflavin does not appear to be related to caloric intake or to muscular activity, but there does seem to be a relationship to body weight. The Food and Nutrition Board of the National Research Council in 1958 recommended 1.5 mg. for women and 1.8 mg. for men as a daily requirement for optimal nutrition. The requirement during pregnancy and lactation is higher (2 to 2.5 mg.). The optimum amount for infants is 0.5 to 0.8 mg. daily and for children 13 to 19 years, 1.9 to 2.5 mg.

Uses. Riboflavin is used to prevent the development of deficiency states and also to treat them. It is used along with niacin in the treatment of pellagra.

Preparation, dosage, and administration.

Riboflavin, U.S.P., B.P.* (Lactoflavin). Riboflavin is usually administered orally because it is well absorbed from the gastrointestinal tract. Tablets, 5 and 10 mg., are available for oral administration. *Riboflavin Injection*, U.S.P., 5 and 10 mg. per milliliter, can be given subcutane-

*Spelled Riboflavine in the B.P.

ously. The usual therapeutic daily dose is 5 mg., although 2 to 20 mg. daily may be needed, depending upon the degree of deficiency. Yeast preparations are also given for their riboflavin content.

Methylol Riboflavin° (Hyflavin). This preparation is available in solution for parenteral administration, 10 mg. per milliliter. It possesses the same activity as riboflavin but is preferable for parenteral therapy.

Side effects and toxic effects. Riboflavin is completely nontoxic and reactions to it do not seem to occur. No side effects have been noted after relatively large doses.

Nicotinic Acid (Niacin)

Nicotinic acid	Nicotinamide

Nicotinic acid (niacin) is related chemically to nicotine but possesses none of the latter's pharmacologic properties. Niacin is converted in the body to nicotinamide. Nicotinic acid and nicotinamide are dietary essentials, the lack of which is responsible for the symptoms of pellagra. Pellagra is characterized by disturbances of the gastrointestinal tract, skin, and nervous system. In a milder degree of deficiency, patients are nervous, irritable, have indigestion, diarrhea or constipation, and frequently a certain amount of skin pigmentation.

Pellagra occurs among persons of low economic means and has been seen especially among peoples who eat a good deal of corn (maize) but whose total diet is limited in protein; it is also seen as a result of dietary fads and disease of the gastrointestinal tract in which there is poor intestinal absorption.

Lean meats, poultry, and fish have been found to be a better source of niacin than vegetables and fruits. Milk and eggs are a good source of the precursor substance, tryptophan. Corn contains little tryptophan. The enrichment of white flour has made an appreciable contribution to the increase of niacin in the average diet in this country.

Unlike some of the other water-soluble vitamins, animals as well as man can carry out, to a limited degree, the synthesis of nicotinic acid from the essential amino acid, tryptophan. This finding explains the earlier observation, that on certain types of diet, symptoms of niacin deficiency occur much more readily than on others, even though both types may be equally low in niacin. The explanation is based on the fact

°Described in annual publication of A. M. A. Council on Drugs, N.N.D., 1960.

that the more protective diet, while containing inadequate niacin as such, may be rich in tryptophan, so that the body's need for niacin may be met by converting some of the amino acids. Diets low in both niacin and tryptophan are the most likely to produce clinical deficiency.

Metabolic function. As in the case with riboflavin, a large group of enzymes depend for their function on coenzymes containing niacin. The vital oxidation-reduction coenzymes, diphosphopyridine nucleotide and triphosphopyridine nucleotide, are required for the early reactions of many metabolic pathways. Both contain the nicotinamide molecule as part of their structure.

Ribose-phosphate-phosphate-adenine

This portion of the molecule is in fact believed to function in carrying electrons from the oxidizable compounds to the next step in oxidation, the flavin enzymes. No biologic role of niacin is known except for its presence in the coenzymes, but so many metabolic processes are dependent on the pyridine nucleotides that this is ample to explain the widespread symptoms caused by niacin lack.

Daily requirement. The National Research Council (U.S.A.), in its 1958 revision of Recommended Dietary Allowances, stated the daily niacin requirements in terms of niacin equivalents, assuming that 60 mg. of tryptophan will supply 1 mg. of niacin.* Requirements were estimated on the basis of body weight and caloric intake and then increased by 50 per cent to provide for varying physiologic needs and dietary situations. The requirement for women is given as 17 mg. and for men, 18 to 21 mg., daily. For pregnancy and lactation, 4.4 niacin mg. equivalents are recommended for each 1,000 calories added to the diet and then increased by 50 per cent. For infants, daily recommended intake is 6 to 7 niacin mg. equivalents.

Uses. Both nicotinic acid and nicotinamide are used in the treatment of pellagra, but since pellagra is a disease associated with multiple vitamin deficiencies, riboflavin and thiamine are also indicated. Optimal treatment of the disease must include the administration of all members of the vitamin B complex as well as a diet adequate in animal protein.

Preparation, dosage, and administration.

Nicotinic Acid, U.S.P., B.P. (Niacin). Nicotinic acid is available as a

---

'A diet containing 1,000 mg. of tryptophan can be expected to contribute 17 mg. of niacin. This could be expressed as 17 mg. equivalents.

powder and in tablet form, 25, 50, and 100 mg. for oral administration.

Nicotinic Acid Injection, U.S.P. (This form is available in 10 ml. ampules containing 100 mg. of the drug for parenteral use.

Nicotinamide, U.S.P., B.P. (Niacinamide). Official preparations include tablets, 25, 50, and 100 mg., and ampules containing a solution for injection. The concentration of the solution is 50 or 100 mg. per milliliter.

These vitamins are usually given orally but they may also be given parenterally. The dose for the treatment of pellagra may be as much as 500 mg. daily, by mouth, in divided doses or 100 to 200 mg. by injection. The dose must be determined by the degree of deficiency which is being treated.

Side effects and toxic effects. The administration of large doses of nicotinic acid (especially when given intravenously) causes flushing of the face and neck associated with an unpleasant sensation. This does not occur after the administration of nicotinamide, which is therefore preferred for parenteral administration. In spite of this reaction which is transient, niacin is considered a nontoxic substance.

Pyridoxine Hydrochloride (Vitamin B₆)

Vitamin B_6 occurs as a group of chemically related compounds—pyridoxine, pyridoxal, and pyridoxamine. In the body tissues they can be converted from one form to another. Pyridoxine is changed into pyridoxal, which seems to be especially active. Pyridoxal phosphate functions as a coenzyme and is involved in changing tryptophan to the nicotinamide portion of the pyridine coenzymes. It plays an important role in the metabolism of amino acids and also of fatty acids. It is said to participate in energy transformation in the brain and nerve tissues.

Pork and glandular meats are said to be especially rich in the vitamin B_6 group of enzymes, although they are found in many different foods.

Although no specific deficiency disease has been recognized in man, convulsive disorders have been observed in infants who were fed a diet deficient in vitamin B_6, and adults who have received a vitamin B_6 antagonist have developed seborrheic dermatitis, lesions on mucous membranes, and peripheral neuritis. Patients with an unusual type of hypochromic anemia have responded well to the administration of vitamin B_6.

Daily requirement. The daily human intake of vitamin B_6 should be 1 to 2 mg. This is readily provided in the ordinary adequate diet.

Uses. Pyridoxine hydrochloride is used as an adjunct in the treatment of nausea and vomiting of pregnancy and for the relief of irradiation sickness. It is also used to relieve vitamin B_6 deficiency.

Isoniazid, an antituberculosis drug, acts as an antagonist of vitamin B_6, and when used over a period of time it may produce a vitamin deficiency unless additional amounts of vitamin B_6 are administered.

Preparation, dosage, and administration.

Pyridoxine Hydrochloride, U.S.P. (Beadox Hydrochloride). Official preparations are available in 10, 25, and 50 mg. tablets for oral administration and in solution (concentrations varying from 50 to 100 mg. per milliliter) for intramuscular or intravenous injection. The usual dosage is 5 mg. daily, although as much as 25 to 100 mg. have been administered.

Pantothenic Acid

Pantothenic acid is widely distributed in nature. It is known to prevent nutritional dermatosis in chicks and to promote normal growth in rats. It is believed to be a constituent of an enzyme known as coenzyme A, which plays an important role in the release of energy from carbohydrates, and in the synthesis and degradation of fatty acids, sterols, and steroid hormones. Pantothenic acid is believed to be essential for human beings, although what constitutes the daily requirement is uncertain. An average American diet is said to provide 8.7 mg. daily. *Calcium Pantothenate,* U.S.P., is available in 10 mg. tablets. It is included in many multivitamin preparations. The usual dose is 10 mg.

Biotin

Biotin is a substance believed to play a role in metabolism, probably as a coenzyme. Deficiency states have been reported in man only when fed a diet containing a large amount of raw egg white.* Avidin, a protein found in egg white, binds the biotin and prevents its absorption from the intestine. This results in the development of anorexia, malaise, and dermatitis. Daily administration of 150 to 300 mcg. will prevent the development of these symptoms in human beings. This amount is found in an average American diet.

Choline, Inositol, and Para-aminobenzoic Acid

These compounds have been included in the vitamin B complex but their status is uncertain. Choline and inositol have been found to have a lipotropic (exhibit an affinity for fat) effect. The lipotropic effect of choline was first noted in the liver, and this led to its use for the treatment of fatty infiltration of the liver and other disorders of fat metabolism. However, the evidence to support claims for clinical usefulness is said to be questionable.†

Vitamin B₁₂ and Pteroylglutamic Acid

Vitamin B_{12} and pteroylglutamic acid (folic acid) were discussed in Chapter 14.

---

*National Research Council, Recommended Dietary Allowances, Bulletin 589, 1958, p. 25.
†N.N.D., 1960, p. 710.

Ascorbic Acid (Vitamin C)

Scurvy formerly was common among sailors who were deprived of fresh fruits and vegetables during long voyages. The well-known effects of lemon and orange juices in curing this disease led to attempts to concentrate the active principle by chemical means. Crystalline or ascorbic acid in large amounts has been prepared from Hungarian red pepper. Biologic tests show that ascorbic acid is pure vitamin C. It is synthesized now on a commercial scale. Ascorbic acid is a powerful reducing agent and is therefore sensitive to oxidation. It is relatively stable in an acid medium but quickly oxidized in an alkaline medium. It is believed to be concerned in the oxidation-reduction reactions of all living cells.

However, less that is definite is known about its function than is known about many of the other water-soluble vitamins already discussed. It is concerned with the formation of collagen in all fibrous tissue, including bone, and with the development of teeth, blood vessels, and blood cells. It is believed to stimulate the fibroblasts of connective tissue and thus promote tissue repair and the healing of wounds. It is said to help maintain the integrity of the intercellular substance in the walls of blood vessels, and the capillary fragility associated with scurvy is explained on this basis.

A deficiency in the intake of vitamin C results in scurvy, the chief symptoms of which are spongy, bleeding gums, loosened teeth, hemorrhagic tendencies in regions subjected to trauma or mechanical stress, sore, swollen joints, fatigue, pallor, and anemia. Vitamin C deficiency is thought to be a contributory factor in dental caries, pyorrhea, and certain oral infections.

Foods rich in vitamin C include citrus fruits, oranges, lemons, limes, grapefruit, as well as tomato juice, raw cabbage, broccoli, and strawberries.

Daily requirement. The optimum daily intake of ascorbic acid for an adult male is 75 mg.; for women, 70 mg.; and for infants, 30 mg. During pregnancy and lactation, the requirement may be as much as 100 and 150 mg.

Uses. The specific use of vitamin C is in the prevention and treatment of scurvy and for the subclinical manifestations of this disease. An optimum amount of ascorbic acid should be supplied for individuals of all ages to prevent the development of scurvy. In the absence of vitamin C, changes occur in the collagen of fibrous tissues, in the matrix of tooth substance (dentine), in bone, cartilage, and in the endothelium of blood vessels. Since vitamin C is not stored to any appreciable extent, deficiency can develop easily. Patients who do not eat well or do not receive a diet adequate for their needs or those who must be fed intravenously for a long time may develop a deficiency unless they are given ascorbic acid as a dietary supplement. The vitamin C deficiency may result in delay in the healing of wounds, or it may actually cause a breakdown in the healing process.

The administration of vitamin C, however, is not considered specific treatment for pyorrhea, dental caries, certain gum infections, etc., unless these symptoms are associated with vitamin C deficiency. In fact, bleeding gums are a rather common finding among otherwise healthy individuals; however, vitamin C deficiency to the extent necessary to cause capillary bleeding is quite rare. It is therefore most unreasonable to treat bleeding gums with an increased and supernormal intake of ascorbic acid.

Preparation, dosage, and administration.

Ascorbic Acid, U.S.P., B.P. Ascorbic acid is available in 25, 50, 100, 250, and 500 mg. tablets. A number of multiple-vitamin preparations also contain vitamin C.

Ascorbic Acid Injection, U.S.P. This is a preparation of ascorbic acid suited for parenteral administration.

Ascorbic acid may be given orally because it is well absorbed from the intestinal tract, or the injectable form may be given intramuscularly or added to intravenous fluids. The therapeutic dose for adults is 100 to 150 mg. daily.*

Multiple-vitamin preparations

The daily intake of principal vitamins recommended by the Food and Nutrition Board of the National Research Council is as follows for adults who are normally vigorous and living in a temperate climate: vitamin A, 5,000 units; vitamin D, 400 units; thiamine (vitamin B_1) 1 to 1.6 mg.; riboflavin, 1.5 to 1.8 mg.; nicotinic acid (niacin) 17 to 21 mg. equivalents; ascorbic acid (vitamin C), 70 to 75 mg.

Many of the multiple-vitamin preparations which have come into extensive use in recent years contain amounts of the above vitamins which bear no relation to established therapeutic dosage or to normal daily requirements. In addition, many such preparations contain purified vitamins which are not yet known to be represented by any known deficiency diseases.

Certain multiple-vitamin preparations not only have excessive amounts of each vitamin but also contain vitamins whose importance in human nutrition is open to question. The cost of "overstuffed" vitamin preparations is unnecessarily high. Vitamin requirements may be abnormally high, for a time, in individuals who are acutely and severely ill, but that is another matter.

*N.N.D., 1960, p. 723.

Decavitamin Capsules, U.S.P., and *Decavitamin Tablets*, U.S.P., contain in each capsule or tablet not less than 1.2 mg. (4,000 U.S.P. units) of vitamin A, 10 mcg. (400 U.S.P. units) of vitamin D, 75 mg. of ascorbic acid, 5 mg. of calcium pantothenate, 2 mcg. of cyanocobalamin, 0.25 mg. of folic acid, 10 mg. of nicotinamide, 2 mg. of pyridoxine hydrochloride, 1.2 mg. of riboflavin, and 1 mg. of thiamine hydrochloride. The usual daily dose is 1 capsule or 1 tablet.

Hormones

The hormones are chemical substances produced by the ductless or endocrine glands that act after being secreted into the blood stream.

Specific endocrine substances thus have a widespread effect, acting on many other tissues and organs, and in a general way regulating the rates of certain metabolic processes, such as growth of the body, growth and development of the sex organs, or, as in the case of the pituitary hormones, growth and function of the ductless glands.

One of the major developments of this century in the fields of biology and medicine has been the recognition and then the isolation, purification, and chemical understanding of most of the hormones we now know. In addition, once their chemical structure is known, it becomes hypothetically possible to duplicate them by chemical synthesis, and this has been accomplished for some hormones, although not for all.

Exactly what should be called a hormone and what should not is not well defined. A broad definition could be any chemical substance released by one tissue, circulated by the blood, and having characteristic effects on other tissues. This would include many substances not ordinarily classed as hormones, such as carbon dioxide. In common usage, hormones are confined to those well-recognized and chemically specific products of the various endocrine glands that have specific well-defined physiologic effects on metabolism. The list of major hormones includes the products of the secretions of the anterior and posterior pituitary, the thyroid hormone, insulin and glucogen from the pancreas, epinephrine and norepinephrine from the adrenal medulla, several potent steroids from the adrenal cortex, and the gonadal hormones of both sexes.

In medicine, these substances are used generally in two ways: (1) for replacement when a patient lacks sufficient endogenous hormone, exemplified by the use of insulin in diabetes or the use of adrenal steroids in Addison's disease, and (2) for "pharmacologic" effects beyond those of replacement, exemplified by the use of insulin to produce hypoglycemic shock in schizophrenia or by the use of large doses of the adrenal steroids for their anti-inflammatory effects.

660

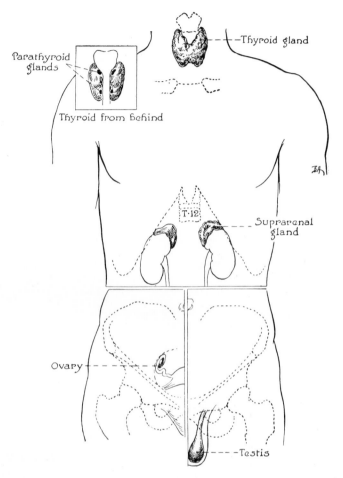

Fig. 42 Location of some of the glands of internal secretion. Why are these structures often called ductless glands? (From McClendon, J. F., and Pettibone, C. J. V.: Physiological Chemistry, St. Louis, The C. V. Mosby Co.)

Pituitary hormones

Because the hormones of the pituitary gland have an important effect in regulating the secretion of the other hormones, it is fitting that they be considered first.

The pituitary body is about the size of a pea and occupies a niche in the sella turcica of the sphenoid bone. It is the coryphaeus (leader) of the endocrine orchestra. It consists of an anterior lobe, a posterior lobe, and a smaller *pars intermedia* composed of secreting cells. The anterior part is particularly important in sustaining the life of the individual. The function of the pars intermedia is not well known. It should be noted that the oral administration of any part of the whole gland is without visible effect because it is destroyed by proteolytic enzymes and the hormones are protein in nature, or at least inseparable from proteins.

Anterior pituitary hormones

Present evidence indicates that a number of factors are concerned in the action of extracts of the anterior lobe of the pituitary gland. How many hormones are secreted by the gland is unknown, but at least six extracts have been prepared in a relatively pure state and they have a markedly specific action.*

*N.N.D., 1960, p. 592.

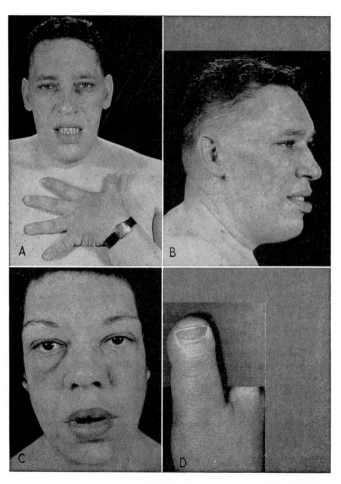

Fig. 43 Acromegaly. **A** and **B,** Note the large and elongated head, large hand, nose, ears, and lips. **C,** Note the coarse features and the increased interdental spaces. **D,** Large blunt-pointed thumb. (From Williams, R. H.: Textbook of Endocrinology, Philadelphia, W. B. Saunders Co.)

1. A growth factor that influences the development of the body. It promotes skeletal, visceral, and general growth of the body. Acromegaly, giantism, and dwarfism are connected with pathology of the anterior lobe of the pituitary gland.

The growth hormone or somatotropin has recently been obtained as a small crystalline protein, but thus far the growth hormone has found no established place in medicine, and its use in various clinical conditions is largely experimental. It tends to increase the blood sugar and antagonize insulin and it may be the "diabetogenic" hormone postulated some years ago.

2. A factor that stimulates the growth and maturation of the ovarian follicle, which in turn brings on the characteristic changes of estrus (menstruation in women)—the follicle-stimulating hormone (FSH). This hormone appears to be a protein or is associated with a protein, but it has not yet been obtained in a highly purified form.

3. A luteinizing hormone (LH), which promotes the development of the corpus luteum, and an interstitial cell-stimulating hormone (ICSH), which stimulates the development of the interstitial cells of the testes and the secretion by them of male sex hormones (androgens).

4. A thyrotropic hormone, which is necessary for normal development and function of the thyroid gland and which, if present in excess, is known to produce hyperthyroidism and an increased size of the gland in laboratory animals.

5. A lactogenic factor, which may play a part in proliferation and secretion of the mammary glands of mammals. This may be identical with the hormone that is responsible for the development of the corpus luteum.

6. The adrenocorticotropic hormone (corticotropin or ACTH), which stimulates the cortex of the adrenal gland.

Although the hormones produced by the anterior lobe of the pituitary gland are important physiologically, a number of reasons explain their limited usefulness. Only in relatively recent times have purified preparations been available, at least for clinical study, and such preparations are both expensive and limited in supply. Increased application of their effects may be expected in the future, however, as chemically defined preparations become available.

The adrenocorticotropic hormone (ACTH) of the anterior pituitary exerts its action primarily on the cells of the adrenal cortex and causes it to secrete its entire spectrum of hormones.

The ultimate effects in the body, therefore, are the effects of the various adrenocortical steroids and, in general, these effects are similar to those of cortisone. Corticotropin is effective only if a functioning adrenal gland is present. Our present source of corticotropin is from the pituitary

Minerals, vitamins, and hormones used as drugs 663

glands of hogs, cattle, and horses in this country and from whales in the Scandinavian countries. The labor involved in the removal of the glands is such that this source is an expensive one. Purification of ACTH from hog pituitary gland has recently led to the analysis of the structure of an active polypeptide, containing 39 amino acids in a known sequence. It is possible that smaller fragments of this large molecule might retain hormonal activity, so the possibility of synthesizing an active ACTH by chemical methods may not lie too far ahead.

During conditions of stress and strain the activity of the adrenal cortex is increased. This is thought to be due to an increased secretion of corticotropin. One explanation for the regulation of corticotropic activity is that during stress, the tissues of the body utilize more of the adrenal hormones than usual, which results in a decreased concentration of the adrenocortical hormones in the blood. This in turn brings about stimulation of cells in the anterior pituitary gland and the production of more corticotropin. On the other hand, when the situation of stress has subsided, the tissues use less adrenocortical hormones, their concentration in the blood increases, and this causes activity of the pituitary gland as well as the adrenal cortex to be decreased.

Absorption. Corticotropin is destroyed by enzymes in the gastrointestinal tract and therefore cannot be given orally. It is absorbed readily from sites of injection when given parenterally (intramuscularly or intravenously). It is said to disappear from the blood rapidly after intravenous injection. Its effects rarely last longer than 6 hours.* This necessitates frequent intramuscular injections, administration by slow intravenous drip, or the use of a preparation that is absorbed slowly. Its effectiveness depends upon the presence of normal adrenal glands capable of responding to the stimulant made by the pituitary gland.

Uses. Corticotropin is used for many of the same conditions for which cortisone and hydrocortisone are used. It has the advantage of rapid absorption and rapid utilization, but it is more expensive than the cortical steroids.

Preparation, dosage, and administration.

Corticotropin Injection, U.S.P. (Acthar). This preparation is marketed as a powder for injection in 10, 25, and 40 U.S.P. units and in solution, 20 to 80 U.S.P. units per milliliter. The average dose of corticotropin for adults is 40 to 50 U.S.P. units daily (up to 100 units) when given intramuscularly. When the drug is administered intravenously, 5 to 20 U.S.P. units are dissolved in 500 ml. of 5 per cent glucose solution or isotonic saline (unless salt is restricted for the patient), and the solution is administered slowly over an 8-hour period.* *Corticotrophin Injection,* B.P.,

*N.N.D., 1960, p. 594.

is administered subcutaneously or intramuscularly in doses of 10 to 25 units every 6 hours.

Repository Corticotropin Injection, U.S.P. (Corticotropin Gel). This is a preparation of corticotropin dissolved in a gelatin solution which results in slow absorption and more satisfactory clinical effect per unit of activity. Repository corticotropin is administered intramuscularly. A daily injection exerts a prolonged and continuous effect. The usual daily intramuscular dose is 40 U.S.P. units.

Sterile Corticotropin Zinc Hydroxide Suspension, U.S.P. This is a preparation of purified corticotropin adsorbed on zinc hydroxide. Absorption after parenteral administration is delayed, and thus its action is prolonged. It is administered intramuscularly and is available as a suspension containing 100 and 200 U.S.P. units in 5 ml. The usual initial dose is 40 U.S.P. units; maintenance dose is 20 U.S.P. units.

Side effects and toxic effects. Effects are much the same as those noted after administration of cortisone or hydrocortisone (pp. 686, 687).

Pituitary gonadotropic hormones

The pituitary gonadotropic hormones are discussed in Chapter 19.

Posterior pituitary hormones

When solutions of extracts of the posterior lobes of the pituitary glands of animals (domestic) are administered parenterally, a number of effects have been observed: (1) stimulation of the uterine muscle (oxytocic effect), (2) promotion of the absorption of water in the renal tubules (antidiuretic effect), and (3) stimulation of the muscle of the superficial blood vessels (pressor effect) and of the intestine.

A great advance in the pharmacology of the posterior lobe has been the recent identification and chemical analysis of two major hormones, obtained from the gland in pure form. These compounds, oxytocin and vasopressin, are both peptides, each containing eight amino acids. After their isolation and determination it proved possible to synthesize them chemically. Availability of the oxytocic and vasopressor pituitary hormones in pure form have cleared up a number of uncertainties about their action and has also opened the door to their better-controlled therapeutic use. It is known, for example, that there is a certain overlap of pharmacologic action even in the pure preparation; pure oxytocin has some vasopressor activity, and vice versa. Vasopressin is also the antidiuretic hormone, its antidiuretic potency being much more marked than its pressor potency. Although therapy still uses mainly the cruder preparations of oxytocic and vasopressor activity, it may be expected that eventually the pure compounds will replace the older extracts.

Oxytocin has been discussed in Chapter 19.

Uses for vasopressin. Vasopressin is used chiefly in the treatment of diabetes insipidus, a condition in which the patient excretes a large amount of urine because sufficient antidiuretic hormone is not secreted. It is also sometimes used for the relief of intestinal gaseous distention. It is rarely used to elevate the blood pressure since more effective drugs are available for this purpose.

Preparation, dosage, and administration.

Posterior Pituitary Injection. This is no longer an official preparation. It contains 10 U.S.P. posterior pituitary units in each milliliter of aqueous solution. The usual dose is 10 U.S.P. units subcutaneously. The preparation contains a mixture of hormones.

Vasopressin Injection, U.S.P., B.P. (Pitressin). This is a purified preparation of antidiuretic and pressor hormone separated from the oxytocic hormone. The usual dose is 1 ml., and it is given subcutaneously or intramuscularly. It contains 20 pressor units per milliliter.

Vasopressin Tannate* (Pitressin Tannate). This compound is marketed in solution for intramuscular injection (5 pressor units per milliliter); 0.3 to 1 ml. (5 to 15 minims) is injected at intervals of 36 to 48 hours. Its effect is more prolonged than that of vasopressin. It cannot be given intravenously.

Posterior Pituitary Powder. This powder is dried pituitary gland, which can be snuffed up into the nose for the relief of diabetes insipidus; it is less expensive than the injectable forms.

Side effects and toxic effects. Vasopressin can cause spasm of coronary arteries and caution is recommended when it is administered to patients with inadequate coronary circulation. Water retention and occasionally water intoxication have been known to occur. The patient with diabetes insipidus will probably have to take the drug the remainder of his life. Large doses may cause intestinal and uterine cramps.

Parathyroid hormone

Lying just above the thyroid, or, in some animals, embodied in it, are a variable number of bean-shaped glands (two pairs in man) known as the parathyroids. Complete removal of the parathyroids results in acute neuromuscular symptoms, known as tetany, which resembles the tetany sometimes seen in young children. The tetany invariably is associated with hypocalcemia. It seems that the glands are concerned with calcium metabolism. The symptoms are twitching spasms, or convulsions, gradual paralysis with dyspnea, and death from exhaustion. Before death usually there are gastrointestinal hemorrhages and hematemesis. At death the intestinal mucosa is congested and the calcium content of the heart, kidney, and other tissues is increased.

*Described in annual publication of A. M. A. Council on Drugs, N.N.D., 1960.

The symptoms of tetany are relieved by the injection of parathyroid extracts and by calcium salts. Because the action of parathyroid hormone is slow, it is usually necessary to administer calcium salts intravenously for rapid relief. Large doses of vitamin D are also useful to relieve tetany and to restore the normal level of calcium in the blood.

The patient should be hospitalized because a frequent check on the blood calcium and phosphate levels is essential. Many disturbances of calcium metabolism are not due to disturbance of the parathyroid function, but hypoparathyroidism is the specific indication for the use of hormonal therapy.

Preparation, dosage, and administration.

Parathyroid Injection, U.S.P. Usual dose is 40 U.S.P. units intramuscularly every 12 hours. One milliliter of the Parathyroid Injection possesses a potency of not less than 100 U.S.P. Parathyroid Units, each unit representing $\frac{1}{100}$ of the amount required to raise the calcium content of 100 ml. of the blood serum of normal dogs 1 mg. within 16 to 18 hours after administration.[*]

Thyroid hormones and drugs used in diseases of the thyroid gland

The thyroid gland stores an iodine-containing protein known as thyroglobulin which is essential for the proper regulation of metabolism. Thyroxin is released from this protein into the blood stream and, in the blood, is transported bound to one of the proteins in the plasma, also a globulin. Thyroxin was isolated by Kendall in 1915, who found that it contained 65 per cent iodine. Thyroxin has been found to exhibit the same physiologic effects as the original protein.

Thyroxin (tetraiodothyronine)

Triiodothyronine

Thyroxin has been known for many years and until recently was regarded as the thyroid hormone or at least the active portion of thyroglobulin.

Within the past few years a closely related compound, identical with

[*]U.S.P. XVI, p. 491.

thyroxin except that it contains one less iodine atom (triiodothyronine or "T3") has been found to be a natural component of thyroid tissue and is even more potent than thyroxin. Although thyroxin is more abundant in man than triiodothyronine, it is not certain which hormone is the dominative one physiologically. Both have essentially the same action.

Physiologic action. Although the exact mechanism of action of the thyroid hormones is not known, their primary effect is on cellular metabolism. They apparently cause all cells to accelerate their rate of metabolism. This is reflected in the way tissues grow and develop. Deficiency causes not only a slowing of growth in the young but also affects many reactions both in the young and in the adult; water and salt metabolism is affected and muscular inefficiency, circulatory disturbances, and disturbance of the central nervous system may be noticed.

Congenital thyroid deficiency results in cretinism, and a deficiency in adults causes myxedema. In these conditions the basal metabolism is subnormal. Preparations of thyroid gland or thyroid hormones act as specifics by supplying the deficient hormones.

The thyroid and other endocrines

The thyroid gland is an important member of the endocrine group and is affected by other endocrine glands, especially by the thyrotropic factor from the anterior lobe of the pituitary. The thyroid also exerts an influence on other endocrines, i.e., the thymus, adrenals, and the gonads. Hyperthyroidism results in increased calcium excretion and also hypertrophic changes in the parathyroid.

Iodine deficiency and its effect on the thyroid gland

The synthesis of the thyroid hormones and their maintenance in the blood in adequate amounts depend in part upon an adequate intake of iodine. Iodine ingested by way of food or water is changed into iodide before reaching the circulation. As such, it is taken up by the thyroid gland. Prolonged iodine deficiency in the diet results in an enlargement of the thyroid gland, known as a simple goiter. When thyroid hormones fail to be synthesized because of a lack of iodine, the anterior lobe of the pituitary is stimulated to increase the secretion of thyrotropic hormone, which in turn causes hypertrophy and hyperplasia (rapid growth and increase of cells) of the gland. This type of goiter can be prevented by providing an adequate supply of iodine for the young. The use of iodized salt is one way of doing it.

Hypothyroid states

Cretinism. Hypothyroidism in the young child is known as cretinism and is characterized by cessation of physical and mental development

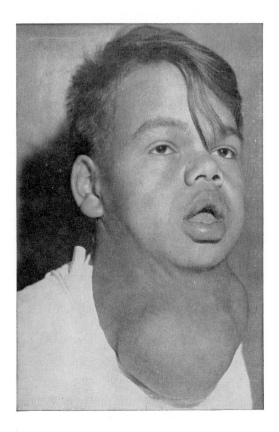

Fig. 44 Goitrous cretin. All cretins do not necessarily have goiters. (From Stanbury, J. B., and Hedge, A. N.: A Family of Goitrous Cretins, J. Clin. Endocrinol. **10:** 1471, 1950.)

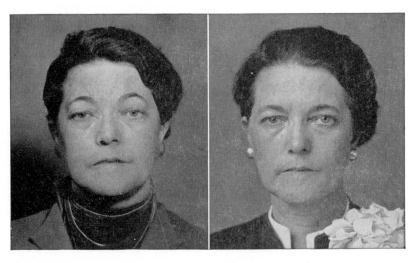

A   B

Fig. 45 Primary myxedema. **A,** Before treatment. **B,** After treatment. (From Perkins, R. F., and Rynearson, E. H.: Endocrine Review: Practical Aspects of Insufficiency of the Anterior Pituitary Gland in the Adult, J. Clin. Endocrinol. **12:** 574, 1952.)

Minerals, vitamins, and hormones used as drugs 669

which leads to dwarfism and idiocy. Cretins usually have thick, coarse skin, a thick tongue, gaping mouth, protruding abdomen, thick, short legs, poorly developed hands and feet, and weak musculature. This condition may result from faulty development or atrophy of the thyroid gland during fetal life. Failure of development of the gland may be due to lack of iodine in the mother.

Myxedema. Hypothyroidism in the adult is called myxedema. Its development is usually insidious and causes a gradual retardation of physical and mental functions. There is a gradual infiltration of the skin, loss of facial lines and facial expression. The formation of a subcutaneous connective tissue causes the hands and face to appear puffy and swollen. The basal metabolic rate becomes subnormal, the hair becomes scanty and coarse, movements become sluggish, and the patient becomes hypersensitive to cold.

Thyroid preparations

Thyroid is a yellowish powder obtained from the thyroid glands of domesticated animals used for food by man.

Thyroid or thyroxin is specific in the treatment of hypothyroid conditions. Patients with cretinism or myxedema will probably require therapy all of their lives. This dosage must be adjusted to the needs of the patient. For most patients an official preparation of thyroid in tablet form is the cheapest and most convenient form and at the same time is very effective. The object of treatment of the patient with myxedema is to rid him of symptoms, not necessarily to raise the metabolic rate to normal. In the treatment of the cretin, however, it may be necessary to raise the metabolic rate to normal or above in order to ensure adequate development. It is most important to start treatment of the cretin very early in life; the sooner the better, which means before the child is 6 months old if at all possible. Otherwise both the physical retardation and mental retardation are likely to be permanent. In myxedema, mental and physical characteristics are restored and complete cure often results.

Thyroid preparations have been used extensively in the treatment of obesity. At best, the use of thyroid is a palliative measure and is not unaccompanied by the danger of inducing severe symptoms of toxicity. Thyroid hormone or thyroid extract should be regarded as a potent substance and should never be used indiscriminately. No one should take it who is not under direct medical supervision. If the obesity is primarily due to hypothyroidism, its use may be indicated, but most authorities agree that obesity usually is due to overeating and must be cured by reducing the caloric intake. The uncontrolled use of the drug has caused death.

Thyroid preparations have also been used in connection with low metabolic levels associated with rheumatoid arthritis, rickets, various skin diseases, and menstrual disturbances. Although thyroid is not considered specific for these conditions, good results have been reported in some cases. Sterility and habitual abortion are sometimes successfully treated with thyroid.

Preparation, dosage, and administration.

Thyroid, U.S.P., B.P. Thyroid is available in tablets containing 15, 30, 60, and 120 mg. each for oral administration. The usual oral dose is 60 mg. (1 gr.), although the dose must be determined by the needs of the patient. Range of dosage for one day may be 30 to 180 mg. or more.

Thyroxine. Thyroxine is no longer an official drug in the United States. It is thought to have little or no advantage over crude preparations of thyroid except that it can be administered parenterally. Since a latent period exists before the drug exhibits its peak effects, there is no advantage in giving the drug parenterally. It is more expensive than thyroid tablets.

Thyroxine Sodium, B.P. This is available in tablet form. The dosage is 0.05 to 0.5 mg. daily. It should be protected from light.

Sodium Levothyroxine, U.S.P. (Synthroid Sodium). This is the sodium salt of the levo isomer of thyroxin. It is more effective than a mixture of D-thyroxine and L-thyroxine. It is given orally. Initial doses range from 0.05 to 0.1 mg. daily. Increase in dosage is made on basis of patient's response. Official tablets are available containing 0.05, 0.1, and 0.2 mg.

Sodium Liothyronine, U.S.P. (Cytomel). This is the active isomer of triiodothyronine. It exhibits a rapid onset of action, but after administration is stopped the duration of effect is correspondingly brief. Five to 25 (up to 50) mcg. are given daily as an initial dose for adults being treated for hypothyroid states. It is available in 5 and 25 mcg. tablets for oral administration.

Side effects and toxic effects. The symptoms of overdosage are, in general, those of hyperthyroidism, viz., palpitation, tachycardia, pain over the heart, dyspnea, nervousness, insomnia, tremor, hyperglycemia, sweating, and loss of weight.

It should be remembered that symptoms come on slowly and may last a long time. It is best, therefore, that a small dose be used at first and the patient be watched closely. One of the first symptoms of overdosage which the nurse may have occasion to note is an increase in the pulse rate. She should always count the pulse before giving the next dose of the drug. In some hospitals it is the rule to *withhold the drug if the pulse rate has reached 100 beats per minute.* In mild cases withdrawal of the drug will result in return to the normal metabolic level. In severe cases it is important to allow the patient to rest in a comfortable position. A sedative also may be indicated.

Minerals, vitamins, and hormones used as drugs 671

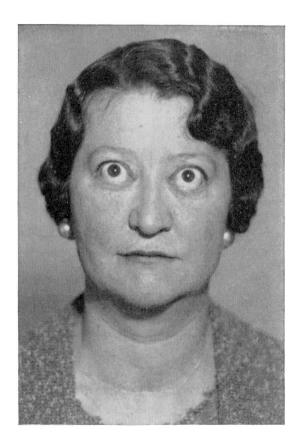

Fig. 46 Patient with exophthalmic goiter. Notice the exophthalmos, the facial expression, and the enlargement of the neck. (From Meakins, J. C.: The Practice of Medicine, St. Louis, The C. V. Mosby Co.)

Hyperthyroid states (thyrotoxicosis)

Excessive formation of the thyroid hormones and their escape into the circulation result in a state of toxicity called thyrotoxicosis. This occurs in the condition known as exophthalmic goiter (Graves' disease), or in some forms of adenomatous goiters.

Hyperthyroidism leads to symptoms quite different from those seen in myxedema. The metabolic rate is increased, sometimes as much as a plus 60 or more. The body temperature frequently is above normal, the pulse rate is fast, and the patient complains of feeling too warm. Other symptoms include restlessness, anxiety, emotional instability, muscle tremor and weakness, sweating, and exophthalmos (protrusion of the eyeballs).

Prior to the advent of antithyroid drugs treatment was more or less limited to a subtotal resection of the hyperactive gland. Since these patients usually are poor operative risks, they may be hospitalized for a time and prepared for surgery by giving them as much mental and physical rest as possible, a diet particularly rich in carbohydrate and vitamins, and iodine. Thyroidectomy is indicated when the pulse has been slowed and the basal metabolic rate lowered to a somewhat stationary level.

Antithyroid drugs provide less rapid control of hyperthyroidism than do surgical measures. Radioactive iodine is less rapid than surgical therapy but it is one of the more effective antithyroid drugs.

Antithyroid drugs

An antithyroid drug is regarded as a chemical agent which lowers the basal metabolic rate by interfering with the formation, release, or action of the hormones made by the thyroid glands. Those which interfere with the synthesis of the thyroid hormones are known as goitrogens. A wide variety of compounds might be included in this category of antithyroid drugs, but only iodine (iodide ion), radioactive iodine, and certain derivatives of thiouracil will be included.

Iodine and iodide

Iodine which has pharmacologic or biochemical significance is either inorganic iodine (iodine ion) or iodine that is bound in organic compounds, e.g., thyroxin. There is thought to be little in common between the physiologic effects of elemental iodine, the iodide ion, and organic compounds which contain iodine in their structure, as is true of thyroxin. Confusion seems to have arisen from the incorrect or loose usage of the word *iodine*.

When elemental iodine is administered locally, a certain proportion of it is converted to iodide and is absorbed. This brings about general systemic effects of iodide. Lugol's solution contains elemental iodine, but it is changed into iodide before absorption. As a result, significant amounts of iodide reach the blood stream and are effective in the treatment of toxic goiter.

Action and result. Iodide is the oldest of the antithyroid drugs. The response of the thyrotoxic patient frequently is remarkable. The metabolic rate falls at about the same rate as occurs after surgical removal of the gland and many of the symptoms of hyperthyroidism are relieved. Maximum effects usually are attained after 10 to 15 days of continuous administration of iodide. Enlargement of the gland and hyperplasia are reduced and the gland rapidly stores colloid which contains highly potent thyroid hormone. The mechanism by which iodide accomplishes its beneficial effect is not fully understood. One explanation is that iodide temporarily promotes storage of hormone in the thyroid gland and at the same time lowers the amount delivered to the circulation. Another hypothesis is that iodide interferes in some way with the action of the thyrotropic hormone or that it diminishes the activity of the anterior lobe of the pituitary gland.

During the time when the metabolic rate is somewhere near the normal range the surgeon may be able to operate upon a patient who is nearly normal instead of on a very sick individual. Unfortunately, the beneficial effects are not prolonged indefinitely. In a few weeks the symptoms are likely to reappear and may be intensified. The thyroid gland has been filled with active hormone which, when released, may plunge the patient into a critical state.

Uses. The chief use of iodide in the treatment of thyrotoxicosis is for preparation of the patient prior to the surgical removal of the thyroid gland. Patients with severe hyperthyroidism are frequently prepared first with propylthiouracil or a related compound, and, during the last part of the treatment, iodide is given to prevent the development of a friable, highly vascular gland which increases the hazards of an operation. A certain number of patients, however, may be controlled and prepared for surgery with iodide alone.

Preparation, dosage, and administration. Convenient preparations are Lugol's solution and saturated solutions of sodium or potassium iodide; 0.3 ml. (0.1 to 1 ml.) of these preparations can be given orally three times a day. They should be well diluted in one-third to one-half glass of milk or some other vehicle that may be preferred by the patient.

Strong Iodine Solution, U.S.P. (Compound Iodine Solution, Lugol's Solution). This preparation contains iodine and potassium iodide. *Aqueous Iodine Solution,* B.P.

Sodium Iodide, U.S.P., B.P.

Potassium Iodide Solution, N.F.; *Potassium Iodide,* B.P. (Saturated Potassium Iodide Solution).

Radioactive iodine

I^{131} is a radioactive isotope of iodine which has given evidence of being useful in medicine. It has a half-life of 8.08 days, which means that at the end of about 8 days 50 per cent of its atoms have undergone disintegration and in another 8 days 50 per cent of the remaining amount has disappeared and so on, until an inappreciable amount remains. The radioactivity of this material is therefore dissipated in a relatively short time. The energy liberated during the period of radioactivity is in the form of beta particles and gamma rays. This radiation brings about the same tissue changes as are secured from radium emanations or from x-rays.

Radioiodine is absorbed rapidly from the stomach, and most of the dose is in the blood within the first hour.[*] The cells of the thyroid gland have an unusual affinity for iodine and will concentrate the element to a marked degree. Radioiodine is useful because it may be located, due to its radioactivity, even when present in extraordinary small amounts. Radioiodine behaves exactly as does ordinary nonradioactive iodine;

[*]Kelsey, M. P., Haines, S. F., and Keating, F. R.: The Treatment of Exophthalmic Goiter With Radioiodine, The Collected Papers of the Mayo Clinic and the Mayo Foundation 41: 202, 1949.

hence an infinitesimal quantity of it can be used to trace or follow the behavior of any amount of ordinary iodine with which it is mixed. Such tiny doses, appropriately called "tracers," when given to a patient, are used to tag all of the ordinary iodine in the patient's body and to permit the observer to trace the behavior of the radioiodine. It has become a useful tool with which to study problems of physiology and disease of the thyroid gland. It is also of value in diagnosing functional states of the thyroid gland, in treating selected cases of cancer of the thyroid gland, and in treating certain cases of hyperthyroidism. Some physicians believe that radioiodine is most effective as a therapeutic agent when used in treatment of patients more than 50 years of age, those who have severe complicating disease, those who have recurrent hyperthyroidism after previous resection of the thyroid, and those who have extremely small glands.

After the oral ingestion of a tracer dose of I^{131}, the following determinations are made: (1) the rate and amount of urinary excretion, (2) the rate and amount of uptake of the radioiodine by the gland, and (3) the rate and degree of incorporation of the radioiodine into the hormonal iodine of the blood. These determinations can be of value because they can be used to help differentiate the patient with a normally functioning thyroid gland from the one with hyperthyroidism or hypothyroidism.

Because radioiodine can be taken by mouth and is collected and concentrated by the thyroid tissue, a much greater degree of irradiation can be secured than is possible with radium or x-ray because of the danger of damaging normal tissue, particularly the skin, when large doses of the latter are used. The results of treatment of the patient with toxic goiter have been encouraging, although the theoretical danger of radiation injury has limited the treatment largely to older patients (beyond the child-bearing period) and to those who are considered poor surgical risks. For the latter type of patient it is thought to be superior treatment to the use of other antithyroid drugs, although it may never be used as widely as certain other antithyroid drugs because of the care and caution with which radioiodine must be handled. However, the chief disadvantage of use of radioiodine is that it may promote the formation of carcinoma. At present this is thought to be possible but unlikely.

When cancer is present in the thyroid gland, the tissue exhibits a variable degree of capacity to collect iodine, depending on the degree of function of the tissue in the tumor. Therefore, the possibility of treating cancer of the thyroid gland with radioiodine appears to be somewhat limited. Metastasis from a malignant tumor of the thyroid gland sometimes can be traced with the use of the Geiger-Müller counter and definite locations of metastatic lesions found. Prolonged treatment with radioiodine may in some cases arrest widespread involvement of this nature.

Preparation, dosage, and administration.

Sodium Radio-Iodide Solution, U.S.P. This is a solution containing iodine[131] suitable for either oral or intravenous administration. Tracer doses range from 1 to 100 microcuries; therapeutic doses, 1 to 100 millicuries. When diagnostic tracer tests are done for evaluation of thyroid function, 1 to 100 microcuries of I[131] are given along with 100 micrograms of nonradioactive sodium iodide as a recommended dosage. This may be given in the morning before breakfast. The test will be invalidated, however, if the patient has been receiving thiouracil or iodine in any form during the preceding week or potassium thiocyanate during the preceding month. Therapeutic dosage is determined by the size of the gland, the severity of the condition being treated, and the results of the preliminary study of the excretion of tracer amounts, or the percentage of the tracer dose observed in the thyroid gland.

Sodium Radio-Iodide Capsules, U.S.P. These are gelatin capsules and contain a radioactive isotope of iodine (I[131]).

Side effects and toxic effects. Although administration of this substance is in one sense very simple, since it can be added to water and given to the patient to swallow as he would a drink of water (for it has no color or taste), on the other hand, the radiation from this substance is dangerous in the same way and to the same extent as are the effects from radium and x-ray. It follows that exposure to radioiodine, like exposure to radium or x-ray, should be avoided or minimized as much as possible. Special precautions must be observed because it is frequently in a form that can be spilled on persons or property. The contamination which may result from spilling a dose of radioiodine or the spilling of urine or other excreta from patients who have received the radioactive substance means that surroundings must be checked and measured with special monitoring instruments, usually by small portable Geiger counters. It is particularly undesirable for nurses and technicians to contaminate their persons with radioiodine, and therefore rubber gloves should be worn whenever the radioiodine is given to patients and during the disposal of their excreta.

Propylthiouracil and related compounds

Propylthiouracil and related compounds interfere with the synthesis of the hormone produced by the thyroid gland. As a result the gland is depleted of hormone, less hormone reaches the tissues of the body, and the rate of metabolism is lowered. Because of the creation of a thyroid hormone deficiency, the thyrotropic hormone made by the anterior lobe of the pituitary gland is increased, and hyperplasia of the thyroid gland occurs. The inhibition of hormone synthesis is sufficiently effective to make these compounds useful in bringing about relief of symptoms of hyperthyroidism. The exact manner in which these drugs prevent synthesis of the thyroid hormone is not known. However, after administration of these compounds is stopped, the thyroid gland rapidly regains its ability to synthesize the hormone as well as to store colloid which contains thyroxin. Propylthiouracil and related compounds are used chiefly to control the signs and symptoms of hyperthyroidism in Graves' disease and in toxic nodular goiter and to prepare the patient who must undergo surgery of the thyroid gland. It is true that the gland is made more friable and vascular with their use, but this is overcome with the simultaneous administration of iodide 10 to 15 days prior to the operation.

Preparation, dosage, and administration. Propylthiouracil and related compounds are readily absorbed from the gastrointestinal tract and are administered by mouth only. Since all have the same mechanism of action, the choice depends on the incidence of side effects and on the duration of action. To ensure adequate and effective therapy, these drugs are administered preferably at evenly spaced intervals during the day. Maintenance doses are determined in accordance with the metabolic rate.

Methylthiouracil, U.S.P., B.P. (Methiacil, Muracil, Thimecil). This drug is marketed in 50 mg. tablets. The usual daily dose is 200 mg. given in divided doses. It may prove useful for patients who are refractory to other antithyroid drugs.

Propylthiouracil, U.S.P., B.P. This preparation is similar to methylthiouracil and is marketed in 50 mg. tablets. The usual daily dose is 100 mg. (75 to 150 mg.). In severe hyperthyroidism, initial doses of 100 mg. every 8 hours may be required. In some instances much larger doses are given.

*Iothiouracil Sodium** (Itrumil Sodium). This drug is said to exert the combined effects of a thiouracil derivative and an iodide. It is available in 50 mg. tablets. Usual daily dose is 150 to 200 mg. in divided doses.

Methimazole, U.S.P. (Tapazole). This is one of the most active of the thyroid-inhibiting drugs. It is marketed in 5 and 10 mg. tablets. Initial doses of 5 to 10 mg. every 8 hours are recommended.

Carbimazole, B.P. This compound is available in 5 mg. tablets. The usual dose is 10 mg. three or four times a day. Claims have been made that this preparation causes less hyperplasia of the thyroid gland than certain of the other preparations of this group of drugs.

Side effects and toxic effects. Drugs of this group vary in their capacity to cause toxic reactions. Thiouracil is the one most likely to cause toxic effects and has been discarded in favor of propylthiouracil and other less toxic substitutes. However, they are all capable of causing

*Described in annual publication of A. M. A. Council on Drugs, N.N.D., 1960.

serious untoward effects, which may include the following: leukopenia, skin rash, drug fever, enlargement of the salivary glands and lymph nodes in the neck, hepatitis, loss of the sense of taste, and edema of the lower extremities. The most grave complication is granulocytopenia. Many of the above-mentioned reactions necessitate the stopping of administration of the drug and the giving of appropriate supportive treatment. Patients should be instructed that if they develop sore throat, a head cold, fever, or malaise they should report the symptoms immediately to their physician. The nurse also should be alert to note warning symptoms. The incidence of untoward reactions is said to be between 3 and 5 per cent. The incidence of agranulocytosis is said to approach 0.5 per cent.* The need for close medical supervision of patients receiving these drugs is obvious.

Hormones of the adrenal gland

The adrenal glands are located just above the kidneys and consist of two parts, the medulla and the cortex. Epinephrine, a secretion of the medullary portion, is discussed in Chapter 10, Autonomic Drugs. The secretion made by the cells of the adrenal cortex is distinctly different from epinephrine. Adrenalectomized animals die within a few days unless they are given injections of adrenal cortex or adrenocortical hormones, whereas removal of the medullary portion of the gland does not necessarily result in death.

Chemistry and function of the adrenal hormones. As an increasing amount of information becomes available about the adrenal gland and its functions, it becomes apparent that its principal function is to deal with emergencies. The medullary portion of the gland functions in emergencies of short duration, whereas the cortex is concerned with emergencies of a more prolonged nature. The cortical hormones function in the regulation of the composition and volume of body fluids and in the mobilization of body energy for cellular work. For example, the adrenal hormones as well as corticotropin from the pituitary gland are not essential for actual cellular oxidation of glucose, but their usefulness is related to the mobilization of glucose from glycogen reserves, the maintenance of blood sugar supported by gluconeogenesis, and rapid utilization of glucose to meet the needs of the body during an emergency.

It is known that the secretory activity of the adrenal cortex is increased during conditions of stress, and there is evidence that cellular utilization of the cortical steroids is also increased during stress. The precise site and method of their action are not known, but it is thought that they exert a supportive effect in a number of body processes. This

*Goodman, L., and Gilman, A.: The Pharmacological Basis of Therapeutics, New York, 1955, The Macmillan Co., p. 1551.

effect has been observed particularly in relation to *electrolyte balance,* the *distribution of body fluids,* and in *carbohydrate metabolism.*

Although a rather large number of steroids have been isolated from the secretion of the cortical portion of the adrenal gland, only a few have been found to have a significant capacity to maintain life in an animal whose adrenal glands have been removed. Among these are desoxycorticosterone, cortisone, hydrocortisone, and a recently isolated steroid first called electrocortin and now known as aldosterone. Note the points of similarity and difference in the accompanying structural formulas.

These as well as a number of other chemically related hormones of the adrenal gland resemble the sex hormones.

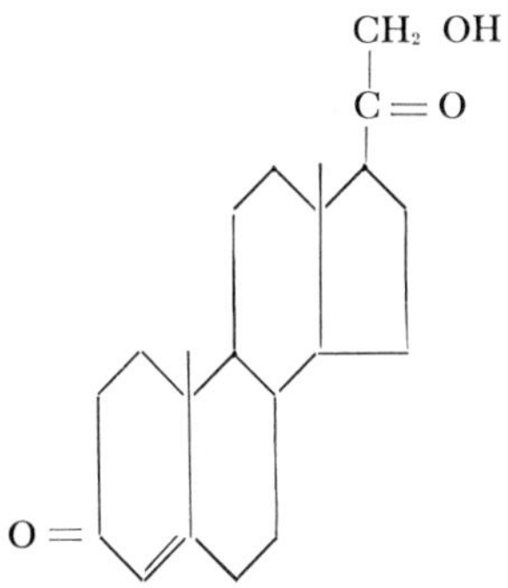

Desoxycorticosterone

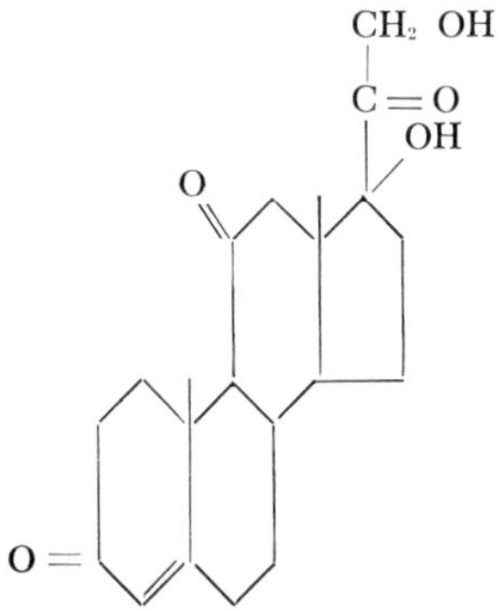

Cortisone

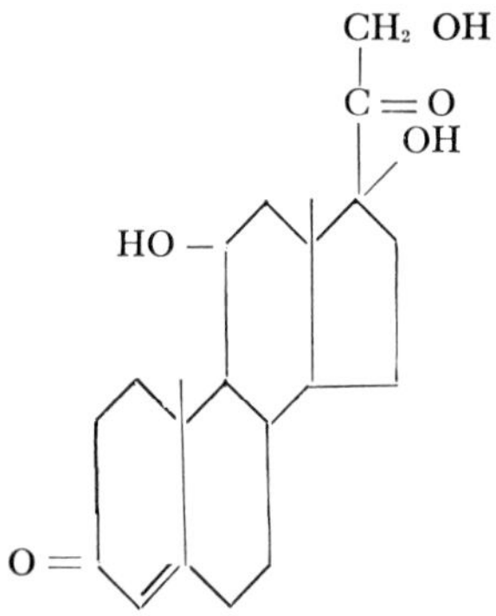

Hydrocortisone

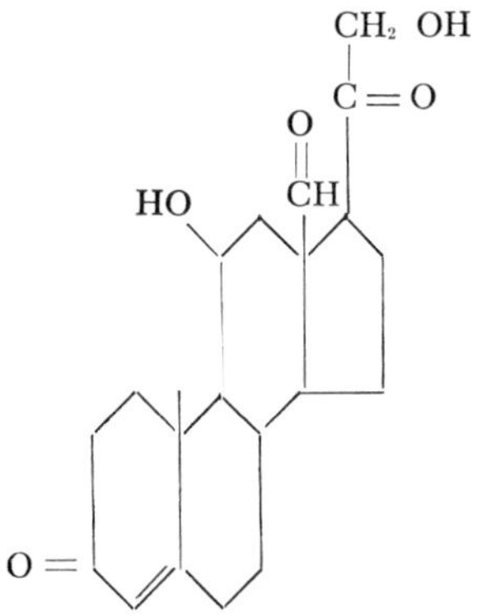

Aldosterone

When crystalline desoxycorticosterone is injected, it is capable of maintaining life, since it is particularly effective in correcting defects in the sodium-potassium balance, but it does not represent full replacement therapy, since it has been noted that patients often show further improvement when they are given additional therapy in the form of preparations of adrenal cortex. Aldosterone has been found to be more effective than desoxycorticosterone in correcting defects of electrolyte metabolism. Moreover, desoxycorticosterone does not correct the abnormalities in carbohydrate metabolism which accompany adrenocortical insufficiency. Patients treated only with desoxycorticosterone are highly affected by states of stress or infections, and a condition known as addisonian crisis may be precipitated.

Adrenal Cortex Injection

Adrenal cortex injection is a sterile solution of a mixture of natural adrenocortical hormones derived from the cortex of adrenal glands of healthy animals used for food by man. This preparation has been used in the prevention and treatment of acute adrenal insufficiency. It is usually administered intramuscularly or intravenously. It is of value in acute stress situations such as are encountered in patients with extensive burns or severe infections. Adrenal cortex injection is expensive, however, and as the availability of the pure adrenocortical steroids has increased, and particularly the availability of the different groups of steroids with their different effects, the use of the whole crude extract has diminished, and it may be anticipated that, like liver extract and other crude preparations, it may soon be completely superseded.

Preparation, dosage, and administration.

Adrenal Cortex Injection, N.F. This preparation is available in 10 and 50 ml. vials. The range of dosage is 10 to 100 ml.

Desoxycorticosterone Acetate (Doca Acetate)

Desoxycorticosterone acetate is a white, crystalline powder, insoluble in water and slightly soluble in vegetable oils. In small amounts it has been isolated from the adrenal cortex and is synthesized as the acetate.

The activity of desoxycorticosterone acetate appears to be limited to the metabolism of sodium, potassium, and water. It promotes the retention of the sodium ions and water and the excretion of potassium. The site of action is seemingly the renal tubule of the kidney where reabsorption is modified.

Patients with chronic adrenal insufficiency, e.g., patients with Addison's disease, may get along satisfactorily with the administration of desoxycorticosterone and sodium chloride. Some physicians prefer to use cortisone and hydrocortisone with sodium chloride along with maintenance doses of desoxycorticosterone. In acute adrenal insufficiency, adrenocortical extract, cortisone, hydrocortisone, and desoxycorticosterone as well as other adrenal steroids may be used.

Preparation, dosage, and administration.

Desoxycorticosterone Acetate, U.S.P. (Doca Acetate, Percorten). *Deoxycortone Acetate,* B.P. This is available as a solution for injection

(5 mg. per milliliter) and in 2 and 5 mg. tablets (buccal). The tablets should be held in the buccal cavity or under the tongue. The solution is given by intramuscular injection.

Desoxycorticosterone Acetate Pellets, N.F. The pellets are available in 75 and 125 mg. quantities for surgical implantation. This form of administration is now seldom used.

Sterile Desoxycorticosterone Trimethylacetate Suspension, U.S.P. This is a microcrystalline suspension of the drug in suspending agents. One injection lasts approximately 6 weeks for the patient with Addison's disease. It is administered intramuscularly. Usual dose is 50 mg.

The maintenance dose of desoxycorticosterone acetate varies from 1 to 7 mg. daily, depending on the response of the patient and the intake of sodium chloride (the higher the intake of salt, the lower the requirement of adrenal steroid).* In the management of an acute crisis, 10 to 15 mg. once or twice a day may be needed along with cortisone or other adrenal steroids. Preparations of desoxycorticosterone do not represent full replacement therapy for adrenal insufficiency.

Side effects and toxic effects. When large doses of desoxycorticosterone are given, patients may develop edema, pulmonary congestion, congestive heart failure, and even death. A fair number of patients develop hypertension after several months or years of receiving this drug. The blood pressure should be taken periodically, and if hypertension develops, the dosage of the steroid and probably also the salt intake should be carefully adjusted. Excessive loss of potassium may account for electrocardiographic changes and sudden attacks of weakness.

Aldosterone

For some years desoxycorticosterone was the only potent steroid available that had selective action in favoring water and salt retention in the patient with Addison's disease, and this hormone, as has been already noted, was lifesaving in the treatment of persons with low or absent adrenal cortical function. Desoxycorticosterone was originally obtained by chemical synthesis and has been found in adrenal glands in only trace levels. There have been reasons to doubt its role as a naturally occurring hormone of importance in regulating salt and water balance. Within the past few years, a new steroid has been discovered in body fluids and in the adrenal gland which seems much more likely to be the natural salt-retaining hormone of the adrenal cortex. This is alderosterone, a compound much more potent in its electrolyte effects than desoxycorticosterone. Although aldosterone has not yet established itself therapeutically in as widely accepted use as DOCA in the past, its increasing use can be anticipated. Preparations of this drug are not commercially avail-

*N.N.D., 1960, p. 531.

able at present. However, a preparation is on the market which appears to block the sodium-retaining effect of aldosterone and is used to relieve edema in patients with cirrhosis of the liver, congestive heart failure, etc. It is a 17-spirolactosteroid sold under the name of Aldactone.

Cortisone and Hydrocortisone

Cortisone and hydrocortisone are adrenal steroids which are particularly concerned with carbohydrate metabolism and are known as glucocorticoids. Cortisone was isolated from the adrenal gland in 1935 and for a time was known simply as Compound E. Hydrocortisone has been known also as Compound F. The activity of these two adrenal steroids is similar, although hydrocortisone is more active possibly and is less irritating to synovial membranes when injected into joint cavities.

Sources. Cortisone is a white, crystalline substance which at the present time is made from an acid obtained from the bile of oxen and sheep. Desoxycholic acid was subjected to some thirty steps whereby changes were made to synthesize the substance now known as 17-hydroxy-11-dehydrocorticosterone. This name was shortened to cortisone. Recently, total synthesis was accomplished. The partial chemical synthesis of hydrocortisone also was achieved soon after that of cortisone. Hydrocortisone, too, is a white, odorless, crystalline powder.

Action and result. Cortisone and hydrocortisone affect carbohydrate, protein, and fat metabolism. They promote glucogenesis, a rise in blood sugar, glycosuria, and a negative nitrogen balance. Large doses over a period of time produce an increased excretion of potassium and retention of sodium. The patient, therefore, must be watched closely to prevent imbalance of electrolytes. These hormones also inhibit activity of the lymphatic system causing lymphopenia and reduction in size of enlarged lymph nodes. Therapeutic doses of cortisone and hydrocortisone depress the function of cells in the adrenal cortex as well as cells of the anterior lobe of the pituitary gland which produce corticotropin. If administration is prolonged and large amounts of these hormones are given, atrophy of the adrenal cortex will develop. The gland usually recovers, fortunately, but permanent damage is always a possibility which must be kept in mind. Administration of the hormones should be withdrawn gradually rather than abruptly, for while termination of their use does not necessarily bring about symptoms of acute adrenal insufficiency, patients are known to experience muscular weakness, lethargy, and exhaustion after administration has been discontinued. Such symptoms are interpreted to mean that there is depression of cortical function.

Both cortisone and hydrocortisone are potent substances which exert widespread physiologic as well as pharmacologic effects in the human body. There is evidence that some of the effects are therapeutically beneficial, others are of no apparent therapeutic significance, and still others are likely to be hazardous to the patient. Although the exact mode of action is unknown, Hench and his associates* were early of the opinion that in diseases which are influenced by cortisone and corticotropin (ACTH), these hormones act as buffer substances against the known or unknown irritant to which the tissues of the body are reacting rather than that they remove the cause of the disease or repair damaged tissues.

"Thus in such conditions as rheumatoid arthritis and rheumatic heart disease, cortisone suppresses the fire; it does not put out the fire (remove the irritant), nor does it repair the fire's damage."*

In other words, cortisone and the closely related hydrocortisone permit the patient to have certain diseases without having the characteristic symptoms thereof or without being injured or destroyed by the disease in some cases at least. In spite of the fact that they do not cure the disease they bring about relief of symptoms in many patients and in addition have provided a remarkable new research tool for medical science.

Uses. Cortisone and hydrocortisone are indicated chiefly for replacement therapy in conditions of adrenal insufficiency, such as may be found after adrenalectomy, Addison's disease, and hypopituitarism. For these conditions these hormones are lifesaving.

To abort attacks of acute gouty arthritis these hormones may be used alone or with colchicine. Corticotropin is thought to be more effective, however, than cortisone.

These hormones are used to relieve allergic manifestations such as may be seen in patients with serum sickness, severe hay fever, status asthmaticus, and exfoliative dermatitis.

Inflammatory conditions of the eye such as uveitis, iritis, acute choroiditis, purulent conjunctivitis, allergic blepharitis, and keratitis are also controlled. More recently, prednisone or prednisolone are considered steroids of choice in treatment of severe ocular inflammation requiring oral therapy.

Cortisone and hydrocortisone have been used extensively for the so-called "collagen" or mesenchymal diseases, such as rheumatoid arthritis, lupus erythematosus, dermatomyositis, and periarteritis nodosa. In these diseases, particularly lupus erythematosus, a sensitivity seems to have been developed following some acute infection, and the brunt of the sensitivity is borne by the connective tissues of the body. Apparently the response of connective tissues to mechanical or chemical injury as well as to states of hypersensitivity such as may be produced by disease or by drugs is somehow altered. The reactivity of the connective

*Hench, P. S., and others: Symposium on Cortisone and ACTH in Clinical Medicine, Proc. Staff Meet. Mayo Clin. **25:** 475, 1950.

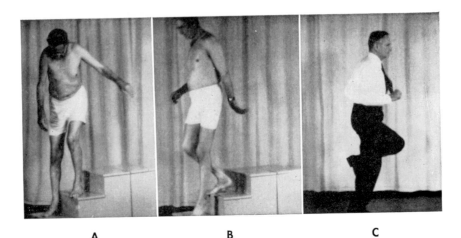

A   B   C

Fig. 47 A, Patient four hours before the first injection of cortisone. Patient is walking down steps unsteadily, with considerable weakness, stiffness, and pain. **B,** Same patient eight days after cortisone injections were begun, walking down stairs normally and without stiffness or pain. **C,** Same patient running easily.

tissue is suppressed regardless of the cause. This effect of cortisone or hydrocortisone seems to explain their capacity to relieve symptoms in a variety of conditions.

In patients with rheumatoid arthritis there is rapid and marked reduction in the symptoms and signs of the disease. Muscle and joint stiffness, muscle tenderness and weakness, and joint swelling and soreness are diminished. The patient getting the drug for the first time usually notices distinct improvement within a few days. Appetite and weight increase, fever, if present, disappears, and the patient feels more energetic. Sedimentation rates usually are reduced or become normal and remain so as long as adequate doses of the hormone are given. Anemic patients usually have a rise in hemoglobin and in the number of red blood cells.

Anatomic changes, however, which have taken place prior to the administration of the hormones are unaffected. Joint deformities which have resulted from damage to bone and cartilage do not improve.* Following the withdrawal of the hormones, symptoms generally reappear within a varying period of time, frequently within a short time.

In acute rheumatic fever the muscle tissue of the heart and connective tissue of the heart valves respond a good deal like other muscle and connective tissues of the body of the patient with rheumatoid arthritis. These hormones suppress the signs and symptoms of the disease, but they neither shorten the natural duration of the disease process nor cure

*Hench, P. S., and others: The Antirheumatic Effects of Cortisone and Pituitary ACTH, Tr. & Stud. Coll. Physicians Philadelphia **18:** 98, 1950.

684

the disease. They do nothing to modify pre-existing valvular damage or hypertrophy of the heart. An adequate evaluation of the role of corticotropin and cortisone in the treatment of rheumatic fever and rheumatic carditis is not possible at the present time.

The need for continued therapy for the patient with rheumatoid arthritis and the effects associated with prolonged administration of large doses make adequate control of symptoms difficult. However, partial relief frequently is possible in a certain percentage of patients without production of undesirable effects.

An aqueous suspension of hydrocortisone acetate may be injected into joint spaces for the local relief of pain and stiffness associated with arthritis and osteoarthritis. It is of some value, particularly for patients who have involvement of only one or two joints. Systemic effects are not observed after intra-articular injection.

Hydrocortisone acetate is useful for topical application for the local management of allergic conditions such as contact dermatitis, allergic eczema, neurodermatitis, and seborrheic dermatitis.

Cortisone and related compounds have been used in the treatment of ulcerative colitis. These compounds suppress the intense inflammatory reaction in the bowel. They do not necessarily cure the condition.

Absorption. Cortisone acetate is absorbed effectively after both oral and intramuscular injection. The response after oral administration is often more rapid than after intramuscular injection, but the effect is less sustained. Since a constant level of the hormone in the tissues is highly desirable, several doses of intramuscular cortisone may be given during the first days of therapy, after which the size of the maintenance dose is determined. After oral administration the absorption of hydrocortisone is highly similar to that of cortisone. Absorption of hydrocortisone from an intramuscular site of injection, however, takes place much more slowly.

Preparation, dosage, and administration.

Cortisone Acetate, U.S.P., B.P. (Cortone Acetate, Cortogen Acetate). Official preparations are available in 25 mg. tablets for oral administration and as a suspension for injection, 25 or 50 mg. per milliliter. There is also available an ophthalmic suspension, 0.5 and 2.5 per cent, and an ophthalmic ointment (1.5 per cent); the latter preparations are no longer official. Cortisone acetate is administered parenterally, orally, or topically. The usual oral dosage is 25 mg. four times a day, and 100 mg. daily by intramuscular injection. However, dosage varies greatly with the nature and severity of the disease being treated and with the responsiveness of the patient. In severe disorders, a common dosage schedule is to give 300 mg. the first day, 200 mg. the second day, and 100 mg. daily thereafter, reducing the dosage gradually to the minimum amount that will bring about the desired effects. Its use in the treatment of acute self-limiting conditions should be discontinued as soon as feasible and dosage must be carefully regulated when used for chronic conditions to avoid undesirable side effects.

Hydrocortisone, U.S.P., B.P. (Cortef, Cortril Hydrocortone). Hydrocortisone is available in 5, 10, and 20 mg. tablets and as a suspension, 2 mg. per milliliter, for oral administration; as a 1 per cent lotion for topical application; and as a solution for injection, 5 to 25 mg. per milliliter. Additional preparations include a cream (1 and 2.5 per cent) and an ointment (1 and 2.5 per cent) for topical application. Hydrocortisone is administered orally, intramuscularly, intravenously, and topically. The dosage of hydrocortisone is said to be about two thirds that of cortisone. Adjustments in dosage are made to meet changes in the needs of the patient. Withdrawal of therapy is sometimes necessary but is avoided when the patient is subjected to additional stress and strain. The usual oral dose is 20 mg. two or three times a day.

Hydrocortisone Acetate, U.S.P., B.P. (Cortef Acetate, Cortril Acetate, Hydrocortone Acetate). This drug is available as a suspension for injection, 25 to 50 mg. per milliliter; as an ophthalmic suspension (0.5 and 2.5 per cent); as an ophthalmic ointment (0.5, 1.5, and 2.5 per cent); and as an ointment for topical application. The dose for intra-articular injection varies greatly with the degree of inflammation, size of the joint, and response of the patient. Doses vary from 5 to 50 mg. Ophthalmic applications also vary but may be used freely since there is no systemic reaction.

Hydrocortisone Sodium Succinate, U.S.P. (Solu-Cortef). This is a highly soluble salt of hydrocortisone which lends itself to parenteral therapy in smaller volumes of diluent. It is recommended for short-term emergency therapy. Dosage and side effects are the same as for hydrocortisone. It is available in vials containing 100 mg. of the powder for injection.

Side effects and toxic effects. Side effects do not often constitute a problem when cortisone or hydrocortisone is given for conditions which are benefited after a short period of administration. This is also true of corticotropin. When large doses or prolonged therapy is necessary, the altered reactions of tissues cells to infections, toxins, and mechanical or chemical injury may bring about serious untoward effects. Healing of wounds may be delayed because of interference with the formation of fibroblasts and their activity in forming ground substance and granulation tissue. Growth of blood vessels into new tissue is also impaired. In patients with peptic ulcer who have been receiving cortisone, neither fever nor abdominal rigidity occurs when perforation of the ulcer and peritonitis develop. Perforation of the bowel has also been reported in patients with chronic ulcerative colitis during treatment with cortisone or corticotropin. Because of the lack of symptoms the diagnosis may be

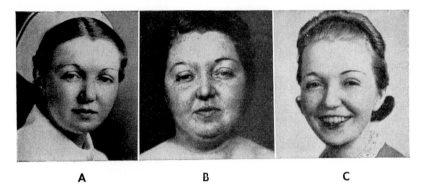

A   B   C

Fig. 48 Cushing's syndrome. Adrenal cortical tumor in a patient 25 years of age. **A,** Before illness. **B,** At height of illness. **C,** One year after removal of the tumor. Overdosage or sustained therapy with cortisone, hydrocortisone, or ACTH may produce symptoms very similar to the naturally occurring Cushing's syndrome. (From Kepler, E. J., Sprague, R. G., Mason, H. L., and Power, M. H.: The Pathologic Physiology of Adrenal Cortical Tumors and Cushing's Syndrome, Recent Progr. Hormone Research **2:** 574, 1948.)

missed and healing may be impaired seriously because of the effect on new scar-forming tissue. This failure of tissue response also explains a breakdown and active manifestation of tuberculosis in persons in whom the infection has been quiescent.

Other side effects which have been noted include amenorrhea, which presumably is due to inhibition of the anterior lobe of the pituitary gland, disorders of calcium metabolism seen particularly after the menopause in women who have developed osteoporosis and spontaneous fractures, and increased incidence of thrombosis and embolic formations. Still other symptoms include those associated with Cushing's syndrome— a rounded contour of the face, hirsutism, purplish or reddish striae of the skin, transient retention of salt and water, and the appearance of edema. Psychic phenomena have also been observed, namely, restlessness, insomnia, euphoria, and even manic states. The psychic status of a patient should, therefore, be considered before these hormones are administered.

Administration of the glucocorticoids may reduce the resistance of the patient to certain infectious processes and to some virus diseases. It is thought, therefore, that acute or subacute infections should be brought under control before starting the administration of these drugs when this is at all feasible. On the other hand, should an infection occur during the course of treatment with these hormones, it may be necessary to increase the dosage to help deal with the added stress occasioned by the infection.

Cortisone and hydrocortisone as well as corticotropin are contraindicated for long-term treatment of patients who have hypertension, cardiovascular-renal disease, or tuberculosis, or for those who exhibit prepsychotic patterns of behavior. In cases of diabetes mellitus, peptic ulcer, and convulsive disorders the need for these hormones must be carefully evaluated in respect to the increased risk that will be present for those who have these complications.

It has become increasingly important to remember that any patient who has received a significant amount of cortisone is likely to have a certain amount of atrophy of the adrenal cortex. The amount of hormone which will produce atrophy is not known; nor is it known how long the atrophy will persist. A patient who must undergo surgery and has received treatment with cortisone should be prepared preoperatively with the administration of cortisone, and its administration should be continued postoperatively in decreasing doses for several days.* The nurse should be alert to pick up this type of information, i.e., she should note whether or not a patient has received treatment with cortisone and, if so, such information should be reported to the physician. It is just possible that it might be overlooked. If patients go to surgery having atrophy of the adrenal gland, it is altogether possible that they will be unable to cope with the stress occasioned by such procedure and death may result.

Some physicians recommend that patients who receive cortisone or corticotropin be given cards similar to those carried by diabetic patients, so that the physician in charge of emergencies may be aware of this fact in the event of an accident.

Newer synthetic corticoids

There is evidence that the compounds already discussed are all natural components of the adrenal gland, although hydrocortisone is considered to be the main steroid found in the blood stream with "corticoid" activity. In recent years, chemical modifications of the basic steroid structure of the corticoids have been made, with the aim of producing more potent and more selectively acting compounds. If an additional double bond is inserted on ring A of cortisone or hydrocortisone, the compounds called prednisone or prednisolone result (see accompanying structural formulas—ring A is the one at lower left of formula).

Prednisone and prednisolone are considerably more active in their anti-inflammatory effect but have little or actually less salt-retaining action as compared to the parent compounds on a weight basis. Hence there is less risk of undesirable side actions related to the retention of salt, hypertension, and formation of edema, when the newer compounds are used for their antirheumatic activity. The addition of a methyl group in the 6 position of ring B of prednisolone produces an even greater effect (see methylprednisolone).

*Priestley, J. T.: Certain Lesions of the Adrenal Glands of Surgical Interest, J. Iowa M. Soc. 44: 407, 1954.

Prednisone (synthetic analogue of cortisone)

Prednisolone (synthetic analogue of hydrocortisone)

Other modifications recently introduced involve adding a fluorine atom in one of the positions (9) of the steroid ring of cortisone and hydrocortisone. This leads to a great increase in both anti-inflammatory and salt-retaining activity. Because the newer fluoro derivatives have such potent salt- and water-retaining action, they have been used less for systemic administration than for topical administration in skin disorders.

9-alpha-fluorohydrocortisone (fludrocortisone)

Methylprednisolone

Preparation, dosage, and administration.

Prednisone, U.S.P., B.P. (Meticorten, Deltasone, Deltra). This drug is available in 1, 2.5, and 5 mg. tablets for oral administration. Dosage varies with the severity of the disease and the response of the patient. A dose of 30 to 50 mg. may be required to suppress severe symptoms, although some physicians prefer to start therapy with a relatively small dose. After 2 to 7 days, dosage is gradually reduced and a maintenance dose established. A dose of 5 to 10 mg. daily may suffice for milder conditions. The daily allotment should be divided into four doses and should be given after meals and at the hour of retirement (with some

Minerals, vitamins, and hormones used as drugs 689

food). Not only the total daily dose but frequently individual doses in the course of the day must be adjusted to meet the needs of the patient. Patients vary in their need and tolerance to all antirheumatic steroids. The nurse should exert great care that the correct dose is given at the right time. When administration of the drug is to be discontinued, it should be withdrawn gradually, and in the event of a medical or surgical emergency or period of unusual stress the drug should be given again to prevent the possibility of acute adrenal insufficiency. This applies to all cortical steroids given for systemic effects.

Prednisolone, U.S.P., B. P. (Meticortelone, Delta Cortef). Prednisolone is available in 1, 2.5, and 5 mg. tablets for oral administration, and as an ointment for topical administration. It has about the same potency as prednisone, and the dosage is approximately the same.

Prednisolone Acetate, U.S.P., B.P. (Sterane). This is marketed as an aqueous suspension, 125 mg. per milliliter, for intramuscular injection. Dosage is the same as for orally administered prednisolone. *Prednisolone Acetate,* B.P., is available in 5 mg. tablets.

Prednisolone Butylacetate* (Hydeltra-T.B.A.). This compound is marketed as a suspension, 20 mg. per milliliter, for injection into joints, bursae, or synovial sheaths. Dosage varies from 4 to 30 mg. Relief of symptoms may not occur for a day or two because the drug is not very soluble.

Methylprednisolone* (Medrol). This drug is available in 2 and 4 mg. tablets for oral administration. Dosage is individually determined, but, in general, it is about two thirds that of either prednisone or prednisolone. Suppressive doses for severe conditions range from 20 to 40 mg. daily; for less severe conditions the initial daily dosage may be from 6 to 20 mg. The daily dose is divided into four parts and is given after meals and at bedtime (with food). The daily maintenance dose is frequently about one half the initial dose.

Prednisolone Phosphate Sodium* (Hydeltrasol). This preparation is more soluble than prednisolone or its acetate or butyl acetate. After parenteral administration it has a rapid onset and short duration of action. It is administered parenterally and topically to the skin, eye, or external ear.

Side effects and toxic effects. Although prednisone, prednisolone, and closely related compounds may achieve their effects with lower dosage, their capacity to produce many of the same side effects as cortisone and hydrocortisone continues to pose problems. A gain in weight, abnormal growth of hair on the face (hypertrichosis), the development of supraclavicular fat pads, increase in blood pressure, euphoria, emotional instability, undue fatigability, and menstrual irregularities are symptoms

*Described in annual publication of A. M. A. Council on Drugs, N.N.D., 1960.

of a developing hypercortisonism which is more difficult to treat than to prevent. Postmenopausal women are especially susceptible to the adrenal steroids and are more likely to develop hypercortisonism than younger women or men. Many physicians recommend that the patient be kept on doses that can be tolerated by the patient even though all the symptoms (rheumatoid arthritis) may not be completely relieved and that the patient have the benefit of other therapy in the form of salicylates, physical therapy, and plenty of rest during both the day and night.

Other synthetic corticoids

Preparation, dosage, and administration.

*Triamcinolone** (Aristocort, Kenacort). This is a potent glucosteroid which is said to produce effects comparable to prednisolone but with lower dosage. It apparently is less likely to produce retention of sodium and water than many of the related compounds and seemingly does not affect excretion of potassium except after large doses. Prolonged use and large doses, however, bring about negative protein and calcium balance and impaired carbohydrate metabolism as well as symptoms of hyperadrenalism. It is administered orally and is available in 1, 2, 4, and 16 mg. tablets. The usual initial dose varies from 8 to 20 mg. daily, given in divided portions. Maintenance dosage is determined in relation to each patient.

*Triamcinolone Acetonide** (Kenalog). This is a derivative of triamcinolone and is suited for topical administration and treatment of acute and chronic dermatoses. It is available as a cream, a lotion, and an ointment (all in a 0.1 per cent concentration).

*Fludrocortisone Acetate** (Florinef Acetate, F-Cortef Acetate). This preparation is marketed as a lotion and as an ointment for topical application. At present it is used primarily for the management of allergic dermatoses. A small quantity is applied to the area of involvement several times a day. Vigorous rubbing at the time of application should be avoided. The part being treated should be carefully cleansed before the application is made. This drug is a derivative of hydrocortisone acetate. It is also marketed as a tablet for oral administration.

*Hydrocortamate Hydrochloride** (Magnacort). This drug is marketed as an ointment for topical application. It is a derivative of hydrocortisone and is used in treatment of dermatoses having an allergic or inflammatory basis. The ointment is applied to the infected areas two or three times a day.

All of the adrenal steroids which are used clinically have distinctive and individual qualities. Cortisone is still useful and in some cases is thought to be preferable to other steroids. It is the least costly to syn-

*Described in annual publication of A. M. A. Council on Drugs, N.N.D., 1960.

thesize.* Hydrocortisone is superior to cortisone, especially for local injection into joints, etc. Fludrocortisone is said to have an anti-inflammatory effect approximately 10 times greater than cortisone (weight-to-weight basis) but an even greater effect than cortisone on the retention of water and salt. Its systemic usefulness is under investigation. It may be useful in the treatment of adrenal insufficiency associated with Addison's disease. For prolonged systemic administration when it is important to avoid disturbances produced by loss of potassium or retention of sodium and to minimize the amount of steroid used, some authorities consider prednisone or prednisolone the steroid of choice.

The production of new synthetic compounds has demonstrated that the steroid molecule can be altered to produce compounds with more selective effects and has paved the way for the synthesis of compounds with even greater selectivity of effects.

Insulin

The discovery of insulin begins with Johann Conrad Brunner (1653-1727), the discoverer of Brunner's glands in the duodenum. In 1683 he made incisions in the pancreas of a dog, after which the dog had extreme thirst and polyuria. Brunner suggested that there is a connection between the pancreas and diabetes. This seems to have been a pioneer experiment on the internal secretions of the pancreas.

In 1889 von Mering and Minkowski showed that removal of the pancreas from dogs produced symptoms identical with diabetes mellitus. In 1906 Minkowski showed that this experimental diabetes could be prevented by pancreatic grafts. This work practically proved that the pancreas produces an internal secretion or hormone that controls carbohydrate metabolism. Corroborative findings soon followed. Partial removal of the pancreas produces a mild diabetes in animals, and transfusion of normal blood ameliorates the symptoms. In autopsy of many diabetic patients, changes in the islets were found. This indicated that the hormone was produced in the islets. Repeated attempts to isolate the hormone failed until Banting and Best in 1921 isolated it in sufficiently pure state to permit its use in diabetic patients. The difficulty in isolating it lay in the fact that pancreatic enzymes destroy insulin. Banting and Best focused their attention on the islets, and to avoid the interfering influence of protein-digesting enzymes of the gland, ligated the pancreatic ducts, and also worked with early fetal pancreas. In both cases trypsin production in the gland is markedly reduced or absent, while it is believed that the islets of Langerhans are functioning. Extracts from such pancreas were found to cause a great reduction of blood sugar.

*Ward, E. E., and others: Prednisone in Rheumatoid Arthritis, Metabolic and Clinical Effects, Ann. Rheumat. Dis., p. 145, June, 1958.

Repeated daily injections permitted animals with the pancreas removed to live beyond the span of life usual under such conditions. Later, methods were developed for the extraction of insulin from adult pancreas, and continuous improvement in the method of extraction has been made. Insulin is now prepared from mammalian pancreas (sheep, hogs, cattle).

Chemistry of insulin. The active material in insulin is a protein which upon hydrolysis yields a number of amino acids. In its crystalline state it appears to be chemically linked with certain metals (zinc, nickel, cadmium, or cobalt). Normal pancreatic tissue is rich in zinc, a fact that may be of significance in the natural storage of the hormone. Insulin keeps rather well in a slightly acidified state but is unstable in dilute alkali. Slight changes in its chemical structure greatly change its behavior and for this reason it cannot be given by mouth.

One of the major advances in our knowledge of insulin came within the last few years, when an English group headed by Frederick Sanger determined the complete amino acid sequence of insulin. Insulin, as a result of this work for which Sanger received the Nobel prize, is known to consist of two polypeptide chains and to consist of 48 amino acids, the exact sequence of which is known. There are slight differences in the order of amino acids in insulin from different species of animals.

Action and result. Since relatively small amounts of insulin are necessary in the body tissues, it is thought that insulin acts as a catalyst in cellular metabolism.

Carbohydrate metabolism is controlled by a finely balanced interaction of a number of endocrine factors (adrenal, anterior pituitary, thyroid, and insulin), but the particular phase of carbohydrate metabolism which is affected by insulin is not entirely known. When insulin is injected hypodermically, however, it produces a rapid lowering of the blood sugar. This effect is produced in both normal and diabetic patients. Moderate amounts of insulin in the diabetic animal promote the storage of carbohydrate in the liver and also in the muscle cells, particularly after the feeding of carbohydrate. In the normal animal, there is also an increase in the deposit of muscle glycogen but apparently no increase in the level of liver glycogen.* In both the normal and the diabetic individual the oxygen consumption increases and the respiratory quotient rises.

Diabetes mellitus. Diabetes mellitus is a disease of metabolism characterized particularly by an inability to utilize carbohydrate. The blood sugar becomes elevated, and when it exceeds a certain amount, the excess is excreted by the kidney (glycosuria). Symptoms include increased appetite, thirst, weight loss, increased urine output, weakness, and itch-

---

*Best, C., and Taylor, N.: The Pharmacological Basis of Medical Practice, Baltimore, 1955, Williams & Wilkins Co., p. 669.

ing (pruritus vulvae). In diabetes mellitus there is a failure to store glycogen in the liver, although the conversion of glycogen back to glucose or the formation of glucose from other substances (gluconeogenesis) is not necessarily impaired. As a result, the level of blood sugar rapidly rises. This derangement of carbohydrate metabolism results in an abnormally high metabolism of proteins and fats. The normal short-chained fatty acids, which result from oxidation of fatty acids, accumulate faster than the muscle cells can oxidize them, resulting in the development of ketosis and acidosis. The course of untreated diabetes mellitus is progressive. The symptoms of diabetic coma and acidosis are directly or indirectly due to the accumulation of acetone, beta-hydroxybutyric acid, and diacetic acid. Respirations become rapid and deep, the breath has an acetone odor, the blood sugar is elevated, the patient becomes dehydrated, and stupor and coma develop unless treatment is promptly started.

Therapeutic uses of insulin. Insulin is a specific in the treatment of diabetic coma and acidosis. The administration of glucose intravenously often accompanies the administration of the insulin, although not all physicians advocate that glucose be used early in the treatment of acidosis. Glucose and insulin promote the formation and retention of glycogen in the liver and the oxidation of fat in the liver is arrested. Therefore, the rate of formation of acetone bodies is slowed and the acidosis is checked. Other supportive measures such as the restoration of the fluid and electrolyte balance of the body are exceedingly important.

Insulin has its principal use in the control of symptoms of diabetes mellitus, when this disease cannot be satisfactory controlled by a dietetic regimen alone. Certain mild cases of the disease can be treated by diet alone, but many patients require insulin in order to live active and useful lives. The dosage must be determined for each individual patient and can best be done when the patient is under the direct observation of the physician for a period of time. A number of factors determine the amount of insulin needed by the patient, and this means that a patient's needs are not always constant. Adjustments in dosage may be necessary if infection is present, if the patient has an anesthetic, if emotional strain and stress are present, or if his amount of activity is increased or decreased.

It is important that the symptoms of diabetes be adequately controlled because the more nearly the blood chemistry of the diabetic patient is restored to normal, the more normal his metabolism and nutrition will be and the less degenerative damage will occur in organs such as the eye and the heart.

Insulin has been used also in some hospitals for the purpose of producing hypoglycemic shock for its effect on the patient with schizophre-

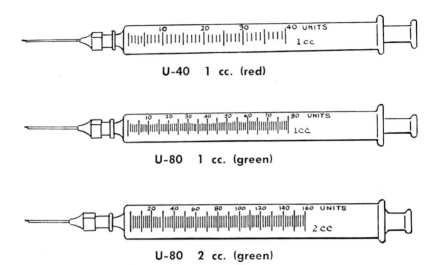

U-40   1 cc. (red)

U-80   1 cc. (green)

U-80   2 cc. (green)

Fig. 49 Insulin syringes. The first or uppermost syringe is used only for U-40 insulin (40 units of insulin in 1 cc. [ml.]). It is scaled in red. The next syringe is used for U-80 only and is scaled in green. The third syringe is also scaled in green and is used only for U-80 insulin. The latter syringe is suited for use when unusually large doses of insulin must be given.

nia. It is a dangerous treatment with a relatively high mortality and should be used only by those who are well equipped, qualified, and familiar with the procedure. It has been replaced, to a great extent, by electroshock therapy.

Preparation, dosage, and administration. A number of different types of insulin preparations are used in medicine. All preparations have the same fundamental pharmacologic action. Differences are those related to the time and duration of absorption of the injected insulin into the circulation, providing faster or slower, shorter or more prolonged effects.

Insulin is given subcutaneously into the loose connective tissues of the body, usually into the arms or thighs. It cannot be given by mouth because it is destroyed by digestive enzymes. Regular insulin is usually given about 20 minutes before meals. It is somewhat irritating, and since the tissues of the diabetic patient are likely to be less resistant to the invasion of pathogenic organisms than normal tissue, the technic used in administration of insulin should be flawless. The same site of injection should not be used repeatedly, but a plan of rotation should be followed so that the same site is not used oftener than once a month.

There is no average dose of insulin for the diabetic; each patient's needs must be determined individually. Unless complications are present, insulin should not be used if the patient's glucose tolerance is suffi-

Minerals, vitamins, and hormones used as drugs   695

ciently high to permit him to have a diet sufficient for light work.

Dosage of insulin is expressed in units rather than in milliliters or minims. Insulin injection is so standardized that each milliliter contains 20, 40, 80, or 100 U.S.P. units per milliliter. One insulin unit will, on the average, promote the metabolism of approximately 1.5 Gm. of dextrose.*
In order to estimate the necessary insulin dosage for the patient, the physician must know how much dextrose will be obtained from the diet and what the patient's glucose tolerance is, i.e., how much insulin the patient is able to make for himself. Insulin must be regularly administered and must be accompanied by carefully estimated diets of known composition.

Insulin Injection, U.S.P., B.P. This is an acidified aqueous solution of the active principle of the pancreas which affects the metabolism of glucose. This preparation is marketed in 10 ml. vials in strengths of 40, 80, 100, and 500 U.S.P. units per milliliter of the injection. The maximum degree of lowering of the blood sugar occurs in 2 or 3 hours. The onset of its activity is 1 hour, and the duration of activity in 6 to 8 hours.

Protamine Zinc Insulin Suspension, U.S.P.; *Protamine Zinc Insulin Injection*, B.P. This is a preparation of insulin to which has been added an appropriate amount of protamine and a zinc salt, which has the effect of slowing absorption. The effects produced by protamine zinc insulin are the same as those of insulin except that the blood sugar-lowering action is much more prolonged. It may be used in place of unmodified insulin or in combination with it. The chief indications for its use are in those cases where the unmodified insulin does not provide control of symptoms unless it is given in several daily doses or in cases where lack of control is evidenced by frequent hypoglycemic reactions, ketosis, or pronounced fluctuations in levels of blood sugar. Usually protamine zinc insulin is administered either in the morning, ½ to 1½ hours before breakfast, or in the evening, 1 hour before supper or before retiring. Its maximum blood sugar-lowering action is about 16 to 24 hours after administration. Its onset of action is 4 to 6 hours and its duration of action, 24 to 36 hours or longer.†

Hypoglycemic reactions are recognized less easily than with the regular insulin. Sometimes the main symptom is a feeling of pronounced fatigue out of proportion to the degree of activity. Treatment consists of giving a combination of a rapidly absorbed and a slowly absorbed carbohydrate, something like bread and honey. Protamine insulin is of no value in emergencies such as diabetic coma. A combination of protamine insulin and rapid-acting insulin is frequently necessary if adequate control of symptoms is to be maintained. It is administered subcutaneously, never intravenously. It should be mixed well (but not made to foam)

*N.N.D., 1960, p. 580.
†N.N.D., 1960, p. 583.

before withdrawal from container in order to obtain a uniform suspension. It is available in concentrations of 40 or 80 U.S.P. units of insulin per milliliter of injection.

Globin Zinc Insulin Injection, U.S.P., B.P. This is a preparation of insulin modified by the addition of globin and zinc chloride. The globin is obtained from globin hydrochloride prepared from beef blood. Each milliliter of the finished product contains 40 or 80 units of insulin. The action of this preparation is between that of regular insulin and protamine zinc insulin. The period of maximum effect extends from the eighth to the sixteenth hour after injection.[*] It is beneficial for those patients who require more than a single injection of regular insulin, for those who are sensitive to protamine, and for those whose levels of blood sugar are not satisfactorily controlled by other forms of insulin. It is said to produce fewer local reactions than regular insulin. It should not be given when rapid effects are desired, and it should never be given intravenously. It should be administered only by deep subcutaneous injection. The dosage must be regulated according to the patient's needs. The initial dose may be two thirds to three fourths of the daily dose of regular insulin and then increased gradually as needed.[†]

Isophane Insulin Suspension, U.S.P. (NPH Insulin). This preparation is a modified protamine zinc insulin. N indicates that it is a neutral solution; P stands for protamine zinc insulin; and H means that it originated in Hagedorn's Laboratory.[‡] It is marketed in concentrations of 40 or 80 U.S.P. units per milliliter of suspension. Its action places it between globin insulin and protamine zinc insulin. Its peak effect after subcutaneous injection is reached in 10 to 20 hours, and the duration of its action is 28 to 30 hours.[†] Isophane insulin may be mixed with regular insulin. It is an intermediate-acting insulin preparation and should not be used when a quick-acting insulin is needed. It is given only by subcutaneous injection.

Lente insulins

Lente insulins are a group of newer preparations of insulin. They consist of insulin precipitated with zinc and resuspended in an acetate buffer rather than a phosphate buffer which is usually used in insulin preparations. By varying the way the insulin is prepared it is possible to obtain suspensions which contain particles of different size and form. It has been found that the larger crystals produce a longer but less intense effect, and this preparation is known as ultralente insulin and its action resembles that of protamine zinc insulin. Semilente insulin con-

[*]N.N.D., 1960, p. 583.
[†]N.N.D., 1960, p. 584.
[‡]Goodman, A., and Gilman, A.: The Pharmacological Basis of Therapeutics, New York, 1955, The Macmillan Co., p. 1629.

tains smaller particles and its action falls between that of NPH and crystalline insulin. *Insulin, Zinc Suspension*, U.S.P., B.P. (Lente Insulin) contains a mixture of ultralente and semilente insulins. Lente insulins are available in 40 and 80 units per milliliter of suspension. The duration of lente insulin is much like that of NPH insulin and the two can be used interchangeably. Its characteristics of action place it between regular insulin and protamine zinc insulin.

The principal advantage of the lente insulins is their lack of sensitizing substances such as protamine or globin. They are useful for the treatment of diabetic patients who are allergic to other types of insulin or for those whose disease is difficult to control.

Lente insulins* should be refrigerated and the vials should be rotated and inverted from end to end several times before a dose is withdrawn. A vial should not be shaken vigorously or the suspension made to foam. The injection should be made deep into subcutaneous tissue but not into muscle, and it should never be given intravenously. The usual time of administration is in the morning before breakfast. The dosage must be individualized for each patient. It should not be used in the treatment of acidosis or for conditions that demand a rapid-acting type of insulin.

Symptoms of overdosage. The symptoms of hypoglycemia develop in the patient who is given an overdose of insulin or in the patient with hyperinsulinism due to certain changes in the pancreas. When due to overdose of insulin the fall in blood sugar is in proportion to the amount of insulin given. In man, toxic symptoms occur when the blood sugar falls below 79 mg. per 100 ml. The point at which the symptoms become noticeable varies greatly, however. For each person there is a level at which severe symptoms or the convulsive stage of hypoglycemia is reached. The symptoms of hypoglycemia depend on the speed with which it develops. Symptoms resulting from protamine zinc insulin are especially insidious.

Early symptoms include a feeling of weakness, sweating, nervousness and anxiety, pallor or flushing, and a vague feeling of apprehension. If the patient does not receive treatment, the symptoms may be intensified with the development of aphasia, convulsive seizures, coma, and even death. When the first mild symptoms are noted, the patient should receive treatment at once. Prolonged hypoglycemia is associated with diminished oxygen consumption and irreparable injury of the nervous system. Symptoms of hypoglycemia are quickly relieved by the administration of a soluble carbohydrate in the form of orange juice or two or three lumps of sugar by mouth or a soluble carbohydrate intravenously if the patient is comatose.

Ambulatory patients learn to recognize sudden hunger, sweating, and

*All insulin should be refrigerated.

nervousness as subjective signs of insulin overdosage and learn to carry a few lumps of sugar with them. A night nurse may find a diabetic patient asleep but in a pool of perspiration, a fact which would lead her to suspect that he was having an insulin reaction and that he should be awakened and given treatment.

Other untoward effects. Repeated injections of insulin at the same site may cause local reactions of the subcutaneous tissues. These can be avoided by changing the site of injection.

Some patients experience a disturbance of vision thought to be due to a change in the crystalline lens of the eye. This disappears after a few weeks. Edema of the face and sometimes of the extremities is observed occasionally, especially in young women. This, too, tends to disappear, but if troublesome it may necessitate restriction of sodium chloride and the use of a mild diuretic.

A few patients exhibit allergic reactions in the form of urticaria, redness, and itching in the region where the insulin has been injected. These symptoms can usually be controlled by changing to a different brand of insulin.

An occasional diabetic patient fails to respond to an ordinary therapeutic dose of insulin. In these cases, there has developed what is known as *insulin resistance.* Enormous doses may be required to lower the blood sugar and to prevent acidosis. The cause of this condition is not entirely understood. In some instances it appears to be due to the formation of antibodies and in other cases it is thought to be due to disturbance of the pituitary, adrenal, or thyroid glands. Most patients respond to large doses of insulin and the condition tends to be self-limiting.

Oral hypoglycemic agents

In the early days of insulin therapy many attempts were made to obtain a preparation or modification of insulin active after oral administration. None was successful, and it is unlikely that any can be, since polypeptides and proteins are both susceptible to destruction in the gastrointestinal tract and are poorly absorbed in an intact state.

In recent years, certain drugs have been found which do have blood sugar-lowering or "insulin-like" action when given by mouth. They are principally the group of sulfonylureas. These compounds were originally discovered after observing that some of the antibacterial sulfonamides had hypoglycemic effects. These drugs are sometimes called "oral insulins," although this is definitely incorrect, since, chemically, they are completely different from insulin. They also differ from insulin in origin and mode of action.

The sulfonylureas are thought to act by increasing the pancreas' own ability to secrete insulin. They are most effective therefore in relatively

$$CH_3 - \langle \underline{} \rangle - SO_2 - NH - CO - NH - (CH_2)_3 - CH_3$$

Tolbutamide (Orinase)

$$NH_2 - \langle \underline{} \rangle - SO_2 - NH - CO - NH - (CH_2)_3 - CH_3$$

Carbutamide

mild diabetes when there is still some reserve islet capacity, and they are less effective or ineffective in severe diabetes or juvenile diabetes in which it is presumed that no functional islet tissue is left to respond. It has also been noted that long-continued high doses of the sulfonylureas administered to normal animals can *produce* diabetes, apparently by permanently exhausting the capacity of the islet cells to make insulin.

Although much interest and enthusiasm have greeted this new development and although these drugs have considerable scientific importance, they cannot be said to have fully established themselves, like insulin in the treatment of diabetes. There is no point in using this drug for diabetes, which can be controlled by diet alone. Insulin continues to be indispensable for diabetes complicated by coma and acidosis.

Preparation, dosage, and administration.

Tolbutamide, U.S.P. (Orinase). This drug is marketed in 500 mg. tablets for oral administration. Therapeutic trial with this drug is initiated with 3 Gm. on the first day, 2 Gm. on the second day, 1 Gm. on the third day; then dosage is gradually reduced until the minimum dose has been determined which will provide satisfactory control of blood sugar. Maintenance dosage may vary from 0.5 to 1.5 Gm. per day. The drug is preferably given in divided doses and after meals. Diabetic patients should be under close medical supervision, especially when the drug is first tried, and the patient should be periodically checked thereafter.

Carbutamide. This drug causes allergic reactions in human beings and has not been released for use in the United States.

Side effects and toxic effects. Side effects which have been reported include gastrointestinal upsets, weakness, paresthesia, headache, ringing in the ears, and intolerance to alcohol. A mild type of leukopenia has been reported. It may interfere with some enzymatic reactions in the liver and therefore its use for patients with hepatic damage is not recommended. The incidence of toxicity seems to be low. It is important that the diabetic patient observe dietary restrictions as carefully as when taking insulin. The drug does not cure the diabetes. Some patients develop allergic reactions which may require that administration of the drug be stopped and that therapy with insulin be resumed. Patients should be carefully instructed concerning the limitations of tolbutamide. Overdosage produces characteristic hypoglycemic reactions.

Other hypoglycemic agents

A number of other oral hypoglycemic agents are undergoing investigation. One is chlorpropamide (Diabinese). Chemically, it belongs to the arylsulfonylurea compounds, and many of the same precautions regarding its use are recommended as for tolbutamide.

Phenethylbiguanide (DBI) is a new hypoglycemic agent, but it differs from the sulfonylureas in that it does not stimulate the pancreatic beta cells to secrete insulin. Its mode of action is not known. The chief side effects appear to be gastrointestinal disturbances (nausea and vomiting). Clinical investigation continues to determine its ultimate place in the management of diabetes mellitus.

Questions
for review and study

1 Vitamin D helps to prevent rickets in which of the following ways?
   a. promoting the absorption of calcium from the bowel
   b. stimulating the bone cells to deposit calcium salts
   c. increasing activity of the parathyroid gland
   d. inhibiting activity of cells in the adrenal cortex
2 Preparations of posterior lobe pituitary can be expected to contain which of the following?
   a. growth hormone
   b. antidiuretic hormone
   c. thyrotropic hormone
   d. oxytocic principle
      (1) a and b
      (2) b and c
      (3) b and d
      (4) c and d
3 Which of the following preparations would you expect to see prescribed for a patient with myxedema?
   a. iodized salt
   b. Lugol's solution
   c. radioactive iodine
   d. thyroid tablets
4 Effective therapy with ACTH is dependent upon a normal state of function of which of the following?
   a. thyroid gland
   b. adrenal gland
   c. islands of Langerhans
   d. anterior lobe of pituitary gland
5 Insulin must be administered with a needle for which of the following reasons?

   a. it acts more promptly when given with a needle
   b. oral administration of insulin is most likely to cause gastrointestinal irritation
   c. insulin is subject to destruction by proteolytic enzymes in the digestive tract
   d. insulin is not well absorbed from the gastrointestinal tract
6 Which of the following patients is likely to have prescribed for him a daily dose of ascorbic acid?
   a. a patient recovering from a stroke
   b. a patient recovering from a surgical operation
   c. a patient with acute coronary insufficiency
   d. a patient with pernicious anemia
7 A patient receiving insulin for diabetes mellitus is receiving a form of therapy which can be compared to which of the following?
   a. thyroid for cretinism
   b. streptomycin for tuberculosis
   c. cortisone for rheumatoid arthritis
   d. morphine for severe pain
8 Which of the following constitutes a significant side effect in a patient receiving cortisone?
   a. emotional instability
   b. polyuria
   c. increased appetite
   d. pigmentation of the skin
9 Prednisone differs from cortisone in which of the following respects? It is less likely to:
   a. cause retention of water and salt
   b. inhibit healing of tissues

c. produce symptoms of hypercortisonism
d. bring about depression of the adrenal cortex

10 If one of your patients who has rheumatoid arthritis for which her doctor has prescribed daily doses of aspirin, says to you, "I don't understand why my doctor only gives me aspirin, why can't I have one of the newer medicines like cortisone?" which of the following statements would you consider to be most appropriate and most helpful?

a. cortisone is prescribed by many physicians, but your physician probably wants to take a conservative approach to your problem.
b. cortisone can be a dangerous drug and can produce many undesirable side effects.
c. for the pain associated with rheumatism and arthritis, aspirin is considered one of the safest and best drugs on the market.
d. cortisone is a relatively expensive drug whereas aspirin is inexpensive.

References

American Diabetes Association: Clinical Use of Tolbutamide in Diabetes Mellitus, J. A. M. A. **164**: 1151, 1957.

Beckman, H.: Drugs, Their Nature, Action and Use, Philadelphia, 1958, W. B. Saunders Co.

Best, Charles, and Taylor, Norman: The Physiological Basis of Medical Practice, Baltimore, 1955, Williams & Wilkins Co.

Black, B. M.: An Evaluation of Present Trends in the Treatment of Exophthalmic Goiter, Collected Papers of the Mayo Clinic and the Mayo Foundation **41**: 195, 1949.

Cooper, L. F., Barber, E. M., Mitchell, H. S., and Rynbergen, H. J.: Nutrition in Health and Disease, Philadelphia, 1958, J. B. Lippincott Co.

Council on Foods and Nutrition—Youmans, J. B.: Deficiencies of the Fat Soluble Vitamins, J. A. M. A. **144**: 34, 1950.

Harris, L. J.: Vitamins in Theory and Practice, Cambridge, 1935, University Press.

Kleiner, I. S., and Orten, J. M.: Human Biochemistry, St. Louis, 1958, The C. V. Mosby Co.

National Research Council: Recommended Dietary Allowances, Publication 589, Washington, D. C., 1958.

Nielsen, R. H., and Kirby, T. J.: Tolbutamide for Diabetes Mellitus (editorial), J. A. M. A. **164**: 562, 1957.

Pomeranze, Julius, and others: Phenethylbiguanide, a New Orally Given Hypoglycemic Agent, J. A. M. A. **171**: 252, 1959.

Thyroid and antithyroid drugs

Clark, D. E., Trippel, O. H., and Sheline, G. E.: Diagnostic and Therapeutic Use of Radioactive Iodine, A. M. A. Arch. Int. Med. **87**: 17, 1951.

Drill, V. A. (editor): Pharmacology in Medicine, New York, 1958, McGraw-Hill Book Co., Inc.

Goodman, L., and Gilman, A.: The Pharmacological Basis of Therapeutics, New York, 1955, The Macmillan Co.

Gordon, E. S., and Albright, E. C.: Treatment of Thyrotoxicosis With Radioactive Iodine, J. A. M. A. **143**: 1129, 1950.

Haines, S. F.: Treatment of Exophthalmic Goiter, New York J. Med. **54**: 2175, 1954.

Keating, F. R.: The Medical Use of Radioactive Isotopes, Am. J. M. Sc. **213**: 628, 1947.

Keating, F. R., Haines, S. F., Power, M. H., and Williams, M. M. D.: The Radioiodine-Accumulating Function of the Human Thyroid as a Diagnostic Test in Clinical Medicine, J. Clin. Endocrinol. **10**: 1425, 1950.

Kelsey, M. P., Haines, S. F., and Keating, F. R.: The Treatment of Exophthalmic Goiter With Radio-iodine, the Collected Papers of the Mayo Clinic and the Mayo Foundation **41**: 202, 1949.

Kendall, E. C.: Thyroxine, Am. Chem. Soc. Monographs, New York, 1929, Chemical Catalogue Co.

Owen, C. A.: The Diagnostic Use of Radioactive Isotopes, Radioiodine and Thyroidal Function, Postgrad. Med. **24**: 669, 1958.

Salter, W. T.: A Textbook of Pharmacology, Philadelphia, 1952, W. B. Saunders Co.

Wilkins, L.: The Thyroid Gland; Scient. Am. **202**: 119, March, 1960.

Corticotropin and adrenocortical steroids

Editorial: Effect of Cortisone and Pituitary Adrenocorticotropic Hormone, J. A. M. A. **142**: 730, 1950.

Gordon, D. M., and McClean, J. M.: Effects of Pituitary Adrenocorticotropic Hormone (ACTH) Therapy in Ophthalmologic Conditions, J. A. M. A. **142:** 1271, 1950.

Hampton, P. H., and Kepler, E. J.: Addison's Disease: Treatment and Prognosis, Collected Papers of the Mayo Clinic, Philadelphia, 1941, W. B. Saunders Co.

Hench, P. S., and others: The Effects of the Adrenal Cortical Hormone 17-Hydroxy-11-Dehydrocorticosterone (Compound E) on the Acute Phase of Rheumatic Fever; Preliminary Report, Proc. Staff Meet. Mayo Clin. **24:** 277, 1949.

Hench, P. S., Kendall, E. C., Slocumb, C. H., and Polley, H. F.: The Effect of a Hormone of the Adrenal Cortex (17-Hydroxy-11-Dehydrocorticosterone; Compound E) and of Pituitary Adrenocorticotropic Hormone on Rheumatoid Arthritis; Preliminary Report, Proc. Staff Meet. Mayo Clin. **24:** 181, 1950.

Hench, P. S., and others: Symposium on Cortisone and ACTH in Clinical Medicine, Proc. Staff Meet. Mayo Clin. **25:** 474, 1950.

Hench, P. S., Kendall, E. C., Slocumb, C. H., and Polley, H. F.: The Antirheumatic Effects of Cortisone and Pituitary ACTH, Tr. & Stud. Coll. Physicians Philadelphia **18:** 95, 1950.

Henderson, E. D., and Peterson, C. E.: Hydrocortisone and Prednisolone, Local Injection in Skeletal Diseases, Orthopedics **1:** 6, 1958.

Kendall, E. C.: The Function of the Adrenal Cortex—Collected Papers of the Mayo Clinic, Philadelphia, 1941, W. B. Saunders Co.

Kendall, E. C.: The Story of Cortisone, Hosp. Manage. **70:** 72, 1950.

Kendall, E. C.: Cortisone, Quart. Phi Beta Pi **47:** 187, 1951.

Nielsen, R. H., and Kirby, T. J.: The Modern Treatment of Uveitis, A. M. A. Arch. Ophthal. **58:** 79, 1957.

Priestley, J. T.: Certain Lesions of the Adrenal Glands of Surgical Interest, J. Iowa M. Soc., p. 407, Sept., 1954.

Salassa, R. M., and others: Effects of Aldosterone on Water, Electrolyte and Nitrogen Balance in Addison's Disease, Proc. Staff Meet. Mayo Clin. **32:** 201, 1957.

Slocumb, C. H., and others: Hypercortisonism in Patients With Rheumatoid Arthritis, Postgrad. Med. **25:** 185, 1959.

Sprague, R. G., and others: Observations on the Physiologic Effects of 17-Hydroxy-11-Dehydrocorticosterone, Cortisone and Adrenocorticotropic Hormone (ACTH) in Man, Arch. Int. Med. **85:** 199, 1950.

Ward, L. E., Polley, H. F., Slocumb, C. H., and Hench, R. S.: Cortisone in the Treatment of Rheumatoid Arthritis, J. A. M. A. **152:** 119, 1953.

Ward, L. E., and others: The Effects of Aldosterone (Electrocortin) and of 9α-Fluorohydrocortisone Acetate on Rheumatoid Arthritis: Preliminary Report, Proc. Staff Meet. Mayo Clin. **29:** 649, 1954.

Ward, L. E., and others: Prednisone in Rheumatoid Arthritis, Metabolic and Clinical Effects, Ann. Rheumat. Dis. **17:** 145, 1958.

Wollaeger, E. E.: Untoward Effects of Cortisone and Corticotropin on the Gastrointestinal Tract, Minnesota Med. **37:** 626, 1954.

Chapter 25

Antineoplastic drugs

As malignant diseases have become ever more significant causes of death and disability, chemical agents for the treatment of cancer and related disorders have become increasingly important in therapeutics. The drugs are grouped together in a single chapter because they are employed with the same aim: the pharmacologic eradication or control of malignant tumors. However, it should be pointed out immediately that the various groups of drugs presented act in different ways and that the individual types of tumors may even represent basically different kinds of disorders. It also should be clearly stated that at present there is no known drug that *cures* malignant disease. True cures of malignant tumors are produced only by early surgery and x-ray, and in a varying percentage of cases. The use of drugs—*antimalignant, antineoplastic,* and *carcinostatic* are some of the terms used for this class of drugs—is therefore confined to malignant disease after it has become metastatic and is no longer curative by surgery or to diseases such as leukemia or lymphosarcoma which start out as disseminated malignant processes.

Malignant tumors are those made up of cells that grow rapidly and without the normal controls and restraints to which tissues respond. Such tumors are locally invasive, growing into surrounding tissues and destroying them by pressure or usurping their supply of nutrients and oxygen. Malignant tumors may also metastasize, sending off daughter cells by way of the blood or lymphatic streams, or by the serous fluids in the body cavities, to form new colonies of tumor. Such tumors may arise from cells of virtually any tissue of the body, and, in general, they are always fatal if not totally eradicated by surgery or by irradiation.

Since the basic process of origin of malignant cell growth is not understood, there can be no rationally based pharmacologic treatment. Instead, the types of chemical agents which have been useful have been obtained primarily by empirical screening of many different kinds of compounds. Furthermore, the compounds employed today are not highly selective in the manner that some of the antibacterial agents are, i.e., they are not able to destroy microbial invaders without appreciably harming the host cells. In contrast, many of the effective antineoplastic agents are active because they are toxic to *all rapidly proliferating cells.* Since many normal cells (gastrointestinal and epithelial cells and cells of bone marrow) are also rapidly proliferating, these normal tissues may also be damaged by some of the antineoplastic agents. This means that this group of agents is a comparatively toxic one, and many of the drugs used could not be considered safe enough for use if the type of disease being treated did not itself make the situation desperate.

Classification of drugs used in neoplastic diseases

The antineoplastic drugs can be divided into several large groups, on the basis of their probable manner of action.

The alkylating agents (nitrogen mustards and related compounds). These are compounds that are highly reactive chemically and act by transferring alkyl groups to receptor molecules. It is postulated that they act as anticancer agents by reacting with essential molecules in the cells of the tumor, e.g., nucleic acids. In general, rapidly reproducing cells are sensitive to the alkylating agents so that many of these compounds are also toxic to the gastrointestinal tract and the bone marrow. Important individual examples of this group are mechlorethamine, busulfan, and triethylene melamine.

The antimetabolites. These are compounds the chemical structures of which are close to but not identical with substances normally used by cells for growth and metabolism. Just as sulfanilamide acts as an antimetabolite for the normal bacterial metabolite p-aminobenzoic acid and is thus toxic for certain bacteria, certain artificial relatives ("analogues") of some of the vitamins or the components of nucleic acids can be toxic for rapidly growing human or mammalian cells. Important members of this group are the "antifolic acid agents"—aminopterin and amethopterin. These are compounds resembling folic acid, which are believed to act by "competitively" preventing the conversion of folic acid to a biologically more active derivative. Other antimetabolites are 6-mercaptopurine and 5-fluorouracil. These drugs as a group are also quite toxic to certain normal tissues.

Hormones. The hormones are believed to slow the growth of tumors by making the environment less favorable. Certain tumors of secondary sexual tissue origin, such as prostatic cancer, are somewhat dependent for their growth on a supply of the male sex hormone. If this is removed (as by castration) and, furthermore, if estrogens are added to the environment, the growth of malignant cells of the prostate gland may be slowed. Comparably, some mammary cancers are slowed by the administration of androgenic hormone. A further example, although not so well understood, is the inhibiting effect that adrenocorticotropic hormone (ACTH) has on certain types of leukemia.

Radioisotopes. These are "drugs" that act essentially as x-ray does by liberating cell-destroying ionizing radiation in the vicinity of the tumor. The chemical nature of the radioisotope, however, may take advantage of pharmacologic principles by guaranteeing delivery of the radioactivity to the proper target. Thus radioiodine is used to treat some thyroid cells so that the damaging effects of the radiation are brought to the site desired. Other examples are radioactive phosphate ($P^{32}O_4^{=}$) and colloidal radiogold (Au^{198}).

Miscellaneous. A final group not easily classified in any of the above includes urethane, potassium arsenite, and phenylhydrazine, which have particular uses in reducing the number of neoplastic cells, particularly in abnormal proliferation of leukocytes or erythrocytes.

Neoplastic diseases of blood-forming organs

A number of the drugs mentioned in this chapter are used in treatment of neoplastic conditions which affect the blood and blood-forming tissues. A brief description of several of these disorders follows.

Leukemias. Leukemia is considered by many to be a neoplastic disease which is characterized by excessive production of white blood cells. It affects the bone marrow, lymph nodes, and spleen. For some reason which is not fully understood, the blood-forming tissues produce white blood cells wildly and excessively and the bone marrow becomes infiltrated with abnormal cells. The production of erythrocytes and thrombocytes is reduced and the patient tends to become anemic and to exhibit hemorrhagic tendencies. The type of white cell that predominates in the blood determines the type of leukemia. Myelogenous leukemia means that the type of white cell found most often is a granulocyte or its precursor. Lymphatic leukemia is characterized by a large number of lymphocytes. Both types of leukemia may be acute or chronic. Immature white blood cells are found in the blood of the patient with acute leukemia, whereas more fully matured cells are seen in the case of chronic leukemia. Although the number of white blood cells may be excessive, they afford little protection against infection. Cells other than lymphocytes and granulocytes, but normally found in hematopoietic tissues, may also become active in neoplastic proliferation. The cause of this disorder is not known.

Lymphomas. Lymphomas are tumors that involve the lymph nodes. Lymphosarcoma is a disease in which the lymphocytes multiply excessively and involve the lymph nodes, spleen, and lymphoid tissues of other organs. Almost any part of the body may become involved. Hodgkin's disease also involves lymph nodes as well as nonnodal tissues, but the reticulum cells rather than the lymphocytes are involved. These diseases are usually fatal within a few years at the most. The lymph nodes, liver, and spleen become enlarged in lymphomas. Fever, itching, hemorrhagic tendencies, as well as anemia and thrombocytopenia, present special clinical problems. X-ray therapy is the treatment of choice, although the nitrogen mustards and related compounds are considered valuable as adjunctive forms of treatment.

Polycythemia vera. Polycythemia vera is a disease characterized by excessive formation of erythrocytes, the number per cubic millimeter sometimes being many times the normal number. Increased numbers of leukocytes and thrombocytes are present frequently. Patients with this disease are likely to develop hypertension and are prone to have vascular accidents if the disease is allowed to go untreated.

Some of the most important individual drugs will now be discussed in more detail with reference to clinical indications, method of administration, dosage, and toxicity. It should be emphasized that only the most important drugs of this group will be discussed; many others are under investigation or under clinical trial but it would be premature to present certain ones in this chapter. In cooperation with the National Cancer Institute, Public Health Service, a chemotherapy program is being carried out in which the resources of hospitals, research laboratories, industry, and government have been mobilized in an effort to find effective agents for cancer. Thousands of compounds are being tested annually on laboratory animals, in a search for chemicals with anticancer properties. About 40 substances are approved yearly for clinical trials on human patients.*

Nitrogen mustards and related compounds

Mechlorethamine Hydrochloride (Mustargen Hydrochloride)

The nitrogen mustard that has been used most extensively is mechlorethamine. It is an analogue of sulfur mustard gas used in World War I. In certain respects it has an action on cells of the body similar to that of x-ray. It exerts a selective cytotoxic effect on rapidly growing cells such as those found in blood-forming tissues and malignant tumors. Like other nitrogen mustards and the related compounds it inhibits mitosis by action at some premitotic phase of cell division. There is evidence that such compounds react selectively with certain groups of DNA (desoxyri-

*Pub. Health Rep. 74: 174, 1959.

bonucleic acid) and interfere with the reproduction of cells. As a result, cells may exhibit altered structure of their chromosomes. The normal tissues which react significantly after clinical use of the compounds are those of the bone marrow and the lymphoid organs.

Mechlorethamine is capable of producing severe tissue damage when it comes in direct contact with the skin, eyes, or respiratory tract.

Nitrogen mustard often provides dramatic relief of symptoms (relief of fever, improved appetite and strength, reduction of size of liver and spleen, itching, and pain). The duration of the remission may vary from a few weeks to several months.

Uses. Mechlorethamine is used in the treatment of Hodgkin's disease, certain kinds of lymphosarcoma, bronchogenic carcinoma, certain types of chronic leukemia, lymphoblastomas of the skin, and mycosis fungoides. This is a drug of choice for hospitalized patients when prompt treatment is indicated. It is considered most effective when the disease has become generalized or the patient is refractory to x-ray, but its use in terminal stages of the disease is not thought to be justifiable.

Preparation, dosage, and administration.

Mechlorethamine Hydrochloride for Injection, U.S.P. (Mustargen Hydrochloride). This drug is available in vials containing 10 mg. of the powder and 90 mg. of sodium chloride. Prior to injection the drug is dissolved in 10 ml. of distilled water. It is usually administered intravenously by injecting the solution into the tubing of an intravenous infusion. Dosage is calculated on the basis of body weight (0.1 mg. per kilogram on each of 4 successive days in most cases). The drug is preferably given in divided doses. Single doses of more than 8 to 10 mg. are not recommended.

Side effects and toxic effects. The margin of safety between the therapeutic dose of this drug and the toxic dose is very narrow, necessitating utmost caution in its administration. Thrombosis or thrombophlebitis may occur as a result of its effect on the veins. Leakage of the solution around the needle may cause sloughing of the adjacent tissues. Both the powder and the solution act as a vesicant and strong nasal irritant.

Systemic toxic effects include severe nausea and vomiting and decreased formation of blood cells. Granulocytopenia, lymphopenia, thrombocytopenia, and anemia may occur. Agranulocytosis has been known to develop. The toxic effects are directly proportional to the dosage, and therefore careful calculation of dosage usually will prevent severe reactions. Nausea and vomiting may be prevented by giving the drug late in the day and sedating the patient for the night. Sodium phenobarbital along with chlorpromazine, given intramuscularly, may prove effective.

Additional therapy with this drug should not be undertaken until there is satisfactory recovery in the bone marrow. Subsequent courses of therapy do not, as a rule, produce responses as satisfactory as those of the preceding course.*

Triethylenemelamine (TEM)

Triethylenemelamine is related to the nitrogen mustards and exhibits actions and has uses similar to them (see mechlorethamine). It differs from mechlorethamine in that it can be given orally as well as parenterally, does not produce a blistering effect (vesciant action), and causes less nausea and vomiting; the onset and duration of its action are also more prolonged.

Uses. Although used for many of the same conditions for which mechlorethamine is used, best results have probably been obtained in patients with widely disseminated Hodgkin's disease. Remissions may last from 2 to 14 weeks. During this time the patient has some relief of itching, anorexia, and weakness, and the enlarged lymph nodes and tumor masses decrease in size.

Preparation, dosage, and administration.

Triethylenemelamine, U.S.P. (TEM). This compound is available in 5 mg. tablets for oral administration. The drug is inactivated by the presence of acid and food and therefore should be given an hour or more before breakfast along with 2 Gm. of sodium bicarbonate. The latter substance enhances both absorption and activity of the drug. During initial therapy, 2.5 mg. are given on two successive mornings. If anorexia does not develop a third dose of 2.5 mg. may be prescribed. Whether or not administration is continued depends upon the condition being treated and the response of the patient (condition of the appetite and the blood cell count). Maintenance therapy is sometimes carried out if periodic examinations of the blood can be made. This drug can also be administered intravenously (0.04 mg. per kilogram of body weight) daily for three days.

Side effects and toxic effects. The effects are the same as those for the nitrogen mustards, with the exception that this preparation produces less nausea and vomiting and no vesicant action. Slow onset of action and prolonged effects are its main disadvantages.

Chlorambucil (Leukeran)

Chlorambucil is a derivative of nitrogen mustard and its action and uses are similar to those of mechlorethamine hydrochloride and triethylenemelamine. Chlorambucil is useful in bringing about remissions in neoplastic diseases, especially when there is involvement of the hematopoietic tissues and when the patient has become refractory to radiation therapy. Patients with chronic lymphocytic leukemia may show marked

*N.N.D., 1960, p. 199.

improvement during clinical remissions, i.e., the white blood cell count may be rapidly lowered. Patients with Hodgkin's disease may experience relief of pain, reduction in the size of the liver and spleen, gain in weight, and a general increased sense of well-being.

Uses. Chlorambucil is used as a palliative treatment of chronic lymphocytic leukemia, lymphosarcoma, and Hodgkin's disease. Unfortunately it does not seem to increase the survival time of persons ill with these diseases any better than the nitrogen mustards.

Preparation, dosage, and administration.

*Chlorambucil** (Leukeran). This agent is available in 2 mg. tablets for oral administration. The initial dosage for patients with Hodgkin's disease is 0.2 mg. per kilogram of body weight (10 to 20 mg. in adults), but it is then reduced to a maintenance level after a response is obtained. For patients with leukemia or lymphosarcoma, the dose is usually 0.1 mg. per kilogram of body weight (2 to 6 mg.). It is usually well tolerated.

Side effects and toxic effects. Excessive dosage or prolonged administration may cause severe depression of bone marrow. However, its absorption is said to be more predictable; hence it is easier to handle and produces fewer side effects than some of the other alkylating agents. Patients occasionally complain of gastric distress.

Busulfan (Myleran)

Busulfan is an active alkylating agent which pharmacologically resembles the nitrogen mustards and triethylenemelamine. Its cytotoxic action, however, is restricted chiefly to the cells of the bone marrow. Remission of symptoms is characterized by improved sense of well-being, reduction in the size of the spleen, increase in the hemoglobin level, increase in the erythrocytes, and reduction in the members of circulating white blood cells.

Uses. Busulfan is sometimes preferred to other antineoplastic drugs in the treatment of chronic myelogenous leukemia, because of its depressant effect on the production of granulocytes.

Preparation, dosage, and administration.

Busulfan, U.S.P. (Myleran). This drug is available in 2 mg. tablets for oral administration. The initial dose is usually 2 to 6 mg. daily until clinical improvement occurs. Some physicians prescribe appreciably larger doses but over a relatively short period of time.

Side effects and toxic effects. Busulfan offers the advantages of oral administration and a low incidence of side effects. In addition it can be used in maintenance therapy of ambulatory patients. Overdosage or prolonged administration may produce irreversible damage to cells of the

*Described in annual publication of A. M. A. Council on Drugs, N.N.D., 1960.

bone marrow. Weekly blood examinations (and preferably more often) are recommended. Bleeding tendencies may result from reduced numbers of thrombocytes in the blood.

Triethylene Thiophosphoramide (Thio-Tepa)

Thio-Tepa is one of the alkylating agents which produces effects similar to those produced by nitrogen mustard, triethylenemelamine, and chlorambucil.

Uses. It is used for many of the same conditions for which other drugs belonging to this group of preparations are used. Some authorities prefer not to use Thio-Tepa for the initial treatment of malignant disease but advocate its use only after surgery and radiation therapy are not effective or are not feasible. It is ineffective for acute leukemia.

Preparation, dosage, and administration.

*Thio-Tepa.** This preparation is available in vials containing 15 mg. of powdered drug. The maximum daily dose for initial therapy by intramuscular, intravenous, or intra-arterial injection is 0.2 mg. per kilogram of body weight. The dosage for maintenance therapy is determined by the clinical response of the patient and changes in patient's blood. The powder should be refrigerated, and when solutions are prepared they should be used immediately or discarded. Because this preparation has no vesicant action and because solutions can be prepared at a pH which produces no irritation of tissues, it is suitable for all routes of parenteral administration.

Side effects and toxic effects. Thio-Tepa has a slow onset of action, and immediate side effects such as nausea and vomiting are minimal, although they do occur. It is capable of producing cumulative toxic effects in the blood-forming tissues and therefore caution in its use is recommended. Irreversible aplastic anemia has been known to develop. Further evaluation of this drug is needed to determine its ultimate status in the treatment of neoplastic diseases.

Antimetabolites

Aminopterin

Aminopterin is known as one of the folic acid antagonists. Folic acid is a vitamin which acts as a catalytic agent in the synthesis of nucleic acid, which in turn is an essential component of cellular protein. For this activity, folic acid is converted to a biologically more active form known as folinic acid. Aminopterin blocks the formation of folinic acid from folic acid. Cells are not prevented from going into cell division but prog-

*Council on drugs: J. A. M. A. **172:** 565, 1960.

ress is arrested in the metaphase. Cells undergoing rapid proliferation, such as the white blood cells in the leukemic patient, are particularly affected. This drug also has a damaging effect on embryonic tissue and should not be administered to patients who are pregnant.

Uses. Aminopterin is used in the treatment of acute leukemia in children. In about one third of the cases of acute leukemia seen in children remission is achieved, although it is temporary. Remission is characterized by disappearance of fever, relief of pain in bones, improved appetite, and reduction in the size of enlarged organs such as the liver, spleen, and lymph nodes, and, in general, the child seems to feel better and stronger. The blood picture may become comparatively normal. The drug is used less successfully for adults, for reasons unknown.

Preparation, dosage, and administration.

*Aminopterin Sodium.** This drug is available in 0.5 mg. tablets for oral administration. Dosage for children varies from 0.25 to 0.5 mg., given three to six times a week. It is administered over a period of 3 weeks or more, depending on the response of the patient. When a remission is achieved the patient may be placed on a maintenance dosage or the physician may discontinue the treatment.

Side effects and toxic effects. Toxic effects usually are directly related to dosage. Irreversible depression of all blood cells can develop. The appearance of ulcerations in the mouth or gastrointestinal tract, epigastric pain, diarrhea, hemorrhage (gastrointestinal or cutaneous), or an abrupt drop in the number of leukocytes means that the drug must be discontinued. Frequent examinations of the blood are recommended to detect early signs of developing toxicity.

Resistance to the folic acid antagonists develops rather quickly. A preparation of folinic acid (leucovorin) serves as an antidote in case of overdosage.

Amethopterin (Methotrexate)

Amethopertin is a folic acid antagonist which produces effects similar to aminopterin.

Uses. Its principal use is for the treatment of acute leukemia. It is occasionally used for adults who are refractory to other forms of therapy, but it is used more often for children. In women, it is also used in the treatment of a rare type of cancer known as choriocarcinoma, a tumor composed of cells of fetal origin.

Preparation, dosage, and administration.

Amethopterin (Methotrexate). This compound is available in 2.5 mg. tablets for oral administration. It is usually administered orally since it is readily absorbed from the gastrointestinal tract. A parenteral

*Described in annual publication of A. M. A. Council on Drugs, N.N.D., 1960.

712

preparation is also available in vials containing 5 mg. of the drug. It can be given intramuscularly, intravenously, or intrathecally. Dosage for children varies from 1 to 2.5 mg. daily. The usual daily dose for adults is 5 mg.

Side effects and toxic effects. Although claims have been made that amethopterin is less toxic than aminopterin, some investigators have found that when biologically equivalent doses are given, there is little or no difference in the two drugs from the standpoint of toxicity and therapeutic effectiveness.* (See toxic effects of aminopterin.)

Mercaptopurine (6-Mercaptopurine)

Mercaptopurine acts as an antagonist to certain purines which are constituents of nucleic acids, thus interfering with the formation of nucleic acids. Chemically, mercaptopurine resembles constituents of nucleic acid—adenine and a purine base known as hypoxanthine (see accompanying formulas for similarity in structure). Both of these compounds are needed for the synthesis of nucleic acid by cells; hence they are needed especially when cells are growing and multiplying rapidly. Mercaptopurine resembles adenine and hypoxanthine but it cannot truly take their places, and thus it interferes with certain normal processes.

Mercaptopurine   Adenine   Hypoxanthine

The effects of mercaptopurine can be observed chiefly in the tissues in which there is rapid cellular growth and a high rate of metabolism of nucleic acid, e.g., in the bone marrow and the epithelium of the gastrointestinal tract. As a result of its effects on the bone marrow, there is a reduction in the formation of leukocytes, thrombocytes, and reticulocytes. In the gastrointestinal tract, injury of epithelium results in anorexia, nausea and vomiting, and diarrhea (which may become bloody), and large doses may bring about degenerative changes in the liver.

*Karnofsky, D. A.: Inhibitory Effect of Drugs on Normal and Neoplastic Blood Cell Formation, In Drill, V. A. (editor): Pharmacology in Medicine, New York, 1958, McGraw-Hill Book Co., Inc., p. 734.

Uses. Mercaptopurine is used chiefly for the treatment of acute leukemia in children. Careful use of the drug may bring about remission in the disease and prolongation of life in a fairly large number of patients. Remissions will vary in duration from a few weeks to several months. Leukemia in the adult may also respond to this drug, but the incidence of remissions is lower than for children. The administration of a folic acid antagonist and/or hormone therapy is often considered preferable as an initial form of treatment. When the patient no longer responds satisfactorily, mercaptopurine may be substituted. The reverse is also true, some physicians preferring to employ hormonal treatment as a last resort. Some patients with chronic myelogenous leukemia seem to respond favorably to mercaptopurine, i.e., remissions are produced.

Preparation, dosage, and administration.

Mercaptopurine, U.S.P. (6-Purinethiol). This compound is marketed in 50 mg. tablets for oral administration. Dosage is regulated in accordance with the amount of clinical improvement in the patient and the response made by his blood. The usual initial dose (both for children and adults) is 2.5 mg. per kilogram of body weight daily. Three to six weeks of therapy can be expected to elapse before a remission is achieved.

Side effects and toxic effects. Tolerance develops to the therapeutic effects of this drug. The chief toxic effect is depression of the bone marrow, resulting in marked leukopenia, thrombocytopenia, and anemia. Although it is less toxic to the epithelium of the gastrointestinal tract than the folic acid antagonists, it can cause nausea, vomiting, and diarrhea, and large doses may result in ulcerations of the mucosa, as indicated above. Frequent examinations of the patient's blood during therapy is indicated.

Hormones

The adrenotropic hormone (ACTH) and the cortical hormones made by the adrenal gland are known to inhibit the growth of cells, especially young actively growing and multiplying cells. The mechanism of their action is not known. Prednisone and prednisolone are most frequently used in the treatment of leukemia and lymphomas. Their action is highly similar to that of cortisone, but they cause somewhat less retention of fluid and salt. Prednisone is administered orally in doses of 50 to 100 mg. for adults and 50 mg. for children. This dosage is given daily in divided portions. Critically ill patients may be given ACTH by continuous intravenous infusion.

Temporary remissions are achieved with these hormones in an appreciable number of children who have acute leukemia. Less satisfactory results are obtained in adults. The above-mentioned hormones are also used to produce remissions in patients with Hodgkin's disease, lymphosarcoma, multiple myeloma, and chronic lymphatic leukemia.

The side effects and toxic effects associated with overdosage are presented in Chapter 24.

Hormones that are used in the treatment of cancer of the breast include androgens such as testosterone propionate and fluoxymesterone. Estrogens such as diethylstilbestrol are sometimes administered, provided the patient is well past menopause. Estrogens may increase the growth and metastasis of cancer in women who are still menstruating.

Cancer of the prostate gland in the male is treated with an estrogen such as diethylstilbestrol or by a combination of an orchiectomy and the administration of an estrogen.

A relatively high percentage of patients who have cancer of the breast or cancer of the prostate shows subjective improvement, i.e., the patients have less pain, their appetite improves, and, in general, they feel better. The malignant process may not have changed much, however, although some patients receive benefit for a number of years. For side effects, dosage, etc., see Chapter 19.

Radioactive isotopes

The radiations produced by radioactive isotopes are spoken of as alpha, beta, and gamma rays.* Alpha rays penetrate poorly into tissues, not more than a fraction of a millimeter. Beta rays penetrate tissues to the extent of a few millimeters, whereas gamma rays are highly penetrating radiation. All radioactive isotopes represent a potential hazard to the patient and to all persons who handle the preparations. The cytotoxic action of these preparations is due to their ability to ionize molecules in a cell (by ejecting electrons). Tissues vary in sensitivity to ionizing radiations; cells with a short life and a high rate of reproduction are especially vulnerable. Cells of the body which are particularly affected therefore are the germinal cells of the ovaries and testes, bone marrow, lymphocytes, and the epithelial cells of the gastrointestinal tract. This helps to explain some of the symptoms of "radiation sickness," such as nausea and vomiting, diarrhea, weakness, reduction of cells in the circulating blood, etc. Death may result from depression of the bone marrow, hemorrhage, or infection.

Among the radioactive isotopes used in medicine are sodium radiophosphate, radiogold colloid, and sodium radio-iodide.

*Radiation from radioactive materials is more correctly spoken of as alpha and beta particles and gamma rays.

Sodium Radio-Phosphate (P³²) (Phosphotope)

Sodium radio-phosphate (P³²), when undergoing disintegration, emits only beta rays. The effects produced resemble those of radium or x-ray. It has a half-life of 14.3 days. Like ordinary phosphorus it is incorporated into the nucleoprotein of growing cells and reaches a high level therefore in the rapidly proliferating and neoplastic cells. The cells of the bone marrow are thus subjected to considerable radiation, and large doses may result in severe depression.

Uses. This particular radioactive isotope has been used extensively in the treatment of polycythemia vera. The cells from which the red blood cells develop, as well as other cellular elements of the bone marrow, are depressed. It thus also helps to control excessive formation of white blood cells and thrombocytes and decreases the size of the enlarged liver or spleen. Remissions usually last for a period of months and occasionally for a year or more. They tend to be longer after the use of this preparation than after x-ray or other drugs.

Sodium radio-phosphate (P³²) is also used to produce clinical remissions in chronic myelogenous and chronic lymphatic leukemia. Patients with acute leukemia are not benefited. The drug is excreted in the urine, which necessitates careful disposal of this excretion.

Preparation, dosage, and administration.

Sodium Radiophosphate Solution, U.S.P. (P³², Phosphotope). This radioisotope is administered intravenously or orally in aqueous solution. It is supplied in glass containers but great care must be exercised in handling the material to prevent radiation burns from accidental contact with the skin. Its activity as indicated on the label is expressed in millicuries or microcuries.* It has a half-life of 14.3 days.

For polycythemia vera, the initial dose may vary from 2.5 to 5 mc. (millicuries). After 2 or 3 months an additional dose may be indicated (3 to 4 mc.). For chronic myelogenous leukemia, the dosage is less (1 to 2 mc. in a week). Dosage must be adjusted in accordance with the needs and response of the patient.

Side effects and toxic effects. The indications and contraindications for this form of therapy are much the same as those for x-ray irradiation. This preparation does not cause radiation sickness but it can produce serious depression of the bone marrow. The chief untoward effects are leukopenia, anemia, and thrombocytopenia. Frequent blood examinations are indicated to detect developing states of toxicity. It is relatively inexpensive and usually produces fewer complications than a number of other effective agents.

---

*One microcurie is the quantity of a radioactive material which is breaking down at the rate of approximately two million nuclear disintegrations per minute.

Radiogold Colloid (Aurcoloid)

Radiogold Solution, U.S.P. (Au¹⁹⁸) (Aurcoloid). This radioisotope emits both beta and gamma rays and has a half-life of 3.9 days. It is used to treat recurrent pleural effusion and ascites associated with metastatic malignancy. It does not cure the malignancy, but it contributes to the comfort of the patient by reducing the accumulation of fluid. It is administered by injection into the pleural or peritoneal cavity. Mild radiation sickness may occur after 3 to 4 days, and a decrease in the number of white blood cells may take place.

Sodium Radio-Iodide

Sodium Radio-Iodide Solution, U.S.P. (I¹³¹). Sodium radio-iodide is presented in Chapter 24.

Miscellaneous agents

Actinomycin D

Actinomycin D is an antibiotic that has been under investigation. It appears to be effective in some cases of rare tumors seen in children, such as Wilms' tumor and neuroblastoma.

Urethan (Ethyl Carbamate)

Urethan was originally introduced into medicine as a hypnotic, but it is not considered useful for this purpose. In a manner which is not fully understood, it interferes with cell division, possibly with the metabolism of nucleic acid. It depresses the bone marrow of patients with leukemia and inhibits cell division of neoplastic cells.

Uses. Urethan has been used in the treatment of leukemia, better results having been obtained in chronic myelogenous leukemia than in the lymphatic type. It is also used in the treatment of multiple myeloma. It is of no value in acute leukemia.

Preparation, dosage, and administration.

Urethan, U.S.P.; *Urethane,* B.P. Urethan is available for oral administration in 300 mg. tablets, enteric-coated, and as a solution (10 per cent) for intravenous administration. The usual daily dose is 3 Gm. It is administered after meals in three equal portions. The drug has a cumulative action.

Side effects and toxic effects. Side effects include nausea and vomiting, loss of appetite, and sometimes drowsiness and dizziness. The more toxic effects include severe leukopenia, anemia, hemorrhagic tendencies, and depression of the bone marrow. Hepatitis does not occur often but constitutes a serious complication.

Potassium Arsenite (Fowler's Solution)

Potassium arsenite exerts a comparatively mild depressant action on hematopoietic tissues.

Uses. It is effective in early stages of certain types of myelogenous leukemia, producing temporary clinical remission accompanied by a decreased number of white blood cells, arrest of anemia, and decreased size of the liver and spleen (if they have been enlarged). Continued administration of the drug may keep the patient in a state of remission over a relatively long period of time. When the drug is discontinued, relapse occurs.

Preparation, dosage, and administration.

Potassium Arsenite Solution (Fowler's Solution). This is an aqueous alcoholic solution containing about 1 per cent of arsenic trioxide and potassium bicarbonate. The usual dose is 0.2 ml. (3 minims). It may be prescribed in increasing doses until mild symptoms of overdosage occur. It is gradually decreased until a satisfactory maintenance dose is achieved.

Side effects and toxic effects. Symptoms of overdosage include nausea and vomiting, abdominal cramps, or puffiness under the eyes. Albumin may be present in the urine. Ease of administration and low cost are advantages over a number of other forms of treatment, but it is not widely used.

Phenylhydrazine Hydrochloride

Phenylhydrazine hydrochloride is a potent agent which is destructive to red blood cells. It has been used in the treatment of polycythemia vera. Some patients have responded satisfactorily, although radioactive phosphorus is considered the drug of choice for treatment of this condition. When used it is administered orally (capsules) in doses of 200 mg. daily for several days and then 100 mg. daily until the erythrocyte count and the hemoglobin approach a normal level. The patient is then placed on a maintenance dose. Toxic symptoms include jaundice, severe anemia, disturbances of renal function, skin eruption, and an increased tendency to thrombosis. It is not official in the U.S.P., N.F., or B.P.

References

A. M. A. Council on Drugs: New and Non-official Drugs, Philadelphia, 1960, J. B. Lippincott Co.

Drill, V. A. (editor): Pharmacology in Medicine, New York, 1958, McGraw-Hill Book Co., Inc.

Golbey, R. B.: Chemotherapy of Cancer, Am. J. Nursing 60: 521, 1960.

Hester, H. H.: Today's Treatment of Leukemia, Today's Health 36: 24, 1958.

Holland, J. F.: Chemical Control of Cancer, Pub. Health Rep. 69: 1151, 1954.

Karnofsky, D. A.: Triethylene Melamine in Treatment of Lymphomas and Leukemias, M. Clin. North America, pp. 541-542, 1954.

Karnofsky, D. A.: Chemotherapy of Cancer, CA, Bulletin of Cancer Progress, p. 165, Sept., 1955.

Modell, W. (editor): Drugs of Choice 1960-1961, St. Louis, 1960, The C. V. Mosby Co.

Rhoads, C. P.: Cancer Control—Present and Future, Am. J. Nursing 58: 516, 1958.

Stroebel, C. F., Hall, B. E., and Pease, G. L.: Evaluation of Radiophosphorus Therapy in Primary Polycythemia, J. A. M. A. 146: 1301, 1951.

Wilson, H. E.: Leukemia, Am. J. Nursing 56: 601, 1956.

Chapter 26

Enzymes used as drugs

Enzymes as a group are among the newest agents used in therapy, but it may be anticipated that their application in medicine will increase markedly in future years. As the student will recall from her study of chemistry, enzymes are specific structures that act as catalysts of the many chemical reactions that go on in living systems. Catalysts are substances that accelerate chemical reactions (often stimulating a thousand-fold or greater the speed of reaction) without themselves being used up in the reaction. The catalytic action of enzymes can be illustrated by *catalase,* an enzyme present in many living cells, which speeds up a reaction in which hydrogen peroxide decomposes to form water and oxygen.

$$H_2O_2 \xrightarrow{\text{catalase}} H_2O + \tfrac{1}{2}O_2$$

Catalase permits this reaction (moles of H_2O_2 decomposing per minute) to go on many thousand times the rate that could be observed without catalase; and each molecule of catalase present in solution can stimulate the decomposition of millions of molecules of hydrogen peroxide.

The role of enzymes in living organisms is an important one, because these catalysts of living origin permit the chemical reactions to go on, which make life possible.

One feature of enzymes of great interest to possible pharmacologic application is their specificity. Each separate enzyme catalyzes a distinct chemical reaction or reaction type and the thousands of chemical reactions characteristic of living cells* therefore each require their corresponding enzyme.

Because the usefulness of drugs depends to a large measure on their specificity or selectivity, the high specificity of enzymes in catalyzing a given reaction and in influencing no other is a promising feature. However, their potential usefulness in medicine has been limited by certain

---

*Examples of large groups of reaction types: hydrolysis of peptide bonds in proteins, oxidation of aldehydes to acids, transfer of electrons, and many others.

other properties. The fact that they are proteins means that they need a high degree of purification before administration; and even pure proteins derived from other species may be antigenic and cause toxic reactions of an immunologic type. Also as proteins, most enzymes would need to be given parenterally in order to short-circuit destruction by the protein-digesting enzymes of the gastrointestinal tract. In addition, proteins cannot be synthesized, and the preparation of purified enzymes from natural sources is often a laborious process yielding small amounts of ultimate product. Finally, therapeutic agents which are proteins have the limitation that they do not pass into cells readily, unlike small molecules (which constitute most of the drugs considered elsewhere in this book). A further limitation is that enzymes catalyze single specific chemical reactions and we do not yet understand, if ever we will, disease or symptoms of disease in such simple chemical terms.

Within these limitations, however, certain enzymes have become useful for certain symptomatic purposes: protein-digesting enzymes such as trypsin have been used to remove dead tissue by enzymatic digestion (chemical débridement); enzymes have been used to digest thick purulent exudates the viscosity of which depends on large amounts of this type of nucleic acid. A beginning has also been made in the use of enzymes that can destroy specific toxic or allergenic substances in the body, for example, in the use of penicillinase to remove penicillin from the body fluids of an individual who is suffering an allergic reaction to penicillin. The "detoxifying" action of enzymes has promise because of the specificity of enzymes which might be employed, and it is possible that much wider use will be made of this specific way of removing unwanted drugs or other compounds from the body.

Hyaluronidase (Alidase, Diffusin, Wydase)

Hyaluronic acid is a polysaccharide which constitutes an essential component of intercellular ground substance. It is present in the form of a gel in many parts of body tissues where it serves as an intercellular cement and acts as a barrier to the diffusion of invading substances.

Hyaluronidase is a mucolytic enzyme, prepared from mammalian testes, which is capable of hydrolyzing and depolymerizing hyaluronic acid. It thus acts as a spreading factor to facilitate absorption and distribution of infusions, local anesthetics, and drugs such as penicillin and to increase diffusion and absorption of local accumulations or transudates of blood.

It is especially useful to facilitate administration of fluids by hypodermoclysis. The resulting increased rate of dispersion and absorption of the injected fluid reduces tissue tension and pain. The rate of absorption, however, should not be greater than that of an intravenous infusion. Special care must be exercised for children, to control the speed and total volume administered, to avoid overhydration.

Preparation, dosage, and administration.

Hyaluronidase for Injection, U.S.P. (Alidase, Diffusin, Wydase); *Hyaluronidase,* B.P. This enzyme is available in a stable dried form in vials containing 150 and 1,500 U.S.P. units and in a solution for injection, 150 U.S.P. units in 1 ml. or 1,500 U.S.P. units in 10 ml. A dose of 150 U.S.P. units is dissolved in 1 ml. of isotonic sodium chloride solution and is then added to 1,000 ml. of fluid for hypodermoclysis, or it is injected into the proposed site of the clysis.

Side effects and toxic effects. Hyaluronidase has a low level of toxicity but caution is recommended when it is administered to patients with infections. It should not be injected into or around infected areas since it will produce spread of the infection by the same mechanism of action that causes spread of injected solutions. Patients occasionally exhibit sensitivity to this substance.

Streptodornase

Streptodornase is an enzyme or group of enzymes produced by the growth of hemolytic streptococci. It promotes depolymerization of desoxyribonucleic acid and desoxyribonucleoprotein. These substances occur in degenerating white blood cells and injured tissue cells. Much of the stringy, slimy, viscous material in purulent exudates is due to their presence. Streptodornase changes the thick purulent material to a thin, liquid material, sometimes in a very short time. Fortunately, streptodornase acts on extracellular nucleoprotein and on nuclei of degenerating cells, but it has no effect on nucleoprotein or the nuclei of living cells. The action of this enzyme requires the presence of the magnesium ion but this is freely present in tissues. Activity of the enzyme is inhibited by citrate and heparin. It is most active at a pH between 7 and 8.5. Streptodornase is antigenic, but if used in sufficiently large amounts, the specific antibody does not seem to interfere with the action of the enzyme.

Streptokinase

Streptokinase is an extracellular enzyme activator which is formed during the growth of various groups of hemolytic streptococci, prominent among which are the human strains of Lancefield's Group C. Streptokinase activates a factor present in human plasma, known as *plasmogen.* Plasmogen is present in purulent, serous, and sanguineous exudates and, when activated by streptokinase, it forms an active enzyme, plasmin. Plasmin in turn promotes lysis of fibrin from a gel to a liquid and is accompanied by the formation of large polypeptides. This explains the dissolution of blood clots and fibrinous exudates. Streptokinase is therefore essentially a proteolytic enzyme, active in the solution of fibrin. It exerts its maximal activity between a pH of 7.3 and 7.6

Streptokinase-Streptodornase (Varidase)

This preparation is a mixture of the two enzymes involved which have been described previously. In addition to their proteolytic activity, they are capable of producing two additional reactions. One reaction is local and consists of an outpouring of white blood cells and fluid at the site of application. A pyrogenic effect is sometimes seen, especially when the enzymes are injected into a closed space with limited or delayed drainage. It is thought that the elevation of temperature is due to the absorption of toxic products resulting from activity of the enzymes.

Uses. Streptokinase and streptodornase are used to liquefy coagulated blood and remove clots, and dissolve fibrinous material and purulent accumulations present after trauma or inflammation. The enzyme action thus helps the action of anti-infective forces, such as the action of antibiotics, and encourages the healing of tissues.

Preparation, dosage, and administration.

Streptokinase-Streptodornase * (Varidase). This preparation is available in the form of buccal tablets (10,000 units of streptokinase and 2,500 units of streptodornase); as a powder for topical use (100,000 units of streptokinase and 25,000 units of streptodornase); as a powder for injection (20,000 units of streptokinase and 5,000 units of streptodornase); and as a jelly (100,000 units of streptokinase and 25,000 units of streptodornase). The usefulness of this preparation after intramuscular or buccal administration is not fully established. Varidase is applied topically in the form of wet dressings or as a jelly, or it is injected into cavities. Maximum effects usually occur in 12 to 24 hours. Solutions lose their potency when kept at room temperature but will keep for a week at a temperature of 2° to 10° C.

Side effects and toxic effects. These enzymes are employed as supplements to, rather than as substitutes for, surgical débridement and drainage. They are not recommended for use in the presence of active hemorrhage or acute cellulitis because they may interfere with the clotting of blood or promote the spread of a nonlocalized infection. In the absence of adequate drainage the patient may develop fever, urticaria, nausea, and vomiting when this preparation is injected into a closed cavity. The preparation should not be administered intravenously.

*Council on Drugs: J. A. M. A. **172:** 701, 1960.

Trypsin, Crystalline (Tryptar)

Crystalline trypsin is a purified preparation of the pancreatic enzyme obtained from mammalian pancreatic glands. It exerts a proteolytic action when brought into contact with clotted blood, exudate, and necrotic tissue. It is not harmful to living tissues because of the presence in serum of a specific trypsin inhibitor and other nonspecific inhibitory substances. Crystalline trypsin is useful as an adjunct to surgical treatment of necrotic wounds, abscesses, empyema, sinuses, and fistulas. It is also used to liquefy hematomas and blood clots. It is sometimes employed in the treatment of bronchopulmonary conditions to reduce the viscosity of tenacious secretions which do not respond to expectorant drugs.

It is contraindicated in cases of severe hepatic disease, for use in actively bleeding cavities, and for débridement of ulcerated carcinomas. It should be used with caution in cases of tuberculous empyema.

Preparation, dosage, and administration.

*Trypsin Crystalline** (Tryptar). This preparation is available in the form of buccal tablets, 5 mg.; as a suspension for injection, 5 mg. per milliliter; as a solution for injection, 5 mg. per milliliter; and as a powder in vials containing 25, 50, and 250 mg. Crystalline trypsin is applied to surface lesions either in a dry form by means of a blower or as a freshly prepared solution in the form of wet dressings. For less accessible lesions it may be instilled or used as an irrigant. Solutions or suspensions when given by injection are given by deep intragluteal injection. It should never be given intravenously.

Side effects and toxic effects. Pain and induration may occur at the site of intramuscular injection. Hives and urticaria occur occasionally. A severe burning sensation may be experienced on surface lesions following topical application, and after injection, fever, and an increased heart rate may result. The latter reaction can be prevented by the administration of an antihistamine. Toxic effects are considered negligible when the use of the enzyme is limited to local or topical administration.

Chymotrypsin (Chymar)

Chymotrypsin is another protein-digesting enzyme which is being used to prevent and treat inflammatory reactions causing pain, edema, blood and lymphatic effusions. It is marketed under the name of *Chymar* and is available for intramuscular injection and also for systemic effects in the form of buccal tablets.

Penicillinase (Neutrapen)

As noted in Chapter 8, Anti-infectives–Antibiotics, penicillin is virtually nontoxic to human beings except for hypersensitivity reactions to

*Described in annual publication of A. M. A. Council on Drugs, N.N.D., 1960.

it which are frequent and occasionally severe enough to constitute a considerable hazard in its use. The cortical steroids and the antihistaminics are both useful agents in the treatment of allergic responses to penicillin as to other allergens. A more direct attack is by the use of the enzyme penicillinase. Penicillinase is an enzyme secreted by a number of bacteria, which hydrolyzes a portion of the penicillin molecule and produces a derivative that is inactive as an antibiotic and is believed to have little or no antigenic or allergenic activity. Preliminary reports have suggested that penicillinase, particularly when used early in the course of a penicillin reaction, may be an effective way of relieving symptoms. Adjunctive use of more rapidly acting drugs such as epinephrine is recommended, however.

Preparation, dosage, and administration.

*Penicillinase** (Neutrapen). Penicillinase is available as a lyophilized† stable powder and is marketed in single dose vials containing 800,000 units of the enzyme. It is administered by deep intramuscular injection. The content of the vial is dissolved in 2 ml. of sterile distilled water prior to injection. The dose may be repeated in 3 to 7 days, if necessary.

Side effects and toxic effects. Penicillinase is believed to have a low level of toxicity, but because it is an enzyme and therefore a protein, it is capable of producing allergic reactions, both mild and severe.

*Described in annual publication of the A. M. A. Council on Drugs, N.N.D., 1960.
†Lyophilized means to be dehydrated from a frozen state by means of a vacuum.

References

A. M. A. Council on Drugs: New and Non-official Drugs, Philadelphia, 1960, J. B. Lippincott Co.

Beckman, H.: Drugs, Their Nature, Action and Use, Philadelphia, 1958, W. B. Saunders Co.

Council on Drugs: Buccal and Intramuscular Use of Streptokinase and Streptodornase (Varidase), J. A. M. A. **172:** 701, 1960.

Chapter 27

Serums and vaccines

Immunity is of two kinds, natural and acquired. If an individual is so constituted that the germ of a disease will not grow upon his tissues, or that the toxins of that germ are harmless to him, he is immune to that particular disease. Such immunity is called *natural immunity.*

When natural immunity is not effective and bacteria attack the tissues and live and grow at their expense, the body protects itself by preparing substances destructive to the particular organism making the attack. These substances are called "antibodies." They are present in the blood and other body fluids and are carried to the point of infection by the blood and lymph. The antibodies gradually disappear from the blood, but the body cells have seemingly acquired the ability to resist the same bacteria when they attack the tissues again. Immunity due to these antibodies, as well as the special ability to produce them, is known as *acquired immunity;* and because the individual himself developed the antibodies, the immunity is known as *active immunity.* It is usually present after an attack of an infectious disease such as smallpox, typhoid fever, etc. and may be induced artificially by the injection of substances known as antigens. The antigen may be a suspension of living microorganisms, as, for example, the vaccinia virus, or a suspension of dead microorganisms, as typhoid vaccine; or it may be an extract of the bodies of bacteria, as tuberculosis vaccine or a soluble toxin produced by bacteria, of which diphtheria toxin is an example.

Passive acquired immunity against certain diseases is secured by transferring to a person the blood serum of an animal that has been actively immunized by injections with the specific organisms or toxins of those diseases; it may also be secured by injection of the blood serum of an immune person. Immunity acquired in this way is called passive immunity because the body plays no part in the preparation of the antibodies. The body cells are not prepared to resist infection as they are in active immunity, and as the blood is renewed, the antibodies are lost and the patient is in the same condition as if no antibodies had been administered.

Federal regulations control the manufacture and sale of these potent and, in some cases, dangerous products; firms are licensed under the supervision of the National Institutes of Health of the United States Public Health Service to import, export, or sell these biologic products in interstate commerce.[*]

A number of these products may cause untoward reactions when they are administered as therapeutic or prophylactic agents. Individual sensitivities to animal products, especially horse serum and egg, are primarily responsible for adverse symptoms, and idiosyncrasies toward the products of bacterial metabolism are responsible for the others.[*]

Agents containing antibodies : immune serums

An immune serum is the serum of an animal that has antibodies in the blood stream.

Serum treatment consists of the transfer of the immune serum into the circulation of the patient. This immune serum contains specific antibodies which act upon disease germs.

There are two kinds of immune serums: the naturally produced and the antitoxic.

Naturally produced human serums

These are preparations obtained from normal blood, such as plasma, serum, or globulins or serum from patients who have recovered from a disease and retain the immune bodies in their blood serum.

Immune Serum Globulin, U.S.P. This is a sterile solution of globulins which contain those antibodies normally present in adult human blood. Each lot of the preparation is derived from an original plasma or serum pool which represents at least 1,000 individuals. It is thought to be as useful as convalescent serum and is more readily available. It is useful in the prevention of measles, as well as in the treatment of that disease, and for the prevention of infectious hepatitis.

The dosage varies with a number of factors. It is administered subcutaneously or intramuscularly. The usual prophylactic dose for measles is 0.22 ml. per kilogram of body weight, and the usual dose for modification of measles is 0.045 ml. per kilogram.

Human Gamma Globulin, B.P. This is available in a sterile solution for prevention or attenuation of measles and for the prevention of rubella, poliomyelitis, and infectious hepatitis.

Pertussis Immune Human Serum, U.S.P. This is the liquid or dried serum of blood obtained from donors who have recovered from pertussis (whooping cough) and who for the preceding 7 or more days have been without active clinical manifestations of the disease. The usual

*N.N.D., 1960, p. 619.

intramuscular dose is 20 ml. This is given for three doses with intervals of 1 to 2 days between doses. It may also be given intravenously in doses of 60 ml. and repeated if necessary. The range of dosage is 20 to 100 ml.

Human Scarlet Fever Immune Serum. This is a sterile serum obtained from the blood of a healthy person who has had scarlet fever. For therapeutic use, the usual dose is 20 ml.; for prophylaxis, the dose is 10 ml., given intramuscularly.

Poliomyelitis Immune Globulin (Human). This is a sterile solution of globulins derived from pooled adult human blood. It is also obtained from placental blood.

It is used for the attenuation or prevention of poliomyelitis, measles, and infectious hepatitis. It is administered only by intramuscular injections, preferably in the buttock, using care to avoid accidental intravenous injection. The commercial preparation contains 330 mg. in 2 ml. or 1.65 Gm. in 10 ml. The dosage varies considerably, depending on the purpose of the injection; for protection against paralytic poliomyelitis, the average dose to be injected is calculated on the basis of 0.31 ml. per kilogram of body weight.

Antitoxic serums of animal origin

Antitoxic serums are formed in the body of animals that have been actively immunized by a specific toxin. The animal is then bled and the serum separated from the blood. The serum is purified in most instances to remove inactive substances and to concentrate the antibodies. Antitoxins are given to neutralize the toxins produced in certain diseases.

Horses and rabbits are the animals most often utilized for the artificial production of immune serums. One inoculation with the animal product may sensitize a patient to the blood components of that species, and subsequent inoculations of products from the same animal source may cause serum sickness or anaphylactoid shock. Sensitivity tests to horse serum or other suspected antigens may be done on patients before injection of serums. Temporary desensitization can be induced by repeated injections of minute doses or by the use of alternate routes of administration (i.e., subcutaneous), which ensures slow absorption; prevention of the rapid accumulation of antigen in the circulating blood is essential.†

Diphtheria Antitoxin, U.S.P., B.P. Diphtheria antitoxin is a sterile solution of antitoxic substances obtained from the blood serum or plasma of a healthy animal that has been immunized against diphtheria toxin. It contains not less than 500 antitoxic units per milliliter. It is used to confer a passive immunity to the individual who has been exposed to diphtheria or to the patient ill with the disease. The usual prophylactic dose

°Described in annual publication of A. M. A. Council on Drugs, N.N.D., 1960.
†N.N.D., 1960, p. 620.

is 1,000 units and the therapeutic dose is 20,000 units, although it may range from 10,000 to 80,000 units. It is administered intramuscularly and intravenously.

Mixed Gas Gangrene Antitoxin, B.P. This is a sterile solution of antitoxic substances obtained from the blood of healthy animals that have been immunized against the toxins of *Clostridium perfringens, Clostridium septicum,* and *Clostridium oedematiens.* Usual initial dose (therapeutic or prophylactic) is the contents of one or more packages, given parenterally.

Tetanus Antitoxin, U.S.P., B.P. This antitoxin is prepared from the horse in much the same way as diphtheria antitoxin, but the animal in this case has been immunized against tetanus toxin. Usual therapeutic dose is 40,000 to 50,000 units; usual prophylactic dose, 1,500 units, given parenterally (subcutaneously or intravenously).

Tetanus and Gas Gangrene Antitoxins, N.F. This antitoxin is made by mixing the serums of horses individually immunized to the toxins of tetanus and gas gangrene. Each package of the antitoxins contains not less than 1,500 units of tetanus antitoxin and not less than 2,000 units of each of the other component antitoxins (*Clostridium perfringens* and *Clostridium septicum*). The usual dose is the contents of one or more packages, given parenterally, as a prophylactic measure.

Antigenic agents used to produce active immunity

Vaccines

Vaccines are suspensions of either attenuated or killed microorganisms that are administered for the prevention or treatment or infectious diseases. The viruses for vaccines are commonly grown in chick embryos; this type of vaccine is absolutely contraindicated in persons with a history of hypersensitivity to egg, chicken, or chicken feathers. Vaccines do not afford immediate protection. An interval of days or several weeks elapse between inoculation and the production of antibodies. Because of this, if there is danger of immediate infection and there is a serum available, a prophylactic dose of serum should first be given to afford immediate protection, followed later by the vaccine injection to ensure a prolonged immunity.

Cholera Vaccine, U.S.P., B.P. Cholera vaccine is a sterile suspension of killed cholera vibrios *(Vibrio comma)* in isotonic sodium chloride solution or other suitable diluent. At the time of manufacture, cholera vaccine contains 8 billion cholera organisms in each milliliter of suspension. The usual subcutaneous dose is 0.5 ml., followed by another dose of 1 ml. after a week or 10 days, making a total of two injections.

Influenza Virus Vaccine, Monovalent, Type A* (Asian Strain). This vaccine is a sterile suspension of formaldehyde-killed influenza virus, type A, grown in chick embryos. It is administered subcutaneously in doses of 1 ml. for adults and 0.5 ml. for children from 5 to 12 years of age. For children between 3 months and 5 years, the dose of 0.1 ml. given subcutaneously or intracutaneously is suggested. It is also suggested that these doses for infants and children be repeated within 1 or 2 weeks.

Influenza Virus Vaccine, U.S.P. This vaccine is a suspension of inactivated influenza virus cultivated in chick embryos. Influenza Virus Vaccine is used prophylactically to produce active immunization against influenza. The maximum amount of antibody formation occurs during the second week after vaccination, and the titer remains constant for about one month, after which there is a gradual decline. The vaccine should not be given to persons sensitive to material derived from chick or egg protein. Dosage for prophylactic active immunization is 1 ml. given subcutaneously, followed by 1 ml. in 2 weeks.

Mumps Vaccine.* This vaccine is a sterile suspension of mumps virus grown in chick embryos, inactivated by ultraviolet light or formaldehyde. It is administered subcutaneously in 2 doses of 1 ml. each, given at an interval of 1 to 4 weeks.

Pertussis Vaccine, U.S.P., B.P. (Whooping Cough Vaccine). Pertussis vaccine is a sterile suspension of killed pertussis bacilli. Field Studies show that this vaccine possesses sufficient antigenic value to afford considerable protection against whooping cough. It does not always prevent attacks of the disease, but it lowers the death rate from the disease. The usual dose is three injections of 0.5 to 1 ml. 4 to 6 weeks apart. Pertussis vaccine is given subcutaneously.

Adsorbed Pertussis Vaccine, U.S.P. This is a sterile suspension of the killed pertussis bacilli of a strain or strains selected for high antigenic efficiency and adsorbed or precipitated by the addition of alum, aluminum phosphate, or aluminum hydroxide and resuspended. Because of the adsorption, there is a delay in absorption. The dose is the same as that for Pertussis Vaccine, U.S.P., and is given intramuscularly.

Poliomyelitis Vaccine, U.S.P. Poliomyelitis vaccine is a sterile solution of inactivated poliomyelitis virus of types 1, 2, and 3, grown separately on cultures of monkey kidney tissue. It is administered by subcutaneous injection. It is given in three doses of 1 ml. each; the second injection is given 2 to 6 weeks after the first, and the third injection, 7 months after the second dose.

Rabies Vaccine, U.S.P. This vaccine is a sterile freeze-dried suspension of killed rabies virus prepared from duck embryo or from brain

*Described in annual publication of A. M. A. Council on Drugs, N.N.D., 1960.

tissue of rabbits infected with this virus. The virus obtained from the brain tissue is either attenuated or killed.

The older vaccines made only from nerve tissues sometimes resulted in severe neurologic or paralytic phenomena; such reactions were caused from sensitivity to foreign brain tissue rather than from sensitivity to the virus antigen. Since experiments have shown that the duck embryo contains little, if any, of the "paralytic factor," it is believed that the danger of neurologic side effects is materially reduced by the use of the duck embryo vaccine.

Rabies vaccine is injected subcutaneously for 14 to 21 days. When the killed virus vaccine is administered, 2 ml. of 5 per cent suspension are given daily. When the attenuated virus vaccine is given, 1 ml. of the 5 per cent suspension is administered.

Smallpox Vaccine, U.S.P., B.P. This was the first vaccine prepared. It consists of a glycerinated suspension of vaccinia viruses which have been grown in healthy vaccinated animals of the bovine family or in membranes of the chick embryo. It loses its potency if kept at a temperature above 5° C. Failure of vaccination to "take" is often due to inactive virus. The usual dose is the contents of one container, administered by multiple puncture of the skin.

Typhoid and Paratyphoid Vaccine, U.S.P., B.P. This vaccine is a suspension of the killed typhoid bacilli and the paratyphoid A and B bacilli in suspension in physiologic saline solution. A milliliter of the vaccine contains at least 1,000,000,000 typhoid organisms and at least 250,000,000 of each of the paratyphoid organisms. The dose given subcutaneously is 0.5 ml., to be repeated twice, the interval between doses should be 7 to 28 days. With the use of the mixed vaccine, typhoid and paratyphoid infections may be entirely prevented. Within 12 hours a local reaction develops, and usually there are slight fever and a general lack of energy, which lasts about a day. The patient should avoid activity as much as possible during that period. Immunity lasts for 2 to 4 years.

Typhoid Vaccine, U.S.P. Typhoid vaccine is a sterile suspension of killed typhoid bacilli in physiologic saline solution or other suitable diluent. The vaccine should contain in each milliliter at least 1,000,000,000 typhoid organisms. The usual prophylactic subcutaneous dose is 0.5 ml., to be repeated twice at intervals of 7 to 28 days. Typhoid vaccine is also used in nonspecific protein therapy.

Typhus Vaccine, U.S.P., B.P. Typhus vaccine is a sterile suspension of the killed rickettsial organism of a strain or strains of epidemic typhus rickettsiae cultured in chick embryos. Usual dose, subcutaneously, for active immunization is 1 ml., to be repeated once with a 7- to 10-day interval. The Typhus Vaccine listed in B.P. contains the killed murine typhus rickettsiae as well as the epidemic rickettsiae.

Tuberculosis Vaccine, BCG Vaccine[*]; *Bacillus Calmette-Guérin Vaccine,* B.P. This is a freeze-dried preparation of the culture of an attenuated strain of the bovine tubercle bacillus.

The vaccine is used only in individuals who are negative in their reaction to the tuberculin test. Conversion of negative tuberculin-tested subjects to positive reactors after vaccination is usually considered presumptive evidence that immunity has developed similar to that which follows a naturally resisted or healed primary sensitizing infection.[†] Physicians have a choice either of using the vaccine to reduce the risk of clinical disease or of not using the vaccine and having the tuberculin skin test for early diagnosis and as a guide to the need for further study and treatment.

Tuberculosis vaccine is usually administered by multiple puncture or by intradermal injection. The dose in drops varies, depending on the gauge of the needle or other openings from which the vaccine is deposited on the skin. For example, using the resuspended vaccine (50 mg. per milliliter) 4 drops from a 22-gauge needle would be used for the multiple puncture method. For intradermal injection, 0.1 ml. (equivalent to 0.2 mg.) is further diluted and injected as superficially as possible with a tuberculin syringe and a 26-gauge needle so that a wheal of 8 to 10 mm. is produced.

Yellow Fever Vaccine, U.S.P., B.P. The U.S.P. preparation of this vaccine is the living virus of an attenuated strain of the yellow fever virus, prepared by culturing the virus in the chick embryo. It is dried from the frozen state; the powder is rehydrated immediately before use. It is administered subcutaneously, the usual dose being 0.5 ml.

Toxoids

A toxoid is a toxin modified so that it is nontoxic but still antigenic. Formaldehyde is the agent generally used for the detoxification of toxins. Toxoids are supplied in the plain form and as precipitated and adsorbed preparations. Alum is used for the precipitated products, and aluminum hydroxide and aluminum phosphate are employed to provide an adsorption surface for toxoids. The precipitated and adsorbed products are absorbed more slowly by the circulating and tissue fluids of the body and excreted slowly; therefore, they provide higher immunizing titers than does plain toxoid.[‡]

Diphtheria Toxoid, U.S.P. Diphtheria Toxoid is an aqueous solution of the products of the growth of *Corynebacterium diphtheriae,* so modified by formaldehyde that it has lost its toxic effects for guinea

[*]Described in annual publication of A. M. A. Council on Drugs, N.N.D., 1960.
[†]N.N.D., 1960, p. 635.
[‡]N.N.D., 1960, p. 626.

732

pigs but not its power to produce immunity. One-half or 1 ml. is administered subcutaneously to produce active immunity in three doses with 3- or 4-week intervals between doses. Since some general as well as local reactions are observed in adults and older children, a test dose should be given to determine sensitivity in these persons.

Adsorbed Diphtheria Toxoid, U.S.P. This is a sterile suspension of diphtheria toxoid precipitated or adsorbed by the addition of aluminum hydroxide, aluminum phosphate, or alum. For active immunization it is given subcutaneously, 0.5 or 1 ml., and repeated in 4 to 6 weeks.

Diphtheria Vaccine, B.P. This is prepared from diphtheria toxin and includes alum-precipitated toxoid, purified toxoid, aluminum phosphate, formol toxoid, and toxoid-antitoxin floccules. It is given subcutaneously or intramuscularly.

Tetanus Toxoid, U.S.P.; *Tetanus Vaccine,* B.P. Tetanus toxoid is a sterile solution of the products of growth of *Clostridium tetani,* so modified by formaldehyde that it has lost the ability to cause toxic effects in guinea pigs but retains the property of inducing activity immunity. Usual subcutaneous dose is 0.5 or 1 ml., according to label specifications, repeated three times at intervals of 3 to 4 weeks.

Adsorbed Tetanus Toxoid, U.S.P. This toxoid is tetanus toxoid precipitated or adsorbed by the addition of alum, aluminum hydroxide, or aluminum phosphate. Dosage for active immunization is two injections of 0.5 or 1 ml. at intervals of 4 to 6 weeks, given subcutaneously.

Adsorbed Diphtheria and Tetanus Toxoids and Pertussis Vaccine, U.S.P. This preparation is a sterile mixture of diphtheria toxoid, tetanus toxoid, and pertussis vaccine, adsorbed on aluminum hydroxide, aluminum phosphate, or alum. The antigens are combined in such proportion as to yield a mixture containing one immunizing dose of each in the total dosage prescribed on the label. The dosage is three injections of 0.5 or 1 ml., as specified on the label, 3 to 4 weeks apart. It is administered subcutaneously.

Adsorbed Diphtheria and Tetanus Toxoids, U.S.P. This preparation is a sterile suspension prepared by mixing suitable quantities of the adsorbed forms of diphtheria and tetanus toxoids. Two injections of 0.5 or 1 ml., as specified on the label, are given subcutaneously, 4 to 6 weeks apart.

Diphtheria, Tetanus, and Pertussis Vaccine, B.P. This preparation is administered subcutaneously or intramuscularly in doses of 0.5 or 1 ml. three times at intervals of 4 to 6 weeks.

Agents for cutaneous immunity tests

Diagnostic Diphtheria Toxin, U.S.P.; *Schick Test Toxin,* B.P. This is the toxin for the Schick test which is done to determine the susceptibility of an individual to diphtheria. The toxin that is used is carefully standardized on human beings. The usual dose is 0.1 ml. This is injected intracutaneously, usually on the forearm. If the person is susceptible to diphtheria, i.e., if his blood does not contain a sufficient amount of antitoxin to protect him from the disease, a small area of redness, usually with some infiltration, will occur at the point of injection in 24 to 28 hours. This is known as a positive reaction. It persists about 7 to 10 days and then fades slowly.

Mumps Skin Test Antigen.[*] This agent is a sterile suspension of killed mumps virus. The virus is grown in chick embryos and inactivated by ultraviolet light or formaldehyde. It is used to detect specific skin hypersensitivity to the mumps virus. It may be used to determine susceptibility to mumps or to confirm a tentative diagnosis of the disease.

Mumps skin test antigen is administered intradermally in doses of 0.1 ml., usually on the inner surface of the forearm; the injected area should be observed in 24 to 36 hours.

Old Tuberculin, U.S.P., B.P. (Koch's Tuberculin). Old tuberculin is prepared by filtering a glycerin bouillon culture of the tubercle bacillus through a Berkefeld filter. It contains the toxins of the tubercle bacilli and is used largely in diagnosing tuberculosis. It is given by intracutaneous injection. If the patient has been infected with tuberculosis at some time, there is an area of redness, usually with a papule at the point of application of the tuberculin. The usual dose for diagnostic purposes is 0.0001 ml. A reaction indicates that the patient has at some time been infected with tuberculosis but not necessarily that he has clinical tuberculosis.

Purified Protein Derivative of Tuberculin, U.S.P., B.P. This preparation is a sterile soluble purified product of the growth of the *Mycobacterium tuberculosis* which is prepared in a special liquid medium free from protein. It is used chiefly as a diagnostic aid. Dosage is 0.1 to 0.2 mcg. given intracutaneously.

Allergens

Allergy is a condition of hypersensitiveness to certain antigens; these are usually proteins such as the pollens of plants, the proteins present in the hair or skin of animals or the feathers of fowls, and the proteins of food, serums, bacteria, etc. The person who comes in contact with the proteins to which he is unusually sensitive develops such symptoms as sneezing, coryza, headache, fever, hives, and asthmatic attacks.

Allergens are extracts prepared from the proteins of various substances and are used to determine the susceptibility of the patient to

[*]Described in annual publication of A. M. A. Council on Drugs, N.N.D., 1960.

proteins and to prevent and relieve the conditions caused by hyper-sensitiveness.

The patient's susceptibility is tested by intradermal injection of the allergen. If the patient is sensitive to that particular protein, an urticarial wheal or elevated red spot results.

Prevention and Treatment of Allergy. When the identity of the particular protein causing the symptoms has been determined, the attacks of the disease may frequently be prevented by removing the causative factor; e.g., by omitting certain foods from the diet, by eliminating contact with pet cats and dogs, or by removing the hair mattress or the feather pillows, etc., depending upon the cause of the allergy.

In hay fever the patient may have to be immunized against the specific pollens causing the attack. This process is called desensitization. It consists of a series of ten or more injections of dilute solutions of the specific pollens in graduated strengths given at intervals of about 5 days. The treatment should be begun sufficiently early so that the maximum dose is reached by the time of the first attack of the disease, and this dose is repeated once a week during the pollen season. Immunity lasts only about a year. In some cases of asthma and urticaria the patient may be desensitized to the specific proteins causing their symptoms. Antihistaminic drugs have become prominent in the treatment of allergic manifestations since it was recognized that histamine or a histamine-like substance is released in allergic reactions. For further discussion, see Chapter 12. Cortisone, hydrocortisone, and related compounds have been found to provide symptomatic relief of allergy and allergic manifestations.

Chapter 28

Toxicology

Definitions

Toxicology is the study of poisons, including their action, effects, detection, and treatment of conditions produced by them.

Poison may be defined as any substance which, when applied to the body or introduced into the system in relatively small amounts in whatever manner, causes death or serious bodily harm. It might be added that the substance usually acts chemically and that it can harm an ordinary individual. Most, if not all, drugs can be considered potential poisons.

General symptoms of poisoning

When poisoning is suspected, the nurse should send for the physician. In the meantime, since *time* is such a precious factor, particularly in cases of acute poisoning, she should learn as much about the patient as possible and apply suitable first-aid measures.

There is reason to suspect that a poison has been taken when sudden, violent symptoms occur, such as severe nausea, vomiting, diarrhea, collapse, or convulsions. It is important to find out (if possible) what poison has been taken and how much. Additional information which might prove helpful to the physician in making a diagnosis includes answers to questions or reports of observed phenomena, as follows:

1. Did the symptoms appear suddenly in an otherwise healthy individual? Did a number of persons become ill about the same time (as might happen in food poisoning)?

2. Is there anything unusual about the person, his clothing or his surroundings? Is there evidence of burns about the lips and mouth? Are the gums discolored? Are there needle (hypodermic) pricks, pustules, or scars on the exposed and accessible surfaces of the body? (These may be seen in examination of drug addicts.) Is there any skin rash or discoloration?

3. Note the odor of the breath, the rate of respiration, and any difficulty in respiration. Look for cyanosis.

4. Note the quality and rate of the pulse.

5. If vomitus is seen, what is its appearance and its odor? Is or was vomiting accompanied by diarrhea or abdominal pain?

6. Note any abnormalities of stool and urine; change in color or the presence of blood may be significant.

7. For signs of involvement of the nervous system watch for the presence of excitement, muscular twitching, delirium, difficulty in speech, stupor, coma, constriction or dilatation of the pupils, elevated or subnormal temperature.

The nurse should save all specimens of vomitus, urine, or stool in case the physician wishes to examine them and perhaps turn them over to the proper authority for analysis. This is of particular importance not only in making or confirming a diagnosis but also in the event that the case has medicolegal significance.

Incidence and causes of poisoning

Most poisons are taken accidentally, some are taken with suicidal intent and in a few cases they are administered for homicidal purpose. The advances made in the science of toxicology have discouraged most murderers from using poison to gain their ends. One of the chief causes of accidental death is carbon monoxide poisoning.* Among the agents used for suicide the most popular seem to be carbon monoxide, cyanide, cresol, barbiturates, and bichloride of mercury.

Most children who are poisoned are less than 5 years of age. Poisoning and accidents are responsible for the largest number of deaths in children at the pediatric age group.† The leading causative agent of poisoning of children differs somewhat in different parts of the country, e.g., kerosene is commonly the offending substance in rural areas, but lead and arsenic poisoning is encountered in fruit-growing areas where unwashed fruit, bearing residues of insecticidal sprays, is available to children. Other rather frequent causes of poisoning of children are strychnine, some laxative tablets if taken in large doses, barbiturates, ant poisons, various cleaning agents, sink cleaners, bleaches, paint thinners, silver polish, lye, insecticides, and rodenticides. In the emergency department of a large Midwestern hospital the chief cause of poisoning among children was found to be aspirin. In most cases the children had eaten the sweetened, 1 gr. tablets which they apparently had mistaken for candy.

*Salter, W. T.: A Textbook of Pharmacology, Philadelphia, 1952, W. B. Saunders Co., p. 1189.
†Nelson, Waldo E.: Textbook of Pediatrics, Philadelphia, 1959, W. B. Saunders Co., p. 1378.

Poison control centers

Physicians have long been concerned about the incidence of poisoning, especially among young children, and as a result of such concern the first poison control center was started in Chicago in 1953 as a cooperative and integrated community activity. This idea spread to other cities in many states and similar programs have been started, the administration of which may be the function of the local medical society, a medical school, the health department, a hospital, or a combination of these groups. Their main purpose is to serve as a center from which information about poisons can be obtained. There are now over 200 of these centers in the United States. With thousands of products on the market known only by their trade names, one of the major problems in treating the victim of a supposed poison is the proper identification of the ingredients of the product so that treatment may be adequate or the victim and his family can be assured that the product was harmless. The collection of data which helps to identify a poison is an important contribution of the center, although it has other functions, e.g., data on all cases of poisoning are collected and centrally reported and follow-up visits to homes are often made to help prevent further cases of poisoning.

Classification of poisons

The classification of poisons is as broad as the classification of drugs, since any drug is likely to be a potential poison in the tissues of the right person, and any drug when used in excess amounts is poisonous to almost any person.

Poisons might be classified in various ways. For example, they might be grouped according to chemical classifications as organic and inorganic poisons, as alkaloids, glycosides, and resins, or as acids, alkalies, heavy metals, oxidizing agents, halogenated hydrocarbons, etc.

Another way in which they might be grouped is by locale of exposure, i.e., poisons found in the home, poisons encountered in industry, poisons encountered while camping, etc.

Still another way in which poisons may be classified is according to the organ or tissue of the body in which the most damaging effects are produced. Some poisons injure all cells with which they have contact. Such chemical substances are sometimes called protoplasmic poisons or cytotoxins. Others have more effect on the kidney (nephrotoxins), the liver (hepatotoxins), or on the blood or blood-forming organs.

Poisons that affect chiefly the nervous system are called neurotoxins or neurotropic poisons. They must be studied separately because different symptoms characterize each one. Symptoms of toxicity have been mentioned in connection with each of these drugs as they were presented in previous chapters. Although symptoms of this group of poisons are to some extent specific, it is also true that certain symptoms are encountered repeatedly and are associated with a large number of poisons. Drowsiness, dizziness, headache, delirium, coma, and convulsive seizures always indicate central nervous system involvement. On the other hand, one learns to associate dry mouth, dilated pupils, and difficult swallowing with overdosage of atropine or one of the atropine-like drugs; whereas ringing in the ears, excessive perspiration, gastric upset, etc. are associated with overdosage with salicylates.

Mechanisms of toxic actions of poisons

Poisons produce their injurious effects in a number of ways. Many times the precise mechanism of action is not known, e.g., death may be due to respiratory failure but exactly what happens to cause depression of the respiratory center may not be known.

It is increasingly apparent that the human body is exceedingly dependent upon a constant supply of oxygen if various physiologic functions are to proceed satisfactorily. *Anything* that interferes with the use of oxygen by the cells or with the transportation of oxygen will produce damaging effects in cells and in some cells faster than in others.

Carbon monoxide is one of the most widely distributed toxic agents. It poisons by producing hypoxia and finally asphyxia. Carbon monoxide has a great affinity for the hemoglobin of the blood and forms carboxyhemoglobin. Thus the production of oxyhemoglobin and the free transport of oxygen is interfered with, and oxygen deficiency soon develops in the cells. Unless exposure to the carbon monoxide is terminated, the anoxia may produce serious damage in the brain and death.

The cyanides act somewhat similarily in that they bring about cellular anoxia, but they do so in a different manner. They inactivate certain tissue enzymes so that cells are unable to utilize the oxygen brought by the blood. Death may come very rapidly.

Curare and the curariform drugs in toxic amounts bring about paralysis of the diaphragm, and again the victim dies from lack of oxygen.

Certain drugs have a direct effect on muscle tissue of the body such as that of the myocardium or the smooth muscle of the blood vessels. Death results from the failure of circulation or cardiac arrest. The nitrites, potassium salts, and digitalis drugs may exert toxic effects of this type.

Arsenic is an example of a protoplasmic poison or cytotoxin. Compounds of arsenic inhibit many enzyme systems of cells, especially those that depend on the activity of their free sulfhydryl groups. The arsenic combines with these SH groups and makes them ineffective. Hence extensive tissue damage in the body is brought about.

Methyl alcohol (mentioned under intoxicants) owes its toxic effect to an intermediate product of metabolism-formic acid. This produces a severe acidosis, lowered pH of the blood, reduced cerebral blood flow, and decreased consumption of oxygen by the brain. There is also a selective action on the retinal cells of the eye, but the exact cause of this injury is unknown.

Benzene is an example of a poison that acts by inhibiting the formation of all types of blood cells. In some instances the precursor of one type of blood cell is injured more than another. Depression of the formation of any of the blood cells can cause death.

The strong acids and alkalies denature and destroy cellular proteins. Examples of corrosive acids are hydrochloric, nitric, and sulfuric acids. Sodium, potassium, and ammonium hydroxides are examples of strong or caustic alkalies. Locally, these substances cause destruction of tissue and it is possible for death to be due to the effects of hemorrhage, perforation, or shock or combinations of these complications. Corrosive poisons may also cause death by altering the pH of the blood or other body fluids, or they may produce marked degenerative changes in vital organs such as the liver or the kidney.

Many of the central nervous system depressants cause death by producing excessive depression of respiration and respiratory failure. The general anesthetics, barbiturates, chloral hydrate, and paraldehyde are examples of such drugs.

Central nervous system stimulants such as pentylenetetrazol, strychnine, methylphenidate, and others in toxic amounts cause convulsive seizures, exhaustion, and depression of vital centers. During the convulsive seizure the patient does not breathe adequately and sometimes stops breathing altogether, thereby producing oxygen deficiency which in turn is believed to inhibit activity of vital centers.

First-aid measures for poisoning

As mentioned previously, the duty of the nurse is to send for a physician and, pending his arrival, to ascertain if possible the cause of the symptoms and to apply suitable first-aid measures. The treatment of acute poisoning is always an emergency. Recommendations on first-aid measures for poisoning were made by the Committee on Toxicology of the American Medical Association and are presented on pages 742 and 743.

Treatment of poisoning

Treatment of poisoning includes a number of general principles of action. Under many circumstances good first aid may save the patient's life and make the physician's task easier. To some extent, first aid and the later treatment may overlap. There are many things that may be done for the patient which can be done only under the direction and supervision of a physician, but the more the nurse knows about the poison and what to expect and what to have ready for use, the more help she is to all concerned. Occasionally a nurse must deal with an emergency alone or at best under the direction of a physician she is able to contact by telephone.

When living in or near a city it is faster and more satisfactory to bring a patient to a hospital, clinic, or physician's office than it is to wait for the physician to call at a home. Professional ambulance service, the police, or the fire department will frequently provide transportation, but a family car or that of a neighbor may be a faster way of solving the problem. Treatment of poisoning frequently involves (1) removal of the poison, (2) administration of a suitable antidote, (3) promotion of elimination, and (4) supportive treatment of the patient.

The order of these measures may need to be reversed, depending on the poison taken and the general condition of the patient. Sometimes the prompt removal of the poison is all the treatment that is needed.

Removal of the poison

When poisons are on the external surface of the body, in the nasal or oral cavities or in the eye, attempts to remove them should be made by irrigating with copious amounts of plain water. Acids should then be neutralized with weak bases and bases should be neutralized with weak acids. Toxic oils should be removed with organic solvents or warm, soapy water. If the poison has been swallowed recently, it is advisable to remove it from the stomach as soon as possible to decrease chances of absorption. The simplest way, provided the patient is conscious and co-operative, is to persuade him to drink an excess of tepid water and induce vomiting. Other emetics can be used but some of them must be used with caution. Tepid water with mustard (one teaspoon to a glass), weak salt water, starch water, or weak soap solution can do little harm, although the mustard may accentuate the discomfort of the raw mucous membranes. Copper sulfate is sometimes added to water and used as an emetic, especially for arsenic poisoning, but it has been known to kill infants when the excess cupric ion was not removed. Apomorphine, gr. $\frac{1}{10}$, can be given hypodermically. It acts promptly but tends to be depressing and hence is not widely used. The best emetic is probably the mildest and the one most easily and quickly available.

First-Aid Measures for Poisoning

The following recommendations on first-aid measures for poisoning have been adopted by the Committee on Toxicology. These recommendations are made in response to numerous requests to the American Medical Association for general instructions for poisoning emergencies. They are intended for use in educating the public in what to do when poisoning occurs.

Emergency Telephone Numbers:

PHYSICIAN _____ FIRE DEPT. _____

HOSPITAL _____ (resuscitator)

PHARMACIST _____ POLICE _____

RESCUE SQUADS _____

The aim of first-aid measures is to help prevent absorption of the poison. SPEED is essential. First-aid measures must be started at once. If possible, one person should begin treatment while another calls a physician. When this is not possible, the nature of the poison will determine whether to call a physician first or begin first-aid measures and then notify a physician. Save the poison container and material itself if any remains. If the poison is not known, save a sample of the vomitus.

MEASURES TO BE TAKEN BEFORE ARRIVAL OF PHYSICIAN

I. Swallowed Poisons

Many products used in and around the home, although not labeled "Poison," may be dangerous if taken internally. For example, some medications which are beneficial when used correctly may endanger life if used improperly or in excessive amounts.

In all cases, *except those indicated below*, REMOVE POISON FROM PATIENT'S STOMACH IMMEDIATELY by inducing vomiting. This cannot be overemphasized, for it is the essence of the treatment and is often a life-saving procedure. Prevent chilling by wrapping patient in blankets if necessary. Do not give alcohol in any form.

A. Do Not Induce Vomiting If:

  1. Patient is in coma or unconscious.

  2. Patient is in convulsions.

  3. Patient has swallowed petroleum products (i.e., kerosene, gasoline, lighter fluid).

  4. Patient has swallowed a corrosive poison (symptoms: severe pain, burning sensation in mouth and throat, vomiting. CALL PHYSICIAN IMMEDIATELY.

    (a) Acid and acid-like corrosives: sodium acid sulfate (toilet bowl cleaners), acetic acid (glacial), sulfuric acid, nitric acid, oxalic acid, hydrofluoric acid (rust removers), iodine, silver nitrate (styptic pencil).

    (b) Alkali corrosives: sodium hydroxide-lye (drain cleaners), sodium carbonate (washing soda), ammonia water, sodium hypochlorite (household bleach).

If the patient can swallow after ingesting a *corrosive poison*, the following substances (and amounts) may be given:

For acids: milk, water, or milk of magnesia (1 tablespoon to 1 cup of water).

For alkalis: milk, water, any fruit juice, or vinegar.

For patient 1-5 years old—1 to 2 cups.

For patient 5 years and older—up to 1 quart.

B. Induce Vomiting When Non-corrosive Substances Have Been Swallowed:

  1. Give milk or water (for patient 1-5 years old—1 to 2 cups; for patient over 5 years—up to 1 quart).

  2. Induce vomiting by placing the blunt end of a spoon or your finger at the back of the patient's throat, or by use of this emetic—2 tablespoons of salt in a glass of warm water.

When retching and vomiting begin, place patient face down with head lower than hips. This prevents vomitus from entering the lungs and causing further damage.

II. Inhaled Poisons

1. Carry patient (do not let him walk) to fresh air immediately.
2. Open all doors and windows.
3. Loosen all tight clothing.
4. Apply artificial respiration if breathing has stopped or is irregular.
5. Prevent chilling (wrap patient in blankets).
6. Keep patient as quiet as possible.
7. If patient is convulsing, keep him in bed in a semidark room; avoid jarring or noise.
8. Do not give alcohol in any form.

III. Skin Contamination

1. Drench skin with water (shower, hose, faucet).
2. Apply stream of water on skin while removing clothing.
3. Cleanse skin thoroughly with water; rapidity in washing is most important in reducing extent of injury.

IV. Eye Contamination

1. Hold eyelids open, wash eyes with gentle stream of running water *immediately*. Delay of few seconds greatly increases extent of injury.
2. Continue washing until physician arrives.
3. *Do not use chemicals;* they may increase extent of injury.

V. Injected Poisons (Scorpion and Snake Bites)

1. Make patient lie down as soon as possible.
2. Do not give alcohol in any form.

3. Apply tourniquet above injection site (e.g., between arm or leg and heart). The pulse in vessels below the tourniquet should not disappear, nor should the tourniquet produce a throbbing sensation. Tourniquet should be loosened for 1 minute every 15 minutes.
4. Apply ice-pack to the site of the bite.
5. Carry patient to physician or hospital; DO NOT LET HIM WALK.

VI. Chemical Burns

1. Wash with large quantities of running water (except those caused by phosphorus).
2. Immediately cover with loosely applied clean cloth.
3. Avoid use of ointments, greases, powders, and other drugs in first-aid treatment of burns.
4. Treat shock by keeping patient flat, keeping him warm, and reassuring him until arrival of physician.

MEASURES TO PREVENT POISONING ACCIDENTS

A. Keep all drugs, poisonous substances, and household chemicals out of the reach of children
B. Do not store nonedible products on shelves used for storing food.
C. Keep all poisonous substances in their original containers; do not transfer to unlabeled containers.
D. When medicines are discarded, destroy them. Do not throw them where they might be reached by children or pets.
E. When giving flavored and/or brightly colored medicine to children, *always* refer to it as medicine—*never* as candy.
F. Do not take or give medicine in the dark.
G. READ LABELS before using chemical products.

From Council on Drugs, J. A. M. A. **165**: 686, 1957.

Use of the stomach tube to remove poisons can be hazardous. Especially is this so if there is (1) danger of perforating a corroded esophagus or stomach, (2) danger of aspirating the poison, as there may be when the person has swallowed kerosene, or (3) danger of precipitating a convulsive seizure such as might occur in strychnine poisoning.

Use of the stomach tube is probably preferable in many cases to the use of emetics, because the tube has greater efficiency in emptying the stomach and because less prostration is likely to follow its use than when the patient is made to vomit. The stomach tube, however, usually is passed by the physician and there are times when there is need for more prompt evacuation of the stomach, as indicated under first-aid measures.

Administration of suitable antidote

After the stomach has been emptied, it is necessary to administer the proper antidote. An *antidote* is any agent used to counteract the action of a poison. There are three kinds of antidotes: (1) physical or mechanical, (2) chemical, and (3) physiologic.

A *physical antidote* is one that envelops or mixes with the poison and prevents its absorption, soothes, and protects the tissues and may aid in removal of the poison.

Demulcents, emollients, emetics, cathartics, and the stomach tube are used as physical antidotes.

Milk, white of egg, boiled starch or porridge, gruels, barley water, mashed potato, and mucilage of acacia are suitable demulcents. Fixed oils such as olive, cottonseed, cod liver, or liquid petrolatum may be used, but in cases where the poison is soluble in the oil, like cantharides or phosphorus, the stomach should be emptied after giving the oil.

A *chemical antidote* is one that reacts with the poison and neutralizes it. Common salt (sodium chloride) is an excellent antidote for silver nitrate. The products formed, silver chloride and sodium nitrate, are both harmless. Magnesium oxide, milk of magnesia, or baking soda are chemical antidotes for acids. In general, it is to be remembered that alkalies counteract acids and vice versa. *Care should be used when sodium bicarbonate is given because if too much gas results from the reaction, the pressure may rupture the corroded stomach.* For this reason, milk of magnesia or calcium carbonate may be preferable. Lemon juice, grapefruit juice, and vinegar are suitable weak acids to neutralize strong bases. Poisoning with irritant metallic salts is best treated with albumin in the form of white of egg, an insoluble albuminate being formed. The antidote for the vegetable alkaloids such as morphine, atropine, or strychnine is tannic acid or potassium permanganate. Both the tannic acid and the potassium permanganate (1:2,000) may be used to wash out the patient's stomach. The tannic acid may be conveniently obtained from strong green tea and it brings about precipitation of the alkaloids while the potassium permanganate brings about oxidation of the alkaloids.

Chemical antidotes act only on such portions of the poison as have not been absorbed, and must be given promptly. They are frequently added to the lavage solution.

A *physiologic antidote* is one that produces the opposite systemic effect from that of the poison. If a person has taken or been given too much pilocarpine, the sweating is readily counteracted by the hypodermic use of atropine ($\frac{1}{60}$ to $\frac{1}{30}$ gr.). Caffeine is a physiologic antidote for morphine and sedatives like pentobarbital, and an anesthetic is an antidote for strychnine poisoning. If there are spasms, use ether first, a sedative later.

Antidote kit

The following materials have been suggested to cope with poison emergencies. Others may be added. (See Table 15.) A nurse is many times responsible for keeping up the supplies and for seeing that clear legible labels are maintained.

Alcohol
Amyl nitrite pearls
Apomorphine tablets, 2 mg.
Aromatic spirit of ammonia
Atropine tablets, 1 mg.
Bicarbonate of sodium
Caffeine-sodium benzoate
Calcium gluconate, 10%, ampules
Charcoal, activated
Chloroform
Cupric sulfate, powdered
Dextrose, 50%, ampules
Epinephrine tablets, 1 mg.
Ephedrine hydrochloride, 16 mg. tablets
Limewater
Magnesia, calcined

Methylene blue, 50 ml., 1% in 1.8% sodium sulfate
Metrazol, 10%, 1 ml. ampules
Morphine sulfate tablets, 10 mg.
Nalorphine, 10 mg. in 2 ampules
Nitrite of sodium, 2%, 10 ml. ampules
Olive oil
Pentobarbital sodium, 0.5 Gm. ampules
Picrotoxin, 3%, 20 ml.
Potassium permanganate, 1% solution, to be diluted 20 times
Thiosulfate of sodium, 30%, 10 ml. ampules
Tincture of iodine
Whisky

Also a hypodermic syringe in good order and a stomach tube with a funnel should be available. The following can be secured usually at the home of the patient: boiled water, hot, strong black coffee, eggs, hot-water bottles, milk, mustard, salt, starch, tea, and vinegar.

Table 15

Some specific poisons, symptoms, and emergency treatment

Poison	Symptoms	Treatment
Acids (e.g., hydrochloric or nitric)	Parts in contact with acid are first white, later colored (brown or yellow) Pain in throat, esophagus, and stomach; dysphagia, diarrhea, shock, circulatory collapse Death may be due to asphyxia from edema of glottis	Avoid stomach tube, emesis, and solutions of carbonate, e.g., soda bicarbonate Give milk of magnesia, aluminum hydroxide, mild soap solution, plenty of milk, or water with egg white Copious amounts of water Keep patient warm and quiet
Arsenic (found in weed killers, insecticides, sheep-dip, rodenticides, etc.)	Rapidity of onset of symptoms related to whether or not poison is taken with food Odor of garlic on breath and stools Faintness, nausea, difficulty in swallowing, extreme thirst, severe vomiting, gastric pain, "rice water" stools, oliguria, albuminuria, cold, clammy skin Collapse and death	Universal antidote 5 to 6 teaspoonfuls followed by repeated lavage with warm or weak sodium bicarbonate solution; or by an emetic (warm water, salt water, or mustard water) repeated until vomiting occurs Intravenous fluids Sedation, analgesics Dimercaprol (BAL) (see p. 749) Keep patient warm
Carbon monoxide (present in coal gas, illuminating gas, exhaust gas from motor cars, etc.)	Symptoms vary with concentration of carbon monoxide in blood Headache, dizziness, impaired hearing and vision, drowsiness, confusion, loss of consciousness Slow respiration, rapid pulse Coma, cherry-red lips and nails	Remove patient to fresh air; artificial respiration; high concentration of oxygen along with 5 to 10% carbon dioxide to promote deep breathing Artificial respiration Bed rest for 48 hr. Keep patient warm
Carbon tetrachloride (found in some dry-cleaning fluids and in some home fire extinguishers)	*When inhaled:* headache, nausea, vomiting, diarrhea, jaundice, oliguria, albuminuria, dark-colored urine *When swallowed:* headache, nausea, vomiting, sometimes blood in vomitus, abdominal pain, disturbance of hearing and vision, jaundice, profuse diarrhea, albuminuria, anuria	Remove patient from poisoned atmosphere; administer oxygen or oxygen with carbon dioxide Simple emetics to produce repeated vomiting if lavage not available; if possible, lavage followed by saline cathartic High-protein, high-carbohydrate, high-calcium diet General supportive measures
Chlorophenothane (dichlorodiphenyltrichloroethane, or D.D.T.)	Headache, nausea, vomiting, diarrhea; paresthesis of lips and tongue, numbness of extremities, malaise, sore throat Coarse tremor, convulsions, respiratory failure	Induce vomiting or use gastric lavage if convulsions do not threaten Give saline cathartic, force fluids, give strong tea or coffee Avoid fats, fat solvents, and epinephrine Wash contaminated skin areas with soap and water

Table 15—Cont'd

Poison	Symptoms	Treatment
Cyanides	An odor of oil of bitter almonds on breath; headache, rapid breathing, dyspnea, palpitation of heart, feeling of tightness in chest, cyanosis, convulsions Death may come within few minutes	Prompt treatment sometimes successful Amyl nitrite (several pearls broken into gauze and given by inhalation), followed by 1% sodium nitrite intravenously slowly, "in 10 ml. doses, to a total of 50 ml. in an hours,"* and this followed by slow intravenous administration of sodium thiosulfate (50 ml. of a 50% solution) Oxygen and blood transfusion may be indicated
Fluoride (found in insecticides)	Nausea, vomiting, abdominal pain, diarrhea, muscle weakness, difficult swallowing, facial paralysis, inability to speak, convulsions at times, respiratory failure and circulatory collapse	Give emetic containing soluble calcium salts (calcium lactate or gluconate) or use plenty of warm water and follow with plenty of milk Preferable to lavage promptly with 1% calcium chloride to inactivate fluoride General supportive measures
Hydrocarbons (present in kerosene, gasoline, naphtha, cleaning fluids, etc.)	Symptoms of intoxication similar to those of alcohol, burning sensation in mouth, esophagus, and stomach Vomiting, dizziness, tremor, muscle cramps, confusion, fever Cold, clammy skin, weak pulse, thirst, unconsciousness, coma Death due to respiratory failure	Emetics and lavage usually avoided unless large amounts swallowed; saline cathartics after small amounts taken Some authorities recommend large doses of mineral oil for severe poisoning, followed by lavage with 1% or 2% sodium bicarbonate solution† General supportive measures
Iodine	Brown-stained lips, tongue, and mouth, which are painful Odor of iodine in vomitus Intense thirst, fainting attacks, giddiness, vomiting, burning, abdominal pain, diarrhea, shock	Give promptly plenty of water, with starch or flour or mashed potatoes Gastric lavage if possible with thin, cooked suspension of starch or 5% sodium thiosulfite solution Give drinks of milk or white of egg, with water

(Continued on next page.)

---

*Sollmann, T.: A Manual of Pharmacology, Philadelphia, 1957, W. B. Saunders Co., p. 987.
†Lucas, G. H. W.: The Symptoms and Treatment of Acute Poisoning, Chicago, 1953, The Macmillan Co., p. 219.

Table 15—Cont'd

Poison	Symptoms	Treatment
Lye (a severe caustic)	Severe burning pain in mouth, throat, and stomach Strong soapy taste in mouth Early violent vomiting with mucus and blood in vomitus Mucous membranes become white and swollen; lips and tongue swell; throat may become constricted Respirations difficult Skin cold and clammy Pulse rapid Violent purging Great anxiety	Emetics and lavage frequently not recommended Give large amounts of water containing weak acids, lemon, vinegar, lime juice, etc., later give demulcents white of egg, gruel, olive oil or salad oil Analgesics, parenteral fluids
Mercury and its compounds	Burning sensation of throat Nausea and vomiting (vomitus blue if antiseptic tablets of bichloride used) Sense of constriction in throat and esophagus Ashen-gray color of mucous membranes which have been in contact with poison Bloody, profuse diarrhea, with shreds of mucous membrane in stool and vomitus Shock, albuminuria, and hematuria During acute phase, pain and prostration; late, progressive uremia	Preferably give 5 to 6 heaping teaspoonfuls of universal antidote and then lavage with 5% sodium formaldehyde sulfoxylate solution followed by sodium bicarbonate solution If not feasible, give emetic of mustard water or salt water until vomiting has occurred repeatedly Give milk and egg white in water Dimercaprol indicated (see p. 749) Parenteral fluids Keep patient warm Recovery depends on dose taken, amount of absorption, and amount of kidney damage
Nicotine (Black Leaf 40 contains about 40 per cent nicotine sulfate)	Burning sensation in mouth and throat, increased flow of saliva, abdominal pain, vomiting, diarrhea, headache, sweating, confusion, weakness, dilatation of pupils, faintness, death from respiratory paralysis	Universal antidote 6 to 8 teaspoonfuls; lavage with 0.5% tannic acid or 1:5,000 potassium permanganate Artificial respirations Wash contaminated skin with cold water
Paris green (copper arsenite and copper acetate)	Vomiting of green material followed by gastric and abdominal pain; diarrhea with dark and sometimes bloody stools; metallic taste; neuromuscular weakness Thirst, oliguria, anuria Cold, clammy skin Coma, convulsions, death	Potassium ferrocyanide 10 gr. in water as soon as possible (forms an insoluble salt of copper), followed by lavage with sodium bicarbonate solution or a mustard-water emetic until stomach cleansed Demulcents (milk, egg white in water, gelatin, etc.) Supportive measures

Table 15—Cont'd

Poison	Symptoms	Treatment
Phenolic compounds (carbolic acid, cresol, Lysol, creosote)	Corrosion of mucous membranes that have come in contact with poison Severe pain, vomiting, bloody diarrhea, headache, dizziness Cold, clammy skin Oliguria, hematuria, unconsciousness, slow respiration, respiratory failure Urine dark and turns very dark on exposure to air	Of utmost importance to remove poison before absorption, prompt lavage with olive oil which is a good solvent;* leave some oil in stomach after lavage; give egg white and milk for demulcent effect Parenteral fluids, oxygen, carbon dioxide, analgesics Other supportive measures Phenol on skin can be removed with 50% solution of alcohol, followed by thorough rinsing with water, or wash external burns with olive oil or castor oil
Quaternary, ammonium compounds (e.g., Zephiran)	Burning pain in the mouth and throat, nausea and vomiting, apprehension and restlessness muscle weakness, collapse, coma, sometimes convulsions	Induce vomiting or use gastric lavage if it can be done promptly; mild soap solution will serve as antidote for unabsorbed portions Give cathartic

*Nelson, Waldo E.: Mitchell-Nelson Textbook of Pediatrics, Philadelphia, 1959, W. B. Saunders Company, p. 1391.

Universal antidote

This old and widely advocated antidote consists of 1 part of tannic acid, 1 part of magnesium oxide, and 2 parts of activated medicinal charcoal. The magnesium oxide neutralizes acid without forming gas, the tannic acid brings about the formation of insoluble salts (of alkaloids and metals), while the charcoal is an excellent adsorbent of a variety of substances. The recommended dosage is ½ ounce or 4 to 5 heaping teaspoons. The preparation is light and fluffy and must be stirred into a glass of water so as to form a thin paste before it is swallowed. It can be swallowed quickly following the ingestion of certain poisons but should be removed by emesis or lavage before the stomach content has time to pass into the intestine.

Dimercaprol, U.S.P. (BAL)

Dimercaprol was developed in the course of World War II as an antidote for the arsenic-containing blister gas, Lewisite; hence the name "BAL" for "British Anti-Lewisite." It was used to decontaminate the skin and eyes of persons who had been in contact with the gas, but later it

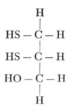

was found to be of value in treatment of various forms of arsenic poisoning.

Dimercaprol is a colorless liquid with a rather offensive odor. It is dispensed in 10 per cent solution in peanut oil for intramuscular injection. One milliliter contains 100 mg.

Arsenic compounds produce their toxic effects by combining with the sulfhydryl groups of enzymes which are necessary for normal metabolism. As a result, the processes of oxidation and reduction in the tissues are seriously hindered. BAL interferes with this combination, forms a stable combination with the arsenic, and hastens its excretion from the body.

BAL is also indicated in the treatment of gold and mercury poisoning. Treatment should begin as soon as possible after poisoning has occurred.

Results in the treatment of other heavy metal poisoning are disappointing or inconclusive.* Although the toxicitiy of BAL is less among patients suffering from arsenic, gold, or mercury poisoning than among persons in normal condition, doses of 300 mg. may cause the following symptoms: nausea and vomiting, headache, a burning sensation of the mouth, throat, and eyes, a constricting sensation in the chest, and muscular aching and tingling in the extremities.

In the treatment of arsenic or gold poisoning, the dose is 2.5 to 3 mg. of dimercaprol per kilogram of body weight, given intramuscularly every 4 hours the first two days, reduced to 4 injections and 2 injections on the third and fourth days, and then daily until recovery takes place. In mild cases the dose may be reduced. In mercury poisoning the dosage is sometimes increased.

Promotion of elimination

Promotion of elimination may be accomplished by the use of certain cathartics, such as saline cathartics, or castor oil, or by rectal irrigation. After gastric lavage, 1 ounce of 50 per cent magnesium sulfate sometimes is left in the stomach and plenty of water then is given. Magnesium sulfate helps to cleanse the lower part of the bowel. In case of anuria, the use of an artificial kidney may tide the patient over a serious crisis.

*N.N.R., 1960, p. 438.

Supportive care of the patient

In an effort to find the right antidote for a poison, the most important aspect of care of the patient may be overlooked. Sometimes the greatest need of the patient is met by giving artificial respiration. Shock is an important factor to be considered. Intravenous administration of physiologic saline or glucose solution is important for the maintenance of adequate circulation and for the replacement of fluid which may be lost due to diarrhea from gastrointestinal irritation. Attention to fluid needs may also help to conserve kidney and liver function, particularly in the presence of certain poisons. Sometimes depressant drugs are indicated, sometimes stimulants. Often attention must be given to keeping the patient warm and, if stuporous or comatose, to see that his position is changed periodically to prevent development of hypostatic pneumonia.

Under some circumstances the nurse must help friends and relatives of the patient to understand that his strength will be unnecessarily depleted by too many individuals fussing over him. On the other hand, one or two cooperative members of the family may be able to help a great deal.

Poisonous foods

Many foods, because of their content of inherently poisonous chemicals (mushrooms and other fungi) or the presence of bacterial exotoxins, produce symptoms of poisoning when eaten. The symptoms are diverse but intense gastrointestinal irritation is common to all of them, and they may therefore be appropriately classed as irritants. Mushroom poisoning arises through mistaking various fungi, such as poisonous mushrooms, toadstools, and truffles, for edible varieties. The toxin of many of these plants is muscarine, a deadly alkaloidal poison, which causes violent vomiting, colic, thirst, dyspnea, paralysis, and death. Many of the cases of food poisoning seen especially in the warm season of the year are due to soluble exotoxins which result from bacterial contamination of the food. Foods that seem prone to cause symptoms of poisoning, are corned beef, sausage, pickled or decaying fish, shellfish, ham, home-canned vegetables, salads, whipped cream, and custards. Poisoning is more likely to occur, especially from salads, whipped cream, and custards, when large amounts are made at one time and are improperly prepared and refrigerated. The treatment of food poisoning, from whatever cause, is prompt evacuation of the stomach, preferably by stomach tube. In the process of this evacuation plenty of water is used and tannic acid or strong tea is administered; a large dose of magnesium sulfate or castor oil is given to empty the bowel and prevent absorption therefrom. Morphine may be given for the abdominal pain, and stimulants may be indicated if there is prostration.

Questions

for review and study

Single choice

Encircle the answer of your choice.

1 Which of the following conditions would lead you to suspect acute poisoning?
a. gradual loss of weight
b. anorexia, undue lassitude
c. onset of sudden violent symptoms
d. weakness, anemia, headache

2 Which of the following factors is likely to be the crucial one in the successful treatment of early and acute poisoning?
a. amount of supportive treatment
b. immediate removal of poison from the body
c. control of shock
d. administration of the right antidote

3 Which of the following kinds of antidotes are represented when sodium chloride solution is used in the treatment of silver nitrate poisoning?
a. chemical
b. physical
c. universal
d. physiologic

4 If you were working in the chemistry laboratory of the school of nursing and splashed some hydrochloric acid in your eye, what is the *first* thing you would do?
a. rush to the emergency room
b. search for a weak base and instill some in your eye.
c. neutralize the acid with solution of sodium hydroxide
d. wash eye with copious amounts of plain water

5 BAL (British Anti-Lewisite) is a recommended antidote for poisoning due to:
a. hydrocarbons
b. strong acids
c. phenolic compounds
d. certain heavy metals

6 Death from carbon monoxide is likely to be due to:
a. changes in bone marrow
b. damage to liver and kidney
c. depression of heart
d. anoxia

7 Death from a poison like methyl alcohol is likely to be due to:
a. destruction in the kidney
b. perforation, hemorrhage, or both
c. acidosis
d. depression of the respiratory center

8 Which of the following kinds of foods are *least* likely to be a source of bacterial contamination and food poisoning?
a. lobster salad
b. boiled dinner of cabbage, meat, and potatoes
c. chicken salad, Boston cream pie
d. ham sandwiches, iced tea

9 Which of the following statements best explains why children are often poisoned by medicines left around the house?
a. children are naturally curious about things
b. children mistake sweet-tasting tablets or pills for candy
c. children like to explore new things with their mouths
d. children like to imitate other members of the household

10 Which of the following would you do if present at the scene of a poisoning and the patient had been vomiting?
a. note odor and color of the vomitus before flushing down the toilet
b. save a specimen of vomitus and add a preservative if possible
c. save a specimen of vomitus (an early one if possible) for the doctor
d. discard emesis as fast as possible to avoid offense to the patient

References

A. M. A. Council on Drugs: New and Non-official Drugs, Philadelphia, 1960, J. B. Lippincott Co.

Adams, E.: Poisons, Scient. Am. **201**: 76, Nov., 1959.

Beckman, Harry: Pharmacology in Clinical Practice, Philadelphia, 1952, W. B. Saunders Co.

Brookes, V. J., and Jacobs, M. B.: Poisons, Properties, Chemical Identification, Symptoms, and Emergency Treatment, New York, 1958, D. Van Nostrand Co., Inc.

Gleason, M. N., Gosselin, R. E., and Hodge, H. C.: Clinical Toxicology of Commercial Products, Baltimore, 1957, Williams & Wilkins Co.

Keehn, Robert J.: Home Accidents Resulting From Gas, Am. J. Nursing **55**: 720-721, 1955.

Lawson, W. R., and Gemsch, R. D.: The Minnesota Poison Information Center Network, Minnesota Med. **41**: 767, 1958.

Lucas, G. H. W.: The Symptoms and Treatment of Acute Poisoning, New York, 1953, The Macmillan Co.

Nelson, Waldo E.: Textbook of Pediatrics, Philadelphia, 1959, W. B. Saunders Co.

Press, E.: Poison Control Centers, Nursing Outlook 5: 29, 1957.

Price, E. C.: A Remote Village, a Neighborhood Nurse, and an Antidotes Chart, Am. J. Nursing 59: 688, 1959.

Salter, William T.: A Textbook of Pharmacology, Philadelphia, 1952, W. B. Saunders Co.

Sollmann, Torald: A Manual of Pharmacology, Philadelphia, 1957, W. B. Saunders Co.

Tonyan, A.: The Nurse's Part in Poison Control, Am. J. Nursing 58: 96, 1958.

Chapter 29

History of materia medica

The story of materia medica is as old as the story of man, for sickness has been man's heritage from the beginning of time and the search for ways and means to combat disease has been one of his earliest and most persistent activities. Early man's first experiments in dealing with disease were suggested by the belief common to all primitive people that the world in which they live teems with invisible spirits, some of whom are good and some bad. Whatever puzzled them in nature was attributed to these supernatural agencies, and it followed that disease was at first thought to be an evil spirit or the work of such a spirit. If this supposition were true, the logical treatment was to placate the invader by burnt offerings or to frighten it away by resorting to hideous noises or by administering foul-tasting substances, these measures being designed to make the body an uncomfortable habitat for the spirit. The search for obnoxious materials led man to experiment with herbs of the field and the forest, and as the knowledge gained from experience increased, the rudiments of materia medica were assembled. These intuitive efforts of man led to some valuable discoveries. Savages in separated countries know the properties of the most fatal arrow poisons, such as curare, veratrine, and ouabain, as well as the virtues of drugs like opium, hashish hemp, and tobacco. Centuries ago the Indians of Peru discovered the value of cinchona bark for the treatment and prevention of malaria, and the natives of Brazil knew the worth of ipecac for amebic dysentery. The victims of leprosy in the Far East believed that they received relief by rubbing their wounds with chaulmoogra oil, and for some time chaulmoogra oil was used in the treatment of leprosy. The Indians of our own country used arbutus for rheumatism; lobelia for coughs and colds; wild sage tea, goldenseal, and flowering dogwood for fevers; elders, wild cherry, and sumac for colds and quinsies; inhalations of pennyroyal for headache; sassafras leaves for wounds and felons, and the roots of sassafras for cooling and purifying the blood.

As the medical lore accumulated, there appeared individuals who demonstrated a special talent for herb-doctoring, bone-setting, and rude surgery and who employed it as a means of earning a livelihood. They were either the wisewomen who sought by their art to lessen the hardships and dangers of childbirth, or certain men of superior intelligence and cunning, who, appreciating the credulity of the rank and file, made use of incantations and charms in their therapeutics and established themselves in the community in the role of priest and physician. These nature healers soon perceived not only what substances are good and what are harmful but that a number of poisons are also remedies under certain conditions. This drug and poison lore was the beginning of materia medica and medicine.

Ancient period

Egypt

The oldest phase of medicine is the Egyptian. The main sources of data are the medical papyri, the most important of which is the Ebers papyrus, written in the sixteenth century B.C. It is a scroll twenty-two yards long and about twelve inches wide and contains a collection of prescriptions and formulas covering a wide range of uses. Included among them are many invocations and conjuring forms for driving away disease, as well as specific recipes, calling in many instances for drugs which are in common use today, e.g., aloes, castor oil, figs, vinegar, turpentine, opium, wormwood, peppermint, and squill.

Among the mineral and metal substances were iron, copper sulfate, magnesia, niter, sodium carbonate, and salt, and precious stones ground into powder.

The animal preparations included such substances as lizards' blood, swine's teeth, putrid meat, stinking fat, milk, goose grease, asses' hoofs, animal fats, excreta of various animals and flies (a soothing syrup for babies was made of the latter), and such ingredients as the thigh bone of a hanged man or the moss grown on a human skull.

The prescriptions called for purges, headache remedies, tonics, hair restorers, and remedies for hookworm, tapeworm, and intestinal worms, to be put up in the form of pills, powders, infusions, decoctions, gargles, salves, plasters, poultices and confections. Over 700 drugs are mentioned and one prescription required 35 ingredients.

As the inclusion of invocations and charms in the prescriptions would imply, medicine was closely allied with religion, as it was to remain for many centuries. The doctors were all priests paid out of the royal treasury, but they were allowed to take fees also.

Greece

The pharmaceutic history of Greece begins with legends regarding gods and goddesses. The reputed activities of these mythical characters are so inextricably woven with the authentic doings of real men and women that it is often hard to determine where legend ends and history begins. The story goes, however, that Chiron, the centaur, originated the pharmaceutic art and imparted his valuable knowledge to Aesculapius, son of Apollo. Aesculapius, with the aid of his daughters Hygeia and Panacea, in turn taught mortals the art of healing, but he became so successful in combating disease that he incurred the wrath of Pluto, god of the underworld, because he was diminishing too greatly the number of shades received in Hades. Pluto prevailed upon almighty Zeus to destroy Aesculapius with a thunderbolt, but upon the intercession of Apollo, Zeus deified him as the god of healing. His mortal followers in time made up the organized guild of physicians called Aesclepiades. They built temples in his honor in which they practiced their art and increased their knowledge of healing. These temples were situated in hills or mountains, usually near mineral springs, and were managed by trained priests. Hence they were virtually sanatoriums or hospitals for the sick. The patient was received by the physician priests and, after spiritual purification by prayers and sacrifice, was further cleansed by a bath from the mineral springs, catharsis, massage, and inunction, and encouraged with medicated wines and soft music to sleep and to dream. The priest then interpreted the dream as a message from Morpheus, and offered medical advice accordingly. If the treatment was a success and the patient recovered, a votive tablet giving the history of the case and the treatment was hung in the temple where anyone who wished might consult it. In this way, a considerable body of empirical knowledge was assembled and these Temples of Health took on some of the characteristics of a medical school. The most celebrated ones were at Cnidus and Cos.

The most famous representative of the Aesclepiades was Hippocrates, who was born in the Island of Cos 460 B.C., of a long line of priest physicians, and was reputed by popular tradition to be the seventeenth in direct descent from Aesculapius. Hippocrates pursued his early studies at Cos and Cnidus but later came under the influence of the great thinkers and philosophers of the period and soon began to give to medicine their scientific and ethical ideas. He denounced the belief in the supernatural origin of disease and the use of charms, incantations, and other superstitious devices of priestcraft and substituted the doctrine that disease was due to natural causes and that knowledge of it would be gained only through the study of the natural laws. He taught the use of the senses in collecting data for diagnosis, and the use of inductive reasoning in arriving at diagnostic conclusions.

His therapeutic measures were decidedly modern. He believed that the body has great power to recuperate and that the role of the physician should be simply to aid Nature in her work. His treatment consisted usually of fresh air, good food, purgation, bloodletting, massage, and hydrotherapy. Although he mentioned over 400 drugs in his writings, he used only a few of the important ones, among them opium. His preparations included foments, poultices, gargles, suppositories, pills, lozenges, ointments, cerates, and inhalations.

Hippocrates is called the Father of Medicine because his influence has extended through the ensuing ages and his teachings established the sound principles which control the practice of medicine to the present day.

Another early Greek physician was Dioscorides, who was an authority on materia medica. He described 600 plants and plant principles of which no less than 74 are in use today. His work was the chief source of pharmaceutic knowledge of antiquity.

Rome

After the Roman conquest of Greece, Greek medicine migrated to Rome. The most famous Greek physician of this period was Galen (A.D. 131-201). He based his teachings and practice largely upon the work of Hippocrates and established a system of medicine and pharmacy which made him the supreme authority for several hundred years. He originated many preparations of vegetable drugs, which even now are spoken of as galenicals, and was the first to prepare rosewater ointment or cold cream.

Medieval period (A.D. 400 to 1500)

Early period—the Dark Ages—A.D. 400-1100

The term Middle Ages is given to that period of European history that lies between what are known as ancient and modern times, extending from about the middle of the fifth to the middle of the fifteenth century. The historical event that marked the close of ancient times was the decline and fall of the Roman Empire. This process extended over three or four centuries, during which period successive hordes of Germanic barbarians poured in from the north and east and overran Western Europe. They succeeded gradually in wresting the territory piecemeal from the Romans and in setting up their own tribal organizations. This process of dismemberment of the Roman Empire was completed in the fifth century and was followed by a period of about six hundred years known as the Dark Ages, because during this time the old civilization was largely destroyed and there was little progress in learning. The German tribes were slowly learning to combine their primitive institutions with those of Rome and were assimilating the first rudiments of culture through their contact with the Latins. Wars between the tribes were frequent and served to stifle all effort along constructive lines. Their medicine was folklore and tradition, the employment of wonder-cures and temple sleeps similar to those of the Greeks before the advent of Hippocrates.

Another important movement at the same time was the spread of Christianity. After three centuries of struggle and persecution, the Christian church triumphed in 311 through a decree of the emperor which made it the official church of Rome. Thereupon, religious orders arose whose members scattered throughout Europe preaching the new doctrine and building monasteries, where they could withdraw from the world and devote their lives to the work of the Church. The monasteries, particularly those of the Benedictines, soon became the repositories of all the learning of the period. The Venerable Bede was a Benedictine. The monks collected all available manuscripts and copied and preserved them. Among other things, they preserved the works on pharmacy and medicine. Since it was part of their religious duty to give aid to the sick and needy, they controlled most of the practice of medicine and disseminated much knowledge of healing. Their treatment was usually good food, quiet, rest, and the administration of decoctions of simples from their gardens. Monastery gardens were an important factor in the development of herbals or books of plant lore, the oldest of which dates 500 years before the invention of printing. Mistletoe was a great panacea. Lycopodium, clover, primrose, henbane, and verbena were common remedies, also wormwood, belladonna, hellebore, and mandragora.

During this period, we have the first record of the use of some of the remedies used in modern practice. In the sixth century, Alexander of Tralles used colchicum for gout, iron for anemia, cantharides as a blister, and rhubarb for dysentery and liver complaints.

Arabian influence

In the eighth century the Arabs spread over the Holy Land, Egypt, North Africa, and Spain and began a supremacy that lasted over 500 years. They were especially interested in medicine, pharmacy, and chemistry, and built hospitals and schools for the pursuit of their study. They carried forward the knowledge obtained from Greece and Rome and preserved the pharmaceutic art from the sixth to the sixteenth centuries. Their medicine was a composite blend of the practice of the Greeks and

758

Jews and of the astrology and occult lore of Egypt and India. The teachings of Hippocrates and Galen, which had been translated into Arabic in the seventh century, furnished much of their material.

The Arabians contributed many new drugs. We are indebted to them for use of senna, camphor, rhubarb, musk, myrrh, cassia, tamarind, nutmeg, cloves, cubeb, aconite, ambergris, cannabis, and sandalwood. They were the originators of syrups, juleps, alcohol, and aromatic water. They introduced into Europe the decimal notation, acquired by them from a now forgotten race in India.

The first great Mohammedan author was Geber, who wrote exclusively on chemistry. He is the reputed discoverer of sulfuric acid, nitric acid, nitrohydrochloric acid, corrosive sublimate, and lunar caustic.

Avicenna was an accomplished physician of the tenth century. He wrote the *Canon*, a miscellaneous collection of past medical lore with his interpretations. His works were considered authoritative in universities as late as 1650.

During this period, pharmacy was practiced somewhat as a profession separate from medicine. The first apothecary shops were established and the first pharmaceutic formulary or set of drug standards was produced. This served as a model for the first London pharmacopoeia. The Arabian pharmacists were called sandalini, and their stocks were regularly inspected and punishment was meted out to those found guilty of selling spurious or deteriorated drugs.

Rise of universities. The word university means an association, and the principal universities of Europe had their origin in the voluntary association of guilds of students banded together for mutual protection and established at some place favorable to the pursuit of their studies. Salerno, which was founded in the eighth century, was the first of the educational institutions of the university type. Others founded later were the University of Paris, 1110; Bologna, 1113; Oxford, 1167; Cambridge, 1209; Padua, 1222; and Naples, 1224. They exerted a great influence upon the development of all science, and especially of medicine and pharmacy. Pharmacy was taught in all as part of the medical course. One of the most eminent pharmaceutic authorities of this period was Nicholas of Salerno, Director of the Medical School. He wrote the *Antidotarium* which was the standard for pharmaceutic preparations for centuries. It contained the basic units of the present apothecaries' system, the grain, scruple, and dram, just as they are used today. At Salerno, the study of anatomy was resumed under a decree which permitted the dissection of a human body every five years. Didactic instruction here was based upon Hippocrates, Galen, Avicenna, and the Antidotary of Nicholas Praepositus. A famous woman physician, Trotula of Salerno, first used mercury in the treatment of syphilis.

Late medieval period

In 1095 occurred the first of the Crusades, which extended over a period of nearly 200 years, and exerted a profound influence on pharmacy, by bringing about a fusion of Arabian science and learning with the primitive practices based upon folklore and tradition in Central and Northwest Europe. Records of the customhouse of the port of Acri in Italy in the early thirteenth century show large traffic in the various spices, opium, and rhubarb. Venetians brought the first sugar to Europe during the time of the Crusades. It was costly and was used exclusively as medicine, as were most of the spices.

The fourteenth and fifteenth centuries witnessed a great awakening of interest in medicine and pharmacy throughout Europe. The Moors of Spain, who had a great reputation for knowledge and skill in these branches of science, and who had been driven out of Granada by Ferdinand in 1492, scattered over Europe, practicing and teaching. Moreover, during this period, epidemic diseases were very prevalent, especially leprosy, ergotism, and the Black Death. The Black Death (bubonic plague) swept away 25 per cent of the human race or 60 million people during this period. Pharmacies as separate places for compounding and dispensing medicines spread through Europe with great rapidity during the thirteenth century.

In the fifteenth century *alchemy*, brought in by the Arabs, swept over Europe like a conflagration. Alchemy was the search for means of transmuting base metals into gold. The mere desire to discover such a substance gave rise to a universal belief that one existed, and the "philosopher's stone," as this elusive substance came to be known, was as much a reality to the alchemist as the actual substances with which he worked. Gradually belief spread that the philosopher's stone could not only transmute all metals into gold but could also cure all diseases, restore youth, and indefinitely prolong life. It thus became also the Elixir of Life. While the alchemists were carrying on the search for the stone, they made important inventions and discoveries which laid the foundations of the modern science of chemistry. In 1438 printing was invented and the world was flooded with books. One of the earliest printed works extant contains an illustration of a fifteenth-century pharmacy.

Sixteenth century

In the sixteenth century, pharmacy came into its own. Drugs were rare and costly, prescriptions were complex, and special art was required in preparing and keeping the drugs. Formularies appeared in such numbers that a need was felt for an authoritative standard. This was furnished by Valerius Cordus, son of a professor of medicine at Marburg. Cordus collected formulas during twelve years of teaching at Wittenberg and compiled these in manuscript form. The physicians of Nuremberg wished a copy for the local druggists and secured the consent of the senate in 1546 to have it printed. This work of Cordus was the first pharmacopeia to be printed and authorized for use in a community for the sake of uniformity. It drew its material from Greek, Roman, and Arabian sources and quoted freely from Galen, Dioscorides, Avicenna, and Nicholas Praepositus. It contained comparatively few types of preparations, namely, aromatics, opiates, confections, conserves, purges, pills, syrups, plasters, cerates, troches, salves, and oils. Editions were published in Paris, Lyons, Venice, and Antwerp. It held its place till 1666 and was revised five times meanwhile.

The outstanding figure of the sixteenth century was Paracelsus, the son of a German physician and chemist. At the age of sixteen, he began the study of medicine at the University of Basle but soon gave it up to experiment with chemistry and alchemy. He traveled widely, gathering a vast amount of knowledge, especially of folk medicine, from barbers, gypsies, and others with whom he associated. He served some time as a military surgeon in the Low countries and worked in mines in the Tyrol. Here he investigated processes of preparing metals and made experiments as to their medicinal virtues. His cures gained wide publicity and he was called upon to prescribe for many of the great men of his day. In 1526 he was appointed professor of physics and surgery at Basle. Here he inaugurated his career as a teacher by publicly burning the works of Galen and denouncing the Arabian masters whose doctrines were then generally followed. He also flouted tradition by lecturing in German instead of Latin. His defiance of tradition and his arrogant manner aroused the enmity of the other members of the faculty, and he was compelled to leave the university in 1528. He resumed his wanderings. At Salzburg, he gave offense to a prominent physician and was thrown from a window by the man's servants, dying from the fall.

In spite of his objectionable methods, Paracelsus exerted a profound influence upon the medical beliefs of his time and of succeeding centuries. He attacked the weak points of the prevailing system of medicine; he destroyed the "humoral pathology," which taught that diseases were due to an excess or deficiency of the "humors," bile, phlegm, or blood, and substituted the doctrine that diseases were actual entities to be combated with specific remedies. He improved pharmacy and therapeutics, introduced some new remedies such as calomel and sulfur, made some new chemical compounds, and strove to reduce the overdosing then practiced.

Seventeenth century

In 1618 the first London Pharmacopoeia appeared. It was chiefly a compilation of older authorities. It was sponsored by the London College of Physicians and its use was made obligatory throughout the British realm by a decree of King James. It was very large compared with the modern pharmacopeia, containing 1,028 simple drugs and 932 preparations and compounds. The most complex preparation contained 130 ingredients. One substance listed was usnea. This was moss from the skull of a man who died a violent death. It was not hard to obtain in England in those days because the bodies of criminals who had been executed were suspended in chains in public places as a warning to other criminals, and the exposure was conducive to growth of moss on the skull.

Great interest was displayed in chemistry and pharmacy in this century, and many preparations originated then which are still in use. Among them were the infusion of senna or black draught, the alcoholic tincture of opium or laudanum, the compound tincture of benzoin, the balsams of Peru and Tolu, guaiacum, sarsaparilla, and jalap. In 1638 cinchoma was imported by the Countess of Cinchoma, wife of the Viceroy of Peru, who had been cured of a severe intermittent fever by its use. Coca was likewise introduced from Peru, and ipecac found its way into Europe and was used with such skill by a certain quack named Helvetius that Louis XIV paid him $4,000 for his secret.

Eighteenth century

The eighteenth century likewise witnessed great progress in pharmacy. A German practitioner by the name of Hoffmann originated the elixir of orange and Hoffmann's anodyne. A Berlin apothecary identified magnesia, the alums, the potassa and soda and discovered beet sugar. A French pharmacist published an essay entitled "The Superstitions Concerning the Philosopher's Stone" and thereby helped divert alchemy into more profitable channels. In 1775 Louis XVI paid nearly $5,000 to a certain Madame Nouffer for a celebrated cure for tapeworm. She inherited the secret from her husband, a Swiss physician. The drug proved to be male fern, commonly known since Galen.

Inoculation against smallpox was introduced in the latter part of the eighteenth century by Edward Jenner, an English physician. He had been studying for years on the subject of smallpox, swinepox, and cowpox and the development of the two latter diseases when communicated to man and had noticed that milkmaids who were frequently infected with cowpox were immune to smallpox. He finally inoculated his own son with swinepox and ascertained that the child was proof against smallpox. He made his first public inoculation with vaccine on May 14,

1796, and within a year had won the confidence of the physicians in his theory of immunization.

In 1785 the infusion of digitalis was introduced by William Withering of England for the treatment of heart disease. The foxglove is carved on Withering's monument.

Dover's powder had its origin about this time. Thomas Dover administered the drug in doses of 60 grains and claimed to have given 100 grains. This was equivalent to 10 grains of opium and 10 grains of ipecac. The pharmacists in filling his prescriptions usually advised patients first to make their wills.

A great number of important pharmacopeias and works of reference appeared during the century. One of particular interest was the dispensatory of the London hospitals, St. Thomas', Guy's and St. Bartholomew's, 1741. It listed viper's flesh as an ingredient of one preparation and wood lice of several. Dried horses' hoofs were used to check the spitting of blood. The motto of the book was, "Prepare to die, for behold, Death and Judgment is at hand."

Nineteenth century

During this century, chemistry gradually takes its place as a highly specialized science, with pharmaceutic chemistry as an important subdivision. The first great pharmaceutic discovery was that of the alkaloid morphine obtained from opium by a German apothecary, Serturner, in 1815. This was the first active principle to be isolated and led to enthusiastic research on many vegetable drugs. The result was the discovery of quinine, strychnine, and veratrine by Pelletier and Caventou; of emetine by Pelletier and Majendie; of atropine by Brandes, and of codeine by Robiquet. All of these men were pharmacists. Their discoveries made it possible to administer drugs in a form which was attractive and palatable and which made possible the accurate study of dosage.

In 1842 Dr. Crawford W. Long of Georgia first used ether as a general anesthetic, and in 1847 Sir J. T. Simpson used chloroform for the same purpose.

About 1856 appeared the first of the numerous coal-tar products. Perkin, in a vain attempt to produce synthetic quinine, discovered instead the first coal-tar dye, called after him "Perkin's purple" or mauve. This led to the preparation in the laboratory of a great family of remedial agents, some of which, such as salicylic and benzoic acids, duplicated products previously obtained from natural sources, and others of which were new to science, for example, acetanilid and antipyrine.

The discovery of so many new drugs and the invention of new and convenient dosage forms led to the establishment of large-scale manufacturing plants which took over much of the work formerly done by the pharmacist with his mortar and pestle.

This century witnessed also the initial appearance of the important national pharmacopeias. The French Codex was first to be produced. It was issued in 1818 and contained one remarkable item, a formula for an extract of opium in which the preparation was to be boiled incessantly for six months and the water lost by evaporation to be constantly replaced. The first pharmacopeia for the United States appeared in 1820, the national standard for Great Britain in 1864 to replace those of London, Edinburgh, and Dublin, and that for Germany in 1872, superseding nearly a score of local volumes.

Fewer drugs were prescribed, and such prescriptions as were given were accompanied with greater knowledge of their expected action. In other words, rational medicine began to replace empiricism. During this period purging and bloodletting became less popular and definite action toward exposing harmful patent medicines and nostrums was taken.

More recent progress

Great progress has been made in pharmacy and medicine since this century began. In pharmacy, growth has been chiefly along the lines of strengthening and improving the work of the professional organizations such as the American Pharmaceutical Association and the National Association of Retail Druggists, and with the promotion of legislation controlling the manufacture and sale of drugs. The most important acts were the Food and Drug Acts of 1906 and 1938 and the Harrison Anti-Narcotic Act of 1914.

It is said that more progress has probably been made during the past 50 years than in all the years prior to that time. As far as therapeutics is concerned this is largely due to changes in the concept of the cause of disease. When it was believed that evil spirits caused disease, the treatment given was highly varied and used in the hope that one of the measures resorted to would be the right one. Since the acceptance of the germ theory there has been a rapid advancement in scientific method of research. Such method has been greatly aided by animal experimentation, appropriation of money for research work, efforts of public health organizations to educate the public and to collect valuable vital statistics.

Of interest to both pharmacy and medicine are the many biologic preparations such as the vaccines, antitoxins, and serums now in common use and the valuable group of anesthetics which is constantly growing, through the isolation and duplication in the laboratory of more and more of the potent vegetable substances found in nature. The introduction into medicine by the German physician Ehrlich in 1907 of salvarsan, the great specific for syphilis, and the discovery by Banting in 1922 of insulin for the treatment of diabetes constitute two of the epoch-making events of the century.

With the increased knowledge of drugs has grown an increasing awareness of implications in their misuse and overuse. Among other trends in modern medicine is the use of other therapeutic agencies either to supplement drug therapy or to replace it. Such therapies would include vitamin therapy, diet therapy, and various kinds of physical therapy.

To discover chemotherapeutic agents which will be effective in every infectious disease is one of the goals of research workers in medicine. However, for years there were only a few chemicals which acted as specifics. Among the most important were quinine for malaria and the arsenicals for syphilis. In the last few years several remarkable chemotherapeutic agents have changed chemical therapy tremendously. Infections which a few years ago took a tremendous toll in sickness and deaths are now well controlled by the sulfonamides, penicillin, and other antibiotics. In 1908 sulfanilamide was first prepared by Gelmo, a German organic chemist, who was investigating azo dyes. It was not until 1932, however, that its possible therapeutic value was realized. In 1932 prontosil was patented in Germany by Klorer and Mietzsch. A German worker, Domagk, is credited with the discovery of the therapeutic value of prontosil. In 1932 Domagk observed that mice with streptococcic septicemia could be protected by prontosil. It was later shown that prontosil breaks down into para-amino benzene sulfonamide, which is the effective substance. In the next few years more and more interest was aroused in these drugs, and today they have a rightful place as some of our most important drugs. Para-amino benzene sulfonamide was accepted by the Council on Pharmacy and Chemistry of the American Medical Association for inclusion in N.N.R. in 1937, at which time the name of sulfanilamide was suggested for it. Since then many new sulfonamide derivatives have been tried, and a few of them have become well established in drug therapy.

The story of the recent development of antibacterial agents of biologic origin or antibiotics is one of the most interesting new developments in pharmacy. In 1929 Dr. Alexander Fleming at the University of London noted that a mold which contaminated a plate of staphylococci produced a zone of inhibition around it in which the staphylococci did not grow. Fleming found that the mold, *Penicillium notatum*, secreted into its medium an antibiotic agent, which he named penicillin. He found it was not toxic to animals, did not hurt white blood cells, and that it inhibited the growth of certain gram-positive pathogens. He used broth containing penicillin clinically on several cases of skin infections with favorable results. However, little was done clinically about it for the next 10 years.

In 1939 Rene J. Dubos of the Rockefeller Institute for Medical Research published the results of experiments done on certain bacteria found in the soil. Dubos acted on the assumption that all organic matter added to the soil would eventually undergo decomposition by microorganisms. Samples of soil were incubated for a few weeks to bring about decomposition of most of the organic matter present. Then cultures of staphylococci, Group A hemolytic streptococci, and pneumococci were added to the soil at intervals.

After two years, a gram-positive, spore-bearing aerobic bacillus capable of lyzing the living cells of many gram-positive bacteria was isolated from the soil. The soil bacillus, called *Bacillus brevis*, produced a substance destructive to certain gram-positive bacteria. The destructive substance could be extracted from the bacteria. It was named tyrothricin and was later shown to be composed of two substances, gramicidin and tyrocidine. Gramicidin is much more effective than tyrocidine therapeutically. Unfortunately, gramicidin is hemolytic and so must be used only for local infections, never where it can get in contact with the blood.

Our story now turns back to penicillin. In 1938 Dr. Howard Florey at Oxford University began to study penicillin and other naturally occurring antibacterial agents. Dr. Florey and his associates are responsible for the isolation of penicillin, its assay and dosage, and for proof of its usefulness clinically. The first patient was treated with penicillin early in 1941. Because of World War II it was impossible to start large-scale production in England. Dr. Florey came to the United States in 1941 and asked for the help of the National Research Council in studying penicillin. Production was soon started in the United States, and the first patient in this country was treated with penicillin in March, 1942. Since that time a number of new antibiotics, streptomycin, dihydrostreptomycin, chloramphenicol, chlortetracycline, oxytetracycline, tetracycline, and many others have been added to the physician's armamentarium.

It should be noted that obtaining antibacterial agents from natural sources is not a new procedure. There are many such substances throughout the plant and animal kingdoms. Quinine, which is produced by a plant, has been used for many years. One of the most important factors in discovering chemotherapeutic agents is that they give to research workers important clues for the understanding of chemotherapeutic agents. When the action of a chemotherapeutic agent is understood, whether it be of chemical origin (as are the sulfonamides) or biologic origin (as is penicillin), the making of new chemotherapeutic agents and the proper use of those already known will be best accomplished.

In 1935 a series of events occurred which were to have far-reaching significance. Dr. E. C. Kendall and associates, of the Mayo Foundation,

Dr. Wintersteiner and Dr. Pfiffner, of Columbia University, and Prof. Reichstein, of Switzerland, independently isolated a group of crystalline substances from the cortex of the adrenal gland. Continued effort resulted in the discovery of the chemical structure of these compounds. Among these new products was one which proved to be 17-hydroxy-11-dehydrocorticosterone. The name of this compound was shortened to cortisone. It was first used in medicine in 1948. It appears to have opened a new era in medical science. More recently (1950) hydrocortisone and (1954) aldosterone have been isolated and identified.

In 1955 the announcement of a new poliomyelitis vaccine focuses the attention of the world upon another achievement which gives promise of bringing great benefit to mankind.

An overwhelming number of drugs have been synthesized. Many new preparations are being made available, e.g., new antineoplastic drugs, hormonal agents, and anti-infectives, to mention a few. Scientists are challenged to formulate laws and theories of how drugs act. In this area there is much that is unknown.

References

Dubos, R. J.: Studies on a Bactericidal Agent Extracted From a Soil Bacillus, J. Exper. Med. 70: 1, 1939.

Dubos, R. J.: Antimicrobial Agents of Biologic Origin, J. A. M. A. 124: 633, 1944.

Editorial: The History of Penicillin, J. A. M. A. 126: 170, 1944.

Sellew, G., and Ebel, M. E.: A History of Nursing, St. Louis, 1955, The C. V. Mosby Co.

Silverman, Milton: Magic in a Bottle, New York, 1948, The Macmillan Co.

Sokoloff, Boris: The Miracle Drugs, Chicago, 1949, Ziff-Davis Publishing Co.

Woodham-Smith, Cecil: Florence Nightingale, New York, 1951, McGraw-Hill Book Co., Inc.

Glossary

absorbent a medicine or substance that absorbs liquids or other secretion products; a substance that takes in or sucks up, e.g., a blotter absorbs ink.

acapnia a condition of diminished CO_2 in the blood, with decreased respiration.

acidosis condition of decreased alkalinity in the body, caused by excess formation of acid or by depletion of base.

acromegaly a disease of man, manifested by giantism, due to a tumor of the pituitary gland with increased secretion therefrom.

actinomyces moldlike, parasitic fungi.

adrenergic sympathomimetic

adsorbent a substance that gathers up another substance on its surface in a condensed layer.

aerosol a medicine mixed with air for inhalation or insufflation.

ampule a small glass vial.

analeptic a drug that produces wakefulness; arouses from unconsciousness.

analgesic a medicine that is used to relieve pain—acetanilid, acetylsalicylic acid, acetophenetidin, antipyrine, colchicum (gout and rheumatism), opium.

anaphylactic pertaining to the increased susceptibility to a foreign protein following subsequent absorption of the same protein.

androgen a male sex hormone.

anemia deficiency of the hemoglobin of the blood.

anesthetic (general) a medicine that produces total loss of consciousness and insensibility to pain—alcohol, ether, chloroform, nitrogen monoxide, ethylene; loss of sensation.

anesthetic (local) a medicine that diminishes the sensibility of the part to which it is applied—camphor, cocaine, ethyl, chloride, procaine, phenol, metycaine.

anhidrotic a medicine that decreases the amount of perspiration—belladonna, hyoscyamus, stramonium, atropine.

anorexia loss or lack of appetite.

anoxemia deficiency of oxygen in the blood.

anthelmintic drug used in the treatment of worms.

antibiotic against life; but restricted in use to antibacterial agents of microbial origin.

anticholinergic opposes the action of cholinergic drugs (parasympatholytic).

antiemetics a medicine that stops vomiting.

antipyretic a medicine that decreases the body temperature, relieves fever.

antiscorbutic relating to the property of preventing scurvy.

antiseptic a medicine that retards the growth of microorganisms.

antitoxin a chemical (or chemicals) produced by the living body which reacts with and alters to the point of being innocuous; a poison or toxin.

aromatic a medicine that has a spicy odor and stimulant properties—anise, cardamom seed, cariander, fennel, zingiber.

arteriosclerosis scarring or hardening of arteries as a result of disease in the arterial walls.

asepsis condition of freedom from microbial contamination; absence of sepsis.

astringent a medicine that contracts tissue and decreases the size of vessels.

ataraxic (ataractic) a drug that produces calm and composure (tranquilizer).

atonic (or atony) lack of tone.

atretic (or atresic) without a usual opening; imperforate.

atrophy shrinkage and wasting of tissues.

autolysis autodigestion.

bactericidal refers to an agent that brings about death of bacteria.

bacteriostasis a condition in which bacteria are prevented from growing and spreading. Adjective *bacteriostatic* is more general in its meaning than antiseptic.

bacteroides small, anaerobic, gram-negative rods commonly found in feces.

bradycardia slow rate of the heart.

calorie a unit of heat used frequently to express the fuel value of food; it is the heat required to raise the temperature of 1 ml. of water 1° C. (from 0° C. to 1° C.). The Calorie ("large calorie") is the heat required to increase the temperature of 1,000

768

grams of water one degree (from 0° to 1° C.).

carcinomatous relating to malignant cancer of epithelial cells.

cardiac decompensation a condition in which the heart is failing to maintain adequate circulation.

cardiotonic a drug that produces a favorable effect on the heart; acts like a tonic.

carminative a medicine that brings about expulsion of gas from the stomach and intestines.

carotenemia an excessive amount of a pigment called carotene in the blood. Carotene, is found in carrots and egg yolk.

centrifuge a device for separating parts by a rapid rotary motion (e.g., cream from milk), which depends on the centrifugal forces of rotary motion.

cervical referring to the neck of any structure, e.g., neck of the uterus.

chemotherapy the use of chemical agents in the treatment of disease; the chemical substance exerts a specific toxic effect on the microorganisms rather than on the tissues of the patient.

colloid a gluelike or gelatinous substance; a particle that does not dissolve but is held in suspension.

colloidal suspension a mixture in which particles are held in suspension, such as drops of fat in milk, gas bubbles in foam, etc.; the forms and surfaces of the particles change easily with the forces acting on them and are not rigid as in crystals.

condiment a substance used to make food more appetizing—allium, caraway, cinnamon, clove, fennel, ginger, myristica, pimenta, piper, *sinapis nigra.*

congener a drug that belongs to a group of compounds having the same parent substance; the ataractics belonging to the phenothiazine group might be described as congeners, one of another.

cortex the outer portion of a gland or structure; the rind or bark.

cycloplegia paralysis of the muscle of accommodation in the eye (ciliary muscle); this causes blurred vision.

cystine an amino acid which forms one of the components of proteins and contains sulfur.

cystitis inflammation of the urinary bladder.

demulcent (emollient) a medicine that protects and soothes the surface to which it is applied.

deodorant a medicine or substance that absorbs, masks, or destroys undesirable odors

depilatory a substance used to remove hair.

desquamate to scale off or peel off (as in the scaling off of the skin in scarlet fever).

detergent a medicine used as a cleansing agent—soaps, tincture of green soap; decreases surface tension.

diabetes insipidus a disease in which the patient suffers from great thirst, drinks a great deal, and has a large urine output.

digestant a medicine that aids digestion.

disinfectant (germicide) a medicine that destroys microorganisms.

diuresis rapid secretion of urine; stimulation of formation of urine.

diuretic a drug that increases the quantity of urine secreted.

dyspnea difficult or labored breathing.

emetic a substance that causes vomiting.

empiric that which is based on experience rather than on scientific proof.

emulsifier a substance used to form an emulsion with a fixed oil.

endemic habitual, established incidence of disease in a locality.

endoderm the innermost layer of cells, e.g., of an embryo.

endometrium the mucous membrane lining of the uterus.

enucleate to remove the nucleus or center.

enzyme an organic substance, produced in living cells, that affects the speed of a chemical action; thus pepsin, produced by the lining of the stomach, accelerates the digestion (hydrolysis) of proteins.

epidemic a widely prevalent disease, such as an epidemic of cholera.

epiphyses the end portion of long bones, which develops separately from the shaft.

escharotic (caustic) a medicine that chemically destroys the tissue with which it comes in contact.

estrogen a generic term for many compounds that have estrogenic activity, i.e., produce effects like estrin.

etiology the science of causes, as of a disease.

eugenics the science of improving the human race through its offspring.

eunuch an unsexed (castrated) man

exacerbation an increase or aggravation of a process, as a fever, rapid pulse, anemia, or pain.

exophthalmic associated with protruding eyeballs, as may be seen in certain patients with hyperthyroidism.

expectorant a medicine that increases or modifies bronchial secretion.

fertilization the union of a male element (e.g., a spermatozoon in animals, pollen in plants) with the female reproductive cell (the egg or ovum in animals, the ovule in plants), which starts the development of a new individual.

fetal pertaining to the fetus, the young of an animal while still in the womb.

flaccid soft, relaxed; flaccid paralysis is associated with soft musculature.

fluoroscope an instrument for observing objects in surroundings not ordinarily visible except to roentgen rays; e.g., a patient may swallow barium sulfate and the movements of his stomach can be observed with a fluoroscope.

formication sensation as if ants were creeping on the body.

fungicide a substance that is able to destroy a fungus.

gene the factor or differential substance in a germ cell (or other cell) that determines a given character.

genetics genetics is the science that deals with the resemblances and the differences exhibited among organisms related by descent.

germinal pertaining to a germ or germ cell.

gestation period of pregnancy; phenomena of pregnancy.

glycemia the presence of sugar (glucose) in the blood; hyperglycemia, an excessive amount of sugar in the blood; hypoglycemia, an unusually low concentration of sugar in the blood.

glycogenolysis the conversion of glycogen into glucose.

glyconeogenesis formation of glucose from other than carbohydrate molecules.

gonadotropic having an affinity or tropism for the testis or ovary.

griping a sharp, cramping pain in the bowel.

hemolytic pertaining to the property of rupture of the red blood corpuscles.

histology the science of the minute structure and function of the tissues of the body; microscopic anatomy and physiology.

homozygous breeding true to type.

hormone a chemical product manufactured by some tissue, such as a gland, which, carried by the blood, acts as a messenger and controls other tissues, as by stimulation or depression; growth, sex characteristics, effects on the heartbeat are instances of such control.

hydrogen ion concentration hydrogen ions (H+) are formed by acids and give acids their acid character; the concentration of these ions in the blood or other liquids has a vital effect on all life processes.

hydrostatic pertaining to the pressure exerted by liquids and on liquids; medically also— stagnation of fluid.

hyperplasia abnormal multiplication of cells; rapid growth.

hypertrophy increased size due to growth, which is greater than usual and may be abnormal.

hypophysectomy removal of the hypophysis or pituitary gland, a small gland at the base of the brain.

hypostatic pneumonia a pneumonia resulting from a patient remaining in one position over a long period of time.

icterus; jaundice deposit of bile pigments in the skin, giving it a deep yellow color.

ileus severe colic from intestinal obstruction.

indolent painless, slow healing.

infundibular pertaining to a funnel-shaped passage; applied to the passage of the pituitary extending down from the brain to certain portions of the kidney, part of the nose, etc.

interstitial structures, such as cells, lying between other structures; a supporting framework of tissue within an organ.

intractable unmanageable, e.g., intractable pain.

in vitro in artificial conditions, resembling those of life, e.g., in a glass vessel or test tube.

in vivo in life; in the body (in contrast to *in vitro*)

keratinize to form a hornlike substance; to harden and to thicken, as said of the skin in the formation of a callus, fingernails, and horns.

keratitis inflammation at the cornea of the eye.

keratolytic a substance that loosens the horny layer of the skin.

keratomalacia softening of the horny (outer) layer of the skin.

kilogram a unit of weight, equal to 1,000 grams, or 2.2 pounds avoirdupois.

labile unstable, liable to change.

larva a stage in insect life during which the "grub" emerges from its egg.

lesion a local abnormality: bruise, wound, scar, inflammation, cavity, etc.

lethargy mental dullness and drowsiness.

leukopenia deficiency in the number of leukocytes.

lockjaw a disease caused by the toxin of tetanus organisms in which the jaws become firmly locked because of muscle spasm.

lyophilized dehydrated from a frozen state by means of a vacuum.

macrophages large white cells of the blood, having the power of ingesting bacteria, débris, etc.

malaise lassitude, fatigue out of proportion to effort expended.

matrix a mold or framework; the intercellular substance of tissues; the womb.

metabolism the sum of the chemical processes by which food is used in the body for the development of heat, the doing of work, the formation of new tissues, etc.

microgram a millionth part of a gram.

millicurie one thousandth of a curie, which is a unit of radiation energy.

milliequivalent one thousandth of an equivalent combining weight of an atom or ion; an equivalent combining weight is the weight of an element (in grams) which will combine with 1.008 Gm. of hydrogen.

miotic a medicine that contracts the pupil of the eye.

morbidity degree of sickness; prevalence of sickness.

moribund in a dying state.

morphology the science of the form and structure of cells and tissues.

motile capable of spontaneous motion.

motor reflex a reflex involving stimulation of a motor nerve; a reflex which produces motion or activity.

mutation an inherited change in the germ plasm, which produces changes in the body.

mydriatic a medicine that dilates the pupil of the eye.

myxedema a condition of a peculiar swelling of tissues, due to thyroid deficiency and associated with low metabolism.

narcolepsy a condition characterized by an inability to remain awake.

narcotic a medicine that produces sleep or stupor and at the same time relieves pain.

necrosis death of cells or tissues.

neuralgia noninflammatory; pain along the course of a nerve.

neurasthenia nervous exhaustion.

neuritis inflammation of a nerve.

nostrum a medicine that authorities recognize as having little or no value (a quack remedy).

ophthalmia severe inflammation of the eye.

ophthalmia neonatorum inflammation in the eyes of the newborn infant.

orthostatic pertaining to the position of the body, e.g., upright position.

osteoporosis rarefaction of bone by enlargement of its cavities or formation of new spaces.

oxytocic ecbolic, parturient; a medicine that stimulates contractions of uterine muscle.

oxyuriasis infestation with pinworms of genus oxyuris.

parasiticides medicines that destroy parasites.

parenteral refers to administration other than by mouth; given with a needle.

paresis a paralytic disease of the brain; a late stage of syphilis.

parkinsonism a condition characterized by muscular rigidity and tremor due to a disturbance in the corpus striatum of the brain.

paroxysm a sudden, violent outburst.

pathogenesis the development of a disease.

pathology the science that studies the changes caused by disease.

peripheral pertaining to the periphery, outside or boundary; the peripheral nervous system is that outside of the skull and spinal canal.

placenta the structure attaching a fetus to the wall of the uterus, where food passes from the mother's blood to that of the fetus; the afterbirth.

planaria a group of flatworms.

plasmodium a microorganism in the blood, causing malaria and similar diseases.

polyneuritis inflammation of more than one peripheral nerve; multiple neuritis.

pressor stimulating; increasing tone (e.g., causing an increase in the blood pressure).

proliferation growth by multiplication of parts, as in cell division.

prophylactic pertaining to prevention of disease.

proteolytic pertaining to the breaking down of proteins, as in digestion.

protozoa animal organisms consisting of single cells.

pruritus an itching sensation.

psychosomatic frequently refers to a disorder affected both by the body (soma) and the mind and emotions (psyche).

pustulant a medicine that produces pustules (pus saco) in the openings of the skin glands.

rachitic pertaining to rickets.

radiopaque not easily penetrated by x-rays.

respiratory depressant a medicine that lowers the activity of the respiratory center and slows respiration; respiratory stimulants, in toxic doses, are respiratory depressants.

respiratory stimulant a medicine that increases the activity of the respiratory center and accelerates respiration.

roentgen rays x-rays; discovered by Dr. Wilhelm Conrad Röntgen.

rubefacient a medicine that produces a reddening of the skin as a result of dilating the vessels.

saline cathartic a medicine that causes evacuation of the bowels by increasing secretion and the amount of water in the intestinal tract.

seminal pertaining to the semen, the sperm, or male reproductive elements.

senility the infirmities of old age.

sequelae sequels or aftereffects.

sol a persistent suspension of minute particles in a liquid; a colloidal suspension of solid, liquid, or gas particles in a liquid, as in milk, foam, etc.

somatic pertaining to the body, as opposed to the germ plasm.

spasticity a tendency to spasm or violent contraction; increased tonus.

spectrum the band of colors produced when white light (such as sunlight) is refracted and dispersed by a prism or similar device; the colors of the rainbow represent a spectrum produced by the refraction and dispersion of sunlight by drops of rain.

sphincters ringlike muscles closing an orifice or passage (as in the intestine).

splanchnic nerve a large and important nerve in the abdomen, enervating the organs of the abdomen.

sporadic occasional, scattered.

stereotropic to see with both eyes; to have focused from both points, as in stereopticon pictures.

steroid a compound with a characteristic chemical structure; the sex hormones, cholesterol, and many hormones of the cortex of the adrenal gland have this type of structure; there are four fused carbon atom rings, three with 6 carbons and one with 5; sharing of carbon atoms occurs between adjacent rings.

stroma the framework of an organ or cell; the matrix.

styptic (hemostatic) a medicine used to check bleeding and hemorrhage.

suppurative pus producing.

symptomatology the combination of symptoms; the symptom complex.

syndrome the complete picture of a disease, including all of the symptoms.

synthetic made in the laboratory; artificially prepared.

tactile by touch.

tenesmus an urgent and distressing desire to empty the bowel or bladder, even though these organs may be empty.

tonus the state of continuous partial contraction of a muscle or muscles; tone; tenseness.

topical medically: local (as topical treatment).

trabeculae partitions (septa) which extend from the enclosing wall or envelope into the enclosed substance.

traumatic pertaining to physical injury, from a blow, pressure, or torsion.

triturated rubbed to a powder.

tropism the tendency of living organisms to move or turn in response to an external stimulus (such as a beam of light, an electric charge, etc.).

urticaria a condition of the skin characterized by wheals surrounded by a red area and associated with sensations of burning and itching, commonly known as "hives."

vesicant a medicine that irritates the skin sufficiently to produce blisters or vesicles.

vibrio a species of microbes.

virilism masculinity; normal in the male but a disease in women, characterized by changes in voice, figure, hair, etc.

viscosity the property of being viscous or sticky, which increases the resistance of a fluid or gas to changes of form.

vulnerary a medicine employed as a healing agent.

xerophthalmia a form of degenerative disease of the eye; atrophy of the conjunctiva.

Index

Abbreviations for orders, prescriptions, and labels, 109, 110-111
Abrasives for cleaning teeth, 370
Absorption, amount and rapidity of, effect on action of drugs, 134
of drug from rectum, 96
and excretion of drugs, relation of dose to, 134
from skin, 492
Acenocoumarol, 470
Acetanilid, 213-215
Acetazolamide as anticonvulsant, 283
as carbonic anhydrase inhibitor, 539
as diuretic, 520-521
as respiratory stimulant, 479-480
Acetomeroctol, 609
Acetophenetidin, 213-215
Acetylation of sulfonamides, 568
Acetylcholine, blocking agents of, 329
formula, 304, 320
muscarinic effects of, 320
nicotinic effects of, 320
in transmission of nerve impulses, 303
Acetylsalicylic acid (see also Salicylates)
analgesic action, 209
combined with other drugs, 213, 214
effects of large doses on respiration, 209
formula, 208
for pain relief, 210

Acetylsalicylic acid—Cont'd
poisoning in children, 212
preparation, dosage, and administration, 211
for rheumatic conditions, dosage, 211
Achlorhydria, agents in diagnosis of, 384
definition, 380
Achromycin (see Tetracyclines)
Achylia gastrica, definition, 380
Acid poisoning, symptoms and treatment, 746
Acid-forming salts as diuretics, 515
Acidity, gastric, diagnostic aids, 384
lowering by drugs, 372-379
Acids, corrosive, toxic action, 740
Acidulin, 380
Acne, bromide, 240
Acridine dyes, 607
Acriflavine, 607
Acromegaly, enlargement of features, 662
ACTH (see Corticotropin)
Acthar, 664
Actinomycin D for tumors in children, 717
Action, drug, 126-136
chemical, 130-132
factors influencing or modifying, 132-135
sites of, 127

Action, drug—Cont'd
systemic, terminology, 128-129
Active constituents of drugs, 35-37
Addiction, barbiturate, 227-228
cocaine, 262
drug, definition, 129
meperidine, 202
methadone, 203
to opiates, results and symptoms, 198-199
role and responsibility of nurse, 199-201
Addition of common fractions, 51
of decimals, 57, 58
Additive action of two antibiotics, definition, 139
effects of drugs, definition, 129
Adenine, formula, 713
Adhesive plaster as skin protective, 503
Administration of drugs, safe, knowledge necessary to, 13
of medicines, 93-125
channels of, 94
to children, 120-123
channels of, 122-123
for local effect, 94
nurse's role, 93
policies and regulations, 112-119
on psychiatric ward, 119-120
route and time of, relation of dose to, 133

Administration of medicines
—Cont'd
student nurse and, 13-14
for systemic effects, 95-
107
Adrenal cortex, activity during stress, 678
hormones of, 678-691
injection, 680
gland, functions, 678
medulla, hormones of, epinephrine and nor-
epinephrine, 307
Adrenalin, 307-311 (see also
Epinephrine)
Adrenaline, 311
Adrenergic blocking agents,
319
drugs, 306-319
definition, 304
Adrenocortical hormones, discovery, 767
in neoplastic diseases,
714
steroids, chemistry, 679
comparison of uses, 691
Adrenocorticotropic hormone
(ACTH), action
of, 663
Adrenotropic hormone
(ACTH) in neo-
plastic diseases,
714
Adsorbed diphtheria and tetanus toxoids and
pertussis vaccine,
733
toxoids, 733
Adsorbents, 402
Aerosols, definition, 94
Aerosporin, 163
Agar for constipation, 391
Age, relation of dose to, 132
Albacide, 499
Albamycin, 161
Albumin, serum, 460
Alchemy, influence on chemistry in fifteenth
century, 760
Alcohol(s), 267-277
amyl, 277
butyl, 277
as disinfectants, 618-619
ethyl, 268-276
absorption and excretion,
270
action and results, 268-
269
concentration in blood
and urine, intoxi-
cation indicated
by, 270, 271

Alcohol(s), ethyl—Cont'd
contraindications, 275-
276
as disinfectant, 618
injection for pain relief,
271
and life span, 276
local action, 268
for peripheral vasodila-
tion, 271
preparation and dosage,
272
systemic action, 268-269
uses, 270-272
as vasodilator, 435
isopropyl, 276-277
methyl (wood), 276
Alcoholics Anonymous, 274
Alcoholism, acute, symptoms
and treatment,
274
amphetamines in treatment
of, 178, 180
chronic, symptoms and
treatment, 274-
275
Aldactone, 522, 682
Aldosterone blocking agents
as diuretics, 522
discovery and use, 681
formula, 679
Alglyn, 376
Alidase, 721-722
Alkagel, 375
Alkalies, caustic, toxic action,
740
Alkaloids, description of, 35
opium, classification, 188-
189
preparation, dosage, and
administration,
194-196
therapeutic uses, 192-193
of Rauwolfia (see Rauwol-
fia alkaloids)
Alkavervir, 439
Alkylating agents for neoplastic diseases,
action of, 705
Allergens, 734-735
Allergic reactions to drug,
definition, 129
to local anesthetics, 260
to penicillin, 147
Allergy, definition, 734
nasal, antihistaminics for,
363
prevention and treatment,
735
Allylmercaptomethyl penicillin, parenteral use,
144

Aloe as cathartic, 399
Alophen pills, 399
Alpha-chymotrypsin in cataract extraction,
539
Alphaprodine hydrochloride,
204
Alseroxylon, 438
Al-U-Creme, 375
Aludrine hydrochloride, 312
Aluminum hydroxide gel, 375-
376
penicillin, dosage, 145
phosphate, 376
solutions, soothing, 495
Alurate, 225
Ambemonium for myasthenia
gravis, 327
Amebiasis and amebicides,
630-637
antibiotics for, 636-637
etiology, 630
extraintestinal, drugs for,
631-633
intestinal, drugs for, 633-
636
Amebic dysentery (see Amebiasis)
Amebicides, 630-637
American Medical Association
Council on Drugs,
functions, 21-22
Amethocaine hydrochloride,
264
Amethopterin for leukemia,
712-713
Aminometradine, 519
Aminophylline, action of, 174
as diuretic, 516
preparation, dosage, and
administration,
435
as respiratory stimulant,
479-480
uses, 435
as vasodilator, 435
Aminopterin for leukemia in
children, 711-712
Aminopyrine, 213-215
poisoning, 214
Aminosalicylic acid for tuberculosis, 579
Amisometradine, 519
Ammoniated mercury oint-
ment, 496
Ammonium chloride or car-
bonate for cough,
484
Amobarbital, dosage and administration, 225
formula, 221

Amodiaquin for malaria, 593, 595
Amphetamine, action and result, 178
  formula, 177, 316
  preparation, dosage, and administration, 178-179
  side effects and contraindications, 179
  source, 177
  sympathomimetic action of, 316
  uses, 178
Amphetamines, 177-181
  adrenergic effects, 316
Amphojel, 375
Amphotericin B, 156
Amphyl, 606
Ampule, withdrawing medication from, 87
Ampules, description of, 43
Amyl alcohol, 277
  nitrite, 433
Amylene hydrate, 256-257
Amytal, 221, 225
Anacin, 214
Anahist, 365
Analeptic, definition, 178
Analeptics for treatment of barbiturate poisoning, 227
Analgesia, stage of, in anesthesia, 245
Analgesics and antipyretics other than salicylates, 213-216
  coal tar, 213
  decrease of uterine motility by, 548
  definition, 187
  ideal, characteristics of, 188
  narcotic, 188-205
    synthetic, 201-205
  nonnarcotic, also antipyretic, 207-216
    synthetic, 207
  for pain of burns, 505
Anaphylactic shock, epinephrine in, 362
Ancient period of medicine, 755-757
Androgens, 560-564
  action and result, 561
  preparation, dosage, and administration, 562-563
  side effects and toxic effects, 563-564
  uses, 562
Andronate, 562
Androsterone, formula, 561

Anectine chloride, 354-355
Anemia, causes, 449
  definition, 448
  drugs for, 449-461
  folic acid for, 458
  histamine in diagnosis of, 360
  hypochromic, iron for, 451
  iron for, 450-454
  pernicious, 455-457
Anesthesia (see also Anesthetics)
  balanced, 242-243
  caudal, 261
  conduction or block, 261
  general, skeletal muscle relaxants as adjunct to, 348, 350
  infiltration, 260
  by injection, 260-261
  preparation of patient by medication, 243-244
  saddle block, 261
  spinal, 261
  stages of, 244-246
  surface, 260
  surgical, stage of, 246
Anesthesin, 267
Anesthetics, 240-267
  barbiturates as, 223
  basal, 256-259
  definitions, 240
  general, 247-256
    action of, 242-243
    ideal, requirements of, 244
    historical points of interest, 241
    by inhalation, methods of administering, 247
  local, action by freezing, 267
    definitions, 259
    epinephrine with, 310, 428
    for eye, 535-536
    methods of administration, 260-261
    miscellaneous, 267
    preliminary medication, 260
    procaine (Novocain), 262-263
    reactions to, 259-260
    slightly soluble, 267
Aneurine hydrochloride, 652
Angina pectoris, 412
  nitrites for, 432
Aniline derivatives, 213-215
Animal antitoxic serums, 728-729

Anionic surface agents, 617-618
Anions, reabsorption of, mechanism, 519
Anoxemia, symptoms, 487
Ansadol, 497
Ansolysen tartrate, 442, 444
Antacids, 372-379
  action of, 373
  classification, 373
  ideal, properties of, 372-379
  nonsystemic, 375-379
  systemic, 373-374
Antagonism, drug, definition, 129
Antagonistic action of two antibiotics, definition, 139
Antagonists of curariform drugs, 352-353
  narcotic, 205-206
Antazoline hydrochloride, 364
Antemetics, 383
Antepar citrate, 626
Anterior pituitary hormones, 662-665
Anthelmintics, 622-630
  good, properties of, 623
Anthracene cathartics, 393-401
Antialdosterone compounds as diuretics, 522
Antianemic drugs, 449-461
Anti-arrhythmic drugs, 424-426
Antibacterial agents, history, 765-766
Antibiosis, definition, 137
Antibiotics, 137-168
  action of, 137
  for amebiasis, 636-637
  for bowel infections, 403
  combination of, action of, 139
  current status of, 138-139
  definition, 566
  effective, characteristics of, 139
  for eye infections, 536-537
  history, 765
  nonsystemic, 166-168
  overuse of, 139
  resistance to, 138
  for skin infections, 496
  for syphilis, 585
  systemic, generally used, 140-155
    occasionally used, 155-165
  for urinary infections, 526-527

Antibodies, agents containing, 727-729
definition, 726
Anticholinergic drugs, belladonna group, 330-336
effects of, 329-330
for relief of symptoms of Parkinson's disease, 343
synthetic substitutes for atropine, 336-343
Anticholinesterase drugs, 324-329
for myasthenia gravis, 327-328
Anticoagulant therapy, contraindications, 472
effective, 471
Anticoagulants, 466-471
Anticonvulsants, 277-284
barbiturates as, 222, 223
bromides as, 279
ideal drug, 278
mechanism of action, 278-279
under investigation, 283
Antidiarrheics, 401-404
Antidiuretics, 523
Antidote kit, 745
universal, 749
Antidotes, chemical, 744-745
kinds and definitions, 744-745
physical, 744
physiologic, 745
poison, 744-750
Antifolic acid agents for neoplastic diseases, action of, 705
Antifungal agents, 497-498
Antigenic agents producing active immunity, 729-733
Antigens, definition, 726
Antihistaminics, 362-367
action of, 362-363
additional listing, 365
for colds, 486
for motion sickness, 366-367
preparation, dosage, and administration, 364-365
side effects, 363
Anti-infectives, anthelmintics and amebicides, 622-637
antibiotics, 137-168
definitions, 600-601
local, antiseptics and disinfectants, 600-620

Anti-infectives—Cont'd
mechanisms of action, 601
other than antibiotics, 566-576
sulfonamide compounds, 566-574
mixtures, 574-575
systemic, 577-598
Antimalarial drugs, 586-596
(see also Malaria)
Antimalignant drugs, 704-718
Antimetabolites for neoplastic diseases, 711-714
action of, 705
Antimony for leishmaniasis, 596
potassium tartrate for schistosomiasis, 629
Antineoplastic drugs, 704-718
Antiprotozoan agents, 586-598
Antipruritics, 501-502
Antipyretic action of salicylates, 209, 210
Antipyretics and analgesics other than salicylates, 213-216
and nonnarcotic analgesics, 207-216
Antipyrine, 213-215
Antiseptic, definition, 600
Antiseptics for intestinal infection, 403
local anti-infectives, 600-620
mercurial, 607-609
in ophthalmology, 537-538
and parasiticides, dermatologic, 495-499
respiratory, 483
urinary, 524-530
Antispasmodics, decrease of uterine motility by, 549
for diarrhea, 404
synthetic substitutes for atropine, 337-343
Antistine phosphate, 364
Antithyroid drugs, 673-678
Antitoxic serums of animal origin, 728-729
Antitussives, 480-483
narcotic, 481
Antrenyl bromide, 341-342
APC capsules, 214
Apomorphine hydrochloride for induction of vomiting, 383
Apothecaries' system, 66-68
conversion to metric system, 75-78

Apothecaries' system, conversion—Cont'd
from one denomination to other within, 75
exercises, 68
Appetite depressants, amphetamines as, 178, 180, 181
stimulants, simple bitters, 369
Apresoline hydrochloride, 440-441
Aprobarbital, 225
Aquasol A, 647
Aqueous solutions, description of, 37
suspensions, description of, 37-38
Arabian influence on medicine in Middle Ages, 758-759
Arabic and Roman numerals, 48-49
Aralen for amebiasis, 632-633
for malaria, 592-593
Aramine bitartrate, 318
Arfonad camphorsulfonate, 446
Argyn, 611
Aristocort, 538, 691
Arithmetic, review of, 47-64
Arlidin hydrochloride, 318
Arrythmias, heart, 413
drugs for, 424-426
Arsenic poisoning, BAL in treatment, 750
symptoms and treatment, 746
toxic action, 739
Arsenicals, organic, for intestinal amebiasis, 633-634
Arsthinol for intestinal amebiasis, 634
Artane hydrochloride, 342-343
Arthritis, rheumatoid, cortisone and hydrocortisone for, 683-685
Ascariasis, drugs for, 626, 627
Ascorbic acid (vitamin C), chemistry and function, 658
daily requirement, 658
preparation, dosage, and administration, 659
uses, 658-659
Aspidium as anthelmintic, 624-625

Aspirin (see Acetylsalicylic acid)
Assay, definition, 19
Asterol dihydrochloride, 497
Asthma, bronchial, epinephrine for relief of, 310
spasm, drugs to relax, 486-490
Astringents for diarrhea, 402-403
mineral and vegetable, 503-504
Atabrine for malaria, 590-591
for tapeworm, 625
Ataractics, 284-296
for itching, 502
and sedatives, distinction between, 284
use, 284
Atarax hydrochloride, 295-296
Atophan, 219
Atrial flutter, 413
Atropa belladonna, 330, 332 (Plate)
Atropine, absorption, distribution, and excretion, 334
as antagonist to choline derivatives, 321, 322, 323, 324, 325, 327
antispasmodic effects and side effects, 337
in bronchitis, 486
central action of, 331
contraindications, 335
formula, 330
as heart stimulant, 413
local action, 331
peripheral action, 331-333
preparation, dosage, and administration, 334
as respiratory stimulant, 479
side effects and toxic effects, 334
source, 330
sulfate, for eye, 334, 534
synthetic substitutes for, antispasmodics, 337-343
mydriatics and cycloplegics, 336-337
uses, 333
Aurcoloid, 717
Aureomycin (see Chlortetracycline; Tetracyclines)

Auricular fibrillation, 413
and flutter, drugs for, 424-425
Autonomic drugs, 302-346
affecting eye, 532-535
classification, 304-305
definition, 304
site of action, 305
ganglia, action of curare on, 350
nervous system, diagram and Plate, 306
divisions, effects produced by, 306
functions, 302
preganglionic and postganglionic fibers of, schematic representation, 305
relation to central nervous system, 302
to digestive tract, 368
sympathetic and parasympathetic divisions, differences between, 303
Avertin, 256-257
Avicenna, 759
Azapetine phosphate, 319
Azo dyes, 607
Azulfidine, 574
for intestinal infection, 403
Azure A carbacrylic resin, 384
Azuresin in diagnosis of achlorhydria, 384

Baciguent (see Bacitracin)
Bacitracin, action, uses, dosage, administration, and effects, 156-157
in ophthalmic ointments, 537
for skin infections, 496
in urinary infections, 527
Bactericides, definition, 600
Bacteriostatic, definition, 600
Baking soda, 374
BAL in treatment of arsenic, gold, and mercury poisoning, 749-750
Balanced anesthesia, 242-243
Balsams, 36
Banthine bromide, 339
Barbital, dosage and administration, 225
formula, 221

Barbitone sodium, 225
Barbiturates, 221-232
absorption, fate, and excretion, 223
action and result, 222
addiction to, 227-228
advantages and disadvantages in use, 228-229
antagonists, 227
choice of, 229
combination of, 229
contraindications, 224
legislation concerning sale and possession of, 229
length of action, 225
poisoning, acute, 226-227
chronic, 227-228
picrotoxin for, 185
as preanesthesia medications, 243
preparation, dosage, and administration, 224, 225
as respiratory depressants, 480
side effects and toxic effects, 224, 226-228
uses, 222-223
Barbituric acid, formula, 221
Barium sulfate in roentgenography of gastrointestinal tract, 385
Basal anesthetics, 256-259
Basaljel, 376
Baths, effects on skin, 506
BCG vaccine, 732
Beadox hydrochloride, 657
Belarsen for intestinal amebiasis, 634
Belladonna (see also Atropine)
for diarrhea, 404
group of cholinergic blocking agents, 330-336
Benactyzine hydrochloride, 296
Benadryl, formula, 362
hydrochloride, 364, 486
Benemid, 218-219
Benylate, 499
Benzalkonium chloride as disinfectant, 616
for eye, 539
Benzathine penicillin G, intramuscular dosage, 144, 145
for syphilis, 585

Benzedrex, 179
    as nasal decongestant, 431
Benzene, toxic action, 740
Benzestrol, 558
Benzethonium chloride as germicide and antiseptic, 617
Benzocaine, 267
Benzoic and salicylic acid ointment, 498
Benzoin tincture, compound, 500
Benzoinated lard, 493
Benzonatate for cough, 481
Benzpyrinium bromide, 328
Benzyl benzoate mixtures, 500
    penicillin, 143
Berocca, 652
Beta-carotene, formula, 645
Betaine hydrochloride, 380
Betalin, 652
Betaxin, 652
Betazole hydrochloride, 384
Bethanechol chloride, 322-323
    formula, 320
Bile and bile salts, 381-382
    ducts, organic iodine compounds in examination of, 385-386
    salts, portal-biliary circulation of, 464 (Plate)
Binders in compressed tablets, use of, 41
Bioassay, definition, 19
Biotin, 657
Bishydroxycoumarin, formula, dosage, and administration, 469
Bismuth compounds as demulcents, 402
    for syphilis, 586
Bistrimate for syphilis, 586
Bistrium chloride, 442, 443
Bitters, simple, 369
Bladder, drugs acting on, 524
Bleeding, capillary, epinephrine in prevention of, 309, 427
Block anesthesia, 261
Blood coagulation, 461-472
    drugs affecting, 447-472
    formation, factors promoting, 449
    physiology, 447-448
    plasma, 459
    pressure (see also Hypertension)

Blood pressure—Cont'd
    determining before administration of antihypertensive drugs, 442, 443
    effect of drugs on, 426
        of ephedrine on, 314, 429
        of levarterenol bitartrate on, 313, 428
    factors modifying, 411
    proteins, 459-460
    supply of heart, 410
    transfusion in anemia, 458
    vessels, action of atropine on, 332
        of caffeine on, 175
        of epinephrine on, 308, 427
        of nicotine on, 344
        of nictonic acid on, 436
        of nitrites on, 432
    drugs affecting, 426-447
    whole, and its constituents, 458-460
Blood-forming organs, neoplastic diseases of, 706-707
Blutene chloride, 462
Body components, normal, as drugs, 638
    inorganic needs, 639-642
    organic needs, 642-700
Bonamine hydrochloride, 367
Boric acid as antiseptic, 619-620
Bornate, 499
Boroglycerin glycerite, 620
Bougies, definition, 44
Bowel function and cathartics, misconceptions, 387
Brain, action of general anesthetics on, 242
    centers, action of drugs on, 171-173
    motor cortex, action of barbiturates on, 222, 229
    stem, action of morphine on, 190
Brand name of drug, 34
Brandy, 272
British Pharmaceutical Codex, 22
    Pharmacopoeia, 22
Bromides, absorption, distribution, and excretion, 238
    action and result, 238
    as anticonvulsants, 279

Bromides—Cont'd
    contraindications, 240
    history, 237
    poisoning, 240
    preparation, dosage, and administration, 239-240
    skin eruption due to, 239, 240
    uses, 239
Bromidrosis, 507
Bromism, 240
Brompheniramine hydrochloride, 365
Bronchial asthma, epinephrine for relief of, 310
    spasm in asthma, drugs to relax, 486-490
Bronchitis, expectorants in relief of, 485, 486
Bulk-forming cathartics, 391-395
Burns, 504-506
    chemical, first-aid treatment, 743
    general treatment, 505-506
    infection in, prevention and treatment, 506
    local treatment, 505
    tissue reaction, 504
Burow's solution, 495
Busulfan for leukemia, 710
Butabarbital sodium, administration and dosage, 225
Butacaine sulfate, 265
Butallylonal, dosage and administration, 225
Butamben picrate, 267
Butazolidin, 215-216
Butesin picrate, 267
    for burns, 506
Butethal, dosage and administration, 225
Butisol, 225
Buttock of child, injections into, 123
    intramuscular injection into, 100, 101
Butyl alcohol, 277
    aminobenzoate, 267
Butyn sulfate, 265

Cade oil, 500
Cafergot, 176, 430
Caffeine, action and result, 175-176
    as diuretic, 515
    formula, 174
    as heart stimulant, 414

Caffeine—Cont'd
  physiologic action, 174
    (Plate)
  preparation, dosage, and
    administration,
    176
  as respiratory stimulant,
    479
  side effects and toxic ef-
    fects, 177
  source, 174
  uses, 176
Calamine lotion, 495
  phenolated, 267
Calciferol, 649
Calcium carbonate, 377-378
  daily requirements, 641
  deficiency, 640
  mandelate for urinary in-
    fections, 528
  preparation, dosage, admin-
    istration, and uses,
    641
Camoquin for malaria, 593
Canada, drug standards in,
    22-23
Canadian drug legislation, 29-
    31
  Food and Drug Act, 29
  Formulary, 22
  nurse and narcotic laws of
    Canada, 30-31
  Opium and Narcotic Act,
    29-30
Cancer of breast and prostate,
    hormones in treat-
    ment, 715
  drugs for control of, 704-
    718
Capacity, table, 72
Capsules, description of, 40
Carbachol, 321-322
  for eye, 533
  formula, 320
Carbacrylamine resins, 523
Carbamide as diuretic, 514
Carbarsone for intestinal ame-
    biasis, 633
Carbetapentane citrate for
    cough, 482
Carbimazole, 677
Carbinoxamine maleate, 365
Carbohydrate metabolism, in-
    sulin and, 693
Carbol-fuchsin solution, 607
Carbolic acid as disinfectant,
    602-603
Carbomycin, 157-158, 585
Carbon dioxide, administra-
    tion, 478

Carbon dioxide—Cont'd
  as respiratory stimulant,
    476, 478
  uses, 478
  monoxide poisoning, symp-
    toms and treat-
    ment, 746
  toxic action, 739
  tetrachloride   poisoning,
    symptoms   and
    treatment, 746
Carbonic anhydrase, action of,
    520
  inhibitors as diuretics,
    519-522
  in ophthalmology, 538-
    539
Carbo-Resin, 523
Carboxide as disinfectant, 620
Carbutamide, drawbacks, 700
  formula, 700
Carcholin (see Carbachol)
Carcinostatic drugs, 704-718
Cardiac effects of chloral hy-
    drate, 235
  of cyclopropane, 255
  of ether, 248
  glycosides, chemistry of,
    414-415
  digitalis series, 415-421
  strophanthin and oua-
    bain, 421-422
Cardiotonics, 414-424
Cardiovascular disease, am-
    phetamine contra-
    indicated in, 178,
    179
  syphilis, penicillin for, 584
  system, action of alcohol
    on, 269
  of morphine on, 191
  effect of salicylates on,
    209
  reactions to local anes-
    thetics, 259
Cardrase, 522, 539
Care of medicines, nursing re-
    sponsibilities in,
    111-112
Carisoprodol, 356
Carmethose, 392-393
Carminatives, 382
Carotene, 644, 645, 646
Carter's pills, 399
Cartridge type container for
    drugs, 43
Cascara sagrada, 398-399
Castellani's paint, 607
Castor oil, 397-398
Catalase, action of, 720
Catalysts, definition, 720

Cathartics, 387-401
  acting by chemical irrita-
    tion, 397-398
  anthracene (emodin), 398-
    401
  bulk-forming, 391-395
  for children, best, 393
  classification, 390-391
  contraindications to use,
    390
  emollient, 395-396
  justifiable use, 389
  nurse's responsibilities in
    relation to use,
    388
  saline, 393-395
Cathomycin, 161
Cation exchange resins as di-
    uretics, 522-523
Cationic agents as antiseptics,
    616-617
Caudal anesthesia, 261
Caustic alkalies, toxic action,
    740
Caustics, 501
Cedilanid, 421
Ceepryn chloride as disinfect-
    ant, 617
Cellothyl, 392
Cellular responses to drugs,
    130
Cellulose, oxidized, 463
Celontin, 283
Central action of drugs, defi-
    nition, 173
  of reserpine, 285
  nervous system, action of
    alcohol on, 268-
    269
  of amphetamines on,
    178, 179, 180, 181
  of atropine on, 331
  of barbiturates on,
    222
  of bromides on, 238
  of caffeine on, 175-
    176
  of   chlorpromazine
    on, 289
  of cocaine on, 261
  of drugs on, 171-
    173
  of ephedrine on, 314
  of ether on, 248
  of ethylene on, 254
  of general anesthet-
    ics on, 242
  of meperidine on,
    201
  of methylphenidate
    hydrochloride on,
    182

Central nervous system, action
—Cont'd
of nicotine on, 344
of pentylenetetrazol
on, 183
of picrotoxin on, 184
of strychnine on, 185
of thiopental sodium
on, 258
of tribromoethanol
on, 256
depressants, 187-296
and stimulants, toxic
actions of, 740
depression, drug-in-
duced, symptoms,
187
reactions to local an-
esthetics, 259
relation of autonomic
nervous system to,
302
stimulants, 173-187
sympathetic suppressants,
ataractics as, con-
cept of, 284
Cerebellum, action of drugs
on, 173
Cerebral cortex, action of
amphetamine on,
178
of caffeine on, 175
of drugs on, 171
Cerebrum, action of atropine
on, 331
of morphine on, 189
Cer-O-Cillin sodium, 144
Cestodes and nematodes,
drugs used against,
624-629
varieties and activities, 623
Cetyl pyridinium chloride as
disinfectant, 617
Charcoal, activated, as adsorbent, 402
Chel-Iron, 453
Chemical action of drugs,
130-131
antidotes, 744-745
assay, definition, 19
burns, first-aid treatment,
743
disinfectants, 601-620
name of drug, 33
Chemistry in nineteenth century, 763-764
Chemotherapeutic agents acting systemically,
577-598
definition, 566
history, 765
for tuberculosis, 577-582

Chemotherapy of ocular infection, 536-538
Children, administration of
medicines to, 120-
123
aspirin overdosage in, 212
dosage for, determination
of, 89-90
reactions to drugs, 123
securing cooperation of,
120-122
Chiniofon, formula, 634
for intestinal amebiasis, 635
Chloral hydrate, 234-236
poisoning, 235
Chlorambucil for neoplastic
diseases, 709-710
Chloramines as disinfectants,
613
Chloramphenicol, 154-155
for eye infections, 537
for syphilis, 585
in urinary infections, 527
Chlorbutanol, 236
Chlorcyclizine hydrochloride,
364
Chloresium as skin protective,
503
Chloretone, 236
Chlorine as disinfectant, 611-
612
Chlorisondamine chloride,
444-445
Chlormerodrin, 518
Chloroform, 251-252
discovery, 241
Chloroguanide, 595
formula, 592
Chloromycetin, 154-155 (see
also Chloram-
phenicol)
Chlorpheniramine maleate,
364
Chlorophenothane poisoning,
symptoms and
treatment, 746
Chlorophyll derivatives, water-soluble, as skin
protectives, 503
Chloroquine for amebiasis,
632-633
formula, 592
for malaria, 592-593, 595,
596
Chlorothen citrate, 365
Chlorothiazide as diuretic,
521-522
as hypotensive agent, 446
Chlorotrianisene, 558
Chlorpheniramine, formula,
362

Chlorprocaine hydrochloride,
264
Chlorpromazine, formula, 289
hydrochloride, 288-290
Chlorpropamide, 701
Chlortetracycline (see also
Tetracyclines)
for syphilis, 585
Chlor-Trimeton, formula, 362
maleate, 364
Chlorzoxazone, 357
Cholecystography, organic
iodine compounds
for, 385-386
Cholera vaccine, 729
Choline, 657
derivatives, 320-324
Cholinergic blocking agents,
belladonna group,
330-336
effects of, 329-330
synthetic substitutes
for atropine, 336-
343
drugs, 319-329
definition, 304
Cholinesterases, action on
acetylcholine, 303
Chorionic gonadotropin, 551,
552
Christianity, spread of, in
Middle Ages,
medicine and, 758
Chymar, 724
Chymotrypsin, 724
Cinchocaine hydrochloride,
265
Cinchophen for gout, 219
Circulatory disease, 412-413
system, action of bromides
on, 238
of drugs on, 408
of ergotamine and er-
gotoxine on, 544
drugs affecting, 408-472
physiology, 408
Citrovorum factor, 458
Clark's rule for dosage for
children, 89
Claviceps purpurea, 542
(Plate)
Clistin, 365
Clopane hydrochloride, 318
Closed method of inhalation
anesthesia, 247
Clotting, blood, drugs inhibit-
ing, 466-471
producing, 462-465
reactions of plasma, 462
CMC cellulose gum, 393
Coagulation, blood, 461-472

Coal tar, 500
   analgesics, 213-215
Cocaine, 261-263
   for eye, 535
   habit, 262
Cocoa butter, 494
   syrup as flavoring agent, 368
Cod liver oil, 647
Codeine, action on central nervous system, 189
   with aspirin, 213
   for cough relief, 190, 193, 481
   formula, 189
   preparation, dosage, and administration, 194
Colace, 397
Colchicine, 217-218
Cold cream, 494
Colds, preparations for, 480-486
Collodion as skin protective, 502
Colloidal silver preparations as antiseptics, 611
Colloids, hydrophilic, for constipation, 391-393
Coloring agents in disguise of unpleasant-tasting drugs, use of, 369
   substances for medicines, 45
Committee on Toxicology of A. M. A., first-aid measures for poisoning, 742-743
Compazine, 291
Complex fractions, 55
Compressed tablets, description of, 40-41
Conduction anesthesia, 261
Congestive heart failure, beneficial effects of digitalis in, 416-417
   pathology, 412
Constipation, cathartics for, 387-401
   causes, 387-388
   in elderly persons, 389
   symptoms and treatment, 388
Conversion from apothecaries' to metric system, and vice versa, 75-78
Convulsion, strychnine, 186, 187

Convulsive seizures, epilepsy, 277-278
Coparaffinate, 497
Copavin, 195
Copper in formation of hemoglobin, 453
Coramine, action, uses, dosage, and administration, 183
   as respiratory stimulant, 479
Cordus, Valerius, author of first pharmacopeia, 761
Corlutone, 559
Corn oil as laxative, 396
Coronary disease, pathology, 412
Corrosive poisons, action of, 740
   sublimate, 608
Corrosives, 501
Cortef acetate, 686
Cortex, cerebral, action of amphetamine on, 178
   of caffeine on, 175
   of drugs on, 171
Corticoids, synthetic, 688-691
Corticotropin, action, 663
   preparation, dosage, and administration, 664-665
   side effects and toxic effects, 686-688
   source, absorption, and uses, 664
Cortisone, absorption, 685
   action and result, 682-683
   formula, 679
   and hydrocortisone, 682-688
   preparation, dosage, and administration, 685
   side effects and toxic effects, 686-688
   source and synthesis, 682
   uses, 683-685
Cortril acetate, 686
Cough, antitussives, 481-482
   causes and treatment, 480-481
   codeine for relief of, 190, 193
   demulcents for, 482-483
   expectorants for relief of, 484-485
   preparations, 480-485
   syrups, 482
Coumadin sodium, 470

Coumarin derivatives, 468-471
   effective anticoagulant therapy with, 471
Council on Drugs of A. M. A., functions, 21-22
Counting pulse of patient on digitalis therapy, 423
Cramps, "night," quinine for, 352
Creamalin, 375
Cresol as disinfectant, 604
Cretinism, 668-670
   treatment, 670
Cross tolerance to drugs, definition, 129
Cryptenamine, 439
Crystodigin, 420
Cumertilin, 518
Cumopyran, 470
Cumulation, drug, definition, 128
Cupron, 453
Curare, absorption and excretion, 350
   action and result, 349-350
   preparation, dosage, and administration, 350-351
   side effects, 351
   source, 349
   toxic action, 739
   uses, 350
Curariform blocking agents, 349-352
   drugs, antagonists of, 352-353
Cushing's syndrome, appearance of patient, 687
Cutaneous disorders, symptoms, 493
   immunity tests, 733-734
Cyanide poisoning, symptoms and treatment, 747
Cyanides, toxic action, 739
Cyanocobalamin, 455-457
   preparations, 456-457
Cyclaine hydrochloride, 265
Cyclamate calcium, 45
   sodium, 45
Cyclamycin, 163
Cyclizine hydrochloride, 366
Cyclobarbital, 225
Cyclobarbitone, 225
Cyclogyl hydrochloride, 337, 535
Cyclomerol, 470
Cyclomethycaine sulfate, 264
Cyclopentolate hydrochloride, 337
   for eye, 535

Cycloplegics and mydriatics, synthetic substitutes for atropine, 336-337
Cyclopropane, 254-255
Cycloserine, 158
for tuberculosis, 581
Cytomel, 671

Danilone, 471
Dapsone, 583
Daranide, 539
Daraprim for malaria, 594-595
Darcil, 145
Dark Ages, medicine in, 757-758
Darvon, 207
Decadron, 538
Decamethonium bromide, 353-354
Decapryn succinate, 364
Decavitamin capsules and tablets, 660
Decholin, 382
Decimal division, definition, 56
form, definition, 57
fractions, 56-59
changing per cent to, 61
point and decimal place, definitions, 57
Decimals, addition and subtraction of, 57, 58
changing fractions to, 59
division of, 58, 59
exercises, 59-60
multiplication of, 58
Decongestants, nasal, 430
Dehydration, treatment, 639
Dehydrocholic acid, 382
Dehydrotachysterol, 649
Delalutin, 560
Delatestryl, 562
Delirium tremens, symptoms and treatment, 275
Delta Cortef, 690
Deltasone, 689
Deltoid muscle, injection into, 100, 101
Deltra, 689
Delvex as anthelmintic, 628-629
Demecarium bromide for eye, 534
Demerol hydrochloride, 201-203
Demulcents, 401-402
for cough, 482-483

Dentrifices, 370
Deodorants, perspiration, 508
Depo-estradiol cyclopentylpropionate, 556
Depolarization, prolongation of, skeletal muscle relaxation by, 353-355
Depressants of central nervous system, 187-296
nonselective, classification, 187
selective, 277-296
toxic action, 740
heart, 424-426
polysynaptic, 355-358
respiratory, 480
Depression of central nervous system by anesthetics, pattern of, 242
drug, definition, 128
Dermatologic agents, 492-508
antipruritics, 501-502
antiseptics and parasiticides, 495-499
astringents, 503
soothing, 493-495
stimulants and irritants, 500
Deserpidine, 288, 438
Deslanoside, preparation, dosage, and administration, 421
Desoxycorticosterone acetate, 680-681
formula, 679
Desoxyephedrine hydrochloride, 180
Desoxyribonucleases as expectorants, 485
Detergents as expectorants, 485
Detoxication, drug, 134, 135
Dexamphetamine sulfate, 180
Dexedrine sulfate, 179-180
Dextran, 460
Dextro amphetamine sulfate, 179-180
propoxyphene hydrochloride, 207
Dextromethorphan for cough, 482
D.H.E.45, 430
Diabetes insipidus, antidiuretics in treatment, 523
vasopressin for, 666
mellitus, characteristics and symptoms, 693
control by insulin, 694

Diabetes mellitus—Cont'd
pancreas and, early experiments, 692
sulfonylureas for, 699-700
Diabetic coma and acidosis, symptoms and treatment, 694
Diabinese, 701
Diagnex blue, 384
Diagnostic aids in gastric acidity, 384
roentgenographic, 385-386
Diamine oxidase, inactivation of histamine by, 361
Diaminodiphenylsulfone (DDS), 583
Diamox as anticonvulsant, 283
as carbonic anhydrase inhibitor, 539
as diuretic, 520-521
as respiratory stimulant, 479-480
Diamthazole dihydrochloride, 497
Diaparene chloride, 617
Diarrhea, adsorbents for, 402
astringents for, 402-403
causes, 401
classification of drugs for, 401
sedatives and antispasmodics for, 404
Dibenamine, 319
Dibenzyline, 319
Dibucaine hydrochloride, 265
Dichlorphenamide, 539
Dicumarol, contraindications, 472
formula, dosage, and administration, 469
Diencephalon, action of barbiturates on, 222
Dienestrol, 557
Diethyl ether, 247-250
Diethylcarbamazine for ascariasis, 627-628
Diethylstilbestrol for cancer of breast and prostate, 715
formula, 553
preparation, dosage, and administration, 557
Diffusin, 721-722
Digestants, 380-382
Digestive tract, action of drugs on, 368

Digilanid, preparation, dosage, and administration, 420

Digitaline Nativelle, 420

Digitalis, absorption, excretion, and administration, 417
action and result, 416-417
compounds, chemistry of, 414
contraindications, 418
introduction in eighteenth century, 763
local irritation due to, 416
poisoning from, 419
preparations, choice of, 418-419
standardization of, 418
purpurea, 416 (Plate)
and quinidine, comparison of effects, 426
series, cardiac glycosides, 415-421
source, 415
systemic effects, 416-417
therapy, nursing care of patients on, 422-424
uses, 417

Digitalization, 418

Digitoxin, formula, 415
preparation, dosage, and administration, 420

Digoxin, preparation, dosage, and administration, 421

Dihydrocodeinone bitartrate, 195
for cough, 481

Dihydromorphinone for cough, 481
hydrochloride, preparation, dosage, and administration, 195

Dihydrostreptomycin, 151-153

Diiodohydroxyquin, formula, 634
for intestinal amebiasis, 635

Diisopropyl fluorophosphate for eye, 534

Dilantin sodium, 279-280

Dilaudid hydrochloride, preparation, dosage, and administration, 195

Diluents in compressed tablets, use of, 41

Dimenformon benzoate, 556

Dimenhydrinate, 366-367

Dimercaprol in treatment of arsenic, gold, and mercury poisoning, 749-750

Dimetane, 365

Dioctyl sodium sulfosuccinate, 396-397

Diodoquin, 635

Diogyn, 556

Dioscorides, 757

Dioxyline phosphate, 435

Di-Paralene hydrochloride, 364

Dipaxin, 471

Diphemanil methylsulfate, 341

Diphenadione, 471

Diphenhydramine, formula, 362
hydrochloride, 364

Diphenylhydantoin, formula, 283
sodium, 279-280

Diphtheria antitoxin, 728
tetanus, and pertussis vaccine, 733
toxin, diagnostic, 733
toxoid, 732, 733
vaccine, 733

Disinfectants (see also Germicides)
chemical, 601-620
definition, 600, 601
evaluation of, criteria, 602

Disintegrators in compressed tablets, use of, 41

Dispensatory of London hospitals, appearance in eighteenth century, 763
of United States of America, 22

Disposable syringes, use of, 43

Distribution of drug through tissues and fluids of body, effect on action, 134

Dithiazanine iodide as anthelmintic, 628-629

Diuretics, 513-523
acidifying, 515
antialdosterone compounds, 522
carbonic anhydrase inhibitors, 519-522
cation exchange resins as, 522-523
mercurial, 517-519
nonmercurial, 519
osmotic, 513-515
zanthine, 515-516

Diuril as diuretic, 521-522
for hypertension, 447

Divinyl ether, 250-251

Division of decimals, 58, 59
of fractions, 53
of mixed number by fraction, 54

Doca acetate, 680-681

Doriden, 233

Dosage for children, determination of, 89-90
forms of drugs, 39-43

Dose of drug, definitions, 132
effect on action, 132-134

Doses from stock solutions, determination of, 86-87
from tablets, determination of, 88-89

Dover's powder, origin in eighteenth century, 763

Doxinate, 397

Doxylamine succinate, 364

Dramamine, 366-367

Drisdol, 649

Drugs (see also Medicine)
action of, 126-136
biological mechanism, 130
on central nervous system, 171-173
chemical, 130-131
competitive inhibition, 131
effects of absorption on, 134
factors that influence or modify, 132-135
addiction, results and symptoms, 198-199
role and responsibility of nurse, 199-201
administration, importance of, 13
memorizing, importance of, 17
central action of, definition, 173
definition, 18
depressing central nervous system, 187-296
detoxication of, 134, 135
distribution through body, effect on action, 134
dosage forms, 39-43
doses of, definitions, 132
elimination from body, 135
fate of, in body, 134-135
for gout, 216-219
legislation, 23-31

Drugs—Cont'd
  listing in N.F., 21
    in N.N.D., 21
    in U.S.P., 20
  local action of, 127
  names of, 33-34
  new, study of, 15, 17
  nurse's attitude toward, 15
  plant, active constituents of, 35-37
  producing systemic effects, administration, 95-107
  pure, definition, 81
    solutions from, preparation of, 82-84
  reactions of children to, 123
  regulation by Harrison Narcotic Act, 26-28
  sites of action, 127
  sources of, 34
  standards in Great Britain and Canada, 22-23
    international, 23
    need for, 19
    in United States, 20-22
  stimulating central nervous system, 173-187
  systemic action, 127-129
    or effects, terminology, 128-129
Durham-Humphrey Law, 24
Dyes, antiseptic, 606-607
Dysmenorrhea, luturin for, 549
Dyspnea, helium-oxygen mixtures for, 490

Echothiophate for eye, 534
Ecolid chloride, 444-445
Edema, control of, by mercurial diuretics, 518
  relief of, by saline cathartics, 393
Edrophonium chloride, 352-353
  in myasthenia gravis, 328
Effervescent sodium phosphate, 394
Egypt, ancient, medicine in, 755
Eighteenth century, pharmacy in, 762-763
Electrocardiogram with diagram of heart showing origin of waves, 411

Elimination of drugs from body, 135
  promotion of, in poisoning, 750
Elixirs, description of, 38
  medicated, dosage range, 39
Elkosin, 573
Emetics, preparation, dosage, and administration, 383
  use, 382
Emetine for amebiasis, 631-632
Emodin cathartics, 398-401
Emollient cathartics, 395-396
Emollients, 493-494
Empiric versus rational medicine, 126-127
Empirin compound, 214
Emulsions, description of, 38
Enteric-coated capsules, description of, 40
Entromone, 552
Enzymatic preparations in ophthalmology, 539
Enzymes, catalytic action of, 720
  definition, 720
  as drugs, 720-725
  as expectorants, 485
  gastric and pancreatic, 381-382
  in medicine, limitations on usefulness, 721
  uses, 721
Ephedrine, 314-316, 429
  action, 314, 429
  formula, 177, 314
  local application to mucous membranes, 429
  preparation, dosage, and administration, 315
  side effects and toxic effects, 316
  source, 314
  uses, 314-315
Epilepsy, diphenylhydantoin sodium for, 279
  grand mal and petit mal, 277
  jacksonian, 278
  phenobarbital for, 223, 229, 230
  psychomotor attacks, 278
  trimethadione for, 282
Epileptic seizures, 277-288
Epinephrine, 307-312, 427-428

Epinephrine—Cont'd
  absorption and excretion, 309
  action, 427
    local, 307
    systemic, 308-309
  contraindications, 428
  fatal dose, 312
  formula, 304
  as heart stimulant, 414
  as histamine antagonist, 362
  hydrochloride for eye, 535
  and norepinephrine, adrenal hormones, 307
  preparation, dosage, and administration, 310-311, 428
  side effects and toxic effects, 311
  source and general characteristics, 307
  uses, 309-310, 427-428
Epsom salt, 394
Equanil as ataractic, 294-295
  as skeletal muscle relaxant, 356
Equivalents in apothecaries' and metric systems, tables of, 76, 77, 79
Ergobasive group of ergot, 543, 544
Ergometrine maleate, dosage and administration, 545
Ergonovine, effect upon uterus, 544
  formula, 543
  maleate, dosage and administration, 545
Ergosterol, 647, 649
Ergot, 542-546
  alkaloids of, groups, action and result, 543-544
    side effects and toxic effects, 545-546
  chemistry of, 542-543
  in obstetrics, preparation, dosage, and administration, 545
  source and constituents, 542
  uses, 544
Ergotamine with caffeine, 176
  and ergotoxine, action on circulatory and sympathetic nervous systems, 544
  on uterus, 543
  preparations for generalized itching, 502

Ergotamine—Cont'd
    tartrate, action, uses, dosage, and administration, 430
Ergotism, chronic, 545-546
Ergotrate maleate, 545
Eridione, 471
Erythrocin, 154
Erythromycin, absorption, distribution, and excretion, 153
    current status, 138
    for eye infections, 537
    preparation, administration, and dosage, 154
    side effects, 154
    for urinary infections, 527
    uses, 154, 585
Escharotics, 501
Eserine, 324-325
    salicylate for eye, 533
Essence of peppermint, 382
Estinyl, 556
Estradiol, dosage and administration, 556
    formula, 553
Estrogens, 552-558
    for cancer of breast and prostate, 715
    chemistry, 553
    conjugated, preparation, dosage, and administration, 556-557
    natural, preparation, dosage, and administration, 555-556
    pharmacologic action and result, 554
    side effects and toxic effects, 558
    synthetic, preparation, dosage, and administration, 557-558
    uses, 555
Estrone, dosage and administration, 555
    formula, 553
Etamon chloride, 345
Ethchlorvynol, 232, 502
Ether, advantages and disadvantages, 250
    contraindications, 250
    formula, 247
    history, 241
    local action, 248
    preparation, dosage, and administration, 249
    side effects and toxic effects, 250

Ether—Cont'd
    systemic action, 248-249
    uses, 249
Ethinamate, 233
Ethinyl estradiol, dosage and administration, 556
Ethisterone, dosage and administration, 560
Ethotoin, 281
Ethoxzolamide, 522, 539
Ethyl alcohol (see Alcohol, ethyl)
    biscoumacetate, 470
    carbamate, 717
    chloride, 255-256
        action by freezing, 267
    oxide, 249
Ethylaminobenzoate, 267
Ethylene, 253-254
    oxide as disinfectant, 620
Ethylstilbamine for leishmaniasis, 596
Eucatropine hydrochloride, 337
    for eye, 535
Eugenol, 267
Euphthalmine hydrochloride, 337
    for eye, 535
Evipal sodium, 225, 259
Excitement, stage of, in anesthesia, 245
Excretion of drugs, 135
    absorption and, relation of dose to, 134
    by skin, 493
Exophthalmic goiter, appearance of patient, 672
Exorbin, 379
Expandex, 460
Expectorants, 483-486
    definitions, 483, 484
    sedative, 484-485
    stimulating, 485
    theory of use, 484
Extracts, description and forms of, 39
Eye, anatomy and physiology, 532
    anesthetics for, 535-536
    autonomic drugs affecting, 532-535
    carbonic anhydrase inhibitors affecting, 538-539
    contamination, first-aid treatment, 743
    drops, instillation of, 540
    drugs affecting, 532-540

Eye—Cont'd
    effect of atropine on, 331, 332
        of cocaine on, 262
        of physostigmine on, 324-325
    infection, chemotherapy, 536-538
    instillation of topical preparations, 540
    pupil of, action of morphine on, 190, 197
        effects of ether on, 248
    steroids affecting, 538
    structures of, diagram, 533
Eyeball, anatomy, 532, 533

Fate of drugs in body, 134-135
Fat-soluble vitamins, 644-650
F-Cortef acetate, 691
Fecal moistening agent, 396
Federal Food, Drug, and Cosmetic Act, 23-25
    Trade Commission drug control, 26
Female sex hormones, 559-560
Feosol, 452
Fergon, 452
Ferric ammonium citrate, 452
Ferrocholinate, 453
Ferroglycine sulfate complex, 452
Ferrolip, 453
Ferronord, 452
Ferrous gluconate, 452
    sulfate, 452
Fibers, preganglionic and postganglionic, of autonomic nervous system, schematic representation, 305
Fibrin foam, 462
    formation of, 462
First-aid measures for poisoning, 740, 742-743
Fixed oils, description of, 37
Flavoring agents, 368-369
Flaxedil triethiodide, 351-352
Flexin, 356-357
    for gout, 219
Florantyrone, 382
Florinef acetate, 691
Floropryl, 328-329
    for eye, 534
Fludrocortisone acetate for allergic dermatoses, 691
    formula, 689

Fluid measure, table, 66
Fluidextracts, description and dosage range, 39
Flukes, varieties, 623
Fluorescein sodium for eye, 539
Fluoride in drinking water, reduction of tooth decay by, 371
  poisoning, symptoms and treatment, 747
Fluoxymesterone, 563
Folic acid, 457-458
  antagonists for neoplastic diseases, 711-713
Follicular hormone, activity of, 552-553
Follutein, 552
Folvite, 458
Food and Drug Act, Canadian, 29
  Administration, function of, 25
  Drug, and Cosmetic Act, Federal, 23-25
Foods, poisonous, 751
Formaldehyde as parasiticide, 619
Formalin as germicide, 619
Forthane, 318
Fowler's solution for leukemia, 718
Foxglove, Digitalis purpurea, 416 (Plate)
  purple, preparation, dosage, and administration, 419-420
  white, preparation, dosage, and administration, 420
Fractions, 49-62
  changing to decimals, 59
  common, addition, 51
    changing per cent to, 61
    definition, 49
    raising to higher terms, 50
    subtraction, 52
  comparison of sizes of, 53, 54
  complex, 55
  decimal, 56-59
  division, 53, 54
  equivalent, 50
  exercises, 55-56
  improper, definition, 50
  and mixed numbers, 50-51
  multiplication, 52
    of whole numbers by, 51, 53
  proper, definition, 50

Fried's rule for dosage for infants, 90
Fuadin for schistosomiasis, 629
Fumagillin, 166
  for amebiasis, 636-637
Fumidil, 166, 636
Fungizone, 156
Fungous infections, agents for treatment of, 497-498
Furacin, 496
  for eye infections, 537
Furadantin for urinary infections, 524, 528-529

Galen, 757
Gallamine, triethiodide, 351-352
Gallbladder, organic iodine compounds in examination of, 385-386
Gamma benzene hexachloride, 498, 499
  as scabicide, 499
Gamophen, 604
Ganglionic blocking agents, 343-346, 441-447
  action and effects of, 343
Gantrisin diethanolamine for eye infections, 537
  preparation, dosage, and administration, 572
  as urinary antiseptic, 525
Gargles and mouthwashes, 369-371
Gas gangrene antitoxin, 729
Gases, interchange, in lungs, 477
Gastric acid production, histamine in diagnosis of, 360
  acidity, diagnostic aids, 384
  antacids (see Antacids)
  and pancreatic enzymes, 381-382
Gastrointestinal organs, action of barbiturates on, 222
  drugs affecting, 368-404
  system, action of bromides on, 238
  effect of alcohol on, 269
  tract, action of atropine on, 333
    of ephedrine on, 314
    of morphine on, 191-192

Gastrointestinal tract—Cont'd
  barium sulfate in roentgenographic study of, 385
  demulcents for, 401-402
  effect of ether on, 249
    of physostigmine on, 325
    of salicylates on, 209
Geber, 759
Gelatin capsules, description of, 40
  sponge, absorbable, 462
Gelatine solution, special intravenous, 461
Gelfoam, 462
Gels, description of, 38
Gelusil, 377
Gemonil, 225
General anesthetics (see Anesthetics, general)
Generic name of drug, assignment of, 33
Gentian tincture, compound, 369
  violet as anthelmintic, 628
    as antifungal agent, 497
Gentran, 460
Germicides (see also Disinfectants)
  alcohols, 618-619
  Bard-Parker solution, modifications of, 619
  definition, 600
  mercury, 607
  oxidizing agents, 614-615
  phenol, 603, 606
  satisfactory, characteristics of, 602
  silver compounds, 610
  surface-active agents, 616-618
Gexane, 498, 499
  as scabicide, 499
Gitaligin, 420
Gitalin, preparation, dosage, and administration, 420
Glands, action of atropine on, 332-333
  of epinephrine on, 309
  of internal secretion, diagram, 661
Glauber's salt, 393
Glaucoma, atropine contraindicated in, 335
  isoflurophate for, 329
  physostigmine for, 325
  pilocarpine for, 323
Globin zinc insulin, 697

Globulins, serum, 727, 728
Glomerular filtration in formation of urine, 511-512
Glossary, 768-772
Glucocorticoids, 682
Glucose as diuretic, 514
Glutamic acid hydrochloride, 380
Glutethimide, 233
Glycerin, 493
Glycerol, 493
Glyceryl trinitrate tablets (nitroglycerin), 433
Glycobiarsol for intestinal amebiasis, 634
Glycosides, cardiac, chemistry of, 414-415
    digitalis series, 415-421
    strophanthin and ouabain, 421-422
    description of, 35
Goiter, exophthalmic, appearance of patient, 672
    simple, cause, 668
Goitrous cretin, 669
Gold poisoning, BAL in treatment of, 750
Gonadotropic hormones, pituitary, 550-551
    of placental origin, 551-552
Gout, acute, colchicine for, 217-218
    characteristics of, 216
    chronic, probenecid for, 219
    drugs for, 216-219
    new, 219
    salicylates for, 210
Gram, definition, 73
Grand mal epilepsy, 277
    diphenylhydantoin sodium for, 279
Graves' disease, 672
Great Britain, drug standards in, 22
Greece, ancient, medicine in, 756-757
Griseofulvin, 498
Gum resins, 36
Gums, description of, 36
Gynergen, 430, 502

Habits for nurses in giving medicines, 114
Habituation, drug, definition, 129
Halazone, 613
Halibut liver oil, 647

Halogenated hydroxyquinolines for intestinal amebiasis, 634-636
Halogens as disinfectants, 611-614
Halotestin, 563
Harmonyl, 288, 438
Harrison Narcotic Act, 26-28
Hay fever, antihistaminics for, 363
    desensitization, 735
Heart (see also Cardiac; Cardiovascular)
    action of atropine on, 332
    of epinephrine on, 308
    anatomy and physiology of, 409-411
    arrhythmias, 413
    drugs for, 424-426
    block, 413
    blood supply, 410
    depressants, 424-426
    disease, patients on digitalis therapy, nursing, 422-424
    drugs improving quality of action of, 414-424
    effects of drugs upon, 413-426
    of nicotine on, 344
    failure, congestive, 412
    digitalization for, 418
    muscle, 409-410
    effect of digitalis on, 416
    nerve supply, 410-411
    special tissues of, 409-410
    stimulant, epinephrine as, 310
    stimulants, 413-414
Heavy metals, salts of, as antiseptics, 607-611
Hedulin, 471
Helium, with oxygen for dyspnea, 490
Helminthiasis, therapeutic résumé, 630
    undesirable effects, 622
Helminths, classification, 623
    drugs used against, 622-630
Hemoglobin, physiology, 448
Hemo-Pak, 463
Hemopoietic drugs, 449-461
Hemorrhage, epinephrine in prevention of, 309, 427, 428
Hemostasis, preparations producing, 462-465
Henbane, 330
Heparin antagonist, protamine sulfate, 468
    contraindications, 472

Heparin—Cont'd
    preparation, dosage, and administration, 467
    side effects and toxic effects, 468
    therapy, effective, 471
    uses, 466-467
Heroin addiction, 199
HETP, 328
Hetrazan for ascariasis, 627-628
Hexachlorophene as local anti-infective, 604-605
Hexamethonium chloride, 443-444
Hexestrol, 558
Hexobarbital sodium, 225, 259
Hexocyclium methylsulfate, 342
Hex-O-San, 604
Hexylcaine hydrochloride, 265
Hexylresorcinol as anthelmintic, 627
    as antiseptic, 605
Hinkle's pills, 399
Hippocrates, 756, 757
Histalog, 384
Histamine, action and result, 359-360
    in diagnosis of achlorhydria, 384
    as diagnostic aid, 360-361
    formula, 359
    and hypersensitivity, 360
    preparation, dosage, and administration, 361
    side effects and toxic effects, 361
    uses, 360-361
Histamine-antagonizing drugs, 362-365
Histidine, formula, 359
Histology of kidney, 510-511
History of materia medica, 754-767
    of metric system, 69-70
    of weights and measures, 65
Homatropine hydrobromide, 336-337
    or hydrochloride for eye, 534
    methylbromide, 338
Hormones of adrenal cortex, 678-691
    of medulla, 307
    definition and medical uses, 660
    as drugs, 660-700

Hormones—Cont'd
  follicular, 552-553
  gonadotropic, of placental origin, 551-552
  luteal, 559-560
  for neoplastic diseases, 714-715
    action of, 705
  ovarian, 552
  parathyroid, 666-667
  pituitary, 661-666
    gonadotropic, 550-551
  posterior pituitary, 546-548
  sex, 550-564
  testicular, 560-564
  thyroid, 667-672
  vitamins, and minerals as drugs, 638-700
Hospital application of Harrison Law, 26-27
  formularies, 22
Household measures, 79, 80
Human serums, naturally produced, 727-728
Humorsol for eye, 534
Hyaluronidase in anesthesia of eye, 539
  uses, 721
Hycodan bitartrate, 195
  for cough, 481
Hydantal, 280
Hydeltrasol, 690
Hydeltra-T.B.A., 690
Hydralazine hydrochloride, 440-441
Hydriodic acid syrup, 485
Hydrocarbons, poisoning, symptoms and treatment, 747
Hydrochloric acid for pernicious anemia patients, 457
  preparation, dosage, administration, and uses, 380
Hydrocortamate hydrochloride for allergic dermatoses, 691
Hydrocorten acetate, 686
Hydrocortisone, absorption of, 685
  action and result, 682-683
  and cortisone, 682-688
  formula, 679
  lotion or ointment for pruritus, 502
  preparation, dosage, and administration, 686
  side effects and toxic effects, 686-688
  uses, 683-685

Hydrogen peroxide solution as germicide, 615
Hydrolose, 392
Hydrophilic colloids for constipation, 391-393
  ointment, 494
Hydrous wool fat, 494
Hydroxyprogesterone acetate and caproate, 560
Hydroxyquinolines, halogenated, for intestinal amebiasis, 634-636
Hydroxystilbamidine isethionate for parasitic infestations, 598
Hydroxyzine hydrochloride, 295-296
Hyflavin, 654
Hykinone, 465
Hyoscine (see also Scopolamine)
  formula, 330
  hydrobromide for eye, 534
Hyoscyamine, source, 330
Hyoscyamus, 336
Hypersensitivity, drug, definition, 129
  histamine and, 360
Hypertension, chlorothiazide for, 447
  essential, nitrites for, 433
  ganglionic blocking agents for, 441-447
  hydralazine hydrochloride for, 440-441
  ideal drug for treatment of, 437
  Rauwolfia alkaloids for, 438
  replacement of nitrites by other drugs in, 437
  vasodilators and drugs for, 431-447
  veratrum preparations for, 439-440
Hyperthyroid states, 672
Hypnotics, barbiturates as, use of, 222
  definition, 220
  satisfactory, characteristics of, 220
  and sedatives, barbiturates, 221-232
    differences between, 220
    nonbarbiturate, 232-240
Hypochlorhydria, definition, 380
Hypodermic injection of drugs, 97-99
  in buttock of child, 123

Hypodermic—Cont'd
  needle, insertion into stoppered vial, 87
  use, stock solutions for, determination of dose, 86-87
  tablets for, determination of dose, 88-89
Hypodermoclysis, administration of solutions by, 98
  hyaluronidase as aid in, 722
Hypoglycemia symptoms due to insulin overdosage, 698-699
Hypoglycemic agents, oral, 699-700
Hypotensive agent, chlorothiazide as, 446
  good, characteristics of, 431
Hypothalamus, action of drugs on, 172
  of morphine on, 190
Hypothyroid states, 668-670
Hypoxanthine, formula, 713
Hytakerol, 649

I^{131}, 674-676
Ichthammol, 500
Idiosyncrasy, drug, definition, 129
  opium, 196
Ilidar phosphate, 319
Ilosone, 154
Ilotycin (see Erythromycin)
Imferon, 454
Immune serums, 727-729
Immunity, active, antigenic agents producing, 729
  kinds of, definitions, 726
  tests, cutaneous, 733-734
Indon, 471
Infants, dosage for, Fried's rule, 90
Infections (see also Anti-infectives)
  in burns, prevention and treatment, 506
  ocular, chemotherapy of, 536-538
  skin, antiseptics for, 496-500
  specific, sulfonamides in, 569-570
  urinary, organisms causing, 525
Infiltration anesthesia, 260

Influenza virus vaccine, 730
Infusion, intravenous, 104-106
INH, 580
Inhalation, administering anesthetics by, methods, 247
of drugs, 96
Injection, anesthesia by, 260-261
intracardiac, 107
intradermal or intracutaneous, 96
intramuscular, 98, 100-103
in buttock of child, 123
intraosseous, 107
intrapericardial, 107
intraspinal or intrathecal, 107
intravenous, 103
in children, 123
subcutaneous, 97-99
in children, 123
Inorganic needs of body, 639-642
Inositol, 657
Insomnia, nonbarbiturate sedatives and hypnotics for, 232-237
Instillation of topical preparations in eye, 540
Insulin, action and result, 693
chemistry, 693
in control of diabetes mellitus, 694
discovery, 692
injection, 696
lente, use, 697
overdosage, symptoms, 698-699
preparation, dosage, and administration, 695-697
resistance, 699
syringes, 695
therapeutic uses, 694-695
untoward effects, 699
International drug standards, 23
Intestinal amebiasis, drugs for, 633-636
infections, sulfonamides in, 569-570
Intestine, drugs, acting on, antidiarrheics, 401-404
cathartics, 387-401
Intoxication, acute, symptoms and treatment, 274
indicated by concentration of alcohol in

Intoxication—Cont'd
blood and urine, 270, 271
Intracardiac injection, 107
Intracutaneous injection of drugs, 96
Intradermal injection of drugs, 96
Intramuscular injection of drugs, 98, 100-103
in buttock of child, 123
Intraosseous injection, 107
Intrapericardial injection, 107
Intraspinal injection, 107
Intrathecal injection, 107
Intravenous infusion, 104-106
injection, 103
in children, 123
Inversine hydrochloride, 445-446
Iodeikon, 385
Iodide, action and result, 673
for cough, 485
preparations and uses, 674
Iodine compounds for cholecystography, organic, 385-386
deficiency and its effect on thyroid gland, 668
as disinfectant, 613-614
and iodide, 673-674
poisoning, symptoms and treatment, 747
radioactive, 674-676
tincture in ophthalmology, 538
Iodoalphionic acid, 386
Iodochlorhydroxyquin, formula, 634
for intestinal amebiasis, 635-636
Iodohydroxyquinoline compounds for intestinal amebiasis, 634-636
Iodophors, 614
Iodophthalein sodium, 385
Iopanoic acid, 386
Iophenoxic acid, 386
Iothiouracil sodium, 677
Ipecac for amebiasis, 631
syrup, 485
Ipral sodium, 225
Iron, action and result, 451
compounds, absorption of, 450
loss from body, 451
parenteral administration, 453
toxic symptoms after, 454

Iron—Cont'd
poisoning, 454
preparation, dosage, and administration, 452-454
inorganic, oral administration, precautions, 453
quinine, and strychnine elixir, 369
requirements in man, 450-451
side effects and toxic effects, 454-455
uses, 451-452
Iron-dextran injection, 454
Irritants, skin, 500
Irritation, drug, definition, 128
local, responses of skin to, 500
Isobornyl thiocyanoacetate-technical, 499
Isoflurophate, 328-329
for eye, 534
Isoniazid (INH) for tuberculosis, 579-481
Isonorin sulfate, 312
Iso-Par, 497
Isophane insulin, 697
Isoprenaline sulfate, 312
Isopropyl alcohol, 276-277
as antiseptic, 619
Isoproterenol, 312-313
Isotopes, radioactive, 715-717
Isuprel, 312-313
Itching, drugs for relief of, 501-502
Itrumil sodium, 677

Jacksonian epilepsy, 278
Jarisch-Herxheimer reaction in treatment of syphilis, 585
Jimson weed, 330
Juniper tar, 500

Kanamycin, 159-160, 582
Kantrex, 159-160, 582
Kaolin, 402
Kaopectate, 402
Kenacort, 538, 691
Kenalog, 691
Keratolytic, salicylic acid as, 210, 501
Keratolytics, action of, 501
17-Ketosteroids, 560, 561
Kidney, blood supply, diagram, 512
effect of alcohol on, 270
of ether on, 248

Kidney—Cont'd
    functions, 510
    histology, 510-511
    and urinary tract, drugs affecting, 510-530
Koch's tuberculin, 734
Konakion, 465
Konsyl, 392
Kwell as pediculicide, 498
    as scabicide, 499
Kynex, 573
    as urinary antiseptic, 526, 570, 573

Label on medicine, reading, 113
Lactoflavin, 653
Lanatoside C, preparation, dosage, and administration, 420
Lanolin, 494
Lanoxin, 421
Laudanum, dosage, 193
Laxatives (see Cathartics)
Legislation, drug, 23-31
Leishmaniasis, drugs for, 596, 597, 598
Lente insulins, 697
Leprosy, drugs for treatment of, 582-583
Leptazol injection, 184
Lescapine bromide, 339
Lethal dose, definition, 132
Leucovorin calcium, 458
Leukemia, antimetabolites for, 712-714
    characteristics, 706
Leukeran, 709-710
Leukocytosis, definition, 448
Leukopenia, definition, 448
Levallorphan tartrate, 206
Levarterenol, adrenal hormone, 307
    bitartrate, 313-314, 428-429
        action, 313, 428
        formula, 313
        preparation, dosage, and administration, 313, 428
        side effects and toxic effects, 314
    formula, 304
Levo-Dromoran for cough, 481
    tartrate, 205
Levophed bitartrate (see Levarterenol bitartrate)
Levorphanol tartrate, 205
Lice, agents used to kill, 498-499

Licorice, 400
Lidocaine hydrochloride injection for eye anesthesia, 536
    preparation, dosage, and toxic effects, 266
Life span, alcohol and, 276
Liniments, description of, 43
Lipo-Lutin, 559
Liter, definition, 72
Liver function test, sulfobromophthalein sodium for, 386
    organic iodine compounds in examination of, 385-386
    with stomach, dosage, 457
Local action of drugs, 127
    administration of medicines, 94
    anesthetics (see Anesthetics, local)
    anti-infectives, antiseptics and disinfectants, 600-620
Lorfan tartrate, 206
Lotions, description of, 43
    soothing, dermatologic, 495
Lozenges, description of, 41
Lubricants in compressed tablets, use of, 41
Lugol's solution, 614, 674
Lumbar injection, 107
Luminal (see Phenobarbital)
Lunar caustic, 611
Lungs, gaseous exchange in, 477
    physiology, 476
Luteal hormone, 559-560
Lutocyclol, 560
Lutrexin, 549
Lututrin, decrease of uterine motility by, 549
Lye poisoning, symptoms and treatment, 748
Lymphomas, characteristics and treatment, 706-707
Lyovac Diuril, 447, 522
Lysergic acid, formula, 542
Lysol as disinfectant, 604

Maalox, 379
Magmas, description of, 38
Magnacort, 691
Magnamycin, 157-158
Magnesia, heavy, 378
    light, 378
    magma, 379
Magnesium carbonate, 379
    cathartics, 394

Magnesium—Cont'd
    oxide, 378
    sulfate, decrease of uterine motility by, 550
    trisilicate, 376-377
Malaria, agents for control of, 586-596
    amodiaquin for, 593, 595
    chloroquine for, 592-593, 595, 596
    choice and comparison of drugs for, 595-596
    control of, world-wide problem, 588
    empiric use of quinine for, 126
    ideal drug for, characteristics, 588
    parasites causing, 586-588
    primaquine for, 594, 595
    pyrimethamine for, 594-595
    quinacrine for, 590-591
    quinine for, 588-590
    terminology of drug therapy for, 588
    types of infection, 586
Male fern (aspidium) as anthelmintic, 624-625
    sex hormones, 560-564
Malignant tumors, drugs for control of, 704-718
    origin and growth of, 704
Malpighian body, diagram, 511
    corpuscle, blood supply of, diagram, 512
Mandelamine for urinary infections, 528
Mannitol hexanitrate, 433
Marezine hydrochloride, 366
Materia medica, definition, 18
    history, 754-767
Mathematics for nurses, review of, 47-64
Matromycin, 162
Maximal dose, definition, 132
Measles serums, 727
Measures, household, 79, 80
    weights and, 65-92
        apothecaries' system, 66-68
        conversion from apothecaries' to metric system, and vice versa, 75-78
        exercises, 91
        history of, 65
        metric system, 69-74
Mebaral, 225

Mebroin, 280
Mecamylamine hydrochloride, 445-446
Mechlorethamine hydrochloride, action on cells, 707
    dosage, administration, uses, and toxic effects, 708
Mecholyl bromide, 321
    chloride, 320-321
Meclizine hydrochloride, 367
Mecostin chloride, 350
Medications, orders for, 107-108
    preanesthetic, 243-244
Medicine (see also Drugs)
    administration of (see Administration of medicines)
    Arabian influence, 758-759
    cards accompanying medications, samples, 114
    care of, nursing responsibilities in, 111-112
    coloring substances for, 45
    disagreeable-tasting, administration to children, 122
    Egyptian, 755
    empiric versus rational, 126-136
    Greek, 756-757
    inhalation of, 96
    label, reading, 113
    liquid, pouring, 116
    in medieval period, 757-760
    oral administration, 95
        to children, 122
    parenteral administration, 96-107
    and pharmacy in twentieth century, progress in, 764-767
    for psychiatric patients, administration, 119-120
    recording, 117
    rectal administration, 96
        to children, 123
    Roman, 757
    sublingual administration, 95
    synthetic sweetening agents, 45
    trays with cards, 115
    written orders for, 107-108
Medieval period, medicine in, 757-760

Medrol, 690
Medulla oblongata, action of atropine on, 331
    of caffeine on, 175
    of drugs on, 172
    respiratory center in, physiology, 476
Medullary paralysis, stage of, in anesthesia, 246
Membranes, mucous (see Mucous membranes)
Memorizing important to drug administration, 17
Menadiol sodium diphosphate, 465
Menadione, chemistry, 463
    formula, 469
    preparation and dosage, 464
Menaphthone, 464, 465
Meningococcic meningitis, sulfonamides in, 569
Menopause symptoms, estrogens for, 555
Mental activity, higher, action of drugs on, 171-172
    depression, amphetamines for, 178, 180
Mepacaine hydrochloride, 625
Mepacrine hydrochloride, 591
Mepazine, 293
Meperidine hydrochloride, 201-203
    for pain relief in burns, 505
Mephenesin, 355
Mephentermine sulfate, 317-318
Mephobarbital, dosage and administration, 225
Mephyton, 465
Meprane dipropionate, 558
Meprobamate as ataractic, 294-295, 502
    as skeletal muscle relaxant, 356
Mepyramine maleate, 365
Meralluride injection, 517
Meratran hydrochloride, 181
Merbak, 609
Merbromin, 609
Mercaptomerin sodium, 517
Mercaptopurine, formula, 73
    for leukemia, 713-714
Mercuhydrin injection, 517
Mercumatilin, 518
Mercurial diuretics, 517-519
    preparations, side effects, and contraindications, 518
Mercurochrome, 609

Mercury compounds as antiseptics, 607-609
    in ophthalmology, 538
    ointment, ammoniated, 496
    ointments, antiseptic use, 608
    poisoning, BAL in treatment of, 750
        symptoms and treatment, 748
    preparations, organic, as antiseptics, 609
Merphenyl nitrate basic, 609
Merthiolate, 538, 609
Mesantoin, 280-281
Mesopin, 338
Mestinon for myasthenia gravis, 327
Metabolism, drug, 135
Metals, heavy, salts of, as antiseptics, 607-611
Metamucil, 392
Metandren, 562
Metaphen in ophthalmology, 538
    preparation and use, 609
Meter, definition, 71-72
Methacholine bromide, 321
    chloride, 320-321
    formula, 320
Methadone for cough, 481
    hydrochloride, 203
Methallenestril, 558
Methamphetamine hydrochloride, 180
Methantheline bromide, 339
Methapyrilene hydrochloride, 365
Metharbital, dosage and administration, 225
Methazolamide, 539
Methenamine, 527-528
    mandelate, 528
Methergine maleate, 545
Methiacil, 677
Methimazole, 677
Methionine, 528
Methium chloride, 443-444
Methocarbamol, 357-358
Methocel, 392
Methotrexate for leukemia, 712-713
Methscopolamine bromide, 339
    nitrate, 339
Methsuximide, 283
Methyl alcohol, 276
    toxic action, 740
    salicylate (see also Salicylates)
    as flavoring agent, 210

Methyl salicylate—Cont'd
  formula, 208
  local action, 208
  poisoning in children, 212
  preparation, 211
Methylamphetamine hydro-
    chloride, 180
Methylbenzethonium chloride
    as diaper disin-
    fectant, 617
Methylcellulose for eye, 539
  preparation, dosage, and
    administration,
    392
Methylergonovine maleate
    (methylergomet-
    rine maleate),
    dosage and ad-
    ministration, 545
Methylphenidate, formula,
    181
  hydrochloride, 182
Methyl-phenyl-ethyl hydan-
    toin, 280-281
Methylprednisolone, dosage,
    690
  formula, 689
Methylrosaniline chloride as
    anthelmintic, 628
  as antifungal agent, 497
  preparation and use, 607
Methyltestosterone, 562
Methylthiouracil, 677
Methyprylon, 234
Meticortelone, 690
Meticorten, 689
Metopon hydrochloride, 204
Metrazol, 183-184
  in alcoholism, 273
  as respiratory stimulant,
    479
Metric linear measurement,
    table, 70
  system, 69-74
    advantages over apothe-
      caries' system, 74
    conversion to apothecar-
      ies' system, 75-78
    from one denomination
      to other within,
      75
    exercises, 74
    history, 69-70
Metrology, history of, 65
Metubine iodide, 350
Metycaine hydrochloride, 266
Microorganisms, resistance to
    antibiotics, 138
  source of antibiotics, 137
Middle Ages, medicine in,
    757-760

Midicel, 573
  as urinary antiseptic, 526
Migraine headache, ergota-
    mine tartrate for,
    430
Milibis for intestinal amebi-
    asis, 634
Milk of bismuth, 402
  of magnesia, 379
Milontin, 283
Miltown as ataractic, 294-295,
    502
  as skeletal muscle relaxant,
    356
Mincard, 519
Mineral astringents, 504
  oil, 395-396
Minerals, vitamins, and hor-
    mones as drugs,
    638-700
Minim, definition, 68
Minimal dose, definition, 132
Miotic action of morphine,
    190, 197
  effect of physostigmine, 325
  of pilocarpine, 323
Miracil-D for schistosomiasis,
    629
Mixed numbers, division by
    fraction, 54
  and improper fractions,
    50-51
  multiplication of, 53
Mixtures, definition of, 38
Moderil, 288, 438
Modern Drug Encyclopedia,
    22
Molar solution, definition, 81
Molded tablets, description
    and administra-
    tion of, 41
Morphine, action and result,
    189-192
  addiction, 199
  comparison of alphaprodine
    with, 204
    of levorphanol with, 205
    of meperidine with, 201-
      202
    of methadone with, 203
  constriction of pupil by,
    190, 197
  contraindications, 196
  for cough, 481
  formula, 189
  idiosyncrasy of effect, 196
  lethal dose, 197
  for pain relief in burns,
    505
  poisoning, acute, 196-198
    nalorphine for, 206
    chronic, 198-199

Morphine—Cont'd
  preparation, dosage, and
    administration,
    194
  therapeutic uses, 192-193
  toxic dose, 197
Mosquito, development of
    malarial parasites
    in, 586-587
Motion sickness, antihistamin-
    ics for, 363
  drugs for, 365-367
  nature and cause of, 365-
    366
Mouth, drugs affecting, 368-
    371
Mouthwashes and gargles,
    369-371
Mucotin, 377
Mucous membrane, applica-
    tion of medica-
    tions to, 94
  effects of soaps, 507
  of respiratory tract,
    drugs affecting,
    480-486
  skin and, drugs affecting,
    492-508
Multiple-vitamin preparations,
    659-660
Multiplication of decimals, 58
  of fractions, 52
  of mixed numbers, 53
  of whole number by frac-
    tion, 51, 53
Mumps skin test antigen, 734
  vaccine, 730
Muracil, 677
Muscarinic effects of acetyl-
    choline, 320
Muscle, skeletal (see Skeletal
    muscle)
  smooth, action of atropine
    on, 333
    of epinephrine on, 309
    of morphine on, 191-
      192
    of nitrites on, 432
Muscles, heart, 409-410
  for injection, 100
Muscular relaxation, mecha-
    nism of produc-
    tion of, 348
Mustargen hydrochloride, 707-
    708
Myasthenia gravis, anticho-
    linesterase drugs
    for, 327-328
  neostigmine for, 326-327
  patient before and after
    treatment, 326
  symptoms, 326

792

Mycostatin, 167, 498
Mydriatics and cycloplegics, synthetic substitutes for atropine, 336-337
Myleran, 710
Myocardium, action of caffeine on, 175
Myometrium, action of drugs on, 541-542
response to posterior pituitary extracts, 548
Myoneural blocking agents, 353-355
Mysoline, 283
Mytelase for myasthenia gravis, 327
Myxedema, 669, 670

Nalline hydrochloride, 205-206
Nalorphine hydrochloride, 205-206
Names of drugs, 33-34
Naphuride for trypanosomiasis, 596-597
Narcolepsy, amphetamines in treatment of, 178, 180
Narcotic analgesics, 188-205
synthetic, 201-205
antagonists, 205-206
antitussives, 481
Control Act of 1956, 28
uses of term, 189
Narcotics exempt from Harrison Law, 27
oral prescriptions for, 27
possession of, 28
as preanesthesia medications, 243
regulation by Harrison Act, 26-28
Nasal decongestants, 430
sprays, 483
type of oxygen inhalation apparatus, 489
National Formulary, 21
Nausea and vomiting, relief by drugs, 383
Nebulae, definition, 94
nasal, 483
Nectadon for cough, 482
Needle for intramuscular injection, 100
plastic, for intravenous infusion, 104, 105
Nematodes and cestodes, drugs used against, 624-629
varieties, 623

Nembutal, formula, 221
sodium, 225, 231-232
Neo-Antergan maleate, 365
Neocinchophen for gout, 219
Neodrol, 563
Neohydrin, 518
Neomycin for skin infections, 496
sulfate, 160
for eye infections, 537
in urinary infections, 527
Neonal, 225
Neoplastic diseases of blood-forming organs, 706-707
drugs for, classification, 705-706
Neostam stibamine glucoside for leishmaniasis, 596
Neostibosan for leishmaniasis, 596
Neostigmine, 325-327
bromide for eye, 534
for myasthenia gravis, 326-327
Neo-Synephrine hydrochloride (see Phenylephrine hydrochloride)
Neptazane, 539
Nerve impulses, transmission of, theories, 303-304
supply of heart, 410-411
Nervous system, autonomic, 302-304
central (see Central nervous system)
sympathetic and parasympathetic, 303
systems of body, central and peripheral, action of, 171
Nesacaine hydrochloride, 264
Neurosyphilis, penicillin for, 584
Neutrapen, 148, 724-725
New and Nonofficial Drugs, 21, 23
Niacin (see Nicotinic acid)
Niacinamide, 656
Nicholas of Salerno, 759
Nicotinamide, formula, 654
Nicotine, absorption, action and result, 344
ganglionic blocking agent, 343-345
poisoning, 344-345
symptoms and treatment, 344, 748

Nicotinic acid, daily requirement and uses, 655
formula, 654
metabolic function, 655
preparation, dosage, and administration, 655-656
source, 654
as vasodilator, 436
effects of acetylcholine, 320
"Night cramps," quinine sulfate for, 352
Nikethamide, 183
as respiratory stimulant, 479
Nilevar, 563
Nilodin for schistosomiasis, 629
Nineteenth century, chemistry in, 763-764
Nisentil hydrochloride, 204
Nisulfazole, 574
Nitrates for hypertension (see Nitrites)
Nitrites, action, result, and tolerance, 432
for hypertension, replacement by other drugs, 437
preparation, dosage, and administration, 433-434
side effects and toxic effects, 434
uses, 432-433
Nitrofurantoin for urinary infections, 528-529
Nitrofurazone for eye infections, 537
mustards for neoplastic diseases, action of, 705
and related compounds for neoplastic diseases, 707-711
for skin infections, 496
Nitroglycerin for angina pectoris, 433
Nitromersol, 609
p-Nitrosulfathiazole, 574
Nitrous monoxide (see Nitrous oxide)
oxide, action and result, 252
discovery and history, 241
with ether, 249
preparation, administration, uses, and side effects, 253
Noludar, 234

Norepinephrine and epineph-
  rine, adrenal hor-
  mones, 307
formula, 304
phenylephrine combined
  with, 430
Norethandrolone, 563
Norethindrone, dosage and
  administration,
  560
Norisodrine sulfate, 312
Norlutin, 560
Normacid, 380
Normal components of body
  as drugs, 638
  human plasma, 459
    serum albumin, 460
  solution, definition, 81
Noscapine for cough, 482
Novatophan, 219
Novatrin, 338
Novobiocin, 161
  for urinary infections, 527
Novocain, 263
NPH insulin, 697
Numbers, mixed (see Mixed
  numbers)
Numerals, Arabic and Roman,
  48-49
Nupercaine hydrochloride,
  265
Nurse, approach to patient in
  giving medicine,
  117-118
  attitude toward drugs, 15
  Canadian, and narcotic laws
    of Canada, 30-31
  habits to develop in giving
    medicines, 114
  responsibilities in relation
    to use of cathar-
    tics, 388
  role in administration of
    medicines, 93
  with epilepsy patient,
    283
  and responsibility in drug
    addiction, 199-
    201
  student, drug administra-
    tion and, 13-14
  practical application of
    pharmacology by,
    14
  study of pharmacology,
    16-17
Nursing care of heart patients
  on digitalis ther-
  apy, 422-424

Nursing—Cont'd
  responsibilities relative to
    medicines and
    their administra-
    tion, 111-123
Nystatin, 167, 498

Obesity, amphetamines for,
  178, 180, 181
  thyroid preparations for,
  670
Obstetric sedation and amnesia, barbiturates
  for, 223
Obstetrics, ergot in, preparation, dosage, and
  administration,
  545
  ethylene in, 254
  scopolamine in, 336
Octin hydrochloride, 318
Ocular infection, chemotherapy of, 536-538
Official name of drug, definition, 33
Oil preparations, intramuscular injection of,
  disadvantages,
  100
Oils, description of, 36-37
  fixed, 493
    description of, 37
  volatile, description of, 36
Ointments, descriptions of, 43
  mercurial, antiseptic use,
  608
  ophthalmic, 44
  skin, 494
Old tuberculin, 734
Oleandomycin phosphate, 162
Oleovitamin A, 646
Oleum ricini, 397-398
Olive oil as laxative, 396
Open method of inhalation
  anesthesia, 247
Ophthaine for eye anesthesia,
  536
Ophthalmic ointments, de-
  scription of, 44
Opium, action and result,
  189-192
  assay of, 19
  composition, 188-189
  and its derivatives, 188-201
    side effects and toxic
    effects, 196-199
  preparation, dosage,
    and administra-
    tion, 194-196
  idiosyncrasy, 196

Opium—Cont'd
  and Narcotic Act, Cana-
    dian, 29-30
  poisoning, acute, 196-198
    chronic, 198-199
  poppy, 188 (Plate)
  preparation, dosage, and
    administration,
    193
  as respiratory depressant,
    480
  source, 188
  therapeutic uses, 192-193
  tincture for diarrhea, 404
  tolerance, 195-196
Oral administration of medi-
    cines, 95
  to children, 122
  in relation to meals,
    133
Orders for medications, 107-
  108
Oreton, 562
Organic needs of body, 642-
  700
Organisms, specific, in urinary
    tract, 525
Orientation to pharmacology,
    13-15
Orinase, dosage, and adminis-
    tration, 699-700
  formula, 700
Orthoxine hydrochloride, 318
Osmidrosis, 507
Osmotic diuretics, 513-515
O-syl, 606
Ouabain, 421-422
  poisoning, 422
Ovarian function, hormones
    affecting, 550
  hormones, 552
Ovocylin dipropionate, 556
Ox bile extract, 381
Oxidized cellulose, 463
Oxidizing agents as germi-
    cides, 614-615
Oxycel, 463
Oxygen administration, 488-
    490
  deficiency in body, 487
  high concentrations of, ef-
    fect of, 487
  inhalation apparatus, nasal
    type, 489
  medical uses, 487-488
  and oxygen therapy, 486-
    490
  tent in position, 488
Oxyphenonium bromide, 341-
    342

Oxytetracycline (*see also* Tetracyclines)
for syphilis, 585
Oxytocics, 542-548
Oxytocin, 546-548
chemistry of, 665
injection, 547

P³², 716
Pacatal, 293
Pain relief, alcohol injection for, 271
in burns, 505
by morphine, 189, 192-193
salicylates for, 210
Pamine bromide, 339
Pancreas, early experiments on, 692, 693
Pancreatic and gastric enzymes, 381-382
Pancreatin, 381
Panmycin phosphate, 150
Pantopon, preparation, dosage, and administration, 195
Pantothenic acid, 657
Papaver somniferum, 188 (Plate)
Papaverine, action on blood vessels, 193
on smooth muscle, 189
and uses, 434
formula, 189
hydrochloride, action, 195
dosage and administration, 195, 434
Para-aminobenzoic acid (PABA) combined with sodium salicylate, 213
formula, 568
structure, 131
Para-aminophenol derivatives, 213-215
Para-aminosalicylic acid (PAS), preparation, dosage, and administration, 579
for tuberculosis, 578-579
Paracelsus, 761
Paradione, 282-283
Paraffin, liquid, 396
Paraflex, 357
Paraldehyde, 236-237
Paramethadione, 282-283
Para-Pas, 579
Parasal potassium, 579
Parasites, malarial, 586-588

Parasitic infestations, injuries as result of, 622
Parasiticides and antiseptics, dermatologic, 495-499
Parasympathetic nervous system, effects produced by, 306
and sympathetic divisions of autonomic nervous system, differences between, 303
Parasympatholytic drugs affecting eye, 534-535
effects of, 329-330
Parasympathomimetic drugs, 319-329
affecting eye, 533-534
definition, 303
Parathyroid hormone, 666-667
vaccine, typhoid and, 731
Paredrine as nasal decongestant, 431
Paregoric, dosage, 193
Parenteral administration of drugs, 96-107
Paris green poisoning, symptoms and treatment, 748
Parkinsonism, postencephalitic, amphetamines in treatment of, 178, 180
Parkinson's disease, anticholinergic drugs for, 343
atropine for, 331, 333
Pastes, description, 44
Pathilon chloride, 342
Patient, condition of, relation of dose to, 133
Paveril phosphate, 435
Pectin, kaolin mixture with, 402
Pediculicides, 498
Peganone, 281
Pellagra, 654, 655
Pen Vee, 145
Penicillin, absorption, distribution, and excretion, 142
action and result, 141
aerosol administration, 147
allergic reactions, 147
for burn patients, 506
crystalline, parenteral use of, dosage, 143-144
current status, 138
discovery of, 137
in eye infections, 537

Penicillin—Cont'd
formulas, 140, 141
G, sterile, intramuscular dosage for prolonged action, 144
history, 765-766
intramuscular administration, 146
and prolonged action, dosage, 144-145
intrathecal administration, 147
intravenous administration, 146
kinds of, 140-141
oral administration, 146
dosage, 145-146
organisms resistant to, 143
rarity of toxic reactions to, 134
standardization, 141
subcutaneous injection, 147
for syphilis, 584-585
topical administration, 147
toxicity, 147
in urinary infections, 526
uses, 142-143
Penicillinase, 148
dosage, administration, use, and side effects, 725
Pentaerythritol tetranitrate, 433
Pentobarbital, formula, 221
sodium, action of, 231
preparation, dosage, and administration, 225, 232
Pentobarbitone sodium, 225, 232
Pentolinium tartrate, 444
Pentothal sodium, 225, 257-258
Pentylenetetrazol, 183-184
effectiveness of anticonvulsants measured by, 278
as respiratory stimulant, 479
Peppermint, 382
Pepsin, 381
Peptic ulcer (*see* Ulcer, peptic)
Perazil, 364
Percentage, 60-62
exercises, 62
Percorten, 680
Periclor, 236
Perin, 626
Peripheral circulation, effects of drugs on, 426, 427

Peripheral—Cont'd
vascular disease, effects of nicotine in, 345
sympatholytic drugs for, 319
Peritrate tetranitrate, 433
Pernicious anemia, hydrochloric acid dosage in, 457
pathology, 456
symptoms, 455-456
vitamin B_{12} for, 455-457
Pernoston, 225
Perphenazine, 292
Personality, effect of alcohol on, 269
Perspiration, offensive, treatment, 508
Pertussis serum, 727
vaccine, 730
Petit mal epilepsy, 277
trimethadione for, 282
Petrichloral, 236
Petrogalar, 391
Petrolatum, 494
liquid, 395-396
Petroleum jelly, 494
Phanodorn, 225
Pharmaceutic accessories, 45
chemistry in nineteenth century, 763
preparations, 37-45
Pharmacodynamics, definition, 18
Pharmacognosy, definition, 18
Pharmacology, definition, 18
field of, changes in, 15, 17
orientation to, 13-15
practical application of, by student nurse, 14
scope of, 18-19
study of, methods, 16-17
Pharmacopeia, first, 761
Internationalis, 23
London, first, 762
of United States of America, 20, 22
Pharmacopeias, national, appearance in nineteenth century, 764
Pharmacotherapeutics, definition, 19
Pharmacy, definition, 18
effect of Crusades on, 760
in eighteenth century, 762-763
in late medieval period, 760
and medicine in twentieth century, progress of, 764-767
in seventeenth century, 762

Pharmacy—Cont'd
in sixteenth century, 760-762
Pharmalax, 391
Phelantin, 280
Phemerol chloride as germicide and antiseptic, 617
Phenacemide, 283
Phenacetin, 213-215
Phenergan hydrochloride (see Promethazine hydrochloride)
Phenethylbiguanide, 701
Phenindione derivatives, 471
Pheniramine maleate, 365
Phenmetrazine hydrochloride, 181
Phenobarbital, action and uses, 229
for epilepsy, 223, 229, 230
formula, 221
and phenobarbital sodium, differences, 230, 231
preparation, dosage, and administration, 225, 231
safe anticonvulsant, 279
Phenobarbitone sodium, 225, 231
Phenol derivatives, selected, as germicides, 606
as disinfectant, 602-603
and related compounds as local anti-infectives, 602-606
Phenolated calamine lotion, 267
Phenolic compounds, poisoning, symptoms and treatment, 749
Phenolphthalein as cathartic, 400
Phenothiazine derivatives, 288-294
formula, 289
Phenoxybenzamine, 319
Phenoxymethyl penicillin, dosage, 145
Phensuximide, 283
Phentolamine hydrochloride, 319
Phenurone, 283
Phenyl salicylate, preparation, 211
Phenylazo-diamino-pyridine hydrochloride as urinary analgesic, 529-530
Phenylbutazone, 215-216

Phenylephrine hydrochloride, action and uses, 317, 429
combined with norepinephrine, 430
for eye, 535
formula, 317
preparation, dosage, and administration, 317, 429
source, 316
Phenylhydrazine hydrochloride for polycythemia vera, 718
Phenylmercuric compounds as antiseptics, 609
Phenyl-pyrazolone derivatives, 213-215
Phenytoin sodium, 279-280
Pheochromocytoma, histamine in diagnosis of, 361
sympatholytic drugs in diagnosis of, 319
pHisoderm, soap substitute, 618
pHisoHex, 604-605, 618
Phobex, 296
Phosphaljel, 376
Phospholine iodide for eye, 534
Phospho-soda, 394
Phosphotope, 716
Phthalylsulfathiazole, 573, 574
Physical antidotes, 744
Physicians' Desk Reference to Pharmaceutical Specialties and Biologicals, 22
Formulary, 23
Physiologic action of drug, definition, 128
antidotes, 745
Physostigmine, 324-325
salicylate for eye, 533
Phytonadione, 465
Picrotoxin, 184-185
Pills, description of, 41
Pilocarpine, 323-324
nitrate or hydrochloride for eye, 533
Piperat tartrate, 626
Piperazine estrone sulfate, 557
salts as anthelmintics, 626
Piperocaine hydrochloride, 266
Piperoxan, 319
Pipradrol hydrochloride, 181-182
Pitocin, 547
Pitressin, 666

Pituitary gland, anatomy and physiology, 661
    anterior lobe, factors in, 663
    extracts, 546
    gonadotropic hormones, 550-551
    hormones, anterior, 550-551, 662-665
    posterior, 546-548, 665-666
Pituitrin, obstetrical, 547
Placebos, psychologic implications, 120
Placenta, gonadotropic hormones formed by, 551-552
Placidyl, 232, 502
Plant drugs, active constituents, 35-37
Plantago ovata coating, 392
    seed, 392
Plasma, blood, clotting reactions of, 462
    loss in burns, relief of shock caused by, 505
    physiology, 459
    substitutes, 460-461
    normal human, preparation and use, 459
Plasmin, 722
Plasmogen, 722
Plasters, description of, 44
Plavolex, 460
Plazmoid, 461
Poison control centers, 738
    definition, 736
Poisoning accidents, prevention of, 743
    acid, symptoms and treatment, 746
    aminopyrine, 214
    arsenic, symptoms and treatment, 746
    aspidium, 625
    atropine, 334-335
    barbiturate, acute, 226-227
    chronic, 227-228
    picrotoxin for, 185
    bromide, 240
    caffeine, 177
    carbon monoxide, symptoms and treatment, 746
    tetrachloride, symptoms and treatment, 746
    causes and incidence, 737
    chloral hydrate, 235

Poisoning—Cont'd
    chlorophenothane, symptoms and treatment, 746
    cocaine, 262
    cyanide, symptoms and treatment, 747
    D.D.T., symptoms and treatment, 746
    from depressant drugs, amphetamine in treatment of, 178
    diagnosis, factors in, 736-737
    digitalis, 419
    elimination after, promotion of, 750
    epinephrine, 311
    ergot, 545, 546
    first-aid measures, 740, 742-743
    fluoride, symptoms and treatment, 747
    food, treatment, 751
    gold, BAL in treatment of, 750
    hydrocarbons, symptoms and treatment, 747
    iodine, symptoms and treatment, 747
    iron, 454
    isopropyl alcohol, 277
    lye, symptoms and treatment, 748
    mercury, BAL in treatment of, 750
    symptoms and treatment, 748
    methyl (wood) alcohol, 276
    morphine, acute, 196-198
    nalorphine for, 206
    chronic, 198-199
    nicotine, 344-345
    symptoms and treatment, 748
    nitrite, 434
    opium, acute, 196-198
    chronic, 198-199
    ouabain, 422
    paraldehyde, 237
    Paris green, symptoms and treatment, 748
    phenolic compounds, symptoms and treatment, 749
    physostigmine, 325
    pilocarpine, 324
    quaternary ammonium compounds, symptoms and treatment, 749

Poisoning—Cont'd
    salicylate, 212
    strychnine, 186-187
    supportive care of patient, 751
    symptoms, 736-737
    treatment, 741
Poisonous foods, 751
Poisons, antidotes, 744-750
    classification, 738
    inhaled, first-aid treatment, 743
    injected, first-aid treatment, 743
    mechanisms of toxic actions of, 739-740
    removal of, 741, 744
    specific, symptoms and emergency treatment, table, 746-749
    swallowed, first-aid treatment, 742
Policies and regulations regarding administration of medicines, 112-119
Poliomyelitis serum, 728
    vaccine, 730
Polyamine-methylene resin, 379
Polycythemia, definition, 448
    vera, characteristics, 707
    phenylhydrazine hydrochloride for, 718
    sodium radio-phosphate for, 716
Polymyxin, 163
    B sulfate for eye infections, 537
    in urinary infections, 527
Polysynaptic depressants, 355-358
Polyvinylpyrrolidone, 461
    iodine, 614
Pontocaine hydrochloride, 264
    for eye anesthesia, 536
Portal-biliary circulation of bile salts, 464 (Plate)
Position of patient during intramuscular injection, 101
Posology, definition, 132
Posterior pituitary hormones, 546-548, 665-666
    injection, 546-547
Potassium arsenite for leukemia, 718
    chloride and potassium nitrate as diuretics, 514

Potassium—Cont'd
loss and sodium loss, replacement, 639-640
penicillin G, 143
and O, oral use, 146
for parenteral use, dosage, 143
phenoxyethyl, 140, 145
phenoxymethyl, 145
permanganate as germicide, 615
solution, 498
salts for diuresis, 514
sodium tartrate, 394
Potentiation, drug, definition, 129
Poultices, definition, 45
Povidone-iodine, 614
Powders, description of, 41
nonabsorable, as skin protectives, 503
Pranone, 560
Prantal methylsulfate, 341
Preanesthetic medications, 243-244
barbiturates as, 223
Prednisone and prednisolone, chemistry, 688
formulas, 689
in neoplastic diseases, 714
preparation, dosage, and administration, 689-690
side effects and toxic effects, 690
Pregnancy, changes in uterus in, 541, 542
tests, 552
Preludin, 181
Premarin, 556
Prescriptions, 108-111
abbreviations for, 109, 110-111
typical, example, 108, 109
Primaquine, formula, 592
for malaria, 594, 595
Primidone, 283
Priodax, 386
Priscoline hydrochloride, 319
Privine hydrochloride, adrenergic drug, 318
as nasal decongestant, 431
Pro-Banthine bromide, 340-341
Probarbital sodium, dosage and administration, 225
Probenecid, 218-219

Procainamide hydrochloride, 425-426
Procaine hydrochloride, 263
for eye, anesthesia, 536
penicillin for intramuscular administration and prolonged action, 144-145
G for syphilis, 585
Prochlorperazine, 291
Prodox, 560
Proferrin, 454
Proflavine hemisulfate, 607
Progesterone, chemistry, preparation, dosage, and administration, 559
formula, 559, 561
as respiratory stimulant, 479-480
Progestin, 559
Proguanil, 595
Progynon, 556
Proluton, 559
Promazine hydrochloride, 291-292
Promethazine hydrochloride as antihistaminic, 364
dosage, administration, and side effects, 293
formula, 292
for motion sickness, 364, 366
uses, 293, 364
Promethestrol dipropionate, 558
Promizole, 582, 583
Pronestyl hydrochloride, 425-426
Propadrine hydrochloride as nasal decongestant, 431
Propantheline bromide, 340-341
Proparacaine hydrochloride for eye anesthesia, 536
Propion Gel, 497
Propionate compound, 497
Proportion, ratio and, 62-64
Proprietary name of drug, meaning, 134
Propylhexedrine, 179
Propylthiouracil, preparation, dosage, and administration, 677
and related compounds, 676-678

Prostigmin, 325-327
bromide for eye, 534
Protamine sulfate, heparin antagonist, 468
zinc insulin, 696-697
Protargol, 611
Protectives, skin, 502-503
Proteins, blood, 459-460
Prothromadin, 470
Prothrombin deficiency, causes, 464
Protoveratrine A and B, 439
Protozoan diseases, agents for, 586-598
Provell maleate, 439
Provitamin A, formula, 645
Pruritus, drugs for relief of, 501-502
Psychiatric ward, administration of medicines on, 119-120
Psychiatry, barbiturates in, 223
Psychomotor attacks of epilepsy, 278
Psychotherapy for chronic alcoholism, 274, 275
Psyllium hydrophilic mucilloid, 392
seed, 392
Pteroylglutamic acid, 457
Public Health Service, drug control function of, 26
Pulse, counting, of patient on digitalis therapy, 423
Pupil of eye, action of atropine on, 32
constriction by morphine, 190, 197
effect of ether on, 248
Pure drugs, definition, 81
solutions from, preparation of, 82-84
Purgatives, drastic, contraindicated, 390-391
Purified protein derivative of tuberculin, 734
Purinethiol, 714
Purodigin, 420
Purple foxglove, preparation, dosage, and administration, 419-420
PVP, 461
iodine, 614
Pyrathiazine hydrochloride, 365
Pyrazinamide for tuberculosis, 581

Pyribenzamine citrate, 365
 formula, 362
 hydrochloride, 365, 486
Pyridium as urinary analgesic,
 529-530, 607
Pyridostigmin for myasthenia
 gravis, 327
Pyridoxal, 656
Pyridoxamine, 656
Pyridoxine hydrochloride (vitamin B₆), daily
 requirement and
 uses, 656
 dosage and administra-
 tion, 657
Pyrilamine maleate, 365
Pyrimethamine, formula, 592
 for malaria, 594-595
Pyronil, 365
Pyrrobutamine phosphate, 365
Pyrrolazote, 365

Quaternary ammonium com-
 pounds as anti-
 septics, 616
 poisoning, symptoms
 and treatment,
 749
Quinacrine, action and result,
 590
 formula, 591
 hydrochloride, dosage and
 administration,
 591
 for tapeworm, 625
 side effects and toxic effects, 591
Quinalbarbitone sodium, 225,
 231
Quinidine sulfate, 424-425
Quinine, action and result,
 589
 empiric use, 126
 formula, 591
 for malaria, 588-590
 as muscle relaxant, 352
 preparation, dosage, and
 administration,
 589-590
 side effects and toxic effects, 590
 source, 588
 uses, 589

Rabies vaccine, 730-731
Racephedrine hydrochloride,
 315
Radioactive iodine (radioiodine), 674-676

Radioactive—Cont'd
 isotopes in neoplastic diseases, 715-717
Radiogold colloid for ascites
 in malignant dis-
 ease, 717
Radioisotopes for neoplastic
 diseases, action of,
 706
Ratio and proportion, 62-64
Rational medicine, empiric
 versus, 126-127
Raudixin, 438
Rauwiloid, 438
Rauwolfia alkaloids, 285-288,
 437-438 (see also
 Reserpine)
 action and result, 437
 preparation, dosage, and
 administration,
 438
 source, 285, 437
 side effects, 438
Reactions, drug, in children,
 123
Rectal administration of medicines, 96
 to children, 123
Rectum, absorption of drug
 from, 96
 of child, absorption of drug,
 123
Red blood cells, factors promoting formation
 of, 449
 physiology, 447, 448
 preparations for wound
 healing, 500
Reflex stimulation of respiration, 480
Regitine hydrochloride, 319
Relaxants, skeletal muscle,
 acting centrally,
 355-358
 by prolongation of
 depolarization,
 353-355
 and antagonists, 348-
 358
Relaxin, decrease of uterine
 motility by, 549
Releasin, 549
Replacement therapy, cortisone and hydro-
 cortisone in, 683
 definition, 638
 hormones, 660-700
 inorganic needs, 639-642
 vitamins, 642-660
Reproductive system, drugs
 acting on organs
 of, 541-564

Reproductive system—Cont'd
 of male and female,
 physiology, 541
Rescinnamine, 288, 438
Reserpine, action and result,
 285-286
 effect on Rhesus monkey,
 286, 287
 formula, 285
 for hypertension, 438
 preparation, dosage, and
 administration,
 288, 438
 sedative effect of, 286
 side effects and toxic effects, 288
 source, 285
 uses, 288
Resinat, 379
Resins, description of, 36
Resistance to antibiotics,
 problem of, 138
Resorcinol as antiseptic, 605
 as keratolytic, 501, 605
Respiration, functions of, 477
 physiology, 476
 reflex stimulation, 480
Respiratory antiseptics, 483
 center, action of drugs on,
 172
 of morphine on, 190
 drugs acting on, 477-480
 effects of aspirin on, 209
 of ether on, 248
 physiology, 476
 demulcents, 482-483
 depressants or sedatives,
 480
 stimulants, 476, 477-480
 system, anatomy and physiology, 476-477
 drugs affecting organs of,
 476-490
 tract, action of atropine on,
 331, 332
 drugs affecting mucous
 membrane lining
 of, 480-486
Restrol, 557
Reticular formation, action of,
 172
Rhamnus purshiana, 398
 (Plate)
Rhesus monkey, administration of reserpine
 to, 286, 287
Rheumatoid arthritis, cortisone and hydro-
 cortisone for, 683-
 685
Rhubarb as cathartic, 399

Rhythm, cardiac, disordered, depressants for, 424-426
Riboflavin (vitamin B₂), 652-654
Rickets, vitamin D in prevention of, 648
Ristocetin, 164
Ritalin hydrochloride, 182, 273
Robaxin, 357-358
Rochelle salt, 394
Roentgenographic studies, agents for, 385-386
Rolicton, 519
Roman and Arabic numerals, 48-49
Rome, medicine in, 757
Romilar hydrobromide for cough, 482
Roniacol, 436
Rosaniline dyes as antiseptics, 606-607
Rose water ointment, 494
Route of administration, relation of dose to, 133
Rules for determining dosage for children, 89, 90

Saccharated iron oxide, 454
Saccharin, 45
 sodium, 45
Saddle block anesthesia, 261
Safe administration of drugs, knowledge necessary to, 13
Safety of drug, relative, dosage in relation to, 134
Salamide, 213
Salerno, university at, 759
Salicylamide, 213
Salicylanilide, 497
Salicylates, absorption and excretion, 210
 action and results, 208-210
 analgesic action, 208
 antipyretic action, 209, 210
 drugs combined with, 213
 formulas, 208
 for gout, 217
 overdosage in children, 212
 poisoning, 212
 preparation, dosage, administration, 211
 as respiratory stimulants, 479-480

Salicylates—Cont'd
 side effects and toxic effects, 212
 source, 208
 uses, 210-211
Salicylazosulfapyridine for intestinal infection, 403
 preparation, dosage, and administration, 574
Salicylic acid (see also Salicylates)
 formula, 208
 as keratolytic, 210, 501
 local action, 208
 preparation, 211
Salicylism, 212
Saline cathartics, 393-395
Salinidol, 497
Salol, 403
Salts of heavy metals as antiseptics, 607-611
Scabicides, 499
Scarlet fever serum, 728
 red ointment, 607
Schick test toxin, 733
Schistosomiasis, drugs for, 629
 etiology, 623
Scopolamine, absorption, 334
 action, 335
 formula, 330
 hydrobromide, dosage, 336
 for eye, 534
 preparation, dosage, and administration, 336
 source, 330, 331
 uses, 335-336
Scorpion bites, first-aid treatment, 743
Scurvy, symptoms and treatment, 658
Secobarbital, formula, 221
 sodium, preparation, dosage, and administration, 225, 231
Seconal sodium, 225
Sedation, type produced by reserpine, 286
Sedative, definition, 220
 expectorants, 484-485
Sedatives and ataractics, distinction between, 284
 barbiturates as, 223
 decrease of uterine motility by, 548
 for diarrhea, 404
 and hypnotics, barbiturates, 221-232

Sedatives and hypnotics —Cont'd
 differences between, 220
 nonbarbiturate, 232-240
 nonbarbiturate, for itching, 501
 respiratory, 480
Seidlitz powders, 395
Selective action of drug, definition, 128
Semi-open method of inhalation anesthesia, 247
Senna as cathartic, 400
Seromycin, 158
 for tuberculosis, 581
Serpasil, 285, 438
Serum albumin, 459
Serums, antitoxic, of animal origin, 728-729
 human, naturally produced, 727-728
 immune, 727-729
17-ketosteroids, 560, 561
Seventeenth century, chemistry and pharmacy in, 762
Sex hormones, 550-564
 relation of dose to, 133
Shock due to loss of heat, relief of, 505
 of plasma, relief of, 505-506
 importance in treatment of burns, 504, 505
Side effect or action of drug, definition, 128
Silver, colloidal, preparations of, antiseptic use, 611
 compounds as antiseptics, 610-611
 nitrate, chemistry and use, 610
 in ophthalmology, 537, 538
 protein, strong and mild, 611
Silvol, 611
Sintrom, 470
Sippy powders, 379
Sites of drug action, 127
Sixteenth century, pharmacy in, 760-762
Skeletal muscle, effects of curare on, 349
 of neostigmine on, 325, 326
 of physostigmine on, 324, 325
 relaxants acting centrally, 355-358

Skeletal muscle, relaxants acting—Cont'd
    by prolongation of depolarization, 353-355
    side effects, 348
    and their antagonists, 348-358
    use and action, 348
Skin, absorption from, 492
  antifungal agents, 497-498
  application of medications to, 94
  baths, 506
  contamination, first-aid treatment, 743
  disorders, symptoms, 493
  drugs excreted by, 493
  eruption due to bromide, 239, 240
  infections, antibiotics for, 496-500
  layers of, 492
  lotions and solutions, 495
  and mucous membranes, drugs affecting, 492-508
    itching of, drugs for relief of, 501-502
  ointments, 494
  pediculicides, 498
  protectives, 502-503
  scabicides, 499
  soaps, 507
  stimulants and irritants, 500
Skopolate nitrate, 339
Sleep, barbiturates for, 222
  chloral hydrate for, 234
  drugs producing, 220
  nonbarbiturate sedatives and hypnotics for, 232-237
  paraldehyde for, 237
Smallpox inoculation in eighteenth century, 762
  vaccine, 731
Smoking, excessive, effects of, 344-345
Snake bites, first-aid treatment, 743
Soaps, 507, 617-618
Sodium bicarbonate as mouthwash or gargle, 369
  as systemic antacid, 374
  carboxymethylcellulose, 392-393
  chloride as diuretic, 513-514
  ointment for eye, 539
  solution for intravenous infusion, 106

Sodium—Cont'd
  citrate as anticoagulant, 466
  as systemic antacid, 374
  Diasone, 582, 583
  fluoride in reduction of dental decay, 371
  glucosulfone, 583
  hypochlorite solution as disinfectant, 612
  nitrite, 433
  penicillin G and penicillin O, dosage for parenteral use, 144
  perborate as antiseptic, 615
  as mouthwash, 369-370
  phosphate as cathartic, 394
  and potassium loss, replacement, 639-640
  Promin, 582, 583
  radio-phosphate in neoplastic diseases, 716
  salicylate (see also Salicylates)
    combined with para-aminobenzoic acid, 213
    formula, 208
    for pain relief, 210
    preparation, dosage, and administration, 211
    as sclerosing agent for varicose veins, 210
  Sotradecol, 618
  Sulamyd, 571
  sulfate as cathartic, 393, 395
  sulfoxone, 583
  tetradecyl sulfate, 618
Soluthricin, 168
Solu-Cortef, 686
Solutions, aqueous, description of, 37
  for intravenous infusion, 106
  method of making, 80-85
  molar, definition, 81
  normal, definition, 81
  prepared from pure drugs, 82-84
    from stock solutions, 84-85
  soothing, dermatologic, 495
  stock, definition, 82
    doses from, determination of, 86-87
  and suspensions, 37-39
Soma, 356
Soothing preparations, dermatologic, 493-495
Sources of drugs, 34
Spansules, description of, 40

Sparine hydrochloride, 291-292
Spasm, bronchial, in asthma, drugs to relax, 486-490
Spinal anesthesia, 261
  cord, action of caffeine on, 175
    of drugs on, 173
    of morphine on, 190
    of strychnine on, 185
Spirits, description of, 38
  dosage range, 39
Spiritus frumenti, 272
  vini vitis, 272
Spontin, 164
Sprays, definition, 94
  nasal, 483
Stages of anesthesia, 244-246
Standards, drug (see Drugs, standards)
Stanolone, 563
State laws for drug control, 28
Sterane, 690
Steroids, adrenocortical (see Adrenocortical steroids)
  for bronchial edema in asthma, 486
  estrogens, 553
  in ophthalmology, 538
Stibamine glucoside for leishmaniasis, 596
Stibophen for schistosomiasis, 629
Stigmonene bromide, 328
Stilbamidine for parasitic infestations, 597-598
Stimulants, central nervous system, 173-187
    amphetamines, 177-181
    basis of classification, 173
    caffeine, 174-177
    other than amphetamines, 181-187
    toxic actions, 740
  dermatologic, 500
  heart, 413-414
  respiratory, 476, 477-480
    reflex, 480
Stimulating expectorants, 485
Stimulation by caffeine, diagram, 174
  drug, definition, 128
Stock solutions, definition, 82
  doses from, determination of, 86-87

Stock solutions—Cont'd
  preparation of weaker
    solutions from, 84-
    85
Stomach, drugs affecting, ant-
    acids, 372-379
  antemetics, 383
  carminatives, 382
  diagnostic aids, 384-
    386
  digestants, 380-382
  emetics, 382-383
  types, 371
  hydrochloric acid of, func-
    tions, 380
Stramonium, 336
Streptodornase, action and
    use, 722
Streptohydrazide, 580
Streptokinase, action and use,
    722
Streptokinase-streptodornase,
    dosage, adminis-
    tration, uses, and
    side effects, 723
Streptomycin, absorption, dis-
    tribution, and ex-
    cretion, 151
  for burn patients, 506
  current status, 138
  for eye infections, 537
  with isoniazid for tubercu-
    losis, 580
  preparation, dosage, and
    administration,
    152
  side effects and toxic ef-
    fects, 153
  for urinary infections, 527
  uses, 152
Streptovaracin, 582
Strophanthin, 421
Strychnine convulsion, 186
  treatment, 187
  poisoning, 186-187
  source, action, and uses,
    185
Student nurse (see Nurse,
    student)
Study of pharmacology, meth-
    ods, 16-17
Suavitil, 296
Subarachnoid injection, 107
Subcutaneous injection of
    drugs, 97-99
  in children, 123
Subdural injection, 107
Sublingual administration of
    medicines, 95
Subtraction of common frac-
    tions, 52
  of decimals, 57, 58

Sucaryl calcium, 45
  sodium, 45
Succinylcholine chloride,
    354-355
Succinylsulfathiazole, 573, 574
Sucrose solution as diuretic,
    515
Sulamyd, sodium, 571
  as urinary antiseptic, 526
Sulestrex piperazine, 557
Sulfacetamide, preparation,
    dosage, and ad-
    ministration, 571
  sodium for eye infections,
    537, 571
  as urinary antiseptic, 526
Sulfadiazine for bacillary dys-
    entery and chol-
    era, 403
  formula, 567
  preparation, dosage, and
    administration,
    571
Sulfaethidole, dosage and ad-
    ministration, 573
Sulfaguanidine, 574
Sulfamerazine, preparation,
    dosage, and ad-
    ministration, 572
Sulfamethazine, dosage and
    administration,
    572
Sulfamethizole, dosage and
    administration,
    573
Sulfamethoxypyridazine, ef-
    fects, dosage, and
    administration,
    572-573
  as urinary antiseptic, 526
Sulfanilamide, formula, 567
  structure, 131
Sulfapyridine, dosage and ad-
    ministration, 572
Sulfasuxidine, 574
Sulfathalidine, 574
Sulfinpyrazone for gout, 219
Sulfisomidine, dosage, admin-
    istration, and uses,
    573
Sulfisoxazole diethanolamine
    for eye infections,
    537
  preparation, dosage, and
    administration,
    572
  as urinary antiseptic, 525
Sulfobromophthalein sodium
    for liver function
    test, 386

Sulfonamide compounds, 566-
    574
  mixtures, 574-575
Sulfonamides, absorption, dif-
    fusion, and excre-
    tion, 568-569
  action, 131
  and result, 567-568
  for bacillary dysentery, 403
  chemistry, 567
  for eye infections, 537
  formula, 568
  preparation, dosage, and
    administration,
    571-574
  resistance of organisms to,
    570
  side effects and toxic ef-
    fects, 575-576
  for urinary infections, 525-
    526
  uses, 569-570
Sulfones, action and results,
    582
  preparation, dosage, and
    administration,
    583
Sulfonylureas for diabetes,
    699-700
Sulfur ointment, 498
Sul-Spansion, 573
Sul-Spantab, 573
Sumycin, 150
Sunburn, 506
Superinfections, cause of, 138
  with penicillin therapy,
    147, 148
  with tetracyclines, 150, 151
Suppositories, description and
    forms of, 44
Suramin for trypanosomiasis,
    596-597
Surfacaine, 264
Surface anesthesia, 260
Surface-active agents, 616-618
Surgical anesthesia, stage of,
    246
Surgi-Cen, 604
Surital sodium, 259
Suspensions, aqueous, descrip-
    tion of, 37-38
  and solutions, 37-39
Sweetening agents, synthetic,
    45
Sympathetic ganglia, blockage
    in, symptoms,
    441-442
  nervous system, effects pro-
    duced by, 306

Sympathetic—Cont'd
  and parasympathetic divisions of autonomic nervous system, differences between, 303
Sympathin, definition, 304
Sympatholytic drugs, 319
Sympathomimetic amines, 177-181
  drugs, 306-319
  affecting eye, 535
Syncelose, 392
Syncillin, 140, 145
Syncurine, 353-354
Synergism, drug, definition, 128
Synergistic action of two antibiotics, definition, 139
Synestrol, 557
Synkamin, 465
Synkayvite sodium diphosphate, 465
Synthetic sweetening agents, 45
Synthroid sodium, 671
Syntocinon, 547
Syphilis, antibiotics other than penicillin in treatment of, 585
  bismuth compounds for, 586
  drugs for, 583-586
  Jarisch-Herxheimer reaction, 585
  penicillin treatment, 584-585
  prognosis and treatment, 583-584
Syringes, disposable, use of, 43
  for drug administration, 97
  insulin, 695
Syrups, description of, 37
  in expectorants, 484, 485
  as flavoring agents, 368
Systemic action of drugs, 127-129
  administration of medicines, 95-107
  anti-infectives, 577-598

Tablet triturates, description and administration of, 41
Tablets, description of, 40-41
  doses from, determination of, 88-89
  in making solutions, 81

Tace, 558
Tagathen, 365
Tannic acid for diarrhea, 402, 403
  glycerite as astringent, 504
Tannins, 36
Tapazole, 677
Tapeworms, varieties and activities, 623
Tars for skin disorders, 500
Tartar emetic for schistosomiasis, 629
Telepaque, 386
TEM, 709
Temaril, 502
Temperament of patient, relation of dose to, 133
Tensilon chloride, 352-353
  in myasthenia gravis, 328
TEPP, 328
Teridax, 386
Terpin hydrate in bronchitis, 485
  dosage, 194
Terramycin (see also Tetracyclines)
  for syphilis, 585
Tessalon for cough, 481
Testosterone, chemistry, 560
  formula, 561
  preparation, dosage, and administration, 562, 563
Tetanus antitoxin, 729
  toxoid and tetanus vaccine, 733
Tetracaine hydrochloride for eye anesthesia, 536
  preparation and dosage, 264
Tetrachloroethylene as anthelmintic, 627-628
Tetracyclines, absorption, distribution, and excretion, 149
  action, 149
  current status, 138
  dosage and administration, 150
  for eye infections, 537
  formulas, 149
  preparations, 150
  side effects and toxic effects, 151
  in urinary infections, 527
  uses, 149

Tetraethylammonium chloride, action, uses, dosage, and administration, 345
  as ganglionic blocking agent, 441
Tetraiodothyronine, formula, 667
Tetrex, 150
Thalamus, action of drugs on, 172
Theelin, dosage and administration, 555
  formula, 553
Thenylene hydrochloride, 365
Theobroma oil, 494
Theobromine, action of, 174
  formula, 174
Theophylline, action of, 174
  as diuretic, 516
  formula, 174
Therapeutic action of drug, definition, 128
Thiamine (vitamin B$_1$), daily requirement, source, and role, 651
  uses, preparation, dosage, and administration, 652
Thiamylal sodium, 259
Thiazolsulfone, 583
Thimecil, 677
Thimerosal, 609
  in ophthalmology, 538
Thiocarbanidin, 582
Thiocyanates for hypertension, 436-437
  toxicity, 437
Thiomerin sodium, 517
Thiopental sodium, 225, 257-258
Thiopentone, 258
  sodium, 225
Thiosulfil, 573
Thio-Tepa, 711
Thiouracil, toxic effects, 677
Thonzylamine hydrochloride, 365
Thorazine hydrochloride, 288-290
Thorn apple, 330
Thrombin, formation of, 462
  as hemostatic, 463
Thromboplastin, formation of, 462
Thylose sodium, 393
Thymol as antiseptic, 606
Thyroid gland, diseases of, drugs for, 673-678

Thyroid gland—Cont'd
  effect of iodine deficiency on, 668
  and other endocrines, 668
  hormones, 667-672
  physiologic action, 668
  preparations, 670-671
Thyrotoxicosis, 672
Thyroxin, formula, 667
  for hypothyroidism, 670
  preparations, 671
Time of administration, relation of dose to, 133
Tinctures, description of, 38
  dosage range, 39
Tissues, action of burns on, 504
Tobacco, effects of, 344-345
Toclase for cough, 482
Tolazoline hydrochloride, 319
Tolbutamide, 700
Tolerance, drug, definition, 129
Tolonium chloride, 462
Tooth powders, 370
Toxic actions of poisons, mechanisms of, 739-740
  dose, definition, 132
  stage of anesthesia, 246
Toxicology, 736-751 (see also Poisoning; Poisons)
  Committee on, of A. M. A., first-aid measures for poisoning, 742-743
  definition, 19, 736
Toxins, detoxification of, 732
Toxoids, 732-733
Trade-mark name of drug, 34
Tral, 342
Tranquilizers, 284-296
Transfusion, blood, in anemia, 458
Trematodes, drugs used against, 629
  varieties and activities, 623
Triacetyloleandomycin, 163
Triamcinolone, 691
Tribromoethanol, 256-257
Tricoloid chloride, 342
Tricyclamol chloride, 342
Tridione, 281-282
Triethylene thiophosphoramide for neoplastic disease, 711

Triethylenemelamine for Hodgkin's disease, 709
Trihexethyl chloride, 342
Trihexyphenidyl hydrochloride, 342-343
Triiodothyronine, formula, 667
Trilafon, 292
Trimethadione, 281-282
Trimethaphan camphorsulfonate, 446
Trimeton maleate, 365
Tripelennamine citrate, 365
  formula, 362
  hydrochloride, 365
Triphenylmethane dyes as antiseptics, 606-607
Trisulfapyrimidines, 575
Troches, description of, 41
Tromexan ethyl acetate, 470
Troxidone, 282
Trypanosomiasis, drugs for, 596-597
Tryparsamide for trypanosomiasis, 597
Trypsin, crystalline, dosage, administration, and side effects, 724
Tryptar, 724
Tubadill injection, 350
Tuberculin syringe, 97
Tuberculosis, chemotherapeutic agents for treatment of, 577-582
  diagnostic agents, 734
  streptomycin for, 152
  vaccine, 732
Tubex-sterile needle units, 42
Tubocurarine chloride, 350
Tubular reabsorption in formation of urine, 512
  secretion in formation of urine, 513
Tuinal, 229
Tumors, malignant, drugs for, 704-718
Typhoid vaccine, 731
Typhus vaccine, 731
Tyrothricin, action, dosage, and administration, 168
  for eye infections, 537
  for skin infections, 496

Ulcer, peptic, antacids in treatment, 372-379
  characteristics of ideal drug for, 338
  drugs in treatment, types, 372
  etiology, 371
Ultandren, 563
Undecoylium chloride-iodine, 614
Unidigin, 420
United States drug legislation, 23-29
  standards in, 20-22
  Pharmacopeia, 20, 22
Unitensen, 439
Universal antidote, 749
Universities, rise of, in Middle Ages, 759
Untoward effect or action of drug, definition, 128
Urea as diuretic, 514
Urecholine chloride, 322-323, 443, 524
Urethan in neoplastic diseases, 717
Uricosuric agents for gout, 216
Urinary antiseptics, 524-530
  tract infections, sulfonamides in, 570
  organs of, and kidney, drugs affecting, 510-530
  specific organisms in, 525
Urine, drugs to increase flow (see Diuretics)
  excretion of, 510, 511
  volume and composition of, factors influencing, 511-513
Urotropin as urinary antiseptic, 527-528
Urticaria in patients sensitive to penicillin, 148
U.S.P., 20, 22
Uterus, action of atropine on, 333
  of ergot alkaloids on, 543, 544
  drugs acting upon, 542-564
  effect of posterior pituitary and oxytocin injections on, 547
  motility of, drugs decreasing, 548-550
  increasing, 542-548
  physiology, 541-542

804

Vaccines, 729-732
Vallestril, 558
Valmid, 233
Vancocin, 165
Vancomycin, 165
Varidase, 723
Vascular effects of smoking, 345
Vasoconstrictor action of epinephrine, 309, 428
Vasoconstrictors, 427-431
nasal, 431
Vasodilators and drugs for hypertension, 431-447
Vasopressin, chemistry, 546, 665
uses and side effects, 666
Vasospasm, sympatholytic drugs for, 319
Vasoxyl hydrochloride, 318
V-Cillin, 145
Vehicle for disagreeable-tasting medicine for administration to children, 122
Veins for injection, 103
Ventricular tachycardia, procainamide hydrochloride for, 426
Veralba, 439
Veratrum preparations, 439-440
Veriloid, 439
Veronal, 225
Vesicants, 501
Vials, description of, 43
Vinactane sulfate, 166
Vinethene, 250
Vinyl ether, 250-251
Viocin sulfate, 166
Vioform, formula, 634
for intestinal amebiasis, 635-636
for skin infections, 496
Viomycin sulfate, 166
for tuberculosis, 581
Viosterol, 649
Virac, 614
Vitamin A, 644-647
and vitamins A and D combined, 646-647
B complex, 650
B₁ (see Thiamine)
B₂ (see Riboflavin)

Vitamin—Cont'd
B₆ (see Pyridoxine hydrochloride)
B₁₂, 455-457
with intrinsic factor concentrate, 457
C (see Ascorbic acid)
D, 647-650
combined with vitamin A, 646-647
E, source, 650
K, 463-465
formula, 469
K-like compounds, formula, 463
Vitamins, 642-660
deficiencies, causes, 642-643
fat-soluble, 644-650
functions, 642
medical use, 643
minerals, and hormones as drugs, 638-700
multiple, preparations, 659-660
potency, 644
present status, 643
water-soluble, 650-660
Volatile oils, description, 36
Vomiting, causes and control, 383
induction of, 382-383
Vonedrine as nasal decongestant, 431
Vulneraries, 500

Warfarin sodium, 470
Water as diuretic, 513
fluoridation of, to reduce dental decay, 371
loss, replacement of, 639
Waters, description of, 37
Water-soluble vitamins, 650-660
Weight, body, relation of dose to, 132
table, 66, 73
Weights and measures, 65-92
apothecaries' system, 66-68
conversion from apothecaries' to metric system and vice versa, 75-78
exercises, 91
history of, 65
metric system, 69-74

Wescodyne, 614
Whisky, 272
White blood cells, physiology, 448
foxglove, preparation, dosage, and administration, 420
ointment, 494
Whitfield's ointment, 498
Whole blood and its constituents, 458-460
Wines, 272-273
Wintergreen oil, 211
Wood alcohol, 276
Worms, classification, 623
drugs used against, 622-630
Wyamine sulfate, 317-318
as nasal decongestant, 431
Wydase, 721-722

Xanthine diuretics, 515-516
Xanthines, circulatory effects, 435-437
formulas, 174
side effects and toxic effects, 516
Xeroform for skin infections, 496
Xylocaine hydrochloride for eye anesthesia, 536
preparation, dosage, and toxic effects, 266

Yatren for intestinal amebiasis, 635
Yellow fever vaccine, 732
ointment, 494
Young's rule for dosage for children, 90

Zanchol, 382
Zephiran chloride as disinfectant, 616
Zinc oxide ointment, 494, 495
peroxide, medicinal, as wound disinfectant, 615
stearate, 495
sulfate in ophthalmology, 538
Zoxazolamine, 356-357
for gout, 219